INTENSIVE NEUROSURGERY BOARD REVIEW

Neurological Surgery Q&A

Thomas G. Psarros, MD

Shawn P. Moore, MD

INTENSIVE NEUROSURGERY BOARD REVIEW

Neurological Surgery Q&A

THOMAS G. PSARROS, MD

Chief Resident, Department of Neurological Surgery
University of Texas Southwestern Medical Center
Dallas, Texas

SHAWN P. MOORE, MD

Chief Resident, Department of Neurological Surgery
University of Texas Southwestern Medical Center
Dallas, Texas

Chairman's Note by Duke S. Samson, MD

Foreword by Peter M. Black, MD, PhD

LIPPINCOTT WILLIAMS & WILKINS
A **Wolters Kluwer** Company

Philadelphia • Baltimore • New York • London
Buenos Aires • Hong Kong • Sydney • Tokyo

Acquisitions Editor: Beverly Copland
Development Editor: Kate Heinle
Production Editor: Jennifer Kowalewski
Interior Designer: Janet Bollow Associates
Cover Designer: Leslie Haimes
Compositor: Graphicraft in Quarry Bay, Hong Kong
Printer: Walsworth Publishing in Marceline, MO

Library of Congress Cataloging-in-Publication Data

Psarros, Thomas G.
    Intensive neurosurgery board review : neurological surgery Q & A / Thomas G. Psarros,
Shawn P. Moore ; chairman's note by Duke S. Samson ; foreword by Peter Black.
        p. ; cm.
    Includes bibliographical references and index.
    ISBN-13: 978-1-4051-0479-1 (pbk. : alk. paper)
    ISBN-10: 1-4051-0479-1 (pbk. : alk. paper)
    1. Neurosurgery—Examinations, questions, etc.   I. Moore, Shawn P.   II. Title.
    [DNLM: 1. Neurosurgery—Examination Questions. 2. Nervous
System Diseases—Examination Questions. 3. Neurosurgical Procedures—
Examination Questions.   WL 18.2 P474i 2006]
    RD593.P83 2006
    617.4'8'0076—dc22

                                                                        2005010317

09

Dedication

To my beloved wife, Sandy.
Without her unconditional love and unselfish support,
this book would not be in your hands today.

To my young son, George,
for his constant inspiration and reminders of what really matters.

To my sister, Anna, and my parents, George and Maria,
whose love, unwavering support, and guidance through the years
have made everything possible.

Table of Contents

Chairman's Note

The current generation of neurosurgical residents are especially fortunate in the availability of several formal preparation aids targeted at the written portion of the neurosurgical board examination. "Intensive Neurosurgery Board Review" by Dr. Thomas Psarros is certain to become one of the most valuable of these texts. This work is a well organized compendium of carefully-researched mock examination questions which blanket every aspect of relevant basic and clinical neuro-science. The extensive questions are beneficial not only in probing the reader's understanding, but also by familiarizing him/her with the format and phrasing of the examination. This is an excellent vehicle for rapid and systematic pre-test review as well as an eye-opening refresher for those of us preparing for re-certification.

Duke Samson, MD

Foreword

Neurology and Neurosurgery are among the fastest changing fields in contemporary medicine. Practitioners of these specialties expect to be able to keep up to date in the most recent diagnosis and treatments of the many conditions they treat.

In this comprehensive volume, Dr. Thomas Psarros has developed 1300 questions that cover the entire spectrum of neurological and neurosurgical disease. These include topics in neurobiology, neuroanatomy, neurology, neuropathology, neuroradiology, clinical neurosurgery, and neuroscience. These questions are in the format used by the American Board of Neurological Surgeons. They are generally easy to read and provide a comprehensive review of contemporary clinical neurosurgery and its science.

This book will be useful not only for residents studying for Boards but also for neurosurgeons who are preparing for their re-certification examination and for anyone who wishes to have some sense of contemporary neurosurgery. It is an important and easy way of keeping up with this burgeoning field.

Dr. Psarros has done the field of neurosurgery a great service in preparing this text. It should be part of the library of anyone interested in or involved in neurosurgery.

Peter M. Black, MD, PhD
Franc D. Ingraham Professor of Neurosurgery
Harvard Medical School
Chair, Departments of Neurosurgery
Brigham and Women's Hospital
Children's Hospital Boston
Neurosurgeon-in-Chief
Brigham and Women's Hospital
Boston, MA

Acknowledgments

I am grateful for the assistance of the following people while preparing this text: James L. Fishback, MD, Mark Agostini, MD, G. Lee Pride, Jr., Korgan Koral, MD, Howard Morgan, MD, Carlos L. Perez, MD, Willard D. Thompson, MD, Linda R. Margraf, MD, Scott Clamp, MD, Steven Morgan, MD, Babu Welch, MD, Christopher Madden, MD, Louis A. Whitworth, MD, and the UT Southwestern Department of Neurological Surgery.

I would particularly like to acknowledge the contributions of Dr. Kimmo J. Hatanpaa, MD, PhD, in the Department of Pathology at the University of Texas Southwestern Medical Center for his editorial assistance of Chapter 4, and for graciously providing a large number of the photomicrographs used in Chapters 4 and 8. We are again grateful to James L. Fishback, MD, of the Department of Pathology at the University of Kansas for permitting us to use some of the figures that appeared in our previous book as well as some new ones.

I am also indebted to Suzanne Truex, medical illustrator for the Department of Neurosurgery, who graciously provided most of the photographic or artistic material of this book. Her skill and talent are acknowledged with great appreciation. I would also like to thank Kira Moore, who generously permitted the use of some superb illustrations that appeared in our previous book. I am also thankful for the continued support of my in-laws, George and Despina, during the preparation of this text; their devotion to family is unequaled.

I would also like to thank all of my clinical and basic science colleagues at UT Southwestern who suffered through all the teaching files that were made during the course of this project.

I am especially thankful to the publishers for their continued professionalism, confidence, encouragement, and numerous courtesies, which have made the preparation of this book a satisfying experience.

Thomas G. Psarros, MD

Figure Contributors

Mark Agostini, MD

Assistant Professor
Department of Neurology
University of Texas Southwestern Medical Center
Dallas, Texas

James L. Fishback, MD

Associate Professor and Director of Education
University of Kansas Medical Center
Kansas City, Kansas

Kimmo J. Hatanpaa, MD, PhD

Assistant Professor
Neuropathology Division
Department of Pathology
University of Texas Southwestern Medical Center
Dallas, Texas

Korgun Koral, MD

Assistant Professor
Department of Radiology
University of Texas Southwestern Medical Center
Children's Medical Center
Dallas, Texas

Linda R. Margraf, MD

Professor
Department of Pathology
University of Texas Southwestern Medical Center
Children's Medical Center
Dallas, Texas

Howard Morgan, MD

Professor
Department of Neurological Surgery
University of Texas Southwestern Medical Center
Dallas, Texas

Carlos Perez, MD

Assistant Professor
Neuroradiology Division
Department of Radiology
University of Texas Southwestern Medical Center
Dallas, Texas

G. Lee Pride, Jr., MD

Assistant Professor
Department of Neuroradiology
University of Texas Southwestern Medical Center
Dallas, Texas

Willard D. Thompson, Jr., MD

Neurological Institute of Savannah
Savannah, Georgia

Figure Credits

Mark Agostini, MD: Figures 3.74, 3.76–78, 3.86, 8.30, 8.203, 8.225

James L. Fishback, MD: 4.11, 4.17, 4.19, 4.36, 4.40, 4.58, 4.60, 4.64, 4.70, 4.72, 4.73, 4.81, 4.86, 4.88, 4.89, 4.94, 4.96, 4.101, 4.103, 4.116, 4.122, 4.123–124, 4.125–126, 4.127, 4.128–130, 4.131–132, 4.133, 4.134, 4.135, 4.136, 4.137, 4.138–139, 4.150, 4.151, 4.152, 4.153, 4.154, 4.155, 4.156, 4.170, 4.171, 4.172, 4.173, 4.175, 8.156, 8.218

Kimmo J. Hatanpaa, MD, PhD: 4.3, 4.9, 4.21, 4.26, 4.35, 4.42, 4.52, 4.53, 4.59, 4.61, 4.78, 4.83, 4.90, 4.92, 4.97, 4.110, 4.111, 4.117, 4.118–119, 4.120, 4.136, 4.175, 8.2, 8.10, 8.32–33, 8.55–56, 8.97, 8.102, 8.165, 8.173, 8.190–192, 8.215, 8.219

Korgun Koral, MD: 5.131, 8.85–86, 8.126–127

Linda R. Margraf, MD: 4.54, 4.69, 4.79

Howard Morgan, MD: 5.25, 5.46, 5.77

Carlos Perez, MD: 5.22, 5.58, 5.116, 5.129, 5.137–139, 5.147, 8.44–46, 8.52–54, 8.232, 8.241–242

G. Lee Pride, MD: 2.106–118, 5.6, 5.76, 5.78, 5.84, 5.85, 5.140–141, 8.244

Willard D. Thompson Jr., MD: 5.2, 5.55, 5.64, 5.81, 5.83, 5.87, 5.118, 5.130, 5.132, 8.120–122, 8.133–134, 8.279

Preface

There has been tremendous growth in biomedical knowledge during the last decade that has caused significant changes in medical education. These changes were prompted by the growing body of knowledge acquired by research findings and the realization that students and residents cannot assimilate every factual detail in this expanding body of knowledge. This is especially true with neurosurgical training and the written neurosurgery board examination, which requires knowledge of multiple areas including neuroanatomy, neurobiology, neurology, neuropathology, neuroradiology, neurosurgery, and critical care.

To obtain an adequate understanding of neuroscience while preparing for the neurosurgery written board examination, it is imperative that residents distill from neuroscience those essential elements that have significance for the clinical setting and are often tested. This often requires countless hours and the assimilation of multiple textbooks and core reference articles, which can be a daunting task, to say the least, for busy neurosurgical residents. For these reasons, we have attempted to break down those aspects of medical neuroscience that are often contained within the written neurosurgical examination in the form of a textbook and a supplemental question-and-answer book.

With this book, our intention is not to simulate the level of difficulty of the written neurosurgery examination or even to mirror the specifics of the examination but to cover general content areas revealed by the American Board of Neurological Surgery over the past few years. For maximal benefit, we feel that this book should be used as a supplement to our first book, entitled *The Definitive Neurological Surgery Board Review*, although the large number of questions, bulky discussions, and large number of figures and tables in this text will certainly provide a valuable single resource in your preparatory efforts.

This text is primarily intended for the use of neurosurgery residents, although it may appeal to medical students and residents in other subspecialties as well. Additionally, some sections of this book may prove valuable to practicing neurosurgeons preparing for the oral neurosurgery board examination. It is composed of 1300 multiple-choice questions in eight sections: Neurobiology (100 questions), Neuroanatomy (175 questions), Neurology (175 questions), Neuropathology (175 questions), Neuroradiology (175 questions), Neurosurgery (100 questions), Critical Care and Clinical Skills (100 questions), and a Multidisciplinary Self-Assessment Examination (300 questions). All questions are accompanied by in-depth answers that have been referenced to major texts or articles. Various high-yield topics have been reiterated in various sections of this book to enhance learning. The book includes a total of 291 figures and tables, the majority of which do not appear in our first book. Although every attempt was made to ensure the clarity and accuracy of the questions and answers, the reader is referred to the multiple referenced textbooks for further clarification or detail should the need arise.

We wish you luck during your preparatory efforts for the Neurosurgery Written Board Examination.

Thomas G. Psarros, MD

Neurobiology Questions

QUESTIONS 1–8

Directions: The questions below consist of lettered headings followed by a set of numbered items. For each numbered item, select one heading with which it is most closely associated. Each lettered heading may be used once, more than once, or not at all.

- **A.** Apoptosis
- **B.** Necrosis
- **C.** Both
- **D.** None of the above

1. Chromatin condensation and fragmentation, dilation and blebbing of the nuclear membrane, and cellular shrinkage

2. Mobilizes the immune system

3. The mechanism of cell death after radiation therapy

4. Type of cell death detected by the annexin V/propidium iodide assay

5. Pharmacologic strategies that inhibit caspase 8 may decrease this form of cell death

6. Rapid cell lysis

7. Translocation of phosphatidylserine to the outer plasma membrane is an early characteristic of this mode of cell death

8. DNA ladder formation on gel electrophoresis

End of set

9. Which of the following ion channels is partly responsible for carrying current during the repolarization phase in cochlear hair cells?

- **A.** Na^+ channel
- **B.** Ca^{2+} channel
- **C.** Ca^{2+}-sensitive K^+ channel
- **D.** Cl^- channel
- **E.** Mg^{2+} channel

10. Which of the following causes an increase in decerebrate rigidity?

- **A.** Sectioning the dorsal roots
- **B.** Chemically inactivating the lateral vestibular nucleus
- **C.** Sectioning the γ motor neurons
- **D.** Activating the medullary reticular formation
- **E.** Destruction of the flocculonodular lobe of the cerebellum

11. Neurotransmitter release at the synaptic terminal is triggered mainly by which ion?

- **A.** Na^+
- **B.** K^+
- **C.** Cl^-
- **D.** Ca^{2+}
- **E.** Mg^{2+}

12. Which of the following would hyperpolarize a resting neuron?

- **A.** Increase in Cl^- conductance
- **B.** Increase in Na^+ conductance
- **C.** Increase in Ca^{2+} conductance
- **D.** Decrease in K^+ conductance
- **E.** Increase in K^+ conductance

13. Which of the following would increase conduction velocity in an axon?

- **1.** Increasing the diameter of an axon
- **2.** Increasing the transmembrane resistance (R_m)
- **3.** Decreasing the capacitance of the membrane (C_m)
- **4.** Decreasing the membrane length constant (λ)

- **A.** 1, 2, and 3 are correct
- **B.** 1 and 3 are correct
- **C.** 2 and 4 are correct
- **D.** Only 4 is correct
- **E.** All of the above

14. Which of the following about the utricle and saccule is correct?

- **A.** With the head in an upright position, the utricle is oriented vertically on the medial wall of the vestibule
- **B.** They respond to angular acceleration
- **C.** In the utricular macula, the hair cells are arranged with the kinocilium oriented away from the striola
- **D.** The surface of the macula extends into the membranous labyrinth and is bathed in perilymph
- **E.** The tips of the hair cells are covered by the overlying otolithic membrane, which is embedded with calcium carbonate crystals (otoconia)

QUESTIONS 15 AND 16

Scenario: A 52-year-old male underwent subtotal resection of a glioblastoma multiforme originating in the right frontal lobe and extending into the deep nuclei of that hemisphere. Postoperatively, he underwent whole-brain radiation therapy and received 1, 3-*bis*-2-chloroethyl-1-nitrosourea (BCNU). The patient succumbed to his disease process 8 months later.

15. Resistance of this tumor to BCNU may have resulted from

- **A.** A high concentration of O^6-alkylguanine-DNA alkyltransferase (O^6-AGAT) in tumor cells
- **B.** The tumor was in the S phase of the cell cycle (resistant phase) during administration of BCNU
- **C.** The tumor cells lacked topoisomerase II, which causes transient DNA strand breaks during chemotherapy induction
- **D.** The tumor cells lacked cell surface proteins that recognize BCNU
- **E.** An agent that disrupts the blood-brain barrier was not administered concurrently with BCNU

16. Which of the following agents could potentially increase response rates to BCNU chemotherapy?

- **A.** Irinotecan (CPT-11)
- **B.** Tamoxifen
- **C.** Suramin
- **D.** O^6-benzylguanine
- **E.** 1-(2-chloroethyl)-3-cyclohexyl-1-nitrosourea (CCNU)

End of set

17. Experimental studies using the HSV-tk/GCV suicide gene transfer approach in animal models have shown tumor regression and long-term survival in spite of transduction efficiencies of less than 10%. Successful application of suicide gene cancer therapy in these studies despite incomplete delivery of genetic vector to all tumor cells was likely the result of

- **A.** The transfer of phosphorylated GCV (pGCV) into untransduced tumor cells via gap junctions
- **B.** The ensuing inflammatory reaction produced by the viral vector, resulting in the activation of cell death–signaling pathways (Fas/APO-1)
- **C.** The upregulation of p53, which immediately causes release of apoptotic mediators (e.g., caspase 8) from the mitochondria
- **D.** Upregulation of cAMP, a second messenger known to halt tumor proliferation in the G1 phase of the cell cycle
- **E.** Transfer of viral vectors into untransduced tumor cells via clathrin-coated pits

18. What is the only neurotransmitter synthesized in the synaptic vesicle?

- **A.** Dopamine
- **B.** Norepinephrine
- **C.** Acetylcholine
- **D.** Serotonin
- **E.** Substance P

QUESTIONS 19–25

Directions: The questions below consist of lettered headings followed by a set of numbered items. For each numbered item, select one heading with which it is most closely associated. Each lettered heading may be used once, more than once, or not at all.

- **A.** Free nerve endings
- **B.** Meissner's corpuscles
- **C.** Pacinian corpuscles
- **D.** Ruffini's corpuscles
- **E.** Merkel's discs
- **F.** None of the above

19. Most sensitive to skin stretch

20. Particularly sensitive to vibration (600 stimuli/second)

21. Mostly found in clusters at the center of the papillary ridge

22. Provide sharpest resolution of spatial pattern

23. Line the alimentary tract

24. Afferent fibers to the stretch reflex

25. Transmit information about pressure and texture

End of set

26. Which of the following structures is assessed by the doll's eye maneuver?

- **A.** Lateral vestibulospinal tract
- **B.** Medial vestibulospinal tract
- **C.** Vestibular nerve
- **D.** Cerebellum
- **E.** Cerebral cortex

27. Which of the following statements about phototransduction in the retina is correct?

- **A.** Cones perform better than rods in most visual tasks except detection of dim light at night
- **B.** The presence of light results in the opening of sodium channels in the photoreceptors of the retina
- **C.** The flow of sodium into photoreceptor cells is mediated by cAMP channels
- **D.** In the dark, the hyperpolarization of photoreceptor cells of the retina is the result of outward sodium flow
- **E.** Metarhodopsin II, a breakdown product of rhodopsin, deactivates phosphodiesterase molecules

28. Gap junctions close in response to what stimuli?

   A. Decreased concentration of intracellular Ca^{2+}
   B. Increased extracellular K^+ concentration
   C. Elevated intracellular proton concentration
   D. Increased extracellular Ca^{2+} concentration
   E. Gap junctions, unlike ion channels, remain open continuously

29. Unipolar neurons mainly innervate what structure(s)?

   A. Sympathetic nervous system
   B. Exocrine gland secretions and smooth muscle contractility
   C. Cardiac muscle cells (AV node)
   D. Adrenal gland secretions and the renal glomerulus
   E. Small and large bowel muscle contractility

30. Which of the following statements about the cochlea is correct?

   A. High-frequency sounds cause the basilar membrane to vibrate maximally at its apex
   B. Hair cells of the cochlea do not typically adapt to sustained stimuli unless provoked by low-frequency sounds
   C. An endocochlear potential of + 40 mV exists between the perilymph and the endolymph
   D. Deflection of stereocilia in either direction can cause depolarization
   E. The hair cells form chemical synapses with bipolar cells of the spiral ganglion

31. Which of the following statements about olfactory receptors is correct?

   A. An olfactory receptor displays rapid adaptation initially
   B. The life span of olfactory receptor cells is approximately 9 months
   C. A single olfactory receptor cell typically responds to only a single odorant
   D. The receptor potential occurs when Na^+ channels are closed in a manner similar to phototransduction
   E. They are cGMP-regulated

32. Which of the following sensory systems sends signals directly to both the thalamus and cerebral cortex?

   A. Two-point discrimination
   B. Taste
   C. Olfaction
   D. Pain
   E. Balance

QUESTIONS 33–39

Directions: For each question select one or more than one lettered heading (in parentheses) from Figure 1.33–1.39Q with which it is most closely associated. Each lettered heading may be used once, more than once, or not at all.

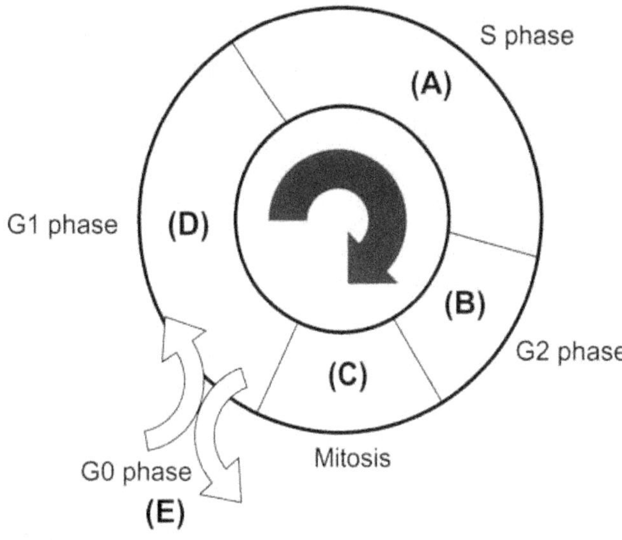

FIGURE 1.33–39Q

33. Cells most sensitive to radiation therapy

34. Nutrient depletion or physical crowding are conditions that encourage cells to move into this phase of the cell cycle

35. Cells can incorporate thymidine analogues into their nuclear DNA

36. Cells most resistant to radiation therapy

37. P15 and p16 cause growth arrest in this cell-cycle phase

38. TP53-dependent growth arrest following DNA damage occurs in this phase

39. Most variable phase of the cell cycle in terms of duration

End of set

40. What is the resting membrane potential for nerve cells?

   A. −100 mV
   B. −90 mV
   C. −80 mV
   D. −65 mV
   E. −40 mV

41. What is the extracellular concentration of Ca^{2+} ions in the brain?

   A. 0.7 mM/L
   B. 2 mM/L
   C. 125 mM/L
   D. 150 mM/L
   E. None of the above

42. Columns of neurons in area 3a of the somatic sensory cortex receive input primarily from what type of receptor(s)?

1. Rapidly adapting skin receptors
2. Slowly and rapidly adapting skin receptors
3. Pressure and joint position receptors
4. Muscle stretch receptors

A. 1, 2, and 3 are correct
B. 1 and 3 are correct
C. 2 and 4 are correct
D. Only 4 is correct
E. All of the above

43. Which of the following is true of action potentials?

1. Action potentials are mediated entirely by changes in K^+ voltage-gated channels
2. The rate of Na^+ influx begins to slow as the membrane potential approaches E_{K+}
3. The threshold for initiating action potentials is usually around +15 mV
4. The falling phase of the action potential is mediated by delayed activation of K^+ conductance

A. 1, 2, and 3 are correct
B. 1 and 3 are correct
C. 2 and 4 are correct
D. Only 4 is correct
E. All of the above

44. Cells with concentric receptive fields along the visual pathway are found in what location(s)?

A. Retina
B. Retina and optic nerve
C. Retina and lateral geniculate nucleus
D. Retina, lateral geniculate nucleus, layer 4 of the visual cortex
E. Cells in the premotor cortex only

45. What is the primary neurotransmitter of the Renshaw cell?

A. Glycine
B. Acetylcholine
C. GABA
D. Serotonin
E. Glutamate

46. A patient with homonymous hemianopsia due to a parietal lesion will have deficient pursuit eye movements _______ of the lesion, resulting in opticokinetic nystagmus. The opticokinetic nystagmus will be decreased when the drum is rotated _________ the side of the lesion.

A. Opposite the side, toward
B. Toward the side, away from
C. Opposite the side, away from
D. Toward the side, toward
E. None of the above

47. All of the following biochemical features regarding receptors for chemical neurotransmitters are correct EXCEPT?

A. They may be membrane-spanning proteins
B. They can work in a direct or indirect fashion to influence synaptic response
C. They can influence cells by activating second messengers, such as cAMP or diacylglycerol
D. They can help reinforce the pathways involved with learning
E. The binding site on the nicotinic acetylcholine receptor usually includes both the α and β subunits

48. All of the following statements about the semicircular canals are correct EXCEPT?

A. The movement of endolymph within each canal is opposite to the direction of head rotation
B. Primary afferent fibers do not discharge after head rotation ceases
C. Linear acceleration of the head is sufficient to activate the posterior semicircular canal
D. The floor of the ampulla contains a ridge of specialized hair cells that is covered by a layer of gelatin called the cupula
E. Hair cells in the horizontal canal are polarized toward the utricle, and those in the anterior and posterior semicircular canals are polarized away from the utricle

49. Slow synaptic transmission between nociceptors and dorsal horn neurons is mediated primarily by what neurotransmitter?

A. Substance P
B. Glutamate
C. Acetylcholine
D. ATP
E. Serotonin

50. A motor unit is composed of

A. A group of α motor neurons to a given muscle
B. A group of α and γ motor neurons to a given muscle
C. A group of α motor neurons to a given muscle and all of the muscle fibers they innervate
D. A group of muscle fibers innervated by a single motor neuron
E. All muscle groups innervated by the ventral root

51. Group 1b sensory fibers from muscle are most sensitive to what sensory modality?

1. Muscle length
2. Deep pressure
3. Rate of change in length
4. Muscle tension

A. 1, 2, and 3 are correct
B. 1 and 3 are correct
C. 2 and 4 are correct
D. Only 4 is correct
E. All of the above are correct

52. Which of the following is a component of the muscle spindle?

1. Intrafusal muscle fibers
2. Annulospiral endings
3. Flower-spray endings
4. γ motor fibers

A. 1, 2, and 3 are correct
B. 1 and 3 are correct
C. 2 and 4 are correct
D. Only 4 is correct
E. All of the above

53. Striking the ligamentum patellae with a reflex hammer results in the activation of which of the following structure(s)?

1. Annulospiral endings
2. Flower spray endings
3. α motor neurons
4. Quadriceps muscle

A. 1, 2, and 3 are correct
B. 1 and 3 are correct
C. 2 and 4 are correct
D. Only 4 is correct
E. All of the above are correct

54. Which of the following statements about neurons is correct?

A. Golgi type I neurons form the short fiber tracts of the brain and spinal cord
B. Golgi type II neurons have long axons that terminate in the neighborhood of the cell body
C. Golgi type I neurons are inhibitory
D. The volume of cytoplasm within the cell body always exceeds that found in the neurites
E. Golgi type II neurons greatly outnumber type I neurons

QUESTIONS 55–59

Directions: The questions below consist of lettered headings followed by a set of numbered items. For each numbered item, select one heading with which it is most closely associated. Each lettered heading may be used once, more than once, or not at all.

A. Kinesin
B. Dynein
C. Dynamin
D. None of the above
E. All of the above

55. Retrograde transport

56. Fast anterograde transport

57. Slow anterograde transport

58. GTP-dependent

59. Binds vinblastine and colchicine to inhibit fast anterograde transport

End of set

60. All of the following are true about GABA-responsive channels EXCEPT?

A. The GABA$_A$ receptor consists of five subunits ($\alpha_2\beta_2\gamma$)
B. Picrotoxin inhibits the GABA$_A$ receptor after binding to the β subunit
C. The GABA$_b$ receptor increases K$^+$ conductance and generates an inhibitory postsynaptic potential (IPSP) after binding baclofen
D. The β subunit of the GABA$_A$ receptor binds benzodiazepines
E. The binding of alcohol, barbiturates, or benzodiazepines to the GABA$_A$ receptor increases Cl$^-$ conductance

61. What ion blocks the ion pore of the N-methyl-D-aspartate (NMDA) glutamate receptor at resting membrane potential?

A. Ca^{2+}
B. Na$^+$
C. K$^+$
D. Mg^{2+}
E. Cl$^-$

QUESTIONS 62–70

Directions: The questions below consist of lettered headings followed by a set of numbered items. For each numbered item, select one heading with which it is most closely associated. Each lettered heading may be used once, more than once, or not at all.

A. Tetrabenazine
B. α-bungarotoxin
C. D-tubocurarine
D. Strychnine
E. Tetanus toxin
F. Cholera toxin
G. Barbiturates
H. Botulinus toxin
I. Pertussis toxin
J. LSD
K. Ondansetron
L. None of the above

62. Inhibits glycine release

63. Binds to α subunit of nicotinic receptors

64. Cleaves the protein synaptobrevin

65. Cleave t-SNAREs and v-SNAREs

66. Selectively activates G$_s$

67. Nondepolarizing inhibitor of nicotinic cholinergic receptors

68. Inactivates G_i

69. Agonist of the 5-HT$_{1C}$ receptor

70. Antagonist of the 5-HT$_3$ (ionotropic) receptor

End of set

71. Clinical evidence of neurologic deficit may not appear until regional blood flow has fallen to 50% or below average levels. At what rate of cerebral blood flow (in mL/100 g/min) does cytotoxic edema develop from failure of the Na$^+$K$^+$-ATPase?

    A. 40–50
    B. 25–30
    C. 16–20
    D. 10–12
    E. < 10

72. Which of the following is believed to be the major vasoactive mediator that plays an integral role in vasomodulation?

    A. Carbon monoxide
    B. Arachidonic acid metabolites
    C. Nitrous oxide
    D. Adenosine
    E. ATP

73. Neural crest cells give rise to all of the following structures EXCEPT?

    A. Ventral root ganglia
    B. Postganglionic cells of the sympathetic and parasympathetic ganglia
    C. Chromaffin cells of the adrenal medulla
    D. Melanocytes
    E. Schwann cells

74. Which of the following are common features of Wallerian degeneration?

    1. Degeneration and phagocytosis of the distal axonal segment
    2. Chromatolysis (peripheralization of rough endoplasmic reticulum with a concomitant increased protein synthesis) due to decreased retrograde neurotrophic factor delivery
    3. Proximal axon segment swelling due to continued anterograde axonal transport
    4. Greater neuronal cell death of postsynaptic neurons in the peripheral nervous system (PNS) than the central nervous system after axotomy

    A. 1, 2, and 3 are correct
    B. 1 and 3 are correct
    C. 2 and 4 are correct
    D. Only 4 is correct
    E. All of the above

QUESTIONS 75–78

Directions: The questions below consist of lettered headings followed by a set of numbered items. For each numbered item, select one heading with which it is most closely associated. Each lettered heading may be used once, more than once, or not at all.

    A. Red muscle fibers
    B. White muscle fibers
    C. Both
    D. None of the above

75. Striated muscle fibers

76. Contain large amounts of mitochondria, contract and relax slowly

77. Aerobic metabolism capacity

78. Contain large stores of glycogen

End of set

QUESTIONS 79–83

Directions: The questions below consist of lettered headings within Figure 1.79–1.83Q, depicting the sarcomere, followed by a set of numbered items. For each numbered item, select one or more than one heading with which it is most closely associated. Each lettered heading may be used once, more than once, or not at all.

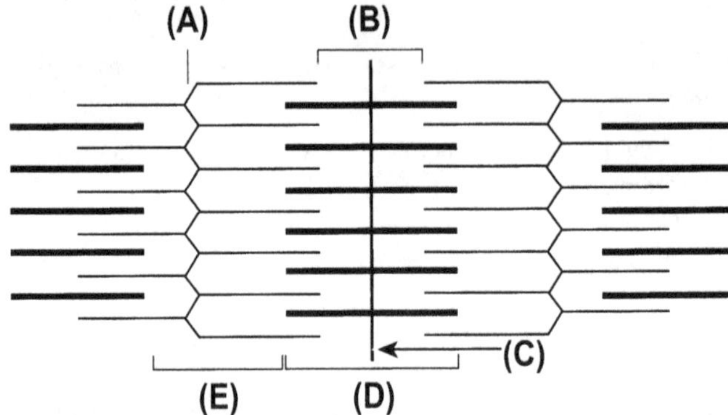

FIGURE 1.79–83Q

79. Composed solely of actin filaments

80. Shortens during muscle contraction

81. H zone

82. A band

83. Z disc

End of set

84. A consulting neuropathologist is asked to determine the gestational age of a stillborn infant thought to have been of approximately 18 weeks' gestational age. What is the best neuroanatomic criterion the pathologist can use to determine the infant's gestational age around this time period?

A. The degree of neural tube closure
B. The pattern of cerebral sulci
C. The extent of myelination
D. The amount of α-fetoprotein in the mother's serum
E. Thickness of the ependymal layer lining the ventricular cavity

85. Which of the following is true regarding cerebrospinal fluid (CSF)?

A. 90% is secreted by the choroid plexus
B. Volatile anesthetic agents and CO_2 increase CSF formation
C. The exit of CSF via the arachnoid villi is volume-dependent
D. About 750 cc of CSF is produced each day
E. Norepinephrine increases the rate of CSF formation

QUESTIONS 86–92

Directions: Match the gestational age with the embryologic milestone using each answer once, more than once, or not at all. Each question has only one correct answer.

A. Day 12
B. Day 14
C. Day 16
D. Day 18
E. Day 21
F. Day 24
G. Day 26
H. None of the above

86. Caudal neuropore closure

87. Notochord begins to develop

88. Neural folds almost fused

89. Rostral neuropore closure

90. Neural groove development

91. Bilaminar disc formed

92. Prosencephalon divides into telencephalon and diencephalon

End of set

93. What neurotransmitter is responsible for generating an excitatory postsynaptic potential (EPSP)?

1. Acetylcholine
2. GABA
3. Glutamate
4. Glycine

A. 1, 2, and 3 are correct
B. 1 and 3 are correct
C. 2 and 4 are correct
D. Only 4 is correct
E. All of the above

94. What occurs during acute metabolic acidosis to maintain the pH homeostasis of the CNS?

1. Compensatory hyperventilation
2. Reduction in CSF pCO_2
3. Paradoxic CSF alkalosis
4. Carbonic anhydrase–catalyzed generation of bicarbonate by the choroid plexus

A. 1, 2, and 3 are correct
B. 1 and 3 are correct
C. 2 and 4 are correct
D. Only 4 is correct
E. All of the above

95. Meningiomas have been shown to be associated with the expression of progesterone receptors. In what part of the tumor cell do they reside?

A. Endoplasmic reticulum
B. Cell membrane
C. Nucleus
D. Ribosomes
E. Golgi complex

QUESTIONS 96–100

Directions: The questions below consist of lettered headings followed by a set of numbered items. For each numbered item, select one heading with which it is most closely associated. Each lettered heading may be used once, more than once, or not at all.

A. G proteins
B. Protein kinase A
C. Protein kinase C
D. Phospholipase C (PLC)
E. Diaglycerol (DAG)
F. Inositol triphosphate (IP_3)
G. cAMP
H. None of the above

96. Binds to smooth endoplastic reticulum, causing release of Ca^{2+} ions

97. Second messenger, which activates protein kinase C

98. Activates protein kinase A

99. Has three subunits termed α, β, and γ

100. Splits PIP_2 into two molecules that act as second messengers

End of set

Neurobiology Answer Key

1. A	21. E	41. B	61. D	81. B
2. B	22. E	42. D	62. E	82. D
3. C	23. A	43. D	63. B	83. A
4. C	24. F	44. C	64. E	84. B
5. A	25. E	45. A	65. H	85. B
6. B	26. C	46. D	66. F	86. G
7. A	27. A	47. E	67. C	87. C
8. A	28. C	48. C	68. I	88. E
9. C	29. B	49. A	69. J	89. F
10. E	30. E	50. D	70. K	90. D
11. D	31. A	51. D	71. D	91. B
12. E	32. C	52. E	72. C	92. H
13. A	33. B, C	53. E	73. A	93. B
14. E	34. E	54. E	74. A	94. A
15. A	35. A	55. B	75. C	95. C
16. D	36. A	56. A	76. A	96. F
17. A	37. D	57. C	77. C	97. E
18. B	38. D	58. C	78. B	98. G
19. D	39. D	59. D	79. E	99. A
20. C	40. D	60. D	80. B, E	100. D

CHAPTER 1

Neurobiology Answers

1-A; 2-B; 3-C; 4-C; 5-A; 6-B; 7-A; 8-A. Cellular injury, including DNA damage induced by radiation or certain chemotherapeutic drugs, can result in either necrosis or apoptosis.

Apoptosis is a form of cell death that serves to eliminate unwanted host cells through preprogrammed mechanisms that result in gene expression and controlled cell death. Apoptosis can be activated by both internal and external stimuli and is characterized by a complex cascade of events that occur within a cell, involving the activation of both upstream (initiator) and downstream (effector) products known as caspases. Two major pathways of caspase-dependent apoptosis have been identified. One pathway is initiated by the formation of a death-inducing cell surface receptor signaling complex (e.g., Fas), leading to aggregation and activation of caspase 8. A second pathway is triggered by intracellular stress, such as DNA damage, and is primarily associated with the activation of caspase 9. During this latter pathway, signals received by the mitochondria (e.g., after DNA injury) stimulate the release of a variety of proapoptotic molecules, including cytochrome c. Release of cytochrome c induces formation of the apoptosome, a multiprotein complex composed of APAF-1, caspase 9, cytochrome c, and ATP. This, in turn, leads to activation of caspase 9 via allosteric regulation by APAF-1. Once activated, the initiator caspases, caspases 8 and 9, activate downstream caspases, such as 3 and 7, by cleavage. These downstream effector caspases, in turn, cleave multiple cellular proteins, triggering a range of apoptotic events such as nuclear membrane blebbing, DNA condensation and fragmentation, and phagocytosis (avoiding an inflammatory response).

Necrosis, on the other hand, results in rapid cell lysis and a widespread inflammatory reaction without the activation of internal cell death pathways. Sometimes it is referred to as "extrinsic cell death," as opposed to apoptosis, which is the result of endogenous cell death pathways. A characteristic biochemical feature of apoptosis is DNA fragmentation into multiple smaller fragments, which are readily detected by agarose gel electrophoresis as a characteristic "DNA ladder" formation. In contrast, necrosis causes random cleavage of DNA, resulting in a diffuse smear on DNA electrophoresis.

The annexin V (AV)/propidium iodide (PI) assay appears to be the most sensitive, specific, and user-friendly method for measuring apoptosis but also concurrently provides quantitative data about the number of vital and necrotic cells. In the early stages of apoptosis, phosphatidyl serine (PS) is externalized to the outer plasma membrane. Fluorescein isothiocyanate (FITC)–labeled AV, in the presence of calcium ions, immediately adheres to PS, which results in green fluorescence of the cells. This binding serves as a specific indicator of early-stage apoptosis in cells whose cell membrane is still intact, as demonstrated by the exclusion of the nuclear stain propidium iodide (PI). In cells that have lost their membrane integrity (necrotic cells), PI readily traverses the leaky membrane and binds to the DNA, inducing red fluorescence of the nucleus. The AV/PI assay can, therefore, not only measure the extent of early apoptosis (AV^+/PI^-) but also concurrently provides information about the number of vital cells (AV^-/PI^-) and necrotic cells (AV^+/PI^+). Of note, differentiating between necrotic (AV^+/PI^+) and late apopfotic (AV^+/PI^+) cells may be difficult with this assay. The terminal deoxynucleotidyl transferase nick-end labeling (TUNEL) method also measures cellular apoptosis (the method traditionally used), but it has proven to be less specific and sensitive and more time-consuming and expensive than the AV/PI assay, as described in the literature (Kandel, pp. 1058–1061; Overbeeke, pp. 115–121; Ross, pp. 41–44; Schwartz, pp. 1268–1279).

9. C. The origin of electrical resonance during hearing has been determined by recording isolated hair cells using voltage-clamp techniques. A positive deflection of the hair bundle or injection of current into the cell with a microelectrode allows K^+ influx into the cell and depolarization. Depolarization opens voltage-sensitive Ca^{2+} channels, which augments depolarization by allowing Ca^{2+} entry into the cell. As Ca^{2+} accumulates in the cytoplasm, it activates Ca^{2+}-sensitive K^+ channels, which along with voltage-sensitive K^+ channels allow for K^+ efflux and repolarization of hair cells (Kandel, pp. 620–622).

10. E. Decerebrate rigidity occurs following isolation of the brainstem from more rostral regions of the brain. This was demonstrated in animals that underwent surgical transection between the superior and inferior colliculi, which resulted in hyperreflexia and increased extensor tone due to loss of descending inhibitory tracts. Transection results in disruption of at least three key descending pathways. First, the lateral vestibular nucleus and pontine reticular formation are released from the inhibitory control of the cerebral cortex, which facilitates extensor motor neurons of the arms and legs. Second, projections from the red nucleus to the spinal cord are disrupted; these normally inhibit extensor motor neurons of the arms and legs. And last, the medullary reticular formation, which also inhibits extensor tone, is inoperative because of the loss of excitatory input from the cerebral cortex. The net effect is profound facilitation of extensor motor neurons of the arms and legs by the lateral vestibular nuclei and pontine reticular formation.

Destruction of the vestibulocerebellum (flocculonodular lobe) also increases contraction of tonic extensors by releasing the lateral vestibular nucleus from tonic inhibition, which facilitates extensor motor neurons of the arms and legs. Sectioning the dorsal roots, chemically inactivating the lateral vestibular nucleus, acute injury in the thoracic spine, and sectioning of the γ motor neurons all decrease decerebrate rigidity.

Patients with significant brain injury above the level of the red nucleus (or at its rostral margin) exhibit a postural state called decorticate rigidity, characterized by contraction of extensors in the legs and flexors of the arms. One reason for this is that the rubrospinal tract in humans projects only as far as the cervical spine, which may counteract vestibulospinal facilitation of arm extensors but not leg extensors (Kandel, pp. 654–656, 717, 841; Greenberg, pp. 118–119; Pritchard, pp. 254–259; Merritt, p. 18).

11. D. The quantal release of neurotransmitter by synaptic vesicles occurs by a specialized method of exocytosis at the active zones of the presynaptic terminal requiring calcium. Synaptic vesicles are bound to cytoskeletal elements near the active zone by synapsins. With depolarization, calcium/calmodulin-dependent protein kinase phosphorylates these synapsin proteins, resulting in the release of the synaptic vesicle (Kandel, pp. 262–274).

12. E. A typical neuron has a resting membrane potential of −65 mV. The equilibrium potential for K^+ is −86 mV, and an increase in conductance of this ion would result in movement of the neurons membrane potential toward −86 mV and hyperpolarization. The E_{Cl}^- (−66 mV) is very similar to the resting membrane potential of a neuron (−65 mV), and an increase in conductance of this anion would not result in any drastic change in the resting membrane potential of a cell. Increasing Na^+ and Ca^{2+} conductance would lead to depolarization of the neuron instead of hyperpolarization (Kandel, pp. 150–170).

13. A. How rapidly an action potential travels through an axon depends on a number of factors, including the internal resistance of an axon (R_i), the transmembrane resistance of the plasma membrane (R_m), (inversely related to the number of ion channels), and membrane capacitance (C_m). To better understand the relationship between these properties, we can use the analogy of a leaky straw. There are two paths that the water can take: one, down the inside of the straw, and the other, through the leaky holes along the straw. How much water flows along each of these paths depends on the relative resistance of each of these pathways, as most of the water will tend to go down the path of least resistance. The same

principles apply to current flowing down an axon. The current can either continue to flow down the axon or exit the axon through a leaky plasma membrane (ion channels). Increasing the diameter of the axon will decrease the R_i and allow the action potential to be conducted down the axon with increased conduction velocity. Increasing the R_m by myelination facilitates flow down the axon as well, just as wrapping tape around a leaky straw would also facilitate water flow down the inside of the straw. The ratio of R_m to R_i is called the membrane length constant (λ) and represents the distance between the point of peak depolarization produced by Na^+ influx and the point where the depolarization has declined to approximately 37% of peak value. λ indicates that Na^+ current is more likely to spread further along the axon if the membrane resistance is higher than the cytoplasmic resistance (increasing λ).

In terms of C_m, this property indicates how well the plasma membrane can hold positive and negative charges. Thinner membranes generally hold charges better than thicker ones because the electrostatic attraction between ions on opposite sides of the plasma membrane increases with decreased membrane thickness. Therefore thinner axons with increased membrane capacitance have decreased conduction velocity because it takes more time for current traveling down an axon to change the electrical potential of the adjacent membrane (and continue current propagation down the axon). The addition of myelin around an axon increases conduction velocity because it decreases C_m (increases membrane thickness). Decreasing the relative refractory period does not affect conduction velocity, but decreasing the diameter of the axon does. In smaller-diameter axons, the resistance of the axoplasm increases, resulting in decreased conduction velocity (Kandel, pp. 147–148; Pritchard, pp. 20–22; Bear, pp. 85–86).

14. E. Refer to Figure 1.14A. The utricle and saccule are located in the vestibule, a large chamber that separates the semicircular canals and the cochlea. The sensory epithelia of the saccule and utricle are called the maculae. Each macula consists of numerous hair cells surrounded by supporting cells resting on a connective tissue base. The orderly arrangement of hair cells within the macula gives the appearance of a curved equatorial line called the striola. In the utricle, the hair cells are arranged with the kinocilium oriented toward the striola, whereas in the saccule, the hair cells are polarized away from the striola. This anatomic polarity ensures that the two otolith organs can respond to linear acceleration or head tilt in any direction. The surface of the macula extends into the membranous labyrinth, which is bathed in endolymph, not perilymph. The macular surface is covered with a gelatinous structure, the otolithic membrane, which has calcium carbonate crystals (otoliths or otoconia) embedded on its surface. Relative movement between the otolithic membrane and the surface of hair cells is the essential macular stimulus, since this produces movement (bending) of hair cells, which results in ionic current flow at the base of hair cells and neurotransmitter release. With the head in a neutral position, the macula of the utricle lies in the horizontal plane (on the floor of the vestibule) and the macula of the saccule lies in the vertical plane (on the medial wall of the vestibule). Linear acceleration is detected by the maculae, whereas angular acceleration is detected by the specialized hair cells of the semicircular canals, called the cristae ampullaris (Kandel, pp. 802–814; Pritchard, pp. 250–253).

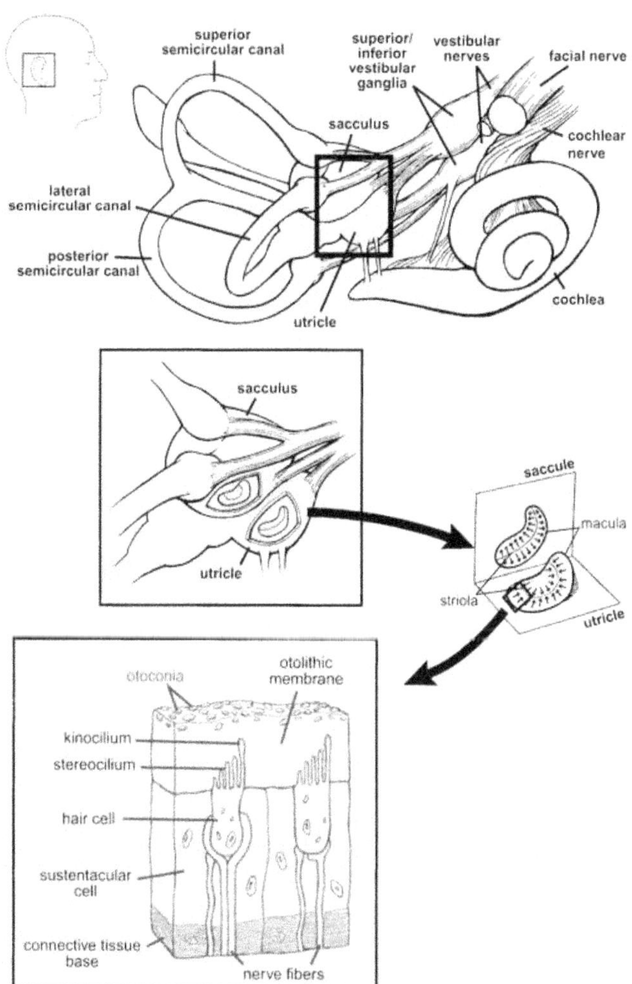

FIGURE 1.14A Otolith organs.

15. A. The nitrosoureas (BCNU, CCNU) are alkylating agents and are the most widely used drugs for patients with malignant brain tumors. They alkylate DNA in multiple locations, primarily on guanine but also on adenine and cytosine. The resultant DNA cross links often produce single- or double-stranded DNA breaks and eventual tumor cell death. O^6-AGAT is a repair enzyme that mediates repair of alkylation products of nitrosoureas. It has been noted that approximately 70% of tumors have high levels of O^6-AGAT and are often resistant to nitrosourea chemotherapy (Bernstein, pp. 231–232).

16. D. Attempts to modify resistance to nitrosoureas are ongoing. As stated in the previous discussion (question 15), O^6-AGAT mediates the repair of alkylating products of nitrosoureas. Inhibition of this repair protein has been the subject of a number of clinical trials using O^6-benzylguanine, a methylating agent. Tamoxifen inhibits protein kinase C, CPT-11 is a topoisomerase I inhibitor, and suramin works by inhibiting growth factors (FGF, IGF-1, PDGF). These agents do not modify resistance to alkylating agents. The addition of CCNU can potentially increase the risk of nitrosourea-induced side effects (Bernstein, pp. 229–332).

17. A. The mechanism whereby untransduced tumor cells die during gene therapy is called the "bystander effect." Until recently, this mechanism was poorly understood; it requires the presence of gap junctions that allow the transfer of toxic metabolites into untransduced tumor cells. In the HSV-tk/GCV approach, the nucleoside analogue GCV becomes cytotoxic after being converted to its triphosphorylated form by HSV-tk and host cellular kinases. It acts as a chain terminator and interrupts DNA synthesis in replicating cells. Phosphorylated GCV can then be transported into surrounding untransduced cells via gap junctions and induce cell death. The degree of bystander effect in individual tumors depends on the cell type and its capability to express gap junctions, the vector used, and the enzymatic activity of the therapeutic gene. The other choices have not been shown to propagate toxicity from transduced to untransduced cells (Bernstein, pp. 280–281).

18. B. Acetylcholine (Ach) is synthesized from choline and acetyl-CoA by the enzyme choline acetyltransferase. ACh is utilized by spinal cord motor neurons at the neuromuscular junction, all preganglionic autonomic neurons, postganglionic parasympathetic neurons, postganglionic sympathetic neurons to sweat glands, and within the nucleus basalis of Meynert. ACh is metabolized in the synaptic cleft by acetylcholinesterase into acetate and choline. Choline is then recycled by reuptake into the terminal bouton via receptor-mediated endocytosis. Dopamine (DA), norepinephrine (NE), and epinephrine are all synthesized from the same precursor molecule, the amino acid L-tyrosine. Tyrosine hydroxylase synthesizes L-DOPA from tyrosine and is the rate-limiting enzyme for both DA and NE synthesis. Aromatic amino acid decarboxylase then synthesizes DA from L-DOPA. Dopamine is synthesized by neurons in the substantia nigra and arcuate nucleus of the hypothalamus and is also active in some mesolimbic and mesocortical tracts. Reserpine prevents the uptake of DA into synaptic vesicles. Dopamine α-hydroxylase is located on the membrane of synaptic vesicles, where it converts DA to NE in the synaptic vesicle itself. NE is the only neurotransmitter that is synthesized within the synaptic vesicle. NE exerts negative feedback on tyrosine hydroxylase. NE is the neurotransmitter of most postganglionic sympathetic neurons and is also found in the locus ceruleus. After NE is released into the synaptic cleft, the termination of its bioactivity is primarily accomplished by reuptake into the presynaptic neuron. NE reuptake is blocked by cocaine. NE is also metabolized by catechol O-methyltransferase (COMT) and monoamine oxidase (MAO) in the cytoplasm of numerous cells. The medications tropolone and selegiline inhibit the enzymes COMT and MAO_B, respectively. Serotonin (an indole) is synthesized from the amino acid tryptophan. Tryptophan is initially converted into 5-hydroxytryptophan by the enzyme tryptophan hydroxylase, which represents the rate-limiting step. Then 5-hydroxytryptophan is converted into serotonin by the enzyme 5-hydroxytryptophan decarboxylase. Serotonergic neurons are primarily found in the raphe nuclei of the brainstem reticular formation. Serotonin reuptake is inhibited by several antidepressants, including the selective serotonin reuptake inhibitors (SSRIs; e.g., fluoxetine) and the tricyclic antidepressants (Kandel, pp. 280–295; Pritchard, pp. 32–45).

19-D; 20-C; 21-E; 22-E; 23-A; 24-F; 25-E. Refer to Figure 1.19–1.25A. Sensory endings of the skin can be classified on a structural basis into encapsulated and nonencapsulated receptors. Nonencapsulated receptors include free nerve endings, Merkel's discs, and hair follicle receptors. Encapsulated endings include Meissner's corpuscles, pacinian corpuscles, and Ruffini's corpuscles. Free nerve endings are widely distributed throughout the body. They line the alimentary tract and are found between epithelial cells of the skin, in the cornea, and in a variety of connective tissues including the dermis, fascia, ligaments, joint capsules, periosteum, and muscle. They are either myelinated or unmyelinated, and

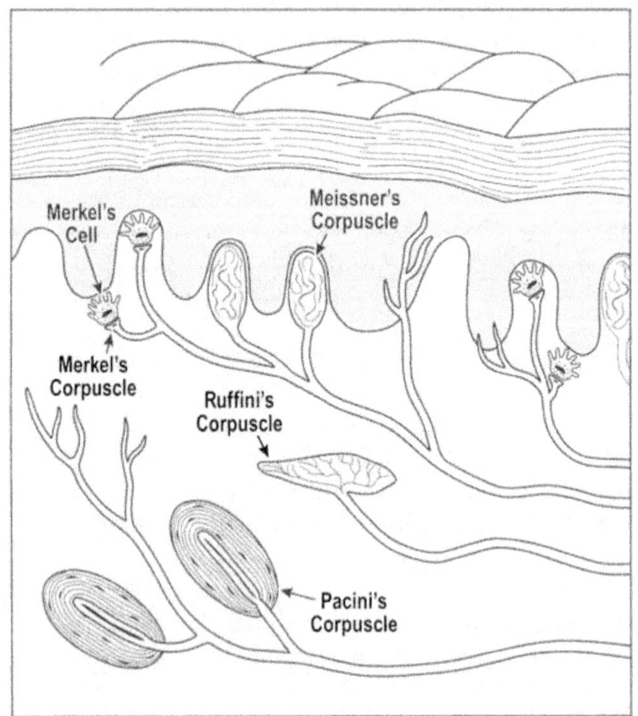

FIGURE 1.19–25A Skin receptors.

most detect pain; however, some detect crude touch, pressure, and tickling sensations. Merkel's discs are found in hairless regions of the body including the fingertips. They terminate in the deeper aspects of the epidermis, are slowly adapting, and transmit information about pressure and texture. Merkel's disc receptors also provide the sharpest resolution of spatial patterns of all the sensory endings of the skin. Meissner's corpuscles also provide sharp resolution of spatial patterns, but the image is generally not as sharp as the one produced by Merkel's endings because they have slightly larger receptive fields. Merkel's discs are normally found in clusters at the center of the papillary ridge. Hair-follicle receptors wind around hair follicles adjacent to a sebaceous gland. Some surround the hair follicle and others run parallel to it. These receptors are rapidly adapting and respond to the bending of hair follicles.

Encapsulated receptors include Meissner's corpuscles, pacinian corpuscles, and Ruffini corpuscles. Meissner's corpuscles are located in the dermal papillae of the skin, especially in the palms and soles of the feet. They are oval in shape and consist of a stack of flattened Schwann cells arranged transversely along their long axis. They are very sensitive to touch (especially stroking, fluttering), are rapidly adapting, and allow people to distinguish between two pointed structures placed together on the skin. Pacinian corpuscles are very similar physiologically to Meissner's corpuscles, are widely distributed, and are numerous in the dermis, subcutaneous tissues, joint capsules, pleura, pericardium, and nipples. Each pacinian corpuscle is ovoid shape, measuring 2 mm long and about 100–500 μm across (largest sensory receptor). The capsule consists of concentric lamellae of flattened cells. A large myelinated nerve enters the corpuscle, loses the myelin sheath, and then passes through the central core before terminating in an expanded fashion. Pacinian corpuscles are rapidly adapting and sensitive mainly to vibration. Ruffini's corpuscle is located in the dermis of hairy areas, is a slowly adapting mechanoreceptor, and responds mainly when the skin is stretched. Muscle spindles and group Ia fibers innervate the afferent limb of the stretch reflex (Kandel, pp. 430–450, 565).

26. C. The doll's eye test assesses the integrity of the vestibulo-ocular reflexes, which include the vestibular labyrinths, vestibular nerves bilaterally, vestibular nuclei, and motor nuclei of the cranial nerves involved with eye movements (nerves III, IV, and VI). The doll's eye maneuver does not test the integrity of the cerebral cortex, cerebellum, or medial and lateral vestibulospinal tracts, as they are not part of the vestibulo-ocular circuit. The vestibulo-ocular reflex stabilizes the eyes during head movements in order to keep an image focused on the retina. Rotation of the head to the right initiates compensatory eye movements to the left as a result of endolymph in the right semicircular canal flowing to the left (toward the utricle). As the endolymph flows through the ampulla, the cupula and underlying stereocilia bend toward the utricle. The resultant depolarization of the receptors causes an increase in the firing of the vestibular nerve, which reaches the vestibular nuclei, which, in turn, project to the motor nuclei of the extraocular muscles. The endolymph in the left (opposite) semicircular canal flows away from the utricle, causing hyperpolarization of hair cells and a lower firing rate of cranial nerves and vestibular nuclei on that side (Kandel, pp. 802–809).

27. A. The absorption of light by the photoreceptor cells of the retina results in a cascade of events (three distinct stages) that leads to a change in ionic fluxes across the plasma membrane of these cells. In rod cells, the visual pigment rhodopsin has two parts. The protein portion, opsin, is embedded in the disc membrane and does not absorb light, whereas the light-absorbing portion, retinal (derivative of vitamin A), can assume several different isomeric conformations, two of which absorb light. In the nonactivated form, rhodopsin contains the 11-*cis* isomer of retinal, which fits into the opsin binding site. In response to light, the 11-*cis* isomer changes to the all-*trans* configuration of rhodopsin, which no longer fits inside the opsin binding site. The opsin then undergoes a conformational change to semistable metarhodopsin II, which triggers the second stage of phototransduction. In this stage, metarhodopsin II activates a large number of phosphodiesterase molecules via an intermediate molecule termed transducin. Transducin, in turn, catalyzes the hydrolysis of cGMP molecules, which are required by cGMP channels for sodium conduction into the cell. This results in less cGMP, and the closure of cGMP-dependent sodium channels (stage 3 of the phototransduction cycle). The light-evoked closing of these channels results in less inward sodium current and, therefore, hyperpolarization of the cell. In the absence of light, cGMP is no longer broken down, sodium channels are reopened, and the cell becomes depolarized again. Cones perform better than rods in all visual tasks except the detection of dim light at night. Cone-mediated vision has higher acuity than rod-mediated vision, provides better resolution of images, and mediates color vision (Kandel, pp. 508–514).

28. C. Gap junctions are sensitive to different modulating factors that control their opening and closing in different tissues. For instance, most gap junctions close in response to lowered cytoplasmic pH or elevated cytoplasmic Ca^{2+}. These two properties serve to decouple damaged cells from other cells, since damaged cells have elevated levels of Ca^{2+} and protons (lower pH). Neurotransmitters released from other cells can also modulate the opening and closing of gap junctions (Kandel, pp. 178–180).

29. B. Unipolar neurons are the simplest in morphology. They have no dendrites and a single axon, which gives rise to multiple processes at the terminal. In humans, they control

exocrine gland secretions and smooth muscle contractility (Martin, p. 2).

30. E. Refer to Figure 1.30A. The hair cells of the cochlea form chemical synapses with bipolar cells of the spiral ganglion. Although the precise neurotransmitter released remains unclear, studies in animals show that transmitter release by hair cells is evoked by presynaptic depolarization and requires the presence of Ca^{2+}, as in most other synapses. The neurotransmitter involved is believed to be glutamate.

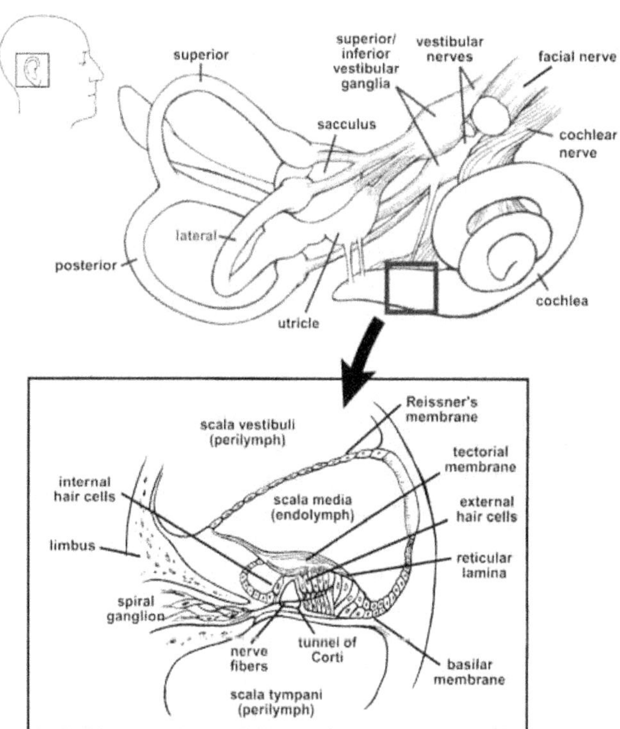

FIGURE 1.30A Cochlea.

The cochlea is a fluid-filled tube coiled $2\frac{1}{2}$ times around itself to resemble a snail shell. Reissner's membrane and the basilar membrane separate the cochlea into three chambers, the scala vestibule (SV), scala tympani (ST), and scala media (SM), which contains the organ of Corti. The SV and ST are filled with perilymph, which resembles CSF, and are continuous with one another at the helicotrema, a small opening located at the apex of the cochlear coil. The SM is filled with endolymph, a clear liquid with high K^+ concentration formed by the stria vascularis. Pressure waves resulting from sound cause the basilar membrane to move up and down, which results in a shearing movement of hair cells against the tectorial membrane. It is the physical bending of the hair cells toward the scala vestibuli that causes them to depolarize (K^+ channels and voltage-sensitive Ca^{2+} channels). Movement in the opposite direction causes hyperpolarization (Ca^{2+}-sensitive K^+ channels) (see discussion for question 9). The different regions of the basilar membrane are sensitive to different frequencies of sound. High frequencies cause the membrane to vibrate maximally at its base, whereas low frequencies cause maximal vibration near the apex. There is a marked difference in ion concentrations between the perilymph of the SV and the endolymph of the SM, which produces an endocochlear potential of +80 mV. Hair cells do adjust to sustained stimuli by a process of adaptation (to either high- or low-frequency sounds), which manifests itself as a progressive decrement in receptor potential during protracted hair-bundle deflection (Pritchard, pp. 229–248; Kandel, pp. 614–624).

31. A. Olfactory receptors (ORs) display rapid adaptation initially and little afterwards. Within the olfactory system, an olfactory stimulus results in the opening of sodium channels, which leads to depolarization and action potentials. These action potentials can increase in frequency to about 20/s. Adenylate cyclase activity catalyzes the formation of cAMP, resulting in opening of many additional channels, which can also increase the rate of discharge in olfactory neurons. Each olfactory neuron is capable of responding to many different odorants, as determined by electrophysiologic studies. The life span of ORs varies from 30 to 120 days in mammalian species. Replacement cells are delivered by mitosis of basal cells. The relatively rapid turnover of ORs makes them partially susceptible to damage after radiation therapy and/or chemotherapeutic agents, which target rapidly dividing cells (Kandel, pp. 626–636; Pritchard, pp. 266–267).

32. C. Taste and sensation from the head are carried to the ventroposterior medial (VPM) nucleus of the thalamus. Sensation and proprioception from the body reach the ventroposterior lateral (VPL) nucleus of the thalamus. The visual system utilizes the lateral geniculate nucleus (LGN) and the auditory system the medial geniculate nucleus (MGN) prior to being relayed to the cortex. Some olfactory information bypasses the thalamus to reach the orbitofrontal cortex, but it should be noted that some projections subserving smell can reach the orbitofrontal cortex via the mediodorsal (MD) thalamic nucleus. The olfactory system, therefore, relies on parallel processing to transmit olfactory inputs to the cortex (Kandel, p. 633).

33-B,C; 34-E; 35-A; 36-A; 37-D; 38-D; 39-D. Cells are most sensitive to radiation during the G2 and M phases of the cell cycle and most resistant in the late S phase. G1 cells have intermediate sensitivity. The precise mechanism(s) accounting for these variations remains unclear, but studies have shown that differences in a cell's ability to repair DNA damage in different phases after radiation may play an important part. In the G1 phase of the cycle, the nucleus has a diploid amount of DNA (2C), which increases to 4C by the end of the S phase. Only cells in the S phase (DNA synthetic phase) are able to incorporate thymidine analogues (bromodeoxyuridine) into their nuclear DNA. Nutrient depletion and crowding can result in the movement of cells into the

quiescent or nonproliferating phase (G0) of the cell cycle; such cells can eventually re-enter the cell cycle at a later point in time. Mitosis is the most easily identifiable stage of the cell cycle by light microscopy. The genes encoding p16 (CDKN2A) and p15 (CDKN2B) map onto chromosome 9p21, a site that is associated with homozygous deletions in high-grade astrocytomas in about two-thirds of gliomas. These proteins act as inhibitors of cyclin-dependent kinases and other pathways during the G1 phase of the cell cycle and help control proliferation at the G1/S phase of the cell cycle. The TP_{53} protein assists in several cellular processes, including cell cycle regulation, response of cells to DNA damage (P_{53}-dependent growth arrest following DNA damage occurs in G1 phase of the cell cycle), cell death, cell differentiation, and neovascularization (WHO, pp. 11–14; Berger, pp. 204–209).

40. D. In resting nerve cells the resting membrane potential is -65 mV. This negative polarity is largely the result of two factors: the selective permeability of the cell membrane to K^+ through voltage-gated channels and the Na^+, K^+ pump, which pumps three Na^+ ions out of the cell for every two K^+ ions that are pumped inside.

In terms of K permeability, as K^+ leaks out of the cell down its concentration gradient, the cell membrane begins to develop a potential difference due to the accumulation of negative charges inside the cell. This eventually slows the continued efflux of K^+ ions out of the cell as a result of the electrostatic attraction between the inside of the cell and positively charged K^+ ions outside the cell. Eventually the rate of K^+ flow inside and outside the cell reaches a state of equilibrium (equilibrium potential for K^+) due to the balancing of the electrical and chemical forces. This produces a net flow of K^+ ions that is zero and a net negative potential difference across the cell membrane. This is called the equilibrium potential for K^+ and can be calculated by the Nernst equation.

$$E = RT/F \log(ion)_{out}/(ion)_{in} = 61 \log(150/5.5) = -86 \text{ mV}$$

Using standard values of concentration gradients (see discussion question 41, $RT/F = 61$), the equilibrium potential for K^+ is -86 mV, which would also be the resting membrane potential across the cell membrane if K^+ were the only ion contributing to the membrane potential. However, rarely does one ion contribute solely to the membrane potential, which is often a combination of multiple ions diffusing through the membrane. For this reason, the Goldman equation was developed to account for the relationship between membrane potential (V) and relative permeability (P) of each population of ion channels. Given this, the resting membrane potential in neurons (-65 mV) is not identical to E_{K+} (-86 mV), since the membrane is slightly permeable to other ions as well.

$$V = 61 \log \frac{P_K^+ (K^+)_{out} + P_{Na+} (Na^+)_{out} + P_{Cl}^- (Cl^-)_{in}}{P_{K+} (K^+)_{in} + P_{Na+} (Na^+)_{in} + P_{Cl}^- (Cl^-)_{out}}$$

The inequality of charge on either side of the cell membrane is also the result of the Na^+, K^+ pump, which is a large membrane-spanning protein with Na^+, K^+, and ATP binding sites. If this pump were not present, the gradient across the cell membrane would eventually dissipate. This pump utilizes one ATP molecule to pump 3 Na^+ ions out of and 2 K^+ ions into the cell. An increase in permeability of Cl^- channels usually has little effect on membrane potential, since the resting potential of a typical neuron (−65 mV) and equilibrium potential for Cl^- (−66 mV) are very similar (Kandel, pp. 125–139).

41. B. Refer to Table 1.41A. Neurons maintain a high concentration of K^+ ions and organic anions inside the cell, and ions such as Na^+, Cl^-, and Ca^{2+} are more highly concentrated outside of the cell (Kandel, pp. 125–139).

TABLE 1.41A   Ion concentrations

IONS	INTRACELLULAR (MM/L)	EXTRACELLULAR (MM/L)	NERNST POTENTIAL (MV)
Na^+	15	150	+60
K^+	150	5.5	−86
Ca^{2+}	0.0001	2	+180
Cl^-	10	125	−66

42. D. Refer to Table 1.42A (Kandel, pp. 456–459).

TABLE 1.42A   Somatic sensory area and receptor type

SOMATIC SENSORY REGION	RECEPTOR TYPE
Area 1	Skin (rapidly adapting)
Area 2	Deep tissue (pressure and joint position) Skin (complex touch)
Area 3a	Deep tissue (muscle stretch receptors)
Area 3b	Skin (slowly and rapidly adapting receptors)

43. D. The rising phase of an action potential is due to a stimulus that results in the activation of voltage-gated Na^+ channels. The rate of Na^+ influx begins to slow as the membrane reaches the membrane potential for Na^+ (not K^+), resulting in a peak amplitude when the Na^+ channels become inactivated. The decline in the action potential is then mediated by the delayed activation of voltage-gated K^+ channels. The efflux of K^+ ions is greatest at the peak of the action potential and begins to decline as the membrane potential approaches the equilibrium potential for K^+. The membrane is, however, briefly hyperpolarized, as K^+ conductance does not return to resting levels until after the membrane voltage has declined below the normal resting potential. The threshold for initiating action potentials may vary but is usually around −50 mV for most mammalian neurons, not +15 mV (Kandel, pp. 150–170; Pritchard, pp. 23–25).

44. C. Both ganglion cells in the retina and the lateral geniculate nucleus are known to have both "on-center" and "off-surround," or concentric, receptive fields. Cells in the optic nerve and premotor cortex are not known to possess such characteristics. Simple cells in layer IV of the visual cortex do not have circular receptive fields but instead respond to stimuli as lines and bars (rectangles) (Kandel, pp. 517–522, 528–529).

45. A. A special class of inhibitory interneurons called Renshaw cells are found in laminae VII and VIII of the spinal cord. These cells have muscarinic cholinergic receptors that receive α–motor-neuron cholinergic collateral projections. The Renshaw cell then exerts a negative feedback on the α motor neuron and other homonymous α motor neurons, called recurrent inhibition. The neurotransmitter released by Renshaw cells is glycine. Renshaw cells also make inhibitory synaptic connections with Ia inhibitory interneurons; this arrangement regulates reciprocal inhibition of antagonistic motor neurons. Renshaw cells receive input from several descending pathways in the spinal cord (Carpenter, pp. 57–79; Kandel, pp. 720–721).

46. D. The precise pathways of the opticokinetic system remain unclear but are believed to be similar to smooth pursuits. The pathway is believed to extend from the visual association areas (18 and 19) to the horizontal gaze center of the abducens nucleus in the pons. The pathway from the left visual association area is believed to terminate in the left pontine gaze center, resulting in pursuit movement of the eyes to the left. Similarly, the right visual association region produces movements to the right. A patient with a pure occipital lobe lesion theoretically should have no difficulty with pursuits, since the pathways originate in more anterior regions. The opticokinetic response should, therefore, be symmetric. A patient with homonymous hemianopsia and a parietal lesion will have deficient pursuit movements to the same side of the lesion, resulting in an asymmetric opticokinetic response (OKN). The opticokinetic response will be decreased when the drum is rotated toward the side of the lesion. Patients with homonymous hemianopsia due to either an optic tract, temporal lobe, or purely occipital lobe lesions should have symmetric opticokinetic responses to both sides. Cogum's dictum can be used to summarize these findings. Homonymous hemianopsia + asymmetric OKN is most likely related to a parietal mass lesion. Homonymous hemianopia + symmetric OKN is most likely a result of an occipital lesion such as stroke (Kline, pp. 16–17).

47. E. Direct receptors like nicotinic ACh receptors are also referred to as ionotropic receptors, which gate ionic current rapidly over only a few milliseconds. The ACh receptor itself is a transmembrane protein composed of five subunits ($\alpha_2\beta\gamma\delta$) with the α subunits representing the binding site for ACh. Receptors that gate ion channels indirectly are called metabotropic receptors and typically produce slower synaptic responses lasting seconds to minutes. Activation of these receptors often requires the production of second messengers such as cAMP and diacylglycerol, ultimately resulting in the modulation of ion channels distinct from the receptor itself. Noradrenergic and serotonergic receptors are examples of indirect receptors. The metabotropic receptors have been shown to influence learning and modulate behavior (Kandel, p. 185).

48. C. Refer to Figure 1.48A. One end of each semicircular canal contains an enlarged region known as the ampulla, where the flow of endolymph serves as a mechanical stimulus for sensory transduction. The floor of the ampulla contains specialized hair cells, the crista ampullaris, and is covered by a gelatinous layer known as the cupula. The stereocilia of the hair cells insert into the cupula. These hair cells are stimulated by changes in endolymph circulation induced by head rotation. The movement of endolymph within each canal is opposite to the direction of head rotation. The response in each pair of semicircular canals (one on each side of the head) is opposite as well. Rotation of the head or angular acceleration is sufficient to stimulate a response in the semicircular canals but insufficient to stimulate the macula of the utricle, which requires linear acceleration. Firing typically ceases once head movement stops. Hair cells in the horizontal canal are polarized toward the utricle, and those in the anterior and posterior semicircular canals are polarized away from the utricle (Kandel, pp. 802–806; Pritchard, pp. 250–253).

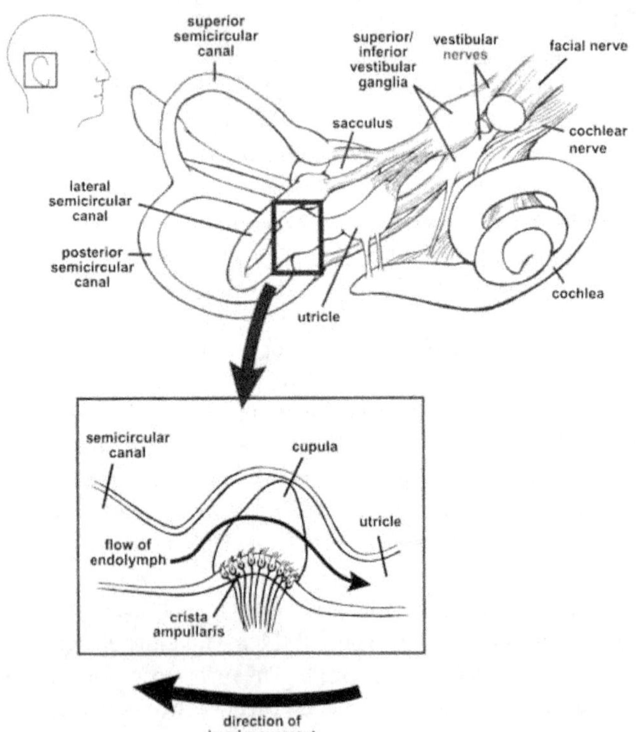

FIGURE 1.48A   Semicircular canals and cupula.

49. A. Slow-excitatory synaptic transmission between nociceptors and dorsal horn neurons in the marginal layer of lamina I and substantia gelatinosa of lamina II is mediated primarily by substance P, released by Aδ and C fibers (Kandel, pp. 477–479).

50. D. The motor unit is the functional unit of muscle contraction; it includes a single motor neuron and all of the muscle fibers it innervates (Kandel, p. 81).

51. D. Refer to Table 1.51A. Sensory fibers from muscle are typically classified according to their diameter. Group Ia sensory fibers (annulospiral endings and flower-spray endings) are between 12 to 20 μm in diameter, myelinated, sensitive to muscle length and rate of change in length, and receive their input from muscle spindles. Group Ib fibers are similar in diameter to group Ia, are also myelinated, and are most sensitive to muscle tension from Golgi tendon organs. Group II sensory fibers receive their input from secondary spindle endings and nonspindle endings and are between 6 to 12 μm in diameter. Secondary spindle endings are sensitive to muscle length and nonspindle endings are sensitive to deep pressure. Group III sensory fibers receive input from free nerve endings, are between 2 to 6 μm in diameter, and are responsive to pain as well as chemical and temperature stimuli. Type IV sensory endings are similar to type III with the exception of being smaller in diameter (0.5 to 2 μm). Intrafusal fibers of muscles spindles are in parallel with extrafusal muscle fibers, whereas Golgi tendon organs (GTOs) are connected in series to skeletal muscle fibers, innervated by Ib sensory afferents, and sensitive to muscle tension, as described above (Kandel, pp. 720–723).

52. E. Refer to Figure 1.52A. Muscle spindles are the sensory receptors of skeletal muscle that signal changes in muscle length. Changes in muscle length are closely associated with changes in the angles of the joints that the muscles cross; thus muscle spindles are capable of sensing relative positions of various body segments. The main components of the muscle spindle include intrafusal muscle fibers with noncontractile central regions, afferent sensory endings originating from the center of the intrafusal fibers (flower-spray and annulospiral nerve endings), and efferent motor fibers (static and dynamic γ motor neurons) (Kandel, pp. 718–719).

53. E. Refer to Figure 1.52A. Striking the ligamentum patellae results in stretching of the intrafusal muscle spindles of the quadriceps muscle. In turn, this causes activation of both annulospiral and flower-spray sensory endings (responsive to stretching around the central region of intrafusal muscle fibers), which are carried to the dorsal horn of the spinal cord within the femoral nerve (L 2, 3, 4). These afferent fibers synapse with large α motor neurons in the anterior gray horns of the spinal cord. Nerve impulses then travel via

TABLE 1.51A   Classification of peripheral sensory fibers

TYPE	VELOCITY (M/S)	STIMULI TRANSDUCED	RECEPTORS
Ia (Aα)	70–120	Muscle length and velocity of contraction	Primary muscle spindle afferents
Ib (Aα)	70–120	Muscle tension	Golgi tendon organ afferents
II (Aβ, Aγ)	30–70	Muscle length, touch, and pressure	Spindle secondaries, Meissner/Merkel/pacinian/Ruffini
III (Aδ)	4–30	Temperature, light touch, stretch, sharp pain	Free nerve endings
IV (C)	0.4–2	Slow/burning pain and some temperature	Free nerve endings

(Reprinted with permission from Moore SP. The Definitive Neurological Surgery Board Review, Table 1.1, p. 10. Blackwell Publishing, 2005.)

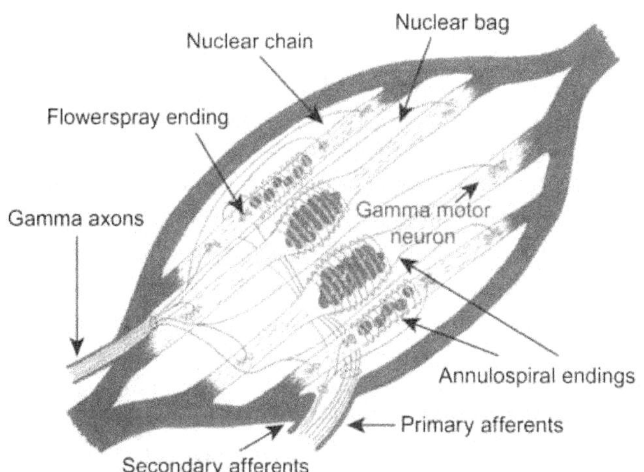

FIGURE 1.52A Muscle spindle. This figure illustrates the structure of the nuclear chain and static nuclear bag fibers. (Reprinted with permission from Moore SP. The Definitive Neurological Surgery Board Review. Malden, MA: Blackwell Publishing, 2005:12, Figure 1.2.)

efferent α motor neurons of the femoral nerve and stimulate the extrafusal fibers of the quadriceps muscle, which contracts. The motor neurons of the antagonist muscles are inhibited. After the muscle contracts, there comes a point at which the intrafusal muscle fibers slacken and are unable to signal any further changes in muscle length, which results in a decreased amount of firing of the afferent sensory fibers (annulospiral and flower spray). At this point, one role of γ motor fibers is to maintain tension on muscle spindle poles during muscle contraction to ensure their firing during movement. The γ motor neurons accomplish this task by terminating as small branches on motor endplates located on both ends of the intrafusal muscle fibers. Stimulation of these motor nerves causes the ends of the intrafusal fibers to contract, which in turn activates sensory endings. Thus, the γ motor neurons provide a mechanism for adjusting the sensitivity of the muscle spindles to keep them under constant tension during muscle movement. In many voluntary movements, the γ motor neurons are activated at the same time as α motor neurons to automatically maintain a level of spindle loading. This is called alpha-gamma coactivation. Under resting conditions, the muscle spindles give rise to afferent nerve impulses at a constant rate, which is not consciously perceived. Although the details remain unclear, it is believed

that this constant baseline firing of muscle spindles helps maintain tone (Kandel, pp. 713–736).

54. E. Golgi type I axons are typically long and include the pyramidal cells of the cerebral cortex, the Purkinje cells of the cerebellar cortex, and the motor cells of the spinal cord. Golgi type II neurons have shorter axons, greatly outnumber type I neurons, and are usually inhibitory. They have short dendrites, which gives them a star-shaped appearance. The volume of cytoplasm in the axons and dendrites usually exceeds the volume in the cell body (Bear, p. 41; Carpenter, pp. 65, 126, 214, 229, 233, 330, 390, 395).

55-B; 56-A; 57-C; 58-C; 59-D. Membranous organelles and secretory vesicles are transported to the axon terminal via fast anterograde axonal transport. This mode of transport is dependent on the protein kinesin and ATP and occurs at a rate of > 400 mm/day. Kinesin binds the organelle or vesicle and then forms intermittent cross bridges with tracks of microtubules, resulting in stepwise transport down the axon. The pharmacologic agents vinblastine and colchicine bind to and interfere with microtubule structure (not kinesin), thereby disrupting fast anterograde transport.

There are several types of slow anterograde axonal transport. Component A utilizes a protein called dynamin, is GTP-dependent, and facilitates transport of cytosolic proteins and cytoskeletal elements. It is much slower than fast anterograde transport, occurring at a rate of 0.2 to 2.5 mm/day. Component B is slightly faster, at 2 to 4 mm/day, and utilizes an actin/myosin motor complex in the transport of cytosolic proteins, actin, and spectrin.

Fast retrograde axonal transport occurs at a rate of > 400 mm/day and is dependent on the protein dynein and hydrolysis of ATP. Retrograde transport facilitates the passage of endosomes from the axon terminal to the neuron soma. Endosomes contain various proteins (such as nerve growth factor) and even pathogens (such as rabies virus or tetanus toxin) that are taken up by the axon terminal via endocytosis (Kandel, pp. 99–103).

60. D. GABA$_A$ receptors consist of five subunits: two α, two β, and one γ subunit (α$_2$β$_2$γ). All three subunits bind GABA, while the α and β subunits bind barbiturates and the γ subunit binds benzodiazepines. After binding GABA, the channel opens and permits the entry of Cl⁻ into the cell, generating an inhibitory postsynaptic potential (IPSP). The binding of neuromodulators such as alcohol, barbiturates, and benzodiazepines increases the GABA-induced Cl⁻ current but does not open the channel directly. Picrotoxin inhibits the GABA$_A$ receptor after binding to the β subunit. The GABA$_B$ receptor increases K⁺ conductance, thus generating an IPSP, and is activated by the agonist baclofen. GABA receptors are highly prevalent throughout the CNS (Kandel, p. 219).

61. D. Glutamate receptors are ionotropic channels that induce EPSPs and include the *N*-methyl-D-aspartate glutamate (NMDA) receptor, the kainate receptor, and the kainate-quisqualate (AMPA) receptor. The NMDA receptor is an ion channel of high conductance that is permeable to Ca²⁺, Na⁺, and K⁺. This receptor contributes only to the later phases of the EPSP because it is active only in the presence of its ligand and membrane depolarization. This channel is unique in this regard because its activity is dependent upon a neurotransmitter and membrane potential. At resting membrane potential, Mg²⁺ blocks the ion pore of the NMDA channel. With membrane depolarization, the Mg²⁺ is displaced from the channel, allowing ion conduction to occur efficiently. The opening of the NMDA channel also requires glycine as a cofactor. The NMDA channel is inhibited by PCP and selectively blocked by APV. This channel is important in long-term potentiation at the neuronal synapse because its activity leads to an increase in cytosolic Ca²⁺ with subsequent activation of second messengers involved with long-lasting synaptic modifications. High levels of glutamate are toxic to neurons, and this toxicity is mediated primarily by the NMDA channel. With excessive levels of glutamate, cytosolic Ca²⁺ increases significantly, activating proteases and phospholipases that generate free radicals toxic to neurons. The non-NMDA glutamate receptors (kainate and AMPA) are permeable to Na⁺ and K⁺ and are responsible for the generation of the early, large component of the EPSP. There are also metabotropic glutamate receptors that act through G proteins and second-messenger systems (Kandel, pp. 219–221).

62-E; 63-B; 64-E; 65-H; 66-F; 67-C; 68-I; 69-J; 70-K. Ion channels conduct ions at extremely high rates, are selective for specific ions, and are regulated or gated. Gated ion channels can be regulated by changes in voltage, chemical transmitters (ligands), and mechanical factors. Ligand-gated channels include glutamatergic channels, cholinergic channels, glycinergic channels, and GABAergic channels. Acetylcholine-activated channels include nicotinic and muscarinic receptors. Nicotinic cholinergic receptors are ionotropic channels that are permeable to Na⁺ and K⁺ and consist of five subunits: two α and the β, γ, and δ subunits ($\alpha_2\beta\gamma\delta$). The α subunit binds a single molecule of ACh, thus requiring two ACh molecules to bind the receptor to elicit channel activation. The snake venom toxin α-bungarotoxin

binds the α subunit as well, effectively inhibiting channel function. Each subunit of the receptor contains four hydrophobic α helices (M1 to M4) that traverse the plasma membrane. Opening of the nicotinic ACh channel results in the generation of a fast excitatory postsynaptic potential (EPSP). Hexamethonium (ganglionic), succinylcholine (depolarizing), and D-tubocurarine (nondepolarizing) represent inhibitors of various nicotinic cholinergic receptors. The nicotinic receptor is found at the neuromuscular junction as well as preganglionic synapses of the autonomic nervous system. The muscarinic cholinergic receptor is a metabotropic receptor that is coupled to G proteins and consists of only two subunits (α and β). This channel is a slow-activating K⁺ channel (M-type channel) that closes when stimulated and results in the generation of a slow EPSP. Muscarinic channels are found throughout the CNS (cerebellum, striatum, cortex, Renshaw cells of the spinal cord) and in autonomic ganglia. These receptors are inhibited by atropine and scopolamine and stimulated by bethanecol (bladder), carbachol (GI tract), pilocarpine (eye), and methacholine.

Glycine is the neurotransmitter released by Renshaw cells (inhibitory interneurons) of the spinal cord (see discussion, question 45). Glycine channels are blocked by strychnine, and glycine release is inhibited by tetanus toxin.

There are five major groups of dopamine and serotonin receptors, all of which are metabotropic. Examples include D1 and D2 receptors, which stimulate and inhibit adenylyl cyclase, respectively. The net effect of D1 receptors is hyperpolarization, while that of D2 receptors is depolarization. The typical antipsychotics selectively inhibit D2 receptors. The majority of serotonin receptors are metabotropic. LSD is an agonist of the 5-HT$_{1C}$ receptor, while ondansetron is an antagonist of the 5-HT$_3$ (ionotropic) receptor. All noradrenergic receptors are metabotropic receptors that utilize G proteins and the second messenger cAMP.

The signal transduction cascade involved in metabotropic receptor activation can be manipulated by cholera toxin, which selectively activates G$_s$, and pertussis toxin which inactivates G$_i$. Tetanus toxin specifically cleaves the protein synaptobrevin, while botulinus toxins cleave t-SNAREs and v-SNAREs, which subsequently results in the inhibition of synaptic vesicle release at the terminal. The docking, fusion, and release of synaptic vesicles appears to involve distinct interactions between vesicle proteins (synaptobrevin and synaptotagmin, v-SNAREs) and proteins of the nerve terminal plasma membrane (syntaxins and neurexins, t-SNAREs) (Kandel, pp. 196–200, 219, 241–243, 1197–1199, 1215–1216).

71. D. Refer to Table 1.71A. Cytotoxic edema refers to swelling of injured neurons, glia, and endothelial cells after hypoxia or global cerebral ischemia. It is the result of ATP-dependent Na⁺/K⁺ pump failure, which allows Na⁺, and therefore water, to accumulate within cells. Vasogenic edema is the most common type of brain edema and is attributed to increased permeability of brain capillary endothelial cells and thus extracellular fluid volume. The white matter is generally affected more than the gray matter because of the tendency of fluid to accumulate adjacent to the white matter tracts (Kandel, p. 1299; Youmans, pp. 1468–1469).

TABLE 1.71A   Cerebral blood flow and clinical manifestations

RATE OF BLOOD FLOW (ML/100 G/MIN)	CLINICAL MANIFESTATIONS
50–60	Normal
25–30	Mild-to-moderate deficit from electrical failure
16–20	Severe deficit from electrical failure
10–12	Deficit from Na^+/K^+-ATPase failure and cytotoxic edema
< 10	Gross metabolic failure/impending death

72. C. As measured by its pivotal vascular actions, nitrous oxide is believed to be the major candidate for vascular modulation. Important actions of this mediator include facilitation of vascular relaxation and prevention of smooth muscle proliferation, platelet and white blood cell adherence, and platelet aggregation. Other important vasomodulators are carbon monoxide, eicosanoids, oxygen-derived free radicals, and endothelin (Youmans, pp. 1469–1474).

73. A. Neural crest cells give rise to the PNS, chromaffin cells of the adrenal medulla, pia, arachnoid, melanocytes, Schwann cells, odontoblasts, certain endocrine cells, cranial nerve sensory ganglia, autonomic ganglia, and dorsal root ganglia, as opposed to the ventral root ganglia (DeMyer, p. 52).

74. A. With axon transection (axotomy), synaptic transmission failure occurs initially, followed by degeneration and phagocytosis of the distal axonal segment, which is called Wallerian degeneration. In addition, the neuronal soma undergoes chromatolysis (peripheralization of rough ER with concomitant increased protein synthesis) due to decreased retrograde neurotrophic factor delivery, and the end of the proximal axon segment swells due to continued anterograde axonal transport. Axotomy also has a negative impact on the postsynaptic neuron and can result in neuronal cell death unless regeneration occurs. Regeneration occurs when axonal sprouts grow from the end of the proximal axonal segment and enter tissue remnants of the distal stump. These sprouts may form new synaptic connections if they eventually reach their targets. Formation of new synapses in this way occurs more effectively in the PNS than the CNS (Kandel, pp. 82–83, 147–148, 1108–1110).

75-C; 76-A; 77-C; 78-B. There are three basic types of striated muscle fibers, including slow-twitch fibers and two types of fast-twitch fibers. Slow-twitch fibers are called type I fibers, or red fibers. Red fibers contain large amounts of mitochondria, due to their high rates of oxidative metabolism, as well as myoglobin, which facilitates oxygen storage for times of increased demand. These fibers contract and relax slowly but are capable of prolonged periods of contraction without fatigue. Fast-twitch fibers are called type II fibers, or white fibers. These fibers generate rapid, short-term contractions. Fast fatigable (type IIB) fibers have large stores of glycogen and utilize anaerobic catabolism for contraction. Lactic acid accumulates rapidly in these fibers, which limits their ability to sustain contraction forces. Fast fatigue-resistant (type IIA) fibers have some aerobic metabolism capacity (less than red fibers, however), and are able to generate rapid contractions, yet maintain them for a period of several minutes. With muscle contraction, weaker motor units are recruited in an orderly fashion before stronger motor units. Synaptic input stimulates smaller cells with higher internal resistances before larger cells, which forms the basis for motor unit recruitment by size (Kandel, pp. 676–682).

79-E; 80-B,E; 81-B; 82-D; 83-A. Refer to Figure 1.79–1.83A. A single muscle cell contains several myofibrils, each of which consists of linear chains of solitary contractile units, or sarcomeres. Myofibrils are connected to one another via desmin intermediate filaments, and this complex is then anchored to the muscle cell sarcolemma by several proteins, including dystrophin. Within the myofibril, each sarcomere is connected to the adjacent sarcomere at the Z disc (A), and actin (thin) filaments radiate from the Z disc toward the center of the sarcomere. Myosin (thick) filaments are found interspersed between adjacent actin filaments. The dark band, or A band (D), is the region of the sarcomere that is composed primarily of myosin filaments. The light band, or I band (E), is the region that is composed solely of actin filaments and is centered on a Z disc. The H zone (B) is the region of the A band where myosin filaments are not overlapped by actin filaments in the resting state, and it is centered on the M line (C). With myofibril contraction, the actin and myosin filaments form successive cross bridges that facilitate sliding across one another. This functionally shortens the sarcomere during contraction and consequently results in H-zone and I-band shortening. This process of muscle contraction requires the presence of cytosolic Ca^{2+}. In the resting state, tropomyosin and a troponin complex (troponins I, C, and T) are bound to actin. After the sarcoplasmic reticulum releases Ca^{2+} in response to an action potential, troponin C binds four molecules of Ca^{2+}, which subsequently relieves the inhibition of the myosin binding site on actin. Myosin heads are then free to bind actin and form cross bridges. The myosin head, which has intrinsic ATPase activity, then rotates, pulling the actin filaments longitudinally and increasing the overlap between the thick and thin filaments. ATP then binds to the myosin head, which stimulates the release of the cross bridge between actin. The subsequent hydrolysis of ATP "cocks" the myosin head, which then forms a second cross bridge, contracts, and further increases the overlap between thick and thin filaments. ADP is released, and the process is repeated as long as ATP and Ca^{2+} are present in the cytosol. In this manner, the myosin heads "walk" along the actin filaments during contraction, effectively shortening the sarcomere and myofibril (Kandel, pp. 676–682).

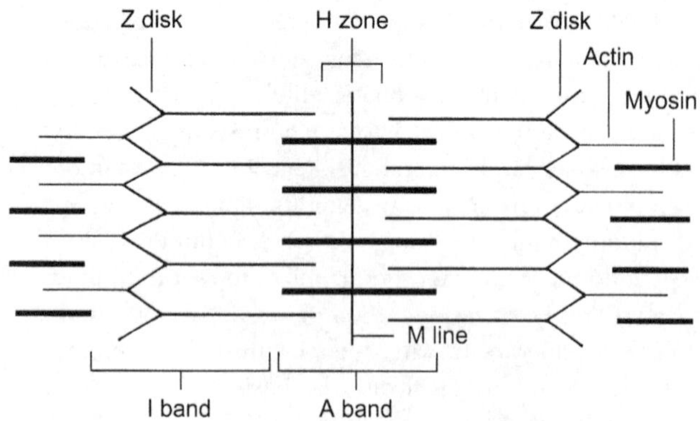

FIGURE 1.79–83A Sarcomere. With sarcomere contraction, the I band and H zone shorten. (Reprinted with permission from Moore SP. The Definitive Neurological Surgery Board Review. Malden, MA: Blackwell Publishing, 2005:11, Figure 1.1.)

84. B. A neuropathologist can best estimate the gestational age by the pattern of cerebral sulci in this case. Before 16 weeks, the interhemispheric and sylvian fissures are present, but the brain remains smooth without any identifiable sulci. After 16 weeks, the sulci begin to appear in a definite sequence (callosal sulcus, parieto-occipital fissure, calcarine sulcus, olfactory sulcus, followed by the central sulcus, precentral sulcus, and postcentral sulcus). If sulcation fails, the cerebral hemispheres remain smooth (lissencephaly),

and contain only four cortical layers, as opposed to the six that are normally present. The timetable for myelination also helps determine gestational age, but most areas of the brain do not myelinate until after birth. The neural tube is generally closed by 18 weeks of gestation, and maternal α-fetoprotein or thickness of the ependymal layer is not a reliable indicator of gestational age (Ellison, pp. 71–76).

85. B. The CSF is a clear fluid containing protein, glucose, K^+, and significantly large amounts of Na^+, which supports the brain and helps cushion it during trauma. About 70% is secreted by the choroid plexus, and the remainder is produced by metabolic water production. The total volume of CSF in humans is about 140 mL, of which about 25 to 30 mL is contained within the ventricular system. Net production is about 400 to 500 mL/day or 0.35 mL/min in humans. The bulk of CSF is returned to the venous system via the arachnoid villi. The exit of CSF is pressure-, not volume-dependent and begins when CSF pressure exceeds venous pressure by 3 to 6 mm Hg of water. Volatile agents and CO_2 increase CSF formation, while carbonic anhydrase inhibitors and norepinephrine reduce CSF formation (Greenberg, pp. 164–165; Carpenter, pp. 9–20).

86-G; 87-C; 88-E; 89-F; 90-D; 91-B; 92-H. Refer to Table 1.86-1.92A (Moore, pp. 60–64, 67–70, 72–73, 84–85).

93. B. A transient postsynaptic membrane depolarization caused by presynaptic release of a neurotransmitter is called an excitatory postsynaptic potential (EPSP). Synaptic activation of ACh-gated and glutamate-gated ion channels causes EPSPs. Synaptic activation of GABA-gated ion channels (Cl^- and K^+-mediated) causes an inhibitory postsynaptic potential (IPSP) (Kandel, pp. 207–218).

TABLE 1.86–92A Gestational age and embryologic milestones

GESTATIONAL AGE	EMBRYOLOGIC MILESTONES
Day 4	12–16 blastomeres present, forming morula
Days 7–14	Process of embryonic implantation complete; process of forming three germ layers begins, although by 14 days, two distinct layers are apparent (bilaminar disc): epiblast and hypoblast
Day 16	Notochord begins to develop and induces overlying ectoderm to proliferate, forming the neural plate
By day 18	Neural groove development along midline of neural plate. Lateral edges of the neural groove are the neural folds
By day 21	Neural folds have begun to approach each other, eventually meeting and forming neural tube; beginning of neural crest development
Day 24	Rostral neuropore closure (lamina terminalis)
Day 26	Caudal neuropore closure
Beginning of fourth week	The portion of neural tube rostral to fourth pair of somites (divides future brain from spinal cord) undergoes a series of dilations and foldings, forming three primary brain vesicles (prosencephalon, mesencephalon, and rhombencephalon)
During fifth week	Prosencephalon divides into telencephalon and diencephalon; rhombencephalon divides into metencephalon and myelencephalon; mesencephalon does not divide

94. A. Despite the absence of large quantities of protein for buffering, CSF pH is maintained in a narrow range, even with major changes in systemic pH. This is emphasized by the fact that the range of CSF pH compatible with life is very narrow (7.19 to 7.38) in comparison to systemic pH (6.9 to 7.8). A number of important mechanisms are involved to achieve this tight balance, which center around the fact that pCO_2 diffuses readily across the blood-brain barrier (BBB), but both bicarbonate and hydrogen ions are relatively impermeable. As a result, the pH of the CSF and brain interstitium is less effectively buffered in acute respiratory acid-base disorders than metabolic ones. For example, acute metabolic acidosis results in compensatory hyperventilation, an immediate reduction in CSF pCO_2, and an increase in CSF pH (paradoxical alkalosis). During respiratory acidosis, compensatory mechanisms such as carbonic anhydrase–catalyzed generation of bicarbonate by the choroid plexus and deamination of glutamic acid typically return CSF and brain interstitial pH toward normal in a matter of hours, not minutes or seconds (Fishman, pp. 135–136; Simmons, pp. 347–348).

95. C. There is evidence of increased growth of meningiomas during various phases of the menstrual cycle and during pregnancy, which has sparked interest in the effects of hormone receptors on meningiomas. Studies have shown that meningiomas express intranuclear, functionally active progesterone receptors, but their precise relationship to tumor growth remains uncertain (Kaye and Laws, pp. 45, 117, 724; Carroll et al., pp. 92–97).

96-F; 97-E; 98-G; 99-A; 100-D. Chemical neurotransmitters can exert their action by two major mechanisms. The first is direct activation of transmitter-gated ion channels (acetylcholine-nicotinic receptor, AMPA, kainate, NMDA glutamate channels, $GABA_A$ and glycine receptors) and the second involves the activation of effector proteins by G protein–coupled receptors (muscarinic receptors, metabotropic glutamate receptors, $GABA_B$, serotonin [5-HT] receptors, D1 receptors, and certain norepinephrine [$\alpha 1$, $\alpha 2$, $\beta 1$, $\beta 2$, $\beta 3$] receptors), as described in questions 60 and 61. G protein–coupled receptors, in turn, exert their effects by two separate mechanisms: either by activating G protein–gated ion channels (distinct from transmitter-gated ion channels described above) or G protein–activating enzymes. Because the former pathway does not involve any other enzymatic intermediaries, it is often referred to as the "shortcut pathway." One example of this is the muscarinic receptors of the heart, which are directly coupled to K^+ channels and explain why K^+ slows the heart rate. Although this "shortcut pathway" is not as fast as transmitter-gated channels, which uses no intermediary between receptor and channel, it is faster than the second-messenger cascades we describe next.

G protein–mediated second messengers activate a variety of downstream mediators to influence downstream events. One pathway involves G protein–mediated activation of the membrane-bound enzyme adenylyl cyclase, which converts ATP to cAMP (activates protein kinase A). Another pathway involves G protein–stimulated activation of phospholipase C (PLC), an enzyme that cleaves PIP_2 into two molecules acting as second messengers: DAG and IP_3. DAG activates protein kinase C, while IP_3 binds to receptors on the smooth endoplastic reticulum to cause discharge of their calcium stores, which activates calcium-calmodulin–dependent protein kinase, or CaMK (Kandel, pp. 196–201, 212–228, 230–250; Bear, pp. 137–147).

Neuroanatomy Questions

1. Regions of the brain devoid of a blood-brain barrier include all the following EXCEPT?

   A. Pineal body
   B. Subfornical organ
   C. Organum vasculosum of the lamina terminalis
   D. Median eminence of the hypothalamus
   E. Habenular nucleus

2. What is the major outflow tract of the basal ganglia?

   A. Lenticular fasciculus (Forel's field H2)
   B. Ansa lenticularis
   C. Thalamic fasciculus (Forel's field H1)
   D. Ansa reticularis
   E. Mammillothalamic tract

3. Injury to Guillain-Mollaret's triangle can produce?

   A. Arm tremor
   B. Torsional nystagmus
   C. Hypotonia
   D. Deafness
   E. Myoclonus

4. Through what structure do fibers from the inferior olives reach the cerebellum?

   A. Superior cerebellar peduncle
   B. Inferior cerebellar peduncle
   C. Middle cerebellar peduncle
   D. Vestibular nucleus
   E. Flocculonodular lobe

5. All of the following are association fibers EXCEPT?

   A. Superior longitudinal fasciculus
   B. Arcuate fasciculus
   C. Uncinate fasciculus
   D. Corona radiata
   E. Cingulum

6. First-order neurons involved in pupillary dilation originate in what structure?

   A. Thalamus
   B. Hypothalamus
   C. Superior colliculus
   D. Superior cervical ganglia
   E. Edinger-Westphal nucleus

7. The basal nucleus (of Meynert) contains what type of neurons?

   A. Cholinergic
   B. Adrenergic
   C. Serotonergic
   D. Dopaminergic
   E. Noradrenergic

8. Beginning the incision for an anterior iliac crest graft approximately 3 cm lateral to the anterior iliac spine attempts to avoid injury of what structure(s)?

   1. Sartorius muscle
   2. Lateral femoral cutaneous nerve
   3. Ilioinguinal ligament
   4. Iliacus muscle

   A. 1, 2, and 3 are correct
   B. 1 and 2 are correct
   C. 2 and 4 are correct
   D. Only 4 is correct
   E. All of the above

QUESTIONS 9–15

Directions: The questions below consist of lettered headings followed by a set of numbered items. For each numbered item, select one heading with which it is most closely associated. Each lettered heading may be used once, more than once, or not at all.

   A. CA1
   B. CA2
   C. CA3
   D. CA4
   E. Indusium griseum
   F. Dentate gyrus
   G. None of the above

9. Mossy fibers originating in the dentate gyrus terminate here

10. Extremely vulnerable to hypoxia

11. Schaffer collaterals project to the pyramidal neurons of this subfield

12. Lies in the concavity of the dentate gyrus

13. Vestigial remnant of hippocampal formation

14. Injury of this sector may produce remote memory problems

15. Largest sector

End of set

16. In normal individuals, the direct and indirect circuits of the basal ganglia are balanced by?

   A. The opposing actions of the dopaminergic nigrostriatal projections on the D1 and D2 receptor subtypes in the putamen

   B. The inhibitory activity of the subthalamic nucleus on the globus pallidus interna

   C. The increased activity of GABAergic neurons in the internal segment of the globus pallidus by the direct pathway

   D. The ascending dopaminergic fibers originating in the midbrain tegmentum and synapsing in the pars compacta of the substantia nigra (influencing D1 and D2 receptors in the globus pallidus)

   E. All of the above

17. A visual lesion producing a central defect in one field with a superior temporal defect in the opposite may be originating in what location?

   A. Anterior chiasm

   B. Occipital lobe

   C. Temporal lobe

   D. Optic nerve

   E. Inferior parietal lobe

18. Fibers from the frontal eye fields pass through the genu of the internal capsule, decussate in the pons, and synapse in what structure involved with saccades?

   A. Medial longitudinal fasciculus (MLF)

   B. Inferior colliculus

   C. Edinger-Westphal nucleus

   D. Solitary nucleus

   E. Paramedian pontine reticular formation (PPRF)

QUESTIONS 19–25

Directions: For each numbered item, select one letter heading (in parenthesis) from Figure 2.19–2.25Q with which it is most closely associated. Each lettered heading may be used once, more than once, or not at all.

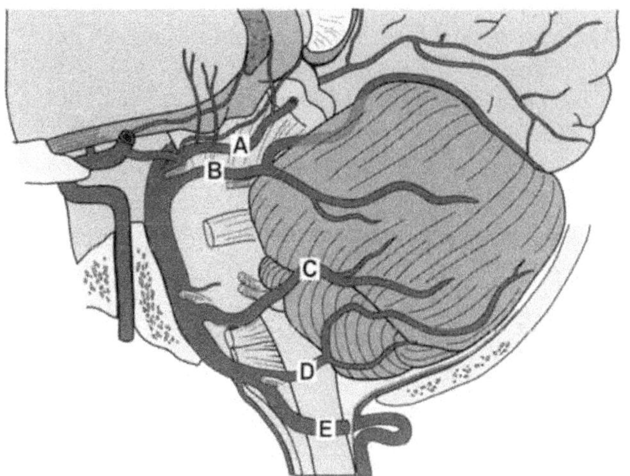

FIGURE 2.19-25Q Posterior circulation.

19. Occlusion of this vessel is the most common cause of lateral medullary (Wallenberg) syndrome

20. Supplies the pyramis, tuber, flocculus, and caudal parts of pontine tegmentum

21. Occlusion can produce contralateral hearing impairment

22. Vessel commonly associated with trigeminal neuralgia

23. Vessel at most risk of injury during Chiari decompression

24. The dentate nucleus is mainly supplied by this vessel

25. Supplies the middle cerebellar peduncle

End of set

26. Fibers passing from the amygdala to the hypothalamus may travel in what fiber bundle?

   A. Stria medullaris

   B. Fornix

   C. Stria terminalis

   D. Medial forebrain bundle

   E. Cingulum

27. A cerebellar glomerulus consists of all of the following EXCEPT?

   A. Climbing fibers

   B. Glial capsule

   C. Dendrites of granule neurons

   D. Axons and dendrites of Golgi type II neurons

   E. Mossy fibers

28. The major site for neuroblast proliferation in the CNS is

   A. Layer III of the cerebral cortex

   B. Periventricular ependymal region

   C. White matter

   D. Spinal cord

   E. Arachnoid layer

29. Which cell represents the only output of the cerebellar cortex?

   A. Granule cell

   B. Golgi cell

   C. Stellate cell

   D. Purkinje cell

   E. Horizontal cell

30. What structures pass through the annulus tendineus (of Zinn)?

1. Ophthalmic vein
2. Lateral rectus muscle
3. Lacrimal branch of ophthalmic nerve
4. Inferior division of oculomotor nerve

A. 1, 2, and 3 are correct
B. 1 and 3 are correct
C. 2 and 4 are correct
D. Only 4 is correct
E. All of the above

QUESTIONS 31–42

Directions: The questions below consist of lettered headings from Figure 2.31–2.42Q followed by a set of numbered items. For each numbered item, select one heading with which it is most closely associated. Each lettered heading may be used once, more than once, or not at all.

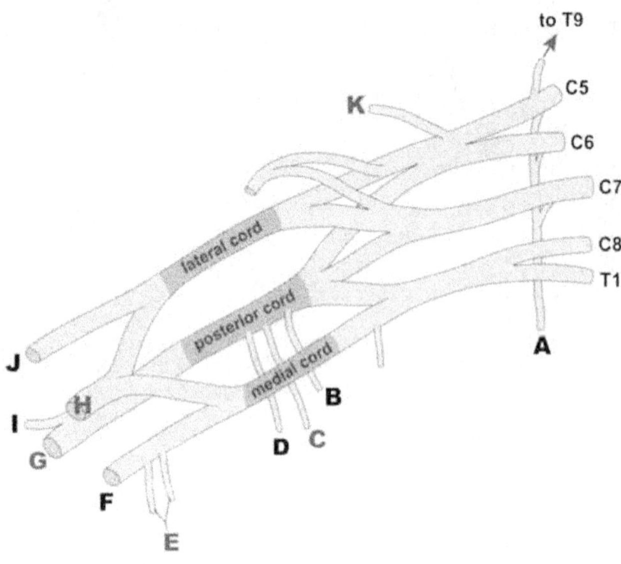

FIGURE 2.31–42Q

31. Nerve supplies muscles that are antagonists to the serratus anterior

32. Injury to this nerve may result in winged scapula

33. Innervates teres minor muscle

34. Injury to this nerve will result in flexion weakness, especially when the forearm is supine

35. Innervates supinator muscle

36. Nerve most commonly affected by entrapment neuropathy

37. A pure lesion of a branch of this nerve can result in weakness of the long flexors of the thumb and index finger (producing a pinch sign) and pronator quadratus

38. Injury of this nerve may occur in Guyan's canal

39. Compression of this nerve may occur by a ligament that bridges the supracondylar process to the medial epicondyle

40. Innervates the interossei muscles

41. Supplies sensation to the anteromedial and posteromedial forearm down to the wrist

42. Entrapment in quadrilateral space

End of set

43. All are features of the cerebral cortex EXCEPT?
A. Vague cytoarchitectural boundaries
B. Laminar arrangement of neurons
C. Conspicuous stripes of unmyelinated fibers
D. Radial or columnar arrangement of neurons
E. Numerous pyramidal cells in layer V of the visual cortex that send fibers to the brainstem for visually directed reflexive eye movements

44. The arcuate fasciculus is composed of association fibers interconnecting which structures?
A. Superior parietal lobule and occipital lobe
B. Superior and middle frontal gyrus and temporal lobe
C. Superior and inferior frontal gyrus and limbic lobe
D. Thalamus and amygdala
E. Orbital frontal gyri and temporal lobe

45. A 27-year-old male presents to the emergency room with ptosis of the right eyelid and pupillary constriction of the same eye, but no gaze palsy or diplopia. The most likely explanation for this is a lesion in what location?
A. CN II
B. CN III
C. CN V
D. CN VII
E. Carotid sympathetic nerve

46. What region(s) of the striate cortex do NOT contain ocular dominance columns?

1. The cortical region representing the blind spot of the retina
2. The cortical region representing the nasal half of the ipsilateral retina
3. The cortical region representing the monocular temporal crescent of the visual field
4. The columnar system, which is mainly concerned with line orientation and retinal position

A. 1, 2, and 3 are correct
B. 1 and 3 are correct
C. 2 and 4 are correct
D. Only 4 is correct
E. All of the above

QUESTIONS 47–51

Directions: The questions below consist of lettered headings (Figure 2.47–2.51Q) followed by a set of numbered items. For each numbered item, select one heading with which it is most closely associated. Each lettered heading may be used once, more than once, or not at all.

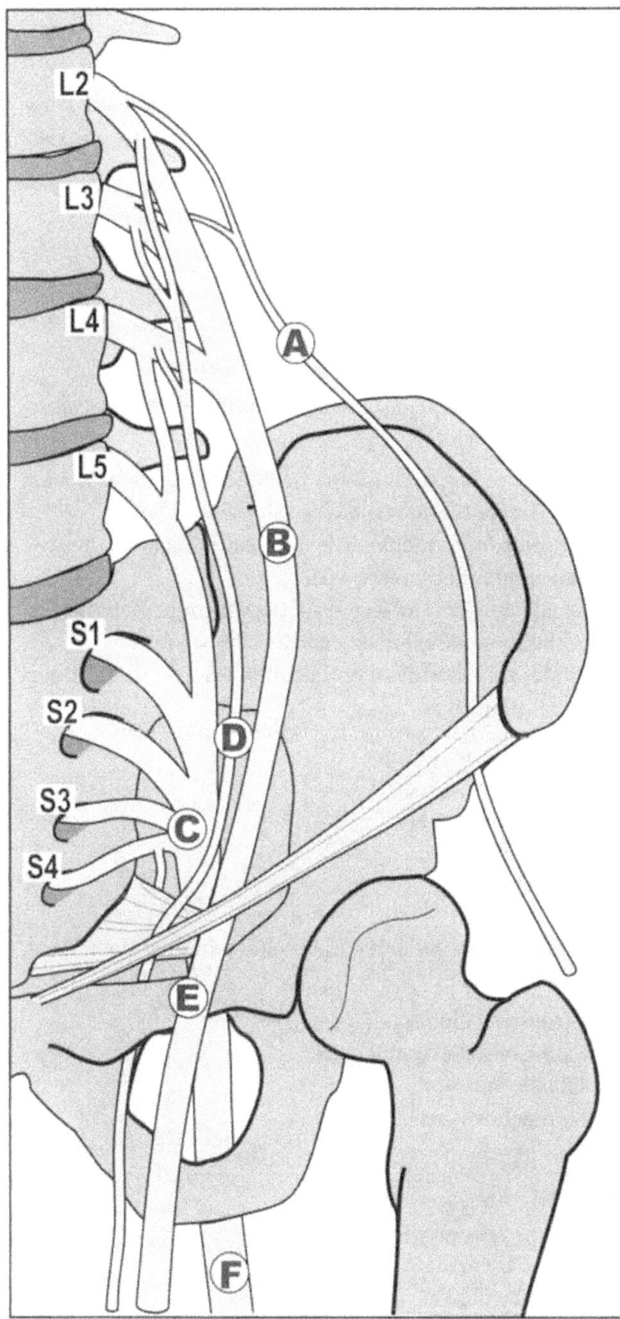

FIGURE 2.47–51Q

47. Prone to injury during obstetric and gynecologic procedures

48. Nerve associated with "meralgia paresthetica"

49. Nerve likely to be damaged by hematoma in the pelvis

50. Diabetic amyotrophy is most likely to affect this site

51. Supplies the pectineus and gracilis muscles

End of set

52. A gray ramus communicans, which extends between a sympathetic trunk ganglion and anterior primary ramus of a spinal nerve, contains which of the following?

    A. General somatic afferent fibers
    B. Myelinated fibers
    C. Preganglionic sympathetic neurons
    D. Fibers that become the enteric nervous system
    E. Adrenergic fibers

53. Muscles that are innervated by the ansa cervicalis include all of the following EXCEPT?

    A. Omohyoid
    B. Geniohyoid
    C. Thyrohyoid
    D. Geniohyoid
    E. Stylohyoid

54. A 46-year-old male with a remote history of a gunshot wound to the face and intravenous drug abuse presents to the emergency room with fevers and swelling on the left side of his neck and face. A CT scan reveals an abscess adjacent to the pterygopalatine fossa. This infection may directly track to all of the following compartments EXCEPT?

    A. Orbital cavity
    B. Nasal cavity
    C. Middle cranial fossa
    D. Inner ear
    E. Oral cavity

QUESTIONS 55–58

Directions: Match the lesion site with the corresponding clinical abnormality. For each numbered item, select one heading with which it is most closely associated. Each lettered heading may be used once, more than once, or not at all.

    A. Marcus-Gunn pupil
    B. Horner's pupil
    C. Adie's pupil (Tonic pupil)
    D. Argyll-Robertson pupil
    E. None of the above

55. Short ciliary nerves

56. Superior cervical ganglion

57. Dorsal midbrain

58. Retina

End of set

59. The term *lentiform nuclei* refers to what structure(s)?

A. Caudate nucleus and globus pallidum

B. Putamen and amygdala

C. Putamen and globus pallidus

D. Caudate nucleus, globus pallidus, and putamen

E. Globus pallidus

60. The subthalamic nucleus (STN) receives its dominant input from which of the following structures?

A. Ventral lateral (VL) nucleus of the thalamus

B. Centromedian (CM) nucleus of the thalamus

C. Lateral globus pallidus

D. Medial globus pallidus

E. Cerebral cortex

61. All of the following are afferent tracts through the inferior cerebellar peduncle EXCEPT?

A. Vestibulocerebellar

B. Olivocerebellar

C. Dorsal spinocerebellar

D. Reticulocerebellar

E. Corticopontocerebellar

62. Axons of which cells leave layer V of the neocortex primarily as projection fibers?

A. Stellate cells

B. Fusiform cells

C. Pyramidal cells

D. Horizontal cells

E. Fusiform cells

63. Which body part has the largest relative representation in the sensorimotor cortex?

A. Genitalia

B. Middle finger

C. Nipple

D. Thumb

E. Index finger

64. A major difference between the archicortex and neocortex includes what?

A. Absence of lamination in the archicortex

B. A six-layer arrangement of the archicortex

C. Presence of a superficial layer of white matter in the archicortex

D. Lack of Betz cells in the archicortex

E. The archicortex has major connections only with the limbic system

65. Which nucleus of the hypothalamus is involved with production of hypothalamic-releasing factors and gives rise to the tuberohypophysial tract?

A. Dorsomedial

B. Suprachiasmatic

C. Arcuate

D. Posterior

E. Preoptic

66. Which of the following constellations about hypothalamic function is/are correct?

1. Lateral and posterior hypothalamic regions concerned with sympathetic responses

2. Anterior and medial hypothalamic regions control parasympathetic responses

3. Localized, bilateral lesions of the ventromedial nucleus in the tuberal region can produce hyperphagia

4. Bilateral posterior hypothalamic lesions can produce poikilothermia

A. 1, 2, and 3 are correct

B. 1 and 3 are correct

C. 2 and 4 are correct

D. Only 4 is correct

E. All of the above

67. The deep peroneal nerve innervates which of the following muscles?

1. Extensor hallucis longus

2. Extensor digitorum longus

3. Tibialis anterior

4. Peroneus longus

A. 1, 2, and 3 are correct

B. 1 and 3 are correct

C. 2 and 4 are correct

D. Only 4 is correct

E. All of the above

68. The posterior limb of the internal capsule contains all the following tracts EXCEPT?

   A. Prefrontal corticopontine
   B. Corticospinal
   C. Corticotectal
   D. Corticorubral
   E. Superior thalamic radiations

69. What is the most common neurotransmitter found in the thalamus?

   A. Glutamate
   B. Aspartate
   C. GABA
   D. Acetylcholine
   E. Substance P

70. Crossed fibers of the optic tract terminate in which layers of the lateral geniculate body?

   A. 2, 4, and 6
   B. 1, 4, and 6
   C. 2, 3, and 5
   D. 1, 3, and 5
   E. 2, 5, and 6

71. Which of the following is NOT a deep nucleus of the cerebellum?

   A. Fastigial
   B. Fusiform
   C. Emboliform
   D. Globose
   E. Dentate

72. How far behind the coronal suture is the motor strip generally located?

   A. 1–2 cm
   B. 2–3 cm
   C. 4–5 cm
   D. 7–8 cm
   E. 9–10 cm

QUESTIONS 73–82

Directions: Match the appropriate cranial nerve (numbered items) with the foramina of the skull base (lettered headings in Figure 2.73–2.82Q) it traverses using each answer once, more than once, or not at all.

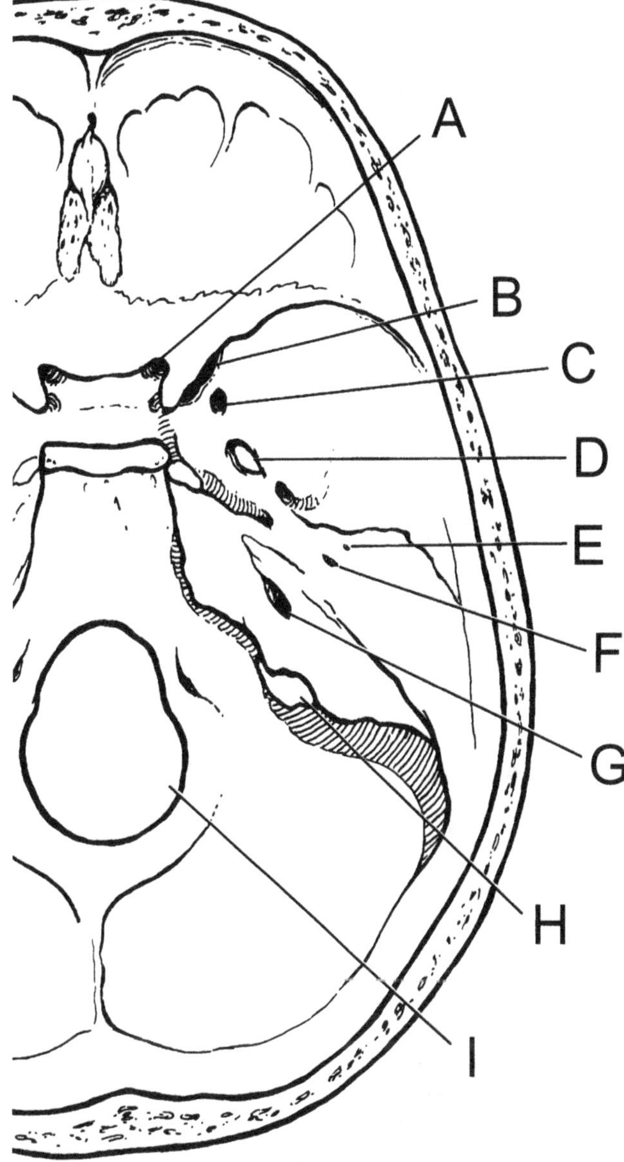

FIGURE 2.73–82Q

73. Injury of the cranial nerve piercing this foramen results in diplopia and weak gaze when looking down and out

74. Nerve that traverses this foramen later joins with the deep petrosal nerve to become the nerve to the pterygoid canal

75. Injury to a small branch of the nerve passing through this canal results in hyperacusis

76. The nerve passing through this foramen innervates the tensor veli palatini muscle

77. The cranial nerve passing through this foramen innervated by the superior salivatory nucleus to produce salivation

78. The nerve passing through this foramen gives rise to general visceral efferent (GVE) fibers that supply the parotid gland

79. The cell bodies of these afferent fibers are located in the nodosal ganglion and enter the skull through this foramen

80. The lesser petrosal nerve traverses this foramen

81. This foramen is traversed by a nerve that gives off the chorda tympani fibers

82. Transmits the ophthalmic vein

End of set

83. A 45-year-old male is found to have diplopia with weakness of downward and medial gaze of the right eye. He also has significant difficulty walking down steps without tilting his head for better visualization. What cranial nerve is most likely affected?

- **A.** Right oculomotor nerve
- **B.** Left oculomotor nerve
- **C.** Left trochlear nerve
- **D.** Right trochlear nerve
- **E.** Right abducens nerve

84. The following statements are true of the corticospinal tract EXCEPT?

- **A.** Approximately 3% of corticospinal fibers originate from Betz pyramidal cells
- **B.** Corticospinal fibers incompletely decussate in the medulla to form a larger lateral corticospinal tract and a smaller anterior corticospinal tract
- **C.** The majority of cervical corticospinal fibers are found medially and sacral fibers are found laterally
- **D.** Corticospinal lesions result in hyperactive tendon jerk reflexes, extensor toe response, and spasticity after a period of hypotonia
- **E.** Terminates primarily on α motor neurons in lamina IX of the spinal cord

85. Papez's circuit includes all of the following structures EXCEPT?

- **A.** Amygdala
- **B.** Fornix
- **C.** Mammillary bodies
- **D.** Cingulate gyrus
- **E.** Hippocampus

86. The predominant type of synapse in the retina is?

- **A.** Electrical
- **B.** Connexin-dependent
- **C.** Chemical
- **D.** Calcium-dependent
- **E.** cAMP-dependent

87. The inner nuclear layer of the retina contains what type of cell(s)?

1. Bipolar cells	**A.** 1, 2, and 3
2. Horizontal cells	**B.** 1 and 3
3. Amacrine cells	**C.** 2 and 4
4. Ganglion cells	**D.** Only 4 is correct
	E. All of the above

QUESTIONS 88–95

Directions: Match the thalamic nucleus (lettered headings in Figure 2.88–2.95Q) with the fibers (numbered items) it receives. Each answer may be used once, more than once, or not at all.

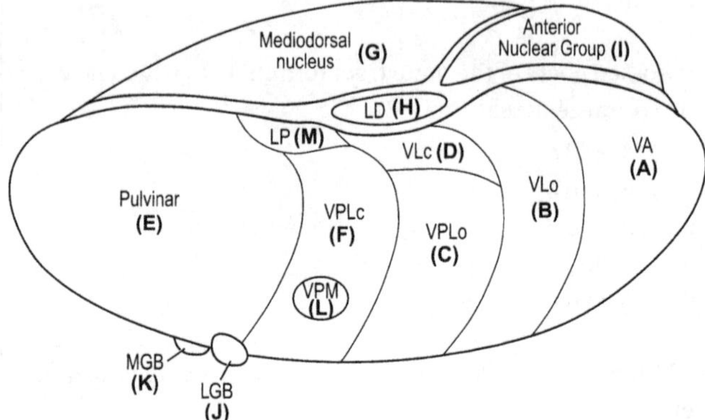

FIGURE 2.88–95Q

88. Area 5

89. Superior colliculus

90. Medial lemniscus

91. Mammillothalamic tract; fornix

92. Inferior colliculus; lateral lemniscus

93. Optic tract

94. Trigeminothalamic tract

95. Cerebellar nuclei

End of set

96. All of the following statements concerning the medulla oblongata are correct EXCEPT?

- **A.** Extends from the pyramidal decussation to the inferior pontine sulcus
- **B.** Receives a portion of its blood supply from the posterior spinal artery
- **C.** Gives rise to GVE fibers that synapse in the otic ganglia
- **D.** Gives rise to the lateral vestibular nucleus
- **E.** Is the origin of GVE fibers that synapse in the sinoatrial and atrioventricular nodes of the heart

97. A 54-year-old male presents with ptosis, miosis, and hemianhydrosis on the left side, loss of vibration sensation in the right leg, loss of pain and temperature on the face, trunk, and extremities on the right, as well as severe ataxia and intention tremor on the left side. The lesion responsible for this constellation of problems is most likely in what location?

   A. Caudal midbrain tegmentum, left side
   B. Rostral medulla, medial zone, right side
   C. Caudal medulla, lateral zone, left side
   D. Pontine isthmus, dorsal lateral region, left side
   E. Posterior limb of the internal capsule

98. An infarct involving the paramedian part of the midbrain would most likely affect what structures?

   1. Oculomotor nerve roots (CN III)
   2. Red nucleus
   3. Dentatorubrothalamic tract
   4. Lateral lemniscus

   A. 1, 2, and 3 are correct
   B. 1 and 3 are correct
   C. 2 and 4 are correct
   D. Only 4 is correct
   E. All of the above

99. All of the following structures are involved with taste sensation EXCEPT?

   A. Cranial nerves VII, IX, and X
   B. Solitary nucleus
   C. Parabrachial nucleus
   D. Hypothalamus
   E. Para bigeminal nucleus

100. For proper motor function, the motor cortex receives inputs from all of the following structures EXCEPT?

   A. Parietal cortex
   B. Basal ganglia
   C. Dentate nucleus
   D. Primary somesthetic area (S I)
   E. Centromedian (CM) nucleus of the thalamus

101. Nitric oxide, a potent second messenger, is synthesized from which of the following?

   A. Lysine
   B. Arginine
   C. Tyrosine
   D. Dopamine
   E. Beta lipoprotein

102. Which of the following fibers violate the Bell-Magendie law?

   A. Peripheral proprioceptive fibers
   B. Unmyelinated C fibers from pelvic viscera
   C. Lower extremity motor fibers to appendicular musculature
   D. General visceral efferent fibers to the proximal GI tract
   E. None of the above

103. Which of the following descending tracts utilizes serotonin as its neurotransmitter?

   A. Tectospinal
   B. Medial longitudinal fasciculus (MLF)
   C. Reticulospinal
   D. Vestibulospinal
   E. Rubrospinal

104. What is the target of substantia nigra efferent fibers?

   A. Thalamus
   B. Internal segment of the globus pallidus
   C. Striatum
   D. A and C
   E. A, B, and C

105. Which of the following structures contains olfactory projections to the hypothalamus?

   A. Lateral olfactory stria
   B. Medial forebrain bundle
   C. Stria medullary thalami
   D. Diagonal band of Broca
   E. Lateral lemniscus

QUESTIONS 106–118

Directions: Match the venous structure with the corresponding letterhead depicted in the angiogram (Figure 2.106–2.118Q).

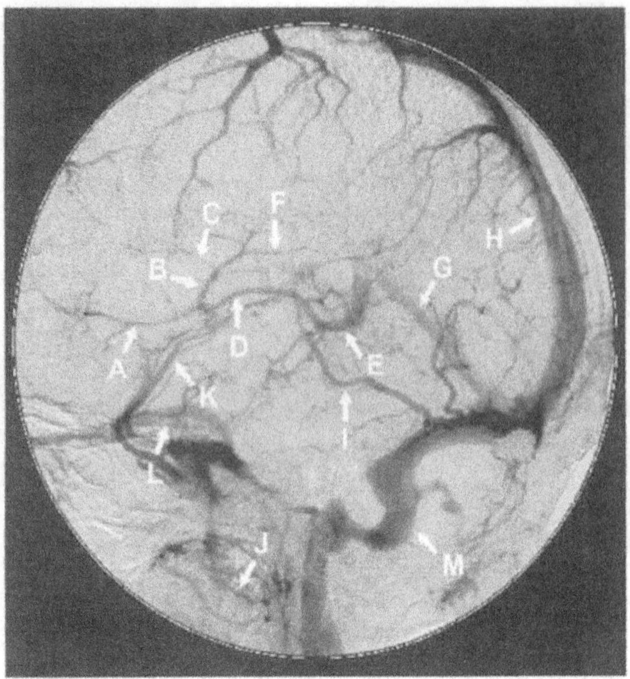

FIGURE 2.106–118Q

106. Vein of Labbé

107. Cavernous sinus

108. Straight sinus

109. Superior sagittal sinus

110. Anterior caudate vein

111. Vein of Galen

112. Internal cerebral vein

113. Pterygoid plexus

114. Thalamostriate vein

115. Anterior septal vein

116. Terminal vein

117. Sigmoid sinus

118. Superficial middle cerebral vein

End of set

119. Which of the following dorsal roots is frequently missing?

    A. C1
    B. C8
    C. T1
    D. T12
    E. S2

120. The junction of the central and peripheral nervous systems occurs at what location?

    A. Dorsal root ganglia
    B. Junction of the dorsal and ventral roots
    C. Ventral horn of the spinal cord and cranial nerves
    D. Site of attachment of nerve roots to spinal cord and brainstem, respectively
    E. Gray rami communicantes

121. A 45-year-old male presents with pain and numbness in the fifth digit of the right hand. These symptoms may occur secondary to a lesion in what location?

    1. Medial cord of the brachial plexus
    2. Ulnar nerve
    3. C8 nerve root
    4. C7 nerve root

    A. 1, 2, and 3 are correct
    B. 1 and 3 are correct
    C. 2 and 4 are correct
    D. Only 4 is correct
    E. All of the above

QUESTIONS 122–124

122. A cadaveric dissection of the posterior fossa is depicted (Figure 2.122–2.124Q). What approach was most likely utilized to obtain this surgical exposure?

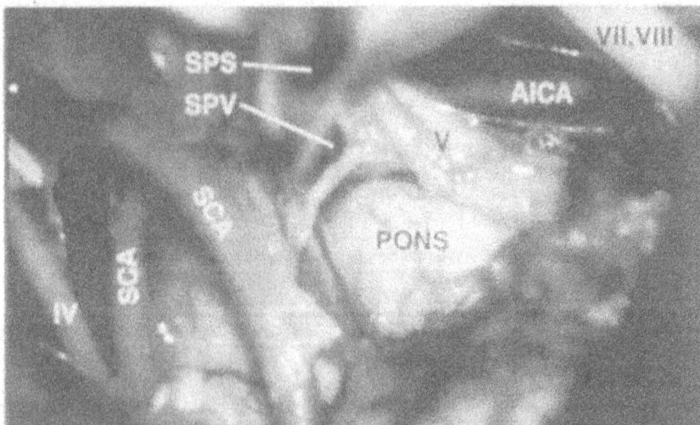

FIGURE 2.122–124Q

    A. Pterional transsylvian
    B. Subtemporal
    C. Midline suboccipital
    D. Infratemporal fossa
    E. Presigmoid transpetrous

123. What cranial nerve is particularly vulnerable to injury during the initial exposure?

    A. IV
    B. V
    C. VI
    D. VII
    E. X

124. What vascular structure is most frequently cauterized and divided to increase exposure during this approach?

A. Inferior petrosal sinus
B. Sigmoid sinus
C. Occipital sinus
D. Superior petrosal sinus
E. Precentral cerebellar vein

End of set

QUESTIONS 125–129

Directions: Match the lesion site with the associated abnormality.

A. Posterior hypothalamus
B. Anterior hypothalamus
C. Lateral hypothalamus
D. None of the above

125. Precocious puberty

126. Starvation

127. Hyperthermia

128. Emotional lethargy, excessive sleepiness, hypothermia

129. Decreased dopamine synthesis

End of set

130. The inferior parietal lobule consists of what gyri?

1. Lingual
2. Angular
3. Lateral occipital gyrus
4. Supramarginal

A. 1, 2, and 3 are correct
B. 1 and 3 are correct
C. 2 and 4 are correct
D. Only 4 is correct
E. All of the above

131. Contractions of the stapedius and tensor tympani muscles are initiated by inputs from what structure?

A. Inferior colliculus
B. Superior temporal gyrus (Heschl's gyrus)
C. Superior olivary nucleus
D. Inner hair cells of the cochlea
E. Cochlear nucleus

132. Root fibers entering the spinal trigeminal tract have definite topographical organization. All of the following are correct about this tract EXCEPT?

A. Fibers of the ophthalmic division are ventral
B. Fibers of the mandibular division are dorsal
C. The fibers of the maxillary division lie in an intermediate location between the mandibular and ophthalmic fibers
D. This tract extends from the trigeminal root entry zone to the uppermost cervical spinal segments
E. Rostrally this tract blends into the solitary nucleus

133. Which of the following is/are secreted by the pineal gland?

1. Serotonin
2. Melatonin
3. Norepinephrine
4. Substance P

A. 1, 2, and 3 are correct
B. 1 and 3 are correct
C. 2 and 4 are correct
D. Only 4 is correct
E. All of the above

134. Which of the following CNS locations contains melanocytes?

1. Ventral medulla
2. Inferior medullary velum
3. Upper spinal cord
4. Habenular nucleus

A. 1, 2, and 3 are correct
B. 1 and 3 are correct
C. 2 and 4 are correct
D. Only 4 is correct
E. All of the above

135. Which of the following structures is formed directly from the embryologic notochord?

A. Nucleus pulposus of the intervertebral disc
B. Vertebral bodies
C. Spinal canal
D. Choroid plexus
E. Dorsal root ganglia

QUESTIONS 136–137

136. The blood supply to the anterior limb of the internal capsule originates from the

A. Anterior choroidal artery
B. Inferolateral artery
C. Recurrent artery of Heubner
D. Tuberoinfundibular artery
E. Basilar communicating artery of Percheron

137. The blood supply to the posterior limb of the internal capsule originates from the

A. Anterior choroidal artery
B. Inferolateral artery
C. Recurrent artery of Heubner
D. Tuberoinfundibular artery
E. Basilar communicating artery of Percheron

End of set

138. Gustatory afferents from CN VII end in what nucleus?

A. Nucleus salivatorius
B. Mesencephalic sensory nucleus
C. Nucleus solitarius
D. Nucleus of Roller
E. Pontine facial nucleus

139. All of the following contain parasympathetic fibers EXCEPT?

 A. CN VII
 B. CN IX
 C. CN X
 D. CN XI
 E. CN III

QUESTIONS 140–148

Directions: Match the following, using each answer only once.

 A. Mainly C5
 B. Thoracodorsal nerve
 C. Axillary nerve
 D. Anterior interosseous nerve
 E. Ulnar nerve
 F. Median nerve
 G. Radial nerve
 H. Suprascapular nerve
 I. Musculocutaneous nerve

140. Abductor pollicis brevis

141. Infraspinatus

142. Deltoid

143. Brachioradialis

144. Biceps

145. Adductor pollicis

146. Pronator quadratus

147. Rhomboid

148. Latissimus dorsi

End of set

QUESTIONS 149–154

Directions: Match the syndrome with the associated clinical findings using each answer once, more than once, or not at all.

 A. Orbitofrontal (frontal pole) syndrome
 B. Frontal convexity syndrome
 C. Medial frontal syndrome
 D. None of the above

149. Mutism, gait disturbance, and incontinence

150. Indifference, apathy, motor preservation, and impersistence

151. Impulsiveness, euphoria, poor judgment

152. Tendency to explore objects orally

153. Apraxia of gait or "magnetic gait"

154. "Salutatory seizures"

End of set

155. The vertebral arteries travel in the transverse foramina of

 A. C6 to C2
 B. C4 to C2
 C. C7 to C1
 D. C7 to C2
 E. C8 to C1

QUESTIONS 156–157

156. A relative afferent pupillary defect is NOT seen with lesions involving the

 A. Retina
 B. Lateral geniculate body
 C. Pretectal nucleus
 D. Optic nerve
 E. Optic chiasm

157. If the left eye shows a relative afferent pupillary defect, the right pupil will

 A. Immediately constrict when the light is swung to the left
 B. Immediately dilate when the light is swung to the right
 C. Dilate when the light is swung from the right eye to the left
 D. Remain unchanged when the light is swung to the left
 E. Remain dilated at all times

End of set

158. Which of the following eye muscles receives contralateral nuclear innervation?

 1. Inferior oblique   A. 1, 2, and 3
 2. Superior rectus   B. 1 and 3
 3. Inferior rectus   C. 2 and 4
 4. Superior oblique   D. Only 4 is correct
                          E. all of the above

159. "Periodic alternating gaze" is usually seen with

 A. Frontal seizure foci
 B. Posterior fossa lesions
 C. Persistent muscle spasms of the face and jaw
 D. Bilateral paramedian pontine reticular formation lesions
 E. Bilateral medial longitudinal fasciculus (MLF) lesions

QUESTIONS 160–168

Directions: For each reflex below, select the nerve that mediates the afferent limb.
   A. CN V1
   B. CN V2
   C. CN V3
   D. CN IX
   E. CN X
   F. None of the above

160. Sneeze reflex

161. Cough reflex

162. Gag reflex

163. Carotid sinus

164. Corneal blink reflex

165. Jaw-jerk reflex

166. Tearing reflex

167. Pupillary light reflex

168. Opticokinetic reflex

End of set

169. Which of the following neurons are cholinergic?
   A. Purkinje neurons of the cerebellum
   B. Substantia innominata
   C. Interneurons of the substantia nigra
   D. Neurons in the ganglionic layer of the retina
   E. Interneurons of the collicular plate

170. A lesion in what location could result in partial bilateral deafness?
   A. Ventral cochlear nucleus
   B. Dorsal cochlear nucleus
   C. Inner hair cells of the retina
   D. Lateral lemniscus
   E. Cochlear nerve

QUESTIONS 171–175

Directions: Match the neurotransmitter with the associated anatomic location using each answer once, more than once, or not at all.
   A. Norepinephrine
   B. Serotonin
   C. Dopamine
   D. Acetylcholine
   E. Glycine
   F. GABA
   G. None of the above

171. Golgi type II interneurons

172. Dorsal raphe nucleus

173. Locus ceruleus

174. Medial raphe nucleus

175. Substantia nigra

End of set

Neuroanatomy Answer Key

1. E	36. H	71. B	106. I	141. H
2. A	37. H	72. C	107. L	142. C
3. E	38. F	73. B	108. G	143. G
4. B	39. H	74. F	109. H	144. I
5. D	40. F	75. G	110. C	145. E
6. B	41. E	76. D	111. E	146. D
7. A	42. I	77. G	112. D	147. A
8. A	43. C	78. H	113. J	148. B
9. C	44. B	79. H	114. B	149. C
10. A	45. E	80. E	115. A	150. B
11. A	46. B	81. G	116. F	151. A
12. D	47. D	82. B	117. M	152. D
13. E	48. A	83. C	118. K	153. C
14. G	49. B	84. E	119. A	154. C
15. A	50. E	85. A	120. D	155. A
16. A	51. D	86. C	121. A	156. B
17. A	52. E	87. A	122. E	157. C
18. E	53. E	88. M	123. A	158. C
19. E	54. D	89. E	124. D	159. B
20. C	55. C	90. F	125. A	160. B
21. B	56. B	91. I	126. C	161. E
22. B	57. D	92. K	127. B	162. D
23. D	58. A	93. J	128. A	163. D
24. B	59. C	94. L	129. D	164. A
25. C	60. C	95. D	130. C	165. C
26. C	61. E	96. D	131. C	166. A
27. A	62. C	97. D	132. E	167. F
28. B	63. D	98. A	133. A	168. F
29. D	64. C	99. E	134. B	169. D
30. C	65. C	100. E	135. A	170. D
31. K	66. E	101. B	136. C	171. F
32. A	67. A	102. B	137. A	172. B
33. I	68. A	103. C	138. C	173. A
34. J	69. C	104. D	139. D	174. B
35. G	70. B	105. B	140. F	175. C

Neuroanatomy Answers

1. E. The pineal body, subfornical organ, organum vasculosum of the lamina terminalis, median eminence of the hypothalamus, neurohypophysis, subcommissural organ, and the area postrema are devoid of a blood-brain barrier and are commonly referred to as circumventricular organs. The habenular nucleus is not a circumventricular organ (Carpenter, pp. 18–20; Kandel, p. 1293).

2. A. The major fibers projecting from the basal ganglia originate in the medial globus pallidus as a fiber tract known as the lenticular fasciculus, or Forel's field H2. Another tract, known as ansa lenticularis, loops around the internal capsule, merges with the lenticular fasciculus in Forel's field H, and continues with the dentatorubrothalamic tract as the thalamic fasciculus (Forel's field H1). These fibers then synapse in the centromedian (CM), ventrolateral (VL), and ventroanterior (VA) nuclei of the thalamus before being relayed to the cerebral cortex. Three other efferent tracts of the basal ganglia include the pallidosubthalamic, pallidohabenular (via the stria medullaris), and pallidotegmental, which terminate in the subthalamic nucleus, habenular nucleus, and midbrain tegmentum, respectively (Carpenter, pp. 341–344).

3. E. Guillain-Mollaret's triangle is a physiologic connection between the red nucleus, inferior olives, and dentate nucleus of the cerebellum. Injury to this pathway has been known to result in palatal myoclonus. This occurs mainly from hypertrophic degeneration of the inferior olive secondary to either red or dentate nucleus damage. Other muscles of branchial origin (face, tongue, vocal cords, and diaphragm) may also be affected. Vascular lesions and multiple sclerosis are common causes of secondary palatal myoclonus that persists during sleep. The etiology of primary myoclonus is unclear and is often associated with bothersome clicking sounds in the ear caused by contractions of the tensor veli palatini (CN V) muscles, which open the eustachian tubes. Primary myoclonus disappears during sleep (Merritt, pp. 666–667; Wilkins, p. 149).

4. B. The fibers exiting the inferior olive are climbing fibers and reach the cerebellum through the inferior cerebellar peduncle. Climbing fibers are excitatory and synapse with Purkinje cells in a distinctive morphologic fashion. They wrap around the cell body and dendrites of Purkinje cells, where numerous synaptic contacts are made. Each climbing fiber contacts 1 to 10 Purkinje cells, and each Purkinje cell receives input from only a single climbing fiber. The response elicited by the interaction between climbing fibers and Purkinje cells is believed to be the most powerful in the CNS and results in a large action potential (complex spike) secondary to Ca^{2+} influx into the Purkinje cell. The other major afferent fibers reaching the cerebellum are mossy fibers, which influence Purkinje cells indirectly through synapses with granule cells (Carpenter, pp. 230–234).

5. D. The corona radiata is made up of projection fibers conveying impulses to subcortical structures including the thalamus, basal ganglia, brainstem, and spinal cord. The superior and inferior longitudinal fasciculus, arcuate fasciculus, uncinate fasciculus, external capsule, and cingulum are six of the more notable association fibers that connect different lobes within the same hemisphere. Commissural fibers connect corresponding regions of the two hemispheres, which include the corpus callosum, anterior commissure, and hippocampal commissure (Carpenter, pp. 33–37).

6. B. First-order neurons involved with pupillary dilation originate in the hypothalamus and descend through the brainstem and cervical spinal cord to the T1-T2 level of the spinal cord. They then synapse on ipsilateral preganglionic sympathetic fibers, exit the cord, travel with the sympathetic fibers as second-order neurons, and synapse on postganglionic sympathetic fibers. The third-order neurons travel with the internal carotid artery to the orbit and innervate the radial smooth muscle of the iris (Kandel, p. 905).

7. A. The basal nucleus (of Meynert) contains neurons with acetylcholine that project to the cingulate gyrus, septal nuclei, and the nucleus of the diagonal band of Broca. Dopaminergic fibers are located mainly in the substantia nigra and ventral tegmental area, which mostly serve the striatum and portions of the frontal lobe. Norepinephrine-containing neurons are found in the locus ceruleus, project to the cerebral cortex, and have been implicated in depression and anxiety disorders (including panic attacks). The raphe nuclei consist of brainstem neurons that contain serotonin, which project rostrally and caudally. The rostrally projecting fibers originate mainly in the midbrain and rostral pons and have been implicated in mood disorders after injury. The descending projections, originating from the caudal pons and medulla, terminate in the medulla, cerebellum, and spinal cord. One function implicated with these descending fibers is the regulation of afferent (nociceptive) information from the periphery (Kandel, pp. 282–297).

8. A. Beginning the incision for an anterior iliac crest graft approximately 3 cm lateral to the anterior iliac spine avoids the attachments of the sartorius muscle and ilioinguinal ligament. The lateral femoral cutaneous nerve courses through this region and is also vulnerable to injury with this approach, but it does not attach to or originate from the iliac crest (Connolly, pp. 818–819).

9-C; 10-A; 11-A; 12-D; 13-E; 14-G; 15-A. Refer to Figure 2.9–2.15A. The hippocampal formation includes the hippocampus, dentate gyrus, and subiculum. The hippocampus and dentate gyrus form interlocking C-shaped structures when viewed in transverse section. Both structures also contain three cortical layers, which is characteristic of the archicortex. The hippocampus is found in the floor of the temporal horn and is composed of the molecular, pyramidal, and polymorphic layers. The neurons of the hippocampus reside in the pyramidal layer and have extensive apical dendrites that project to the molecular layer. Terminal axons from several sources, including the dentate gyrus and entorhinal cortex, synapse with pyramidal cell dendrites in the molecular layer. The polymorphic layer contains basal dendrites and axons of pyramidal cells. The axons of hippocampal pyramidal cells have extensive collateral branching patterns. The hippocampus can be further subdivided into four regions, namely CA1, CA2, CA3, and CA4. CA1 is the largest sector and is continuous with the subiculum, which is located in the parahippocampal gyrus and joins the hippocampal formation to the entorhinal cortex. CA1 is also called Sommer's sector and is extremely vulnerable to hypoxia. The CA2 subfield is a short transitional region between the more extensive CA3 and CA1 subfields. CA3 (harbors largest pyramidal cells of hippocampus) is located at the genu and enters the dentate gyrus and is relatively resistant to hypoxia. CA4 lies in the concavity of the dentate gyrus, and represents the transition zone into this structure.

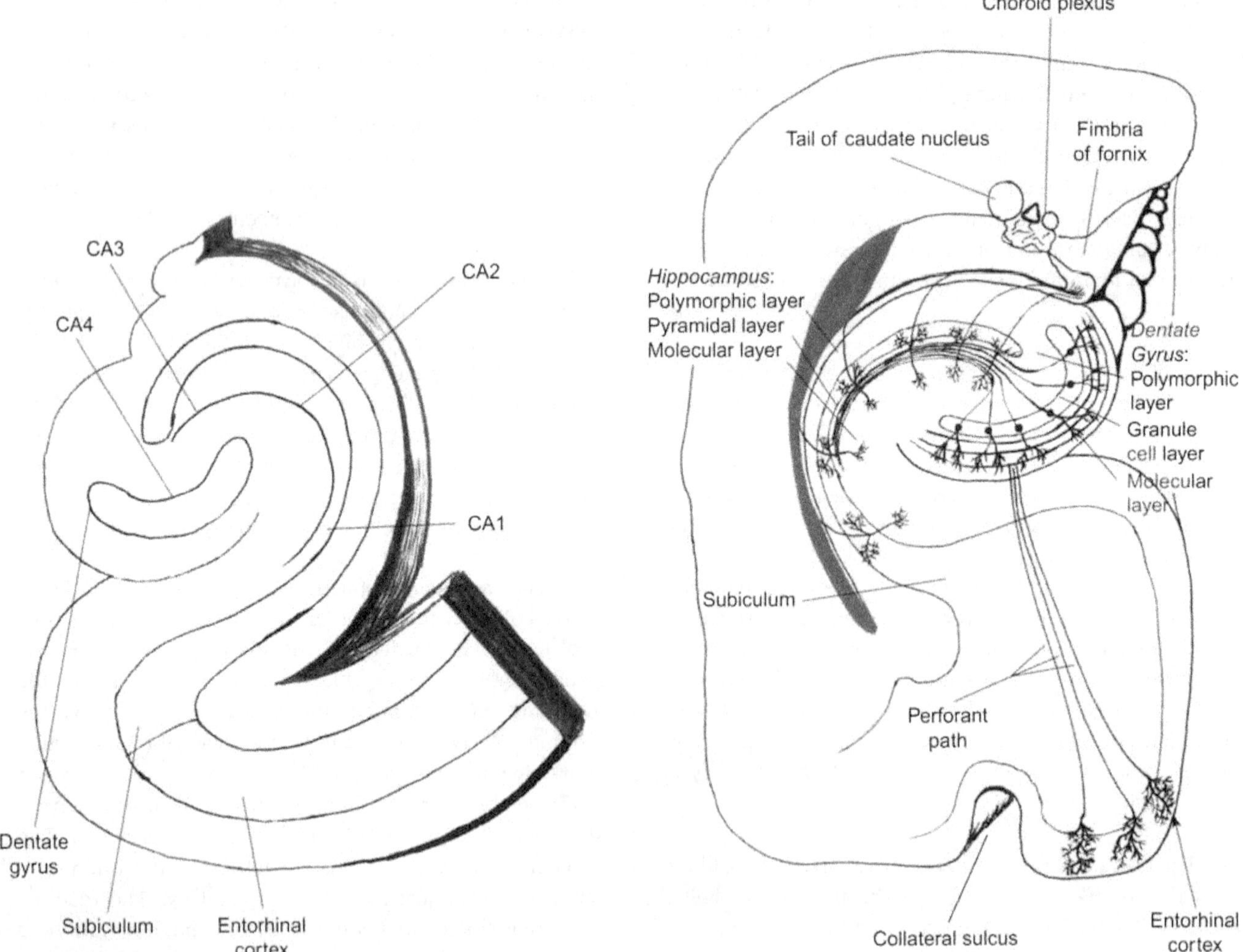

FIGURE 2.9–15A Hippocampus. The four sectors of the hippocampus. Hippocampal formation. The principle intrinsic pathways between the entorhinal cortex, dentate gyrus, subiculum, and hippocampus are depicted. (Reprinted with permission from Moore SP. The Definitive Neurological Surgery Board Review. Malden, MA: Blackwell Publishing, 2005:47, Figures 2.12, 2.13.)

The dentate gyrus also consists of three layers: the molecular, granular, and polymorphic. The granule cells (of the granular layer) have dendritic trees that extend into the molecular layer and axons within the polymorphic layer. The subiculum is located in the superior part of the parahippocampal gyrus and is buried in the ventral bank of the hippocampal fissure. The subiculum forms the transition between the trilaminar hippocampus and the six layers of the entorhinal cortex (area 28); like the dentate gyrus and hippocampus, it also contains three cortical layers: a superficial molecular layer, a deeper polymorphic layer, and a pyramidal layer which lies in between them.

The hippocampus contains three major intrinsic pathways, including the perforant pathway, Schaffer collateral pathway, and mossy fiber pathway. The serial flow of information begins in the entorhinal cortex, which is believed to be the first leg of a multisynaptic loop that flows through the hippocampal formation. Information from the entorhinal cortex (area 28) is first projected to the granule cells of the dentate gyrus via the perforant pathway. It is called the perforant pathway because the fibers perforate the hippocampal formation before reaching the granular cell dendrites of the dentate gyrus (located in the molecular layer). The granule cells of the dentate gyrus, in turn, send a dense projection of axons, or mossy fibers, to the molecular layer of the CA3 subfield, where they synapse on the apical dendrites of pyramidal neurons. Axons from CA3 then bifurcate into two pathways. One pathway enters the alveus to exit the hippocampus in the fibers of the fornix; the other includes Schaffer collaterals, which project to the pyramidal neurons of CA1, which, in turn, project back to the subiculum. Finally, neurons from the subiculum complete this multisynaptic loop through the hippocampal formation by sending axons back to the entorhinal cortex.

These pathways form the intrinsic connections within the hippocampal formation that are involved in long-term potentiation. With long-term potentiation, small stimuli result in increased and prolonged postsynaptic potentials of target neurons (facilitation), and this often involves the NMDA receptor. Long-term potentiation involves depolarization and activation of NMDA receptors and/or voltage dependent calcium channels as well as release of calcium from intracellular stores. This increase in intracellular calcium results in activation of specific intracellular transduction cascades, including gene transduction, resulting in long-lasting modifications of synaptic integrity.

The fornix represents the primary efferent projections of the hippocampal formation (subiculum and hippocampus). The fornix passes under the splenium of the corpus callosum (crura), after which the crura join to form the body of the fornix, which curves around to the rostral thalamus. The body of the fornix then divides into the anterior columns of the fornix that curve ventrally to the foramina of Monro. The fornix then divides into precommissural and postcommissural fibers at the anterior commissure. Precommissural fibers project to the septal nuclei. Postcommissural fibers project to the mammillary body, hypothalamus, septal region, medial frontal cortex, and anterior thalamus. A small number of postcommissural fibers project to the midbrain tegmentum. Collateral projections also exit the fornix at various points along its course and project to neocortical association areas. The majority of fibers that enter the fornix originate in the subiculum, which in turn receives extensive input from the hippocampus and dentate gyrus. The anterior hippocampus also has direct efferent projections to the amygdala. Vestigial remnants of the hippocampal formation include the indusium griseum (supracallosal gyrus), which connects to the dentate gyrus via the fasciolar gyrus. The hippocampus is involved with recent memory and encoding of new memories into long-term storage. Bilateral hippocampal lesions result in marked deficits in short term memory, inability to acquire new information and skills, and mild behavioral changes, while memory for remote events is usually unaffected (Carpenter, pp. 369–376; Kandel, pp. 1259–1260; Pritchard, pp. 377–380).

16. A. The dopaminergic projections of the SN_c to the striatum facilitate movements by influencing the direct and indirect pathways. The nigrostriatal projections to the spiny neurons of the direct pathway (D1 receptors) are excitatory, while the nigrostriatal projections to the spiny neurons of the indirect pathway (D2 receptors) are inhibitory. In normal individuals, the direct and indirect circuits of the basal ganglia are balanced by the opposing actions of these projections on these receptors. The loss of SN_c dopaminergic projections to the striatum results in increased activity of the indirect circuit (and decreased activity of the direct circuit), which accounts for the hypokinetic aspects of Parkinson's disease. It is important to realize, however, that the segregation of the D1 and D2 receptors between the direct and indirect pathways is probably not as strict as described above, but it still serves as a nice framework to explain the differential action of dopamine on striatal output.

The subthalamic nucleus has an excitatory effect on the internal segment of the globus pallidus via the indirect pathway. In normal individuals, the activation of striatal GABAergic neurons inhibits GABAergic neurons within the internal segment of the globus pallidus instead of activating them. The ascending dopaminergic activating system originates in the brainstem reticular activating system and ascends to form multiple supratentorial connections with structures such as the thalamus, hypothalamus, cingulate gyrus, and basal ganglia. Injury of this monoamine pathway has not been shown to result in movement-related disorders; instead, it causes apathetic states such as akinetic mutism (Kandel, pp. 856–864; Youmans, pp. 2673–2674, 2687–2689).

17. A. A visual lesion producing a central defect in one field with a superior temporal defect in the opposite field suggests a lesion near the anterior optic chiasm. This is likely the result of damage to the ipsilateral optic nerve and the fibers that loop forward from the inferonasal retina of the opposite eye (Willebrand's knee). (Brazis, p. 136, Kline, pp. 3, 9).

18. E. Fibers controlling saccades originate in the contralateral frontal eye fields (Brodmann's area 8), pass through the internal capsule, decussate in the pons, and synapse in the paramedian pontine reticular formation (PPRF). Efferent fibers from the PPRF project to the ipsilateral abducens nucleus (VI) and contralateral oculomotor nucleus (III) via the medial longitudinal fasciculus (MLF), which results in saccadic eye movements. Saccades that are organized in the PPRF are usually under the control of the superior colliculus, although some saccadic eye movements occur independently, without collicular influence (Kandel, pp. 789–792).

19-E, 20-C, 21-B, 22-B, 23-D, 24-B, 25-C. The vertebral artery (VA) is generally the largest branch of the subclavian artery; as a variant, the left VA arises from the aortic arch about 4% of the time. There are four segments of the vertebral artery (E). The first courses superiorly and posteriorly to enter the transverse foramen of the sixth cervical vertebral body. The second segment ascends vertically within the transverse foramina, accompanied by a network of sympathetic fibers from the stellate ganglion and a venous plexus. It turns laterally within the transverse process of the axis. The third segment exits the foramen of the axis and curves posteriorly and medially in a groove on the upper surface of the atlas to enter the foramen magnum. The fourth and last segment pierces the dura and joins the opposite VA near the lower pontine border. Branches of the VA include the anterior meningeal artery, which may occasionally feed meningiomas or clival chordomas; the posterior meningeal artery; posterior spinal artery; posterior inferior cerebellar artery (PICA) (D), and the anterior spinal artery. Occlusion of PICA (D) or the vertebral artery (E) may produce the lateral medullary (Wallenberg) syndrome, which is characterized by ipsilateral facial numbness; contralateral trunk numbness; ipsilateral palatal, pharyngeal, and vocal cord paralysis (nucleus ambiguus); ipsilateral Horner's syndrome; vertigo; nausea; vomiting; ipsilateral cerebellar signs; and occasionally hiccups. The most common cause of Wallenberg syndrome is VA occlusion; however, it has classically been described in the literature after PICA occlusion. The PICA vessels are at risk for injury during a Chiari decompression, as they loop around the tonsils.

The characteristic picture of anterior inferior cerebellar artery (AICA) (C) occlusion includes vertigo, nystagmus, nausea and vomiting (vestibular nuclei involvement), ipsilateral facial numbness (trigeminal spinal nucleus and tract), ipsilateral Horner's syndrome (descending sympathetic fibers), contralateral limb numbness (lateral spinothalamic tract), ipsilateral ataxia (middle cerebellar peduncle), and ipsilateral deafness and facial paralysis (lateral pontomedul-

lary tegmentum). It supplies the middle and inferior lateral pontine regions and the anterolateral parts of the cerebellum, which includes the middle cerebellar peduncle, flocculus, pyramis, and tuber. It is the most common vessel compressing the seventh cranial nerve during hemifacial spasm, which occasionally requires surgical decompression.

Occlusion of the SCA (B) is the least common cause of cerebellar infarction, which is characterized by nausea, vomiting, vertigo, nystagmus, ipsilateral Horner's syndrome, ataxia, ipsilateral intention tremor (superior cerebellar peduncle), contralateral limb numbness, contralateral hearing loss (crossed fibers of the lateral lemniscus), and possibly a fourth nerve palsy (pontine tectum). The SCA is the most common nerve compressing the trigeminal nerve in trigeminal neuralgia.

The posterior cerebral arteries (A) are joined by the posterior communicating arteries (PComA) about 1 cm from their origin. The PComA is the major origin of the PCA 15 to 20% of the time and is termed a "fetal" PCA. The PCA comprises the P1 (peduncular), P2 (ambient), P3 (quadrigeminal), and P4 (distal or cortical) segments and their respective branches. Major branches of the PCA include the medial and lateral posterior choroidal arteries; anterior, middle, and posterior temporal arteries; parieto-occipital artery; calcarine artery; as well as the smaller thalamoperforating and thalamogeniculate arteries. The origin of the PComA is the first or second most common location for aneurysm formation, along with the anterior communicating artery (Brazis, pp. 374–377; Kaye and Black, pp. 1603, 1734; Osborn DCA, pp. 153–193; Greenberg, pp. 107–108).

26. C. Afferent connections into the hypothalamus are numerous and complex. Seven of the main pathways are described below.

1. Amygdalohypothalamic fibers pass from the amygdala to the hypothalamus by two pathways: the stria terminalis and a pathway under the lentiform nucleus (ventral amygdalofugal fibers). The stria terminalis arises mainly from the corticomedial part of the amygdala and distributes fibers to the medial preoptic nucleus, anterior hypothalamic nucleus, and ventromedial and arcuate nuclei. Ventral amygdalofugal fibers arise from the basolateral amygdala and pyriform cortex and spread medially and rostrally under the lentiform nucleus to reach the lateral hypothalamus and medial forebrain bundle.

2. Visceral and somatic fibers reach the hypothalamus through collateral branches of the lemniscal tracts and reticular formation.

3. Basal olfactory, septal nuclei, periamygdaloid, and subiculum fibers reach the lateral and preoptic hypothalamic regions via the medial forebrain bundle.

4. Cortical fibers to the hypothalamus arise mainly from the frontal lobe.

5. Hippocampohypothalamic fibers travel through the fornix to the mammillary body.

6. Thalamohypothalamic fibers arise from the dorsomedial and midline thalamic nuclei.

7. Brainstem fibers to the hypothalamus arise from the raphe nuclei of the midbrain, the lateral parabrachial nuclei of the pons, and the locus ceruleus. Brainstem reticular fibers also ascend to the hypothalamus by the mammillary pedicle and dorsal longitudinal fasciculus (Carpenter, pp. 304–307; Kandel, pp. 972–981, 992–993).

27. A. The cerebellar glomeruli have synaptic connections consisting of mossy fiber rosettes, axons of Golgi type II neurons, and dendrites of granule cells. A glial capsule surrounds this conglomeration. The axons of the granule neurons, which enter the molecular layer, provide the output from the glomerulus. Climbing fibers bypass the glomeruli to synapse directly on Purkinje cells (Carpenter, pp. 224–234).

28. B. The major site of neuroblast proliferation in the CNS is the periventricular ependymal surface. After undergoing mitosis, these young neural cells migrate away from the ependyma (Ellison, p. 71).

29. D. Refer to Figure 2.29A. The cerebellar cortex consists of a molecular layer, Purkinje cell layer, and granular layer. The granular layer is deepest and lies just above the central medullary white matter. This layer contains the granule cells, which utilize glutamate as their neurotransmitter and are the only excitatory cells of the cerebellar cortex. Granule cell dendrites terminate in glomeruli, and their axons ascend to the molecular layer of the cerebellum as parallel fibers, which synapse with Purkinje cell dendrites. Golgi type II cells also reside in the granular layer of the cerebellar cortex. These cells are inhibitory (GABA) interneurons; their dendrites contact parallel fibers while their axons terminate in glomeruli. Each glomerulus consists of granule cell dendrites, Golgi cell axons, and a mossy fiber rosette.

The Purkinje cells reside in the middle layer of the cerebellar cortex; they are large cells that project inhibitory fibers (GABA) to the deep cerebellar nuclei and the vestibular nuclei. The Purkinje cell represents the only output of the cerebellar cortex, which is inhibitory. Purkinje cells have extensive dendritic arborizations that extend into the molecular layer and are stimulated by parallel fibers and climbing fibers. Specialized astrocytes, called Bergman cells (Golgi epithelial cells), surround Purkinje cells within the Purkinje cell layer and provide supportive functions.

The molecular layer is the most superficial layer of the cerebellar cortex; it contains stellate cells, basket cells, Purkinje dendrites, and parallel fibers (from granule cells). Stellate cells make synaptic contacts with Purkinje cell dendrites, while basket cells form synapses on Purkinje cell bodies. Both stellate and basket cells are inhibitory and utilize GABA as their neurotransmitter.

Cerebellar cortical input occurs via climbing fibers and mossy fibers. Climbing fibers originate in the inferior olive (olivocerebellars); they ascend to the molecular layer, where they directly stimulate the dendrites of small numbers of Purkinje cells (between one and ten). Climbing fibers are glutamatergic and are the most excitatory fibers of the entire CNS (refer to question 4 discussion). Mossy fibers synapse in glomeruli of the granular layer; they originate from the pontine nuclei, the red nucleus, the spinal cord, the vestibular nuclei, the reticular formation, and deep cerebellar nuclei. These fibers are also excitatory (Glut/Asp) and stimulate granule cell dendrites within the glomerulus. This results in widespread Purkinje cell stimulation (up to 10,000 cells) via the parallel fibers. The locus ceruleus sends noradrenergic projections to the cerebellar cortex, and the raphe nuclei project serotonergic fibers to the cerebellar cortex that end as mossy fibers (Carpenter, pp. 224–233).

30. C. The annulus tendineus (of Zinn) lies at the apex of the periorbita and gives rise to four rectus muscles. The optic nerve, ophthalmic artery, superior and inferior divisions of the oculomotor nerve, abducens nerve, and nasociliary branch of the ophthalmic nerve enter the orbit through the annulus tendineus as they leave the optic canal and superior orbital fissure. The ophthalmic vein and trochlear nerve, as well as the frontal and lacrimal branches of the ophthalmic nerve, pass superiorly to the annulus as they pass through the superior orbital fissure (April, p. 461).

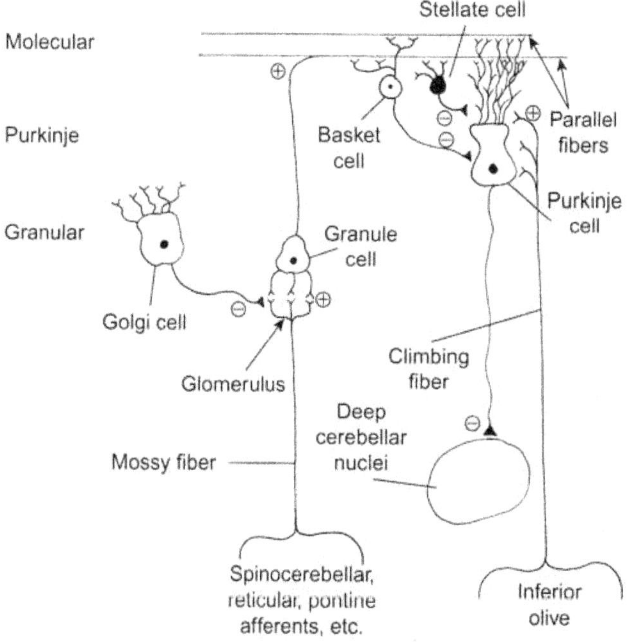

FIGURE 2.29A Cerebellum. This figure illustrates the three layers of the cerebellum and their contents. Climbing fiber and mossy fiber input to the cerebellum is also depicted. (Reprinted with permission from Moore SP. The Definitive Neurological Surgery Board Review. Malden, MA: Blackwell Publishing, 2005:36, Figure 2.6.)

31-K; 32-A; 33-I; 34-J; 35-G; 36-H; 37-H; 38-F; 39-H; 40-F; 41-E; 42-I.
The brachial plexus is formed from the anterior primary rami of segments C5, C6, C7, C8, and T1. It is about 15 cm long in adults and extends from the spinal cord to the axilla. It is divided into five major components, as follows: roots, trunks, divisions, cords, and branches. The fifth and sixth cervical roots unite to form the upper trunk of the plexus, and the eighth cervical and first thoracic spinal roots unite to form the lower trunk. The seventh cervical root emerges as the middle trunk of the plexus. The three trunks then traverse the supraclavicular fossa, behind the axillary artery, and separate into three anterior and three posterior divisions. The three posterior divisions unite behind the axillary artery to form the posterior cord. The anterior divisions of the upper and middle trunks (C5-7) unite to form the lateral cord, whereas the medial cord is formed by the anterior division of the lower trunk (C8-T1). The cords pass through the space formed by the clavicle and first rib and then give off the major terminal branches (peripheral nerves).

The dorsal scapular nerve (K) is a purely motor nerve that arises mainly from the C5 spinal nerve, which courses downward behind the brachial plexus to supply the levator scapulae and major and minor rhomboid muscles. The rhomboids normally elevate and adduct the medial border of the scapula (antagonist to serratus anterior) and, along with the levator scapulae, rotate the scapula so that the inferior angle moves medially. The long thoracic nerve (of Bell, A) is also a purely motor (C5-7) nerve that supplies the serratus anterior muscle, which fixes and stabilizes the scapula against the chest wall. It is tested by observing for scapular winging while the patient pushes and extends the arms against a fixed object. The axillary (circumflex) nerve (I) is a mixed nerve (C5-6) that is one of the terminal branches of the posterior cord. It descends on the subscapularis muscle and then winds around the surgical head of the humerus to supply the deltoid (abduct arm > 90 degrees) and teres minor (lateral arm rotation) muscles. It also sends sensory branches to the joint capsule of the shoulder and upper lateral aspect of the arm superficial to the deltoid muscle. It may be entrapped in the quadrilateral space, an anatomic compartment bounded by the teres major and minor muscles, the long head of the triceps, and neck of the humerus. The musculocutaneous nerve (J, C5-7) arises from the lateral cord of the brachial plexus and supplies the coracobrachialis (adduct arm/flexion forearm), brachialis (flexion forearm), and biceps brachii (flexion and supinate forearm). The musculocutaneous nerve is best tested by having the patient flex the supinated arm against resistance. The musculocutaneous nerve also subserves a sensory function in the lateral forearm that may extend from the elbow to the wrist. The median nerve (H, C5-T1) is formed in the axilla by the joining of the lateral and medial cords of the brachial plexus. The nerve descends down the medial side of the arm in close association with the brachial artery to the cubital fossa. From there, it enters the forearm between the two heads of the

pronator teres muscle and gives off the anterior interosseous nerve. Compression neuropathy of the anterior interosseous nerve can result in weakness in flexion of the distal phalanges of the thumb (weak flexor pollicis longus), index and middle finger (weak flexor digitorum profundus I and II), and pronation (pronator quadratus). In trying to pinch the tips of the index finger and thumb, the terminal phalanges extend instead of the tips and the pulps touch, producing the "pinch sign." There is no sensory loss with anterior interosseous nerve injury. Above the elbow, the median nerve may rarely be compressed by Struthers' ligament, an anatomic structure that bridges the supracondylar process to the medial epicondyle. Patients are usually asymptomatic but occasionally may develop a typical median nerve neuropathy. At the elbow and forearm, the median nerve can potentially be trapped at any of three sites, including behind the lacertus fibrosus (bicipital aponeurosis), between the two heads of the pronator teres muscle, and underneath the fibrous bridge of the flexor digitorum superficialis (sublimis bridge). Pronator teres compression results in vague aching and fatiguing of forearm muscles, with a weak grip and paresthesias in the index finger and thumb. There is often pain with forced pronation, and nocturnal exacerbation is absent. Pain in the palm distinguishes it from carpal tunnel syndrome (CTS), since the median palmar cutaneous branch exits before the transverse carpal ligament and is spared in CTS. The most common median nerve entrapment neuropathy results from compression in the carpal tunnel just distal to the wrist crease. It usually occurs in middle-aged female patients and is bilateral over 50% of the time (worse in dominant hand). The ulnar nerve (F) is the main branch of the medial cord (C8-T1) and supplies no muscles in the arm and only two in the forearm (flexor carpi ulnaris and flexor digitorum profundus III and IV). In the hand it supplies all the muscles except the LOAF muscles (lumbricals I and II, opponens pollicis, flexor pollices brevis, abductor pollices brevis), which are supplied by the median nerve. These include a part of the adductor pollicis that is not supplied by the median nerve, seven interossei (palmar and dorsal), lumbricals III and IV, and the hypothenar muscles (abductor, opponens, and flexor digiti minimi). The ulnar nerve may be entrapped under the arcade of Struthers (distinct from Struthers' ligament) above the elbow and medial to the medial head of the triceps. Entrapment at the elbow may result in tardy ulnar palsy, which can produce pain, numbness and/or tingling in the little finger and ulnar half of the ring finger, elbow pain, and hand weakness. Early symptoms may be purely motor, may be exacerbated by cold, and are often vague and described as loss of finger coordination. Entrapment in the forearm may occur in the cubital tunnel, an anatomic location between the two heads of the flexor carpi ulnaris under the fascial bands connecting these two heads. In the wrist, the ulnar nerve may be compressed in Guyan's canal, the roof of which is formed by the palmar fascia and palmaris brevis, the floor being the flexor retinaculum of the the palm and pisohamate bone. The radial nerve (G) innervates the extensors of the arm, forearm, and wrist. The medial cutaneous nerves of the forearm (E) are two sensory branches that supply various regions of the arm and forearm (Greenberg, pp. 534–543; Brazis, pp. 4–27; Patten, pp. 63, 282–298).

43. C. The cells of the cerebral cortex show both a laminar and radial or columnar arrangement. Several areas of cortex have grossly visible stripes of myelinated fibers, most notably the band of Gennari in layer IV of the occipital cortex. Most cytoarchitectural boundaries are vague rather than sharp. The large pyramidal neurons located in layer V of the visual receptive cortex send axons to the brainstem that mediate visually directed reflex eye movements (Carpenter, pp. 390–433).

44. B. The arcuate fasciculus projects from the superior temporal gyrus (STG) to the superior and middle frontal gyri. More commonly, it is known as the tract that links the receptive area of speech in the superior temporal gyrus (Wernicke's area) with the inferior frontal gyrus (Broca's area). Lesions in this tract often produce conduction aphasia, in which patients have fluent speech with poor repetition of spoken language. Wernicke's aphasia (WA) is a receptive aphasia characterized by poor comprehension of spoken language, neologisms, literal and verbal paraphasias, poor repetition, and a lack of concern regarding the speech problem. Injury to Broca's area results in an executive aphasia characterized by slow and effortful speech, agrammatic sounds, and telegraphic speech. The uncinate fasciculus connects the orbital frontal gyri with the anterior portions of the temporal lobe, while the cingulum connects the medial regions of the frontal and parietal lobes with the parahippocampal and temporal regions. The fibers of the superior and inferior longitudinal fasciculus lie close to the arcuate fasciculus and connect the parietal and occipital lobes with the frontal and temporal lobes, respectively. The anterior commissure (association tract) crosses the midline rostral to the fornix and has two parts: the smaller anterior portion interconnects the olfactory bulbs, and the larger posterior portion interconnects the middle and inferior temporal gyri (Carpenter, pp. 33–37).

45. E. The combination of pupillary constriction and ptosis suggests a Horner's syndrome. Two muscles elevate the eyelid: the levator palpebrae (CN III) and the superior tarsal muscle of Muller (carotid sympathetic nerve). The key to further differentiation is the size of the pupil. A lesion of cranial nerve III may likely result in pupillodilation (due to pupilloconstrictor muscle paralysis), whereas injury to the sympathetic nerve would result in pupil constriction, as seen in this patient. In addition, the ptosis of sympathetic paralysis may improve when the patient volitionally looks up, because the levator palpebrae is the muscle that mediates voluntary upward gaze. The lesion causing injury to the sym-

pathetics may originate in any location along the descending pathways from the hypothalamus through the spinal cord and out through the peripheral pathways along the sympathetic chain and carotid artery (see discussion for question 6) (Brazis, pp. 181–182; Greenberg, p. 578).

46. B. The striate cortex is organized in both vertical and horizontal systems. The vertical or columnar system is mainly concerned with line orientation, retinal position, detection of movements, and ocular dominance. The two regions of the striate cortex that do not contain ocular dominance columns include the region representing the blind spot of the eye and the cortical region representing the monocular temporal crescent of the visual fields (Carpenter, pp. 411–414).

47-D; 48-A; 49-B; 50-E; 51-D. The first clinically relevant branch of the lumbar plexus is the lateral femoral cutaneous nerve of the thigh (A, L2-3), which reaches the thigh by passing under the lateral aspect of the inguinal ligament. Entrapment of this nerve as it enters the thigh can produce a numb, tingling, or burning hypersensitivity over the lateral thigh known as meralgia paresthetica. It is often encountered in obese patients of either sex who have lost a significant amount of weight, or, conversely, can be seen in late pregnancy due to a sagging anterior abdominal wall. This condition often remits on its own, but surgical decompression is sometimes warranted.

The femoral nerve (B, E, L2-4) passes down along the lateral aspect of the psoas muscle and emerges under the inguinal ligament into the femoral triangle. It innervates the iliopsoas (hip flexion), sartorius (hip flexion, thigh eversion), and quadriceps femoris muscles (knee extension). In the abdomen and pelvis, a primary or secondary neoplasm, psoas abscess, or pelvic hematoma may damage the upper portion of this nerve (B). In the femoral ring (E), this nerve is particularly vulnerable to local compression and possibly pressure palsy from diabetes mellitus. Although diabetes can also affect the L2-4 roots of this nerve, diabetic neuropathy of the femoral nerve is most often encountered in the femoral triangle. The patient usually presents with pain that resolves, only to be followed by rapid wasting and weakness of the quadriceps, which makes walking very difficult. Fortunately, the condition eventually improves, although it may take up to 2 years.

The obturator nerve (D, L2-4) lies on the medial side of the iliopsoas muscle and comes into close relationship with the uterus before reaching the obturator foramen. In the pelvis, it is particularly vulnerable to injury during obstetric and gynecologic procedures. This nerve supplies the adductor muscles of the thigh, which includes the pectineus; adductor longus, brevis, and magnus; and gracilis muscles. Its integrity is tested by having the patient hold the legs together against resistance.

The sciatic nerve (C, F) consists of two discrete components invested by the same fascia called the peroneal and tibial nerves. This major nerve may also be damaged in the pelvis by direct spread of neoplasms (along with the femoral nerve), particularly from the rectum or genitourinary tract. In the buttock, misplaced deep intramuscular injections, complicated hip fractures, and penetrating trauma are the most frequent causes of sciatic nerve damage. Misplaced injections can be especially problematic, because they can produce not only significant weakness but also severe causalgic pain over the leg and foot that is often refractory to medications. The superior gluteal neurovascular bundle lies in the superomedial gluteal quadrant. The sciatic nerve and inferior gluteal neurovascular bundle lie in the inferolateral and inferomedial quadrants, respectively. The safest location for intramuscular injection is the superolateral gluteal quadrant. The peroneal nerve is particularly vulnerable to injury as it crosses near the fibular neck, although this nerve is more resilient to injury than the tibial nerve after sciatic nerve injury. The reason for this is not entirely clear (Patten, pp. 299–310; Brazis, pp. 62–65, 73–77; April, p. 584).

52. E. Sympathetic preganglionic fibers originate from the T1 through L2 (thoracolumbar) levels of the spinal cord and pass successively through the ventral roots, anterior primary rami of the spinal nerves, and myelinated white rami communicans before synapsing in the sympathetic chain (composed of paravertebral ganglia and interconnecting fiber bundles). Sympathetic postganglionic fibers from the paravertebral ganglia then may take one of several routes. They may pass back to a spinal nerve along an unmyelinated gray ramus communicans to innervate dermal sweat glands, smooth muscle cells of arterioles, and/or arrector pili muscles of the body and extremities. They may exit the sympathetic ganglia through splanchnic nerves to innervate the abdominal or pelvic viscera or may course up or down the sympathetic chain to synapse with postganglionic neurons located several spinal levels away. Every spinal nerve receives a gray ramus from the sympathetic chain, whereas only spinal levels T1-L2 have white rami communicans (myelinated). Preganglionic sympathetic neurons are cholinergic, whereas the sympathetic postganglionic fibers (some traveling through gray ramus communicans) are adrenergic. Because the paravertebral and prevertebral ganglia are located some distance away from the organ innervated, the sympathetic preganglionic fibers are shorter, whereas postganglionic fibers are longer as compared to the parasympathetic division (April, pp. 28–30).

53. E. The superior ramus of the ansa cervicalis, which arises from C1 and the hypoglossal nerve, innervates the geniohyoid (protracts hyoid) and thyrohyoid (raises larynx) muscles, whereas the inferior ramus, arising from C1-C3, innervates the omohyoid (lowers hyoid) and sternothyroid (lowers larynx) muscles. Since the muscles supplied by the ansa cervicalis often have collateral innervation, sectioning or mobilization of this structure during various surgical pro-

cedures (such as carotid endarterectomy) rarely has clinical consequences. The stylohyoid (elevates and retracts hyoid) muscle is innervated by CN VII (April, p. 512).

54. D. The pterygopalatine fossa harbors many nerves and blood vessels, which directly communicate with various compartments of the face and skull. The pterygopalatine fossa communicates directly with the middle cranial fossa through the foramen rotundum and vidian canal, with the orbital cavity through the inferior orbital fissure, with the nasal cavity via the sphenopalatine foramen, and with the oral cavity by way of the palatine canal. It does not directly communicate with the inner ear (April, pp. 490–491).

55-C; 56-B; 57-D; 58-A. Adie's pupil (dilated pupil) is thought to be due to impaired postganglionic parasympathetics from a viral infection of the ciliary ganglion. Adie's pupil often constricts with dilute (0.1 to 0.125%) pilocarpine, a parasympathomimetic, because of denervation hypersensitivity (normal pupils react to 1% pilocarpine). The Argyll-Robertson pupils are believed to result from disruption of pathways leading to the Edinger-Westphal nucleus, which produces light-near dissociation (pupillary constriction with convergence and absent light response). The Marcus-Gunn pupil is best detected by the swinging flashlight test, as the consensual reflex is stronger than the direct reflex (afferent pupillary defect). It is caused by lesions anterior to the optic chiasm, such as retinal detachment or infarct, optic or retrobulbar neuritis, or trauma to the optic nerve. The presence of the consensual reflex is evidence of a preserved third nerve (with parasympathetics) on the side of the direct reflex. Horner's syndrome (HS) results from interruption of the sympathetic pupillomotor pathways anywhere between the primary motor neuron in the hypothalamus, the second motor neuron in the cervicothoracic junction, and third-order neuron in the superior cervical ganglion. Findings may include miosis, ptosis, enophthalmos, eye hyperemia, or anhidrosis of the face. Cocaine can be used if the diagnosis is in doubt; however, this has no localizing value. Cocaine blocks norepinephrine (NE) reuptake by postganglionic sympathetic fibers at the neuroeffector junction. In HS, no NE is released, so cocaine cannot dilate the eye. If the pupil dilates normally, there is no HS. To differentiate a second-from a third-order neuron injury, administer 1% hydroxyamphetamine, which releases NE from nerve terminals at the neuroeffector junction. This causes pupillary dilation with second-order neuron lesions but not with third-order neuron damage (since third-order neurons do not release NE) (Greenberg, p. 578).

59. C. The term *corpus striatum* refers to the caudate, putamen, and pallidum, whereas the term *striatum* typically includes only the caudate nucleus and putamen. The lentiform nuclei consist of the globus pallidus and putamen, which lie between the internal and extreme capsules and are separated by a curved vertical lamina of white matter called the lateral medullary lamina. Other terms commonly used to refer to the basal ganglia include *neostriatum* (caudate nucleus and putamen), *paleostriatum* (globus pallidus), and *archistriatum* (amygdaloid complex). All the structures mentioned above except for the globus pallidus (and subthalamic nucleus) are believed to have originated from the telencephalon, which is a diencephalic structure (Carpenter, p. 325).

60. C. The largest number of afferent fibers into the STN originate in the lateral pallidal segment. Afferents to the STN from the motor, premotor, and prefrontal cortex are mainly collaterals from other tracts, while a relatively small number of afferents originate from the CM nucleus of the thalamus. Afferents to the STN from the lateral pallidal segment are mainly GABAergic, while most cells of the STN are believed to release glutamate and exert excitatory effects on their targets. The medial globus pallidus is the major outflow site of the basal ganglia, as described in the discussion for question 2 (Carpenter, pp. 347–351).

61. E. The corticopontocerebellar tract consists almost entirely of crossed fibers from the pontine nuclei that transmit impulses from the cerebral cortex to the intermediate and lateral zones of the cerebellum through the middle cerebellar peduncle (brachium pontis). The inferior cerebellar peduncle connects the medulla to the cerebellum and consists of two divisions: the restiform body contains afferent fibers from the olivocerebellar, dorsal spinocerebellar, reticulocerebellar, and cuneocerebellar tracts, while the juxtarestiform body contains both afferent (vestibulocerebellar) and efferent (cerebellovestibular) fibers. The superior cerebellar peduncle (brachium conjuctivum) consists principally of efferents from the cerebellum. Rubral, thalamic, and reticular projections arise from the dentate and interposed nuclei, which exit the cerebellum via the superior cerebellar peduncle. Afferent tracts into the superior cerebellar peduncle include the ventral spinocerebellar, trigeminocerebellar, and tectocerebellar tracts (Kandel, pp. 626–646; Fix, pp. 196–197).

62. C. Refer to Figure 2.62A. The following layers are distinguished in the neocortex in passing from the pial surface toward the white matter:

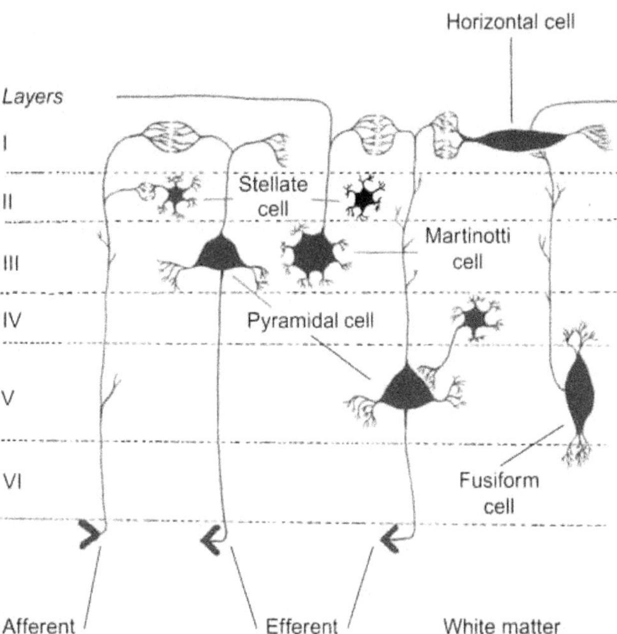

FIGURE 2.62A Layers of the cerebral neocortex. I, plexiform (molecular) layer; II, outer granular layer; III, pyramidal layer; IV, inner granular layer; V, ganglionic layer; VI, multiform cell layer. (Reprinted with permission from Moore SP. The Definitive Neurological Surgery Board Review. Malden, MA: Blackwell Publishing, 2005:49, Figure 2.15.)

Layer I (molecular layer): contains cells with horizontal axons and Golgi type II cells.
Layer II (external granular layer): consists mostly of closely packed granule cells.
Layer III (external pyramidal layer): consists of two sublayers of pyramidal neurons.
Layer IV (internal granular layer): comprises closely packed stellate cells with either short axons ramifying within the layer or larger axons projecting to deeper layers. Myelinated fibers of the external band of Baillarger form a prominent horizontal plexus in this layer.
Layer V (internal pyramidal layer): consists mainly of medium and large pyramidal cells (Betz cells). Apical dendrites of large pyramidal cells project to the molecular layer, while axons mainly leave the cortex as projection fibers.
Layer VI (multiform layer): contains spindle-shaped cells whose long axes are perpendicular to the cortical surface. Axons of these cells also enter the white matter as projection fibers (Carpenter, pp. 390–393).

63. D. Some areas of the body have a greater sensorimotor representation than others. The largest areas involve the tongue, thumb, little finger, and corresponding digits of the foot, as well as the hands and feet in general. The complexity of motor actions of the thumb requires a larger cortical circuitry than the trunk, index finger, nipple, genitalia, and middle finger (Carpenter, pp. 401–404).

64. C. Both the archicortex and neocortex are laminated, contain pyramidal neurons, and have connections with the limbic system. One major difference is that the archicortex has a distinct superficial layer of white matter, in comparison to the neocortex, which has white matter on its inner surface (Carpenter, pp. 390–396).

65. C. The nuclei of the hypothalamus are divided by an imaginary plane formed by the columns of the fornix and mammillothalamic tract into medial and lateral groups. The medial hypothalamic area is again divided into four regions from anterior to posterior: preoptic, supraoptic, tuberal, and mammillary regions. Each of these regions contains a separate subgroup of nuclei.

Medial group
1. Preoptic region: contains the medial preoptic nucleus involved with the release of gonadotropic hormones. This nucleus is sexually dimorphic and requires testosterone for development.
2. Supraoptic region: contains the supraoptic nucleus (synthesizes ADH and oxytocin), paraventricular nucleus (makes and releases ADH, oxytocin, and CRH), anterior nucleus (plays a role in temperature regulation), and suprachiasmatic nucleus (controls circadian rhythms), which lie dorsal to the optic chiasm.
3. Tuberal region: the arcuate nucleus is located in the tuber cinereum; it contains neurons that produce hypothalamic releasing factors and gives rise to the tuberohypophysial tract, which terminates in the hypophyseal portal system of the infundibulum. This nucleus regulates the release of adenohypophyseal hormones into the systemic circulation. The arcuate nucleus, along with the dorsomedial and ventromedial nuclei, lies dorsal to the tuber cinereum and makes up the nuclei adjacent to this structure.
4. Mammillary region: this contains the mammillary and posterior nuclei, which lie dorsal to the mammillary bodies.

The lateral hypothalamic area is traversed by the medial forebrain bundle and includes two major nuclei: the lateral preoptic and lateral hypothalamic nuclei (Carpenter, pp. 297–303).

66. E. The supraoptic and paraventricular nuclei of the hypothalamus synthesize and secrete vasopressin and oxytocin, respectively. The anterior portion of the hypothalamus controls mechanisms that dissipate heat. Stimulation of this area causes dilation of blood vessels and sweating, which lowers body temperature. Stimulation of the posterior hypothalamus results in vasoconstriction of blood vessels, inhibition of sweating, and possibly shivering, which may increase body temperature. The posterior (mainly) and lateral hypothalamic nuclei are also involved with the sympathetic nervous system control. The lateral region of the hypothalamus is sometimes referred to as either the hunger and thirst center, as stimulation can result in increased food and water intake. Stimulation of the medial region of the hypothalamus results in decreased food intake; it is often referred to as the satiety center. The suprachiasmatic nucleus controls circadian rhythms, and the anterior and preoptic nuclei help to control parasympathetic responses as well as gonadotropin secretion (Carpenter, pp. 317–324).

67. A. The sciatic nerve (L4-S3) is the major branch of the sacral plexus and is also the largest nerve in the body. The sciatic nerve consists of the tibial and common peroneal nerves. The tibial nerve (L4-S3) innervates the flexors of the leg, including the semitendinosus, semimembranosus, biceps femoris, gastrocnemius, soleus, flexor hallucis longus, flexor digitorum longus, popliteus, tibialis posterior, and plantaris. The tibial nerve gives rise to the lateral sural cutaneous nerve, which unites with the communicating branch of the peroneal nerve to form the sural nerve. This nerve supplies cutaneous innervation to the lateral inferior leg and lateral foot. The tibial nerve may become entrapped in the tarsal tunnel posterior and inferior to the medial malleolus, which results in pain and paresthesias in the toes and sole of the foot (often sparing the heel because these sensory branches often originate proximal to the tarsal tunnel) and weakness on plantarflexion. The common peroneal nerve (L4-S2) innervates extensors and adductors of the leg (and part of the biceps femoris) and gives rise to the lateral sural cutaneous nerve (to the inferolateral leg), the deep peroneal nerve, and the superficial peroneal nerve. The deep peroneal nerve innervates the foot and toe extensors (tibialis anterior, extensor hallucis longus, extensor digitorum longus) and provides sensation to a small area between the great and second toes. The superficial peroneal nerve innervates the peroneus longus/brevis (foot eversion) and the skin of the distal anterior leg, the dorsum of the foot, and the digits. Lesions of the common peroneal nerve (most common) result in paralysis of dorsiflexion (foot-drop) and foot eversion. The posterior femoral cutaneous nerve (S1-S3) innervates the skin of the inferior buttocks, perineum, posterior thigh, and proximal leg (Greenberg, pp. 522, 544–546).

68. A. Refer to Figure 2.68A. The corticospinal, frontopontine, superior thalamic radiations, and a relatively smaller number of corticotectal and corticorubral fibers run in the posterior limb of the internal capsule. The prefrontal corticopontine tract and anterior thalamic radiations run in the anterior limb of the internal capsule, while the corticobulbar and corticoreticular tracts are contained within the genu of the internal capsule (Carpenter, p. 282).

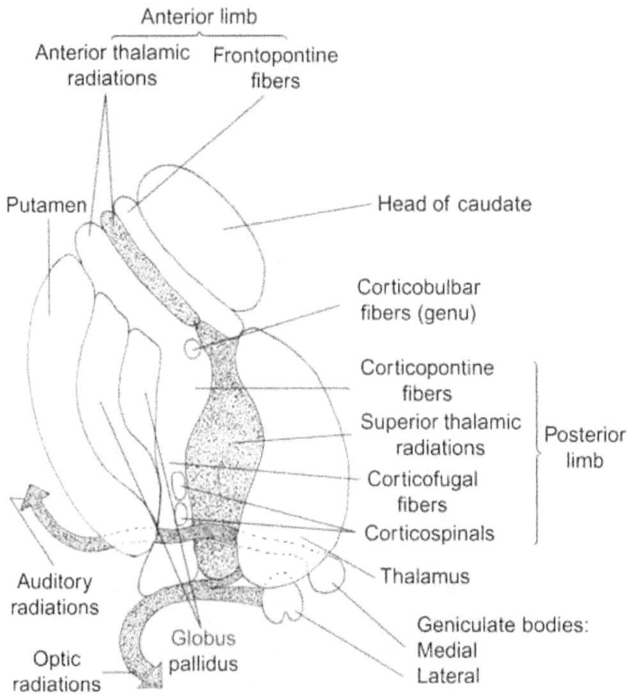

FIGURE 2.68A Internal capsule. The components of the genu and anterior and posterior limbs of the internal capsule are illustrated. (Reprinted with permission from Moore SP. The Definitive Neurological Surgery Board Review. Malden, MA: Blackwell Publishing, 2005:53, Figure 2.18.)

69. C. Although glutamate appears to be the main neurotransmitter of the corticothalamic tracts, the thalamus itself is rich in GABA. Virtually all cells of the thalamus are rich in this neurotransmitter; in primates, the major projections of the medial pallidum to the VA and VL nuclei of the thalamus are GABAergic. Moreover, the projections from the pars reticulata of the substantia nigra to the VA and MD nuclei of the thalamus are also rich in GABA (Carpenter, pp. 278–279).

70. B. The LGN contains six layers, numbered 1 through 6. The ventralmost layers contain large cells and are known as "magnocellular"; they receive their input from M ganglion cells. The dorsal four layers are known as "parvocellular" and receive their input from P ganglion cells. An individual layer receives input from only one eye. Fibers from the contralateral nasal hemiretina synapse in layers 1, 4, and 6, and fibers from the ipsilateral temporal hemiretina synapse in layers 2, 3, and 5 (Kandel, pp. 528–532).

71. B. The cerebellum comprises the fastigial, globose, emboliform, and dentate nuclei. The globose and emboliform nuclei together are known as the interposed nuclei. These nuclei correspond to the three functional divisions of the cerebellum: the vestibulocerebellum, spinocerebellum, and cerebrocerebellum. The vermis projects via the fastigial nucleus to the cortex and brainstem giving rise to the medial descending systems controlling proximal musculature. The intermediate zone of the cerebellum projects via the interposed nuclei to cortical and brainstem regions, which give rise to the lateral descending pathways controlling distal limb muscles. The lateral zone projects to the dentate nucleus, which forms connections with the motor and premotor areas of the cerebral cortex for the planning of voluntary movements (Carpenter, pp. 234–236).

72. C. The motor strip generally lies 4 to 5.4 cm behind the coronal suture (Greenberg, pp. 97–98).

73-B; 74-F; 75-G; 76-D; 77-G; 78-H; 79-H; 80-E; 81-G; 82-B. The oculomotor (CN III), trochlear (CN IV), and abducens nerves (VI) innervate the extraocular muscles and, along with the V_1 and V_2 divisions of CN V, exit the skull base through the superior orbital fissure (B). The trochlear (see question 84 for complete discussion) and abducens nerves provide GSE fibers to the superior oblique and lateral rectus muscles, respectively, while CN III innervates the levator palpebrae superioris, superior rectus, medial rectus, inferior rectus, and inferior oblique muscles. Lesions of CN III will produce lateral strabismus ("wall eyes") with nearly complete ophthalmoplegia of the eye as well as ptosis. The Edinger-Westphal nucleus is the most rostral parasympathetic nucleus, which gives rise to the GVE component of the oculomotor nerve (CN III).

The facial nerve is both a sensory and motor nerve. The main motor nucleus of the facial nerve lies in the reticular formation of the lower pons. Fibers leaving this nucleus course dorsally toward the floor of the fourth ventricle, loop around the abducens nucleus, and slightly indent the floor of the fourth ventricle, forming the facial colliculus. This loop is the internal genu of the facial nerve, which then turns ventrally to emerge on the ventrolateral part of the brainstem at the caudal border of the pons. This nerve then accompanies cranial nerve VIII through the internal auditory canal (G) and petrous temporal bone and exits the skull at the stylomastoid foramen. The nerve to the stapedius muscle is given off prior to exiting the skull, and injury to this small branch can result in hyperacusis. The remaining fibers exit the skull and innervate the frontalis (temporal nerve), orbicularis oculi (zygomatic nerve), buccinator and orbicularis oris (buccal nerve), orbicularis oris (mandibular nerve), platysma (cervical nerve), and occipitalis muscles (posterior auricular nerve). The superior salivatory nucleus (SSN), which supplies the submandibular, salivary, and lacrimal glands, lies posterolaterally to the motor nucleus. The efferents from this nucleus travel via the nervus intermedius and divide in the facial canal into two nerves called the greater petrosal (lacrimal and nasal glands) and the chorda tympani (submandibular gland) nerves. The greater petrosal nerve exits the petrous portion of the temporal bone via the greater superficial petrosal foramen (F) to enter the middle cranial fossa, passes deep to the trigeminal ganglion, traverses the lateral wall of the foramen lacerum, joins with the deep petrosal nerve carrying sympathetic fibers, and becomes the nerve of the pterygoid canal. It then synapses in the pterygopalatine ganglion prior to continuing forward to the lacrimal gland (via V_2 branches) and mucous glands of the nasal and oral cavities. The chorda tympani passes through the petrotympanic fissure to join the lingual branch of the trigeminal nerve (V_3) to supply the submandibular and sublingual glands. Sensation from the anterior two-thirds of the tongue, floor of the mouth, and palate is carried to the solitary nucleus through the geniculate ganglion.

The glossopharyngeal nerve (IX) exits the skull via the jugular foramen (H). The inferior (petrosal) and superior glossopharyngeal ganglia lie within the jugular foramen. The special visceral efferent (SVE) component originates in the nucleus ambiguus, and provides innervation to the stylopharyngeus muscle, which elevates the pharynx during speech and swallowing. CN IX supplies general visceral efferent (GVE) fibers to the parotid gland via way of the tympanic nerve of Jacobson (carrying preganglionic parasympathetic fibers) and the lesser superficial petrosal nerve, which enters the middle cranial fossa lateral to the greater superficial petrosal nerve (E). Postganglionic fibers leave the otic ganglion and travel with the auriculotemporal nerve (of V_3) to innervate the parotid gland and induce salivation. Cranial nerve IX also receives general visceral afferent (GVA) fibers from the carotid body (chemoreceptors) and carotid sinus (baroreceptors) via Hering's nerve, which monitor oxygen tension and arterial blood pressure, respectively. These afferents are relayed to the inferior glossopharyngeal ganglion prior to reaching the nucleus solitarius. The hypothalamus and reticular formation receive afferents from this nucleus to control blood pressure and cardiac output in response to inputs from Hering's nerve. The glossopharyngeal nerve also receives pain and temperature information from the inner surface of the tympanic membrane, skin of the external ear, and posterior third of the tongue. Central processes then transmit information to the spinal trigeminal nucleus via way of the inferior and superior glossopharyngeal ganglia. Taste from the posterior third of the tongue is relayed to the gustatory nucleus of the solitary tract via way of the inferior glossopharyngeal ganglion.

The vagus nerve has three nuclei: the main motor nucleus, the sensory nucleus, and the parasympathetic nucleus. It exits the skull through the jugular foramen (H). The motor nucleus lies deep in the reticular formation and includes the nucleus ambiguus. The motor fibers leave the vagus as three major branches: the pharyngeal, superior laryngeal, and recurrent laryngeal nerves. The pharyngeal branch is the principal motor branch, which enters the pharynx at the upper border of the middle constrictor muscle to supply all the muscles of the pharynx (superior, middle, and inferior constrictors, levator palati, salpingopharyngeus, palatopharyngeus, and palatoglossus) except the stylopharyngeus (IX) and tensor veli palatini (V_3). The superior laryngeal branch leaves the inferior vagal ganglion distal to the pharyngeal

branch and divides into two branches: the internal and external laryngeal nerves. The external laryngeal nerve supplies the inferior constrictor and cricothyroid muscles before sending branches to the pharyngeal plexus and superior cardiac nerve. The internal branch is sensory and receives information from the mucous membranes of the epiglottis, base of the tongue, aryepiglottic folds, and majority of the larynx. It leaves the pharynx by piercing the thyrohyoid membrane and ascends in the neck to join the external branch, which forms the superior laryngeal nerve before passing to the inferior (nodosal) vagal ganglion. Below the vocal cords, sensation is carried by the recurrent laryngeal nerve. Some of these afferent branches also receive input from baroreceptors in the aortic arch and chemoreceptors in the aortic body. The recurrent laryngeal nerve takes a different path on the right and left sides. On the right, it descends anterior to the subclavian artery, loops back under it, and ascends in the groove between the trachea and esophagus. On the left, it descends to the level of the aortic arch, makes a turn underneath it, and ascends between the esophageal-tracheal groove. This nerve supplies the intrinsic muscles of the larynx except for the cricothyroid. The parasympathetic nerve cell bodies are located in the dorsal motor nucleus of the vagus, which is influenced by the hypothalamus, olfactory system, reticular formation, and nucleus solitarius. It is the secretomotor center of the vagus. The efferent fibers are distributed to the involuntary muscles of the bronchi, heart, esophagus, stomach, small intestine, and proximal large intestine. Sensory fibers from the skin of the external ear, external auditory canal, and external surface of the tympanic membrane are carried by the auricular branch, pass to the superior vagal ganglion, and make their way to the spinal trigeminal tract and nucleus before being relayed to the contralateral VPM nucleus of the thalamus and sensory cortex.

The spinal accessory nerve (IX) is a motor nerve that is formed by the union of a cranial and spinal part. It supplies portions of the trapezius and sternocleidomastoid muscles. The spinal component is formed by rootlets from the lateral column of the upper five or six cervical segments that passes to the cranial cavity through the foramen magnum. This nerve then joins the cranial portion within the jugular canal, which it traverses. The hypoglossal nerve (XII) supplies all the muscles of the tongue except for the palatoglossus (X) and exits the skull at the hypoglossal canal adjacent to the foramen magnum.

The ophthalmic artery and central vein of the retina traverse the optic canal (A), while V_2 exits the skull through the foramen rotundum (C) (Wilson-Pauwels, pp. 50–225).

83. C. The trochlear nucleus is located in the tegmentum of the mesencephalon at the level of the inferior colliculus, ventral to the cerebral aqueduct. Axons leaving this nucleus course dorsally around the aqueduct, decussate within the superior medullary velum, and exit the brainstem on the dorsal surface (only cranial nerve to exit the brainstem dorsally and decussate after exiting the brainstem). Since the trochlear nerve crosses to the other side, it innervates the contralateral superior oblique muscle. Of note, the trochlear nerve passes through the cavernous sinus along with cranial nerves III, V_1, sometimes V_2, and VI. Cranial nerves III, V_1, V_2, and IV run along the lateral wall of the sinus, while cranial nerve VI runs more medially and adjacent to the internal carotid artery. Injury to the superior oblique muscle or trochlear nerve results in diplopia, with weakness of downward and medial gaze. Patients have most difficulty walking down stairs, and because of the tendency to tilt the head to compensate for the affected superior oblique muscle, fourth nerve palsies should be included in the differential for torticollis (Wilson-Pauwels, pp. 70–77).

84. E. The corticospinal tracts originate in layer V of the cerebral cortex, pass through the corona radiata and posterior limb of the internal capsule, form the middle third of the cerebral peduncles and the pyramids of the medulla, and terminate primarily on interneurons of lamina VII in the spinal cord. Approximately 40% of corticospinal fibers originate in the parietal lobe, 30% are from the motor cortex (area 4), 30% from the supplementary motor area (area 6), and only 3% originate from the giant Betz pyramidal cells of the motor cortex. Around two-thirds of the corticospinal fibers are myelinated, and there are approximately 1 million corticospinal fibers in each pyramid of the medulla. Corticospinal fibers incompletely decussate in the medulla and form the large crossed lateral corticospinal tract (90% of fibers), the smaller uncrossed anterior corticospinal tract, and the very small uncrossed anterolateral corticospinal tract. The lateral corticospinal tracts descend in the lateral funiculus to all levels of the spinal cord and synapse in laminae IV, V, VI, and VII of the spinal gray. The anterior corticospinal tracts descend adjacent to the anterior median fissure of the spinal cord and terminate primarily in cervical segments. The majority of these fibers (90%) decussate at upper cervical levels of the spinal cord in the anterior white commissure before synapsing in lamina VII of the spinal gray. The uncrossed anterolateral corticospinal tracts (10%) descend ventral to the lateral corticospinal tracts to terminate in the intermediate gray and base of the posterior horns of the spinal cord. A relatively small number of corticospinal fibers synapse directly on motor neurons in the anterior horn of the spinal cord. Within the spinal cord, cervical corticospinal fibers are located medially, and sacral fibers are found laterally. The corticospinal tracts are responsible for voluntary skilled movements of the extremities. Significant corticospinal tract lesions may cause hypotonia followed by hyperactive deep tendon reflexes, extensor toe response (Babinski sign), and loss of superficial abdominal and cremasteric reflexes (Carpenter, pp. 94–97; Martin, pp. 144–145).

85. A. The limbic lobe is not a true lobe of the brain but rather a functional collection of structures that regulates higher activities such as memory and emotion. It does not include the amygdala. Papez's circuit runs from the hippocampus to the fornix to the mammillary body. Fibers are then relayed to the anterior nucleus of the thalamus (through the mammillothalamic tract) to the cingulate gyrus and back to the hippocampus through the cingulate bundle. The term *limbic system* includes the limbic lobe and its associated subcortical nuclei, including the amygdala, hypothalamus, septal, and certain hypothalamic nuclei (Kandel, pp. 986–987; Carpenter, pp. 376, 384–386).

86. C. The retina contains both electrical and chemical synapses. Photoreceptors and horizontal cells are connected to each other via gap junctions, but, as in the rest of the brain, chemical synapses predominate in the retina. Most are calcium-independent and appear to work by cGMP. (See discussion for question 27 in Chapter 1, Neurobiology Answers, for further discussion of phototransduction.) (Kandel, pp. 492–506).

87. A. The innermost retinal cell layer (ganglion cell layer) is named after the retinal output cells. The axons of ganglion cells are unmyelinated, which facilitates light transmission to the photoreceptor layer of the outer retina. The layers superficial to the ganglion cell layer include the inner synaptic (plexiform) layer, inner nuclear layer, outer synaptic (plexiform) layer, and outer nuclear layer. The outer nuclear layer contains the cell bodies of the rods (night vision) and cones (daylight vision). The inner nuclear layer contains the cell bodies of the retinal interneurons, which include the bipolar cells, horizontal cells, and amacrine cells. Bipolar cells link photoreceptors directly with the ganglion cells, while the actions of horizontal and amacrine cells enhance visual contrast through interactions between laterally located photoreceptor cells and bipolar cells. Horizontal cells are located on the outer part of the inner nuclear layer, while amacrine cells are located on the inner portion. Amacrine cells contain dopamine. Müller cells are the principal retinal neuroglial cells (Martin, pp. 164–171; Kandel, p. 515).

88-M; 89-E; 90-F; 91-I; 92-K; 93-J; 94-L; 95-D. Refer to Table 2.88–2.95A (Fix, p. 208; Carpenter, p. 262).

96. D. Refer to Figure 2.96A. The medulla oblongata contains GVE fibers that originate in the inferior salivatory nucleus and gives rise to the fibers that synapse in the otic ganglia to control parotid gland secretion. It also contains the nucleus ambiguus, which gives rise to the vagal preganglionic parasympathetic GVE fibers that synapse in the sinoatrial and atrioventricular nodes of the heart. The medulla extends from the pyramidal decussation to the inferior pontine sulcus and also contains the corticospinal tracts, medial lemniscus, medial longitudinal fasciculus, hypoglossal nuclei, olivary nuclei, spinal lemniscus, spinocerebellar tracts, spinal

TABLE 2.88–95A   Thalamic afferent and efferent connections

THALAMIC NUCLEUS	AFFERENT FIBERS	EFFERENT FIBERS
Anterior nuclear group	Mammillothalamic tract, fornix	Cingulate gyrus
LD	Unclear	Cingulate gyrus
LP	Area 5	Areas 5 and 7
Pulvinar	Superior colliculus	Areas 18 and 19; parietal and temporal neocortex
MGB	Inferior colliculus; lateral lemniscus	Areas 41 and 42
LGB	Optic tract	Area 17
VPM	Trigeminothalamic tracts; gustatory projections (VPM pc)	Areas 3, 1, and 2
VPL	Medial lemniscus; spinothalamic tracts	Areas 3, 1, and 2
VL	Cerebellar nuclei; globus pallidus	Area 4; premotor cortex
VA	Substantia nigra; globus pallidus	Area 6; diffuse frontal

trigeminal tract and nucleus, inferior cerebellar peduncle, dorsal motor nucleus of CN X, solitary tract, CN nuclei of IX to XI (although it also houses portions of CN V and CN VIII), as well as the inferior and medial vestibular nuclei. The lateral vestibular nuclei are mainly in the pons. The medulla receives its blood supply from the posterior spinal artery, anterior spinal artery, PICA, and branches originating from the vertebral arteries (Carpenter, pp. 115–150).

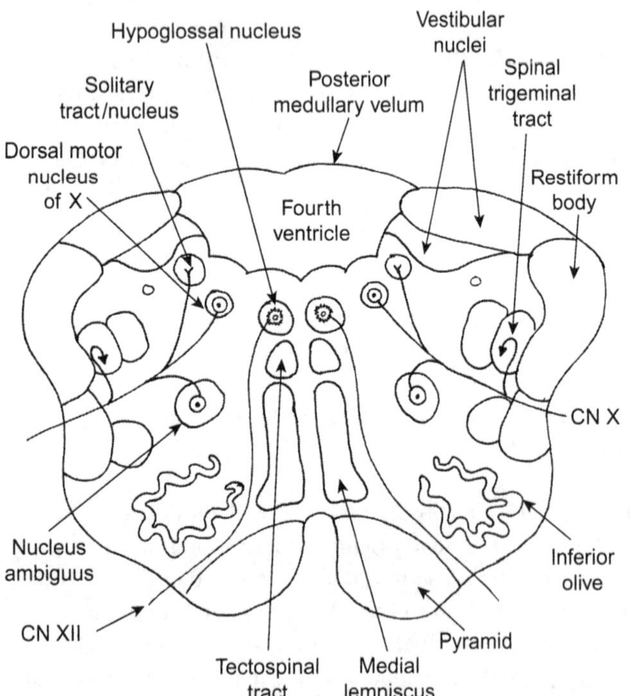

FIGURE 2.96A   Medulla. This represents a transverse section through the rostral medulla at the level of the inferior olive. CN, cranial nerve. (Reprinted with permission from Moore SP. The Definitive Neurological Surgery Board Review. Malden, MA: Blackwell Publishing, 2005:31, Figure 2.3.)

97. D. The most likely cause of the constellation of signs/symptoms reported in this patient is a lesion in the dorsolateral zone of the pontine isthmus on the left side (lateral superior pontine syndrome). Interruption of the descending sympathetic tract resulted in the ipsilateral Horner's syndrome. Involvement of the lateral aspect (includes leg fibers) of the medial lemniscus resulted in loss of vibratory sensation and other dorsal column deficits on the contralateral side. Damage to the trigeminothalamic tract and spinothalamic tracts in this location would account for the contralateral hemianesthesia of the face and body. Disruption of the superior cerebellar peduncle can lead to the severe ataxia and tremor on the ipsilateral side (Carpenter, pp. 151–191; Fix, pp. 184–186).

98. A. Refer to Figure 2.98A. Paramedian midbrain (Benedikt's) syndrome results from occlusion of the paramedian midbrain branches of the PCA and/or basilar artery. Structures affected include the CN III nerve roots (eye abduction and depression due to unopposed action of lateral rectus and superior oblique muscles) as well as the red nucleus and dentatorubrothalamic tract (intention tremor and ataxia). Medial midbrain (Weber's) syndrome results from occlusion of medial midbrain branches, which can result in CN III palsy, corticobulbar tract injury (contralateral facial weakness), and corticospinal tract injury (contralateral hemiparesis or hemiplegia) (Fix, pp. 187–188; Carpenter, pp. 192–223).

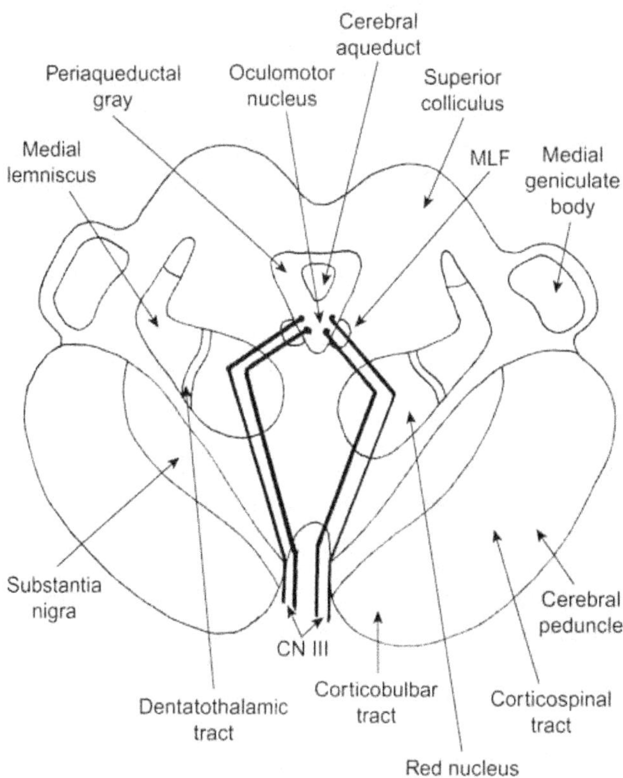

FIGURE 2.98A Mesencephalon. This transverse section illustrates the midbrain at the level of the superior colliculus. CN, cranial nerve; MLF, medial longitudinal fasciculus. (Reprinted with permission from Moore SP. The Definitive Neurological Surgery Board Review. Malden, MA: Blackwell Publishing, 2005:35, Figure 2.5.)

99. E. The gustatory system innervates the special visceral afferent (SVA) modality of taste. Taste buds located on the tongue, epiglottis, and palate are innervated by the SVA fibers of CN VII, IX, and X. First-order neurons are pseudounipolar ganglion cells located in the geniculate ganglion of CNV II, the petrosal ganglion of IX, and the nodose ganglion of X. These fibers project centrally to the solitary nucleus, which then projects, via the central tegmental tract, to the parabrachial nucleus of the pons and VPM nucleus of the thalamus. The parabrachial nucleus then projects to the hypothalamus and amygdala, whereas the VPM projects to gustatory area 43 (parietal operculum) and parainsular cortex. Area 43 then projects via way of the entorhinal cortex to the hippocampal formation. The parabigeminal nucleus functions with the superior colliculus in processina visual information (Fix, pp. 254–256, Carpenter, pp. 137, 140, 143, 171, 271, 418).

100. E. The parafascicular, centromedian, and rostral intralaminar nuclei of the thalamus lie within the internal medullary lamina and are known as the intralaminar nuclei of the thalamus. The parafascicular nucleus of the thalamus lies medial to the centromedian nucleus and ventral to the dorsomedial nuclei of the thalamus. While the projections of the parafascicular and centromedian nuclei of the thalamus

remain ill-defined, the majority are believed to terminate in the striatum. Cells of the centromedian nucleus project principally to the putamen, where they terminate in a mosaic-type pattern, and cells from the parafascicular nucleus project to the caudate nucleus. Few tracts project to both regions of the striatum. The majority of motor activities are influenced by the thalamus, cerebellum, basal ganglia, peripheral receptors, and other cortical areas. The basal ganglia and cerebellum provide priming and feedback functions for smoothly executed movements. Sensory feedback concerning position sense are provided by the dorsal column–medial lemniscus (via the ventral posterior lateral [VPL] nucleus of the thalamus), which is necessary to make both accurate and sequential movements. Complex voluntary motor activity is aided by the premotor region of the posterior parietal region (area 5), which helps with goal-directed movements that require transformation of sensory representations of the environment into limb and hand movements, a process termed sensorimotor transformation (Carpenter, pp. 424–425; Kandel, pp. 756–779).

101. B. Nitric oxide is synthesized from the amino acid arginine by the enzyme nitric oxide synthase (NOS). Nitric oxide easily diffuses across the plasma membrane of target cells. Within target cells, nitric oxide binds guanylyl cyclase to stimulate the production of cGMP. Nitric oxide is synthesized by endothelial cells and then acts upon smooth muscle cells to induce relaxation. Nitric oxide is a potent vasodilator, but it has a short half-life (5 to 10 seconds). Within neurons, NOS is activated by a calcium/calmodulin-dependent enzyme after glutamate binds and activates the NMDA channel (Kandel, p. 295).

102. B. The Bell-Magendie law states that all motor fibers exit the spinal cord via the ventral roots and all sensory fibers enter the spinal cord via the dorsal roots. Unmyelinated C fibers that transmit pain and temperature information from the pelvic viscera reside in the ventral roots from L5 to S3, thus violating the Bell-Magendie law. The cell bodies of these neurons reside in the dorsal root ganglia, like other sensory neurons (DeMyer, p. 55).

103. C. The reticulospinal tracts originate largely in the brainstem reticular formation (pons and medulla) and project to all spinal levels. The raphe nuclei of the reticular formation contain serotonergic projections that compose a portion of the reticulospinal tracts. These serotonergic projections synapse in laminae I, II, and V of the spinal cord (especially cervical levels) to influence afferent nociceptive impulses from the periphery (Carpenter, pp. 101–104).

104. D. Efferent fibers from the substantia nigra project to the striatum (pars compacta efferents) and thalamus (pars reticulata efferents). Nigrothalamic fibers terminate primarily in the VA and MD thalamic nuclei. A small component of efferent fibers from the pars reticulata also project to the pedunculopontine nucleus (Carpenter, pp. 218–220).

105. B. The medial forebrain bundle sends fibers from the basal olfactory regions, the septal nuclei, the periamygdaloid region, and the subiculum to the lateral preoptic and hypothalamic regions (Carpenter, p. 304).

106-I; 107-L; 108-G; 109-H; 110-C; 111-E; 112-D; 113-J; 114-B; 115-A; 116-F; 117-M; 118-K. (Osborn DCA, pp. 217–223).

119. A. The first dorsal root frequently undergoes regression and disappears. The front part of the scalp (forehead) is innervated by CN V: supraorbital and supratrochlear nerves (V_1), zygomaticotemporal nerve (V_2), and the auriculotemporal nerve (V_3). The occipital region is innervated by the greater occipital nerve (C2), the lesser occipital nerve (C2-3), the least occipital nerve (C3), and the great auricular nerve (C2-3) (April, p. 427).

120. D. The Schwann cells and fibrous connective tissue stop abruptly at a site where the nerve roots meet the spinal cord and/or brainstem. Central to this junction, glial connective tissue is composed of oligodendrocytes, whereas in the peripheral nervous system, Schwann cells replace oligodendrocytes. This junction is called the Obersteiner-Redlich zone (DeMyer, p. 59).

121. A. The nerve that innervates the fifth digit, C8, travels through the medial cord of the brachial plexus and down the arm in the ulnar nerve. Therefore, a lesion anywhere along this course may produce pain and numbness in the little finger. The precise localization in this patient would likely require the presence of other concomitant neurologic abnormalities and obtaining nerve conduction or perhaps neuroimaging studies. C7 nerve root abnormalities often cause problems with the third and fourth digits (Brazis, pp. 16–21, 59–60, 72).

122-E; 123-A; 124-D. The majority of posterior circulation aneurysms may be adequately exposed for surgical treatment through either a modification of the transsylvian approach or the far lateral suboccipital approach, which has also been referred to as the Extreme Lateral Inferior Transcondylar Exposure (ELITE). With extensive opening of the posterior lateral portion of the cavernous sinus through a transsylvian approach and by working through the space lateral to the oculomotor nerve, the upper and mid-basilar trunk can be successfully exposed to the level of the anterior inferior cerebellar artery (AICA). The ELITE exposure most often provides satisfactory exposure of the vertebral arteries bilaterally and the lower basilar trunk. The portion of the basilar trunk rostral to AICA origin assumes a distinctly midline location in the majority of circumstances; it becomes increasingly difficult to control and visualize during rostral

dissection due to the prominence of the ventral pons and the envelopment of the basilar artery by the brainstem as it enters the interpeduncular cistern. In select cases (giant aneurysms, cavernomas, or tumors of the dorsolateral pons), additional exposure may be obtained by a presigmoid corridor by removal of a portion of the petrous temporal bone, which may lessen the amount of brainstem or cerebellar retraction, as depicted here. The trochlear nerve (IV) is particularly vulnerable to injury while dividing the tentorium, and the superior petrosal sinus is often cauterized and divided during this exposure in order to mobilize the transverse and sigmoid sinuses (and quadrangular lobe of the cerebellum) as a single unit (Kopitnik, pp. 24–27)

125-A; 126-C; 127-B; 128-A; 129-D. Bilateral lesions of the lateral hypothalamus abolishes the desire to eat, while lesions in the posterior hypothalamus can result in precocious puberty and excessive sleepiness, lethargy, and hypothermia. Lesions of the anterior hypothalamus can result in hyperthermia, while lesions in the arcuate nuclei and paraventricular region can result in decreased dopamine synthesis (Carpenter, pp. 125–129).

130. C. The inferior parietal lobule is composed of two gyri: the angular and supramarginal. The inferior parietal lobule represents a cortical association area, where multisensory signals from adjacent parietal, temporal, and occipital regions converge. The interparietal sulcus divides the parietal lobe into the superior and inferior parietal lobules (Carpenter, p. 27).

131. C. Acoustic reflex mechanisms involve the middle ear muscles, such as the stapedius and tensor tympani. The stapedius muscle (CN VII) serves to dampen the oscillations of the middle ear ossicles in response to loud sounds, while contraction of the tensor tympani muscle (CN V) diminishes the sensitivity of sound by tensing the tympanic membrane. These acoustic reflex mechanisms are initiated by fibers originating in the superior olivary nucleus (Carpenter, p. 159).

132. E. The spinal trigeminal tract merges with the principal sensory nucleus rostrally (not the solitary nucleus), while caudally it blends into the substantia gelatinosa of the first two cervical spinal segments. Fibers of the ophthalmic division are most ventral, fibers of the mandibular division are most dorsal, and fibers from the maxillary division are intermediate (Carpenter, p. 177).

133. A. The best-known pineal secretions are the biogenic amines (serotonin, melatonin, and norepinephrine), but the gland also contains significant concentrations of hypothalamic peptides, such as thyrotropin-releasing hormone, leuteinizing hormone–releasing hormone, and somatostatin. Substance P is not known to be present in high concentrations in the pineal gland (Carpenter, pp. 253–254).

134. B. Melanocytes are located in the leptomeninges are most often located in the ventral medulla and upper levels of the cervical spinal cord (Ellison, pp. 734–737).

135. A. The intervertebral disc is a fibrocartilaginous remnant of the embryologic notochord (Youmans, p. 4327).

136-C; 137-A. The internal capsule is supplied primarily by the lateral lenticulostriate branches from the middle cerebral artery. Additionally, the medial striate artery (of Heubner) supplies the rostromedial parts of the anterior limb of the internal capsule, the genu receives direct branches from the internal carotid artery, while parts of the posterior limb and the entire retrolenticular capsule are supplied by the anterior choroidal artery (Carpenter, p. 448).

138. C. Taste sensation is carried by the facial (VII), glossopharyngeal (IX), and vagus nerves (X). The gustatory afferents end primarily in the nucleus of the tractus solitarius in the medulla (Brazis, p. 273).

139. D. The spinal accessory nerve (XI) does not carry parasympathetic fibers but instead carries branchial motor fibers to the sternocleidomastoid and trapezius muscles (Wilson-Pauwels, p. 205).

140-F; 141-H; 142-C; 143-G; 144-I; 145-E; 146-D; 147-A; 148-B. (Greenberg, pp. 520–521).

149-C; 150-B; 151-A; 152-D; 153-C; 154-C. The orbitofrontal cortex is linked to the limbic and reticular areas; therefore lesions of this area can lead to behavioral abnormalities. Most commonly, orbitofrontal (frontal pole) lesions can result in euphoria, emotional lability, poor judgment and insight, explosiveness, and distractibility. The lateral frontal cortex is linked to motor structures, therefore damage to this area can lead to disturbances of action with apathy, indifference, psychomotor retardation, motor preservation and impersistence, and poor abstraction. The medial frontal syndrome is associated with mutism, gait disturbances, incontinence, "salutatory seizures," "alien hand syndrome," and apraxia of gait or "magnetic gait" (paracentral lobule). Exploring objects orally is a feature of temporal lobe dysfunction (Brazis, pp. 473–474, 509, 522–524).

155. A. The vertebral artery usually travels through the transverse foramina of C6 through C2 prior to exiting the transverse foramen of the axis and curving posteriorly and superiorly in a groove on the upper surface of the atlas (Greenberg, p. 107).

156-B; 157-C. An afferent pupillary defect (Marcus Gunn pupil) can be diagnosed by the "swinging flashlight test." This pupillary sign is characterized by normal bilateral pupillary responses when the normal eye is illuminated, but pupillary dilation occurs when the flashlight is quickly switched to the affected eye. This abnormality may be seen with lesions involving the macula, retina, optic nerve, optic tract, brachium of the superior colliculus, or pretectal nucleus (Kline, pp. 127–128, Brazis, pp. 144–145).

158. C. The superior rectus (medial subnucleus of the oculomotor nucleus, CN III) and superior oblique (trochlear nucleus, CN IV) muscles receive contralateral nuclear innervation (Wilson-Pauwels, pp. 53, 70).

159. B. "Periodic alternating gaze" (PAG) consists of cyclic conjugate lateral deviation of the eyes with compensatory head turning towards the opposite side (1 to 2 minutes), a midline changeover period (10 to 15 seconds), which is followed by conjugate deviation of the eyes toward the other side (with compensatory head turning). It is most common with diseases of the posterior fossa (pontine damage, posterior fossa ischemia, medulloblastoma, and Chiari malformations) (Brazis, pp. 212–213).

160-B; 161-E; 162-D; 163-D; 164-A; 165-C; 166-A; 167-F; 168-F. The trigeminal nerve afferents mediate the tearing and corneal reflex (V_1), sneeze reflex (V_2), and jaw-jerk reflex (V_3). The vagus nerve (X) mediates the afferent limb of the cough reflex, while the glossopharyngeal nerve (IX) mediates the afferent limb of the carotid sinus and gag reflexes. The optic nerve innervates the afferent limb of the pupillary reflex via the Edinger-Westphal nucleus (DeMyer, pp. 171, 176–177).

169. D. The ganglionic cells of the retina are considered to be cholinergic, while some of the neurons of the striatum, dorsal horn, cerebellum, collicular plate, substantia nigra, hypothalamus, pallidum, and anterior perforated substance (substantia innominata) are considered to be GABAergic (DeMyer, pp. 384–385).

170. D. Since the secondary cochlear pathways are both crossed and uncrossed, lesions of one lateral lemniscus can result in partial bilateral deafness. Injury to the inner hair cells of the cochlea, cochlear nerve, or ventral and dorsal cochlear nuclei produces unilateral hearing loss (Brazis, pp. 293–295).

171-F; 172-B; 173-A; 174-B; 175-C. Major sites of origin of the various neurotransmitters are as follows: acetylcholine-gigantocellular complex of the basal forebrain including the basal nucleus (of Meynert); GABA-golgi type II interneurons as well as various areas of the hypothalamus, substantia nigra, cerebellum, dorsal horns, collicular plate, and substantia innominata; dopamine–ventral tegmental region/substantia nigra of midbrain, serotonin–raphe nuclei of midbrain; norepinephrine–locus ceruleus (DeMyer, p. 385; Carpenter, pp. 128, 131).

Neurology Questions

QUESTIONS 1–3

Directions: Match the following questions with the associated syndrome, using each answer only once.

    A. Tolosa-Hunt syndrome
    B. Gradenigo's syndrome
    C. Raeder's syndrome

1. Horner's syndrome and facial numbness

2. Retro- or bital pain and sixth nerve palsy

3. Painful ophthalmoplegia and third, fourth, and fifth nerve palsies

End of set

4. A 56-year-old male with a long history of smoking and hypertension presents to a stroke neurologist with a unique vascular insult involving the cephalad portion of the nucleus ambiguus. Which of the following problems can often be avoided with such an insult?

    A. Palatal paralysis
    B. Pharyngeal paralysis
    C. Laryngeal paralysis
    D. None of the above
    E. All of the above

5. Ipsilateral trapezius and sternocleidomastoid muscle weakness, dysphonia and dysphagia, loss of taste over the posterior third of the tongue, and depressed sensation over the pharynx characterizes what syndrome?

    A. Collet-Sicard syndrome
    B. Vernet's syndrome
    C. Schmidt's syndrome
    D. Garcin syndrome
    E. Weber's syndrome

6. A 7-year-old boy presented to the emergency room with involuntary laughter (gelastic seizures) and precocious puberty. An MRI study of the brain may show a lesion in what location?

    A. Amygdala
    B. Hippocampus
    C. Cingulate gyrus
    D. Hypothalamus
    E. Sella turcica

QUESTIONS 7–9

Scenario: A 52-year-old construction worker noted some weakness in his hands while at work, followed by thickening of his speech and swallowing problems a few months later. Although he complained of generalized fatigue and aching in his upper and lower extremities, no numbness or other sensory abnormalities were noted on physical examination. There were marked fasciculations and atrophy of his arms, legs, and tongue, as well hyperactive reflexes and Babinski signs.

7. The most likely diagnosis in this middle-aged man would be?

    A. Cervical myelopathy
    B. Multiple sclerosis
    C. Myasthenia gravis
    D. Guillain-Barré syndrome
    E. Amyotrophic lateral sclerosis

8. What is the prognosis?

    A. Relatively good with improved blood sugar levels
    B. Often the patient can go into long-term remission with plasmapheresis and steroid treatment
    C. Excellent with anticholinergic medications
    D. Surgery can help prevent neurologic progression
    E. Often fatal within 3–5 years

9. This disease can be associated with what other illness or abnormality?

    A. Infantile spasms
    B. Klüver-Bucy syndrome
    C. Parkinsonism
    D. Down's syndrome
    E. Autonomic nervous system degeneration

End of set

10. *Akinetic mutism* refers to a state in which patients, although seemingly awake, remain motionless and silent. It has commonly been described with lesions involving all of the following structures EXCEPT?

    A. Hypothalamus
    B. Ascending dopaminergic activating system
    C. Cingulate gyrus
    D. Thalamus
    E. Raphe nucleus

11. All of the following are characteristics of *tuberculous* meningitis EXCEPT?

- **A.** The mortality rate is often higher than in bacterial meningitis
- **B.** Treatment initially includes isoniazid, rifampin, pyrazinamide, and ethambutol
- **C.** Treatment, if started early, is effective in preventing poor outcome in the majority of patients
- **D.** The primary focus of infection with tuberculosis is likely from a region outside the brain
- **E.** Bacterial meningitis is marked by basal meningitis, whereas in tuberculosis the base of the brain is relatively spared of infection

12. Gerstmann's syndrome includes all of the following EXCEPT?

- **A.** Finger agnosia
- **B.** Acalculia
- **C.** Agraphia
- **D.** Right and left confusion
- **E.** Anosognosia

13. The biochemical defect in Refsum's disease has been identified as deficiency of what enzyme?

- **A.** Arylsulfatase A
- **B.** Phytanoyl-coenzyme A hydroxylase
- **C.** β-Glucosidase
- **D.** α-Galactosidase
- **E.** Acid ceramidase

QUESTIONS 14–16

Scenario: A 56-year-old female was diagnosed with paranoid schizophrenia and hospitalized. She was started on low-dose risperidone (Risperdal). A few days into her hospitalization, she complained of worsening abdominal pain. On examination, there was no abdominal rigidity, but fever, leukocytosis, diarrhea, hypertension, and tachycardia were noted. Imaging studies of the brain and abdomen were unremarkable.

14. What is the most likely diagnosis?

- **A.** Conversion disorder
- **B.** Schizophrenia with depressive features
- **C.** Acute intermittent porphyria
- **D.** Appendicitis
- **E.** Risperidone-induced infusion syndrome

15. The most reliable test or intervention that confirms this diagnosis would include?

- **A.** Aminolevulinic acid synthase
- **B.** Assay for homocysteine synthetase
- **C.** Assay for porphobilinogen deaminase activity
- **D.** Exploratory celiotomy
- **E.** Discontinuation of the antipsychotic medication with resolution of symptoms

16. The abdominal pain may improve dramatically with what medication?

- **A.** Propranolol
- **B.** Barbiturates
- **C.** Sulfonamides
- **D.** Gabapentin
- **E.** Mercury

End of set

17. All of the following are characteristic of *Diphtheritic* neuropathy EXCEPT?

- **A.** The organism isolated from the larynx and pharynx is frequently *Corynebacterium diphtheriae*
- **B.** The organisms often release an endotoxin that can cause myocarditis or asymmetric neuropathy
- **C.** The neuropathy often begins with impaired visual function
- **D.** Diphtheria and the associated neuropathy can be prevented by immunization
- **E.** It often produces a demyelinating neuropathy

18. The lesion in Korsakoff's psychosis often involves what brain structure?

- **A.** Dorsomedial (DM) nucleus of the thalamus
- **B.** Globose nucleus
- **C.** Amygdala
- **D.** Vermis of the cerebellum
- **E.** Dentate gyrus

19. What is the most common clinical feature of neuroborreliosis?

- **A.** Painful sensory radiculitis that appears about 3 weeks after erythema migrans
- **B.** Cranial mononeuropathy
- **C.** Limb paresis
- **D.** Arthralgia
- **E.** Vertigo

20. Which of the following disorders is not a mitochondrial DNA abnormality?

- **A.** Mitochondrial myopathy, encephalopathy, lactic acidosis, and stroke-like episodes (MELAS)
- **B.** Myoclonic epilepsy with ragged red fibers (MERFF)
- **C.** Leber's hereditary optic neuropathy (LHON)
- **D.** Kearns-Sayre syndrome (KSS)
- **E.** Leigh's disease

QUESTIONS 21–23

Scenario: A 74-year-old male with peripheral vascular disease presents to the emergency room with wild, involuntary left arm flinging. Magnetic resonance imaging (MRI) of the brain reveals ventriculomegaly, diffuse cortical atrophy, and multiple lacunar infarcts.

21. What structure was likely affected to produce this clinical picture?

- **A.** Lateral globus pallidus
- **B.** Subthalamic nucleus
- **C.** Thalamus
- **D.** Red nucleus
- **E.** Caudate nucleus

22. What is the most likely neurotransmitter abnormality in this patient?

- **A.** Dopamine
- **B.** Glutamate
- **C.** GABA
- **D.** Norepinephrine
- **E.** Acetylcholine

23. Treatment may include all of the following EXCEPT?

- **A.** Haloperidol
- **B.** Perphenazine
- **C.** Reserpine
- **D.** Tetrabenazine
- **E.** L-DOPA

End of set

24. Which of the following about Huntington's disease is true?

- **A.** It is a trinucleotide (CAG) repeat disorder that localizes to chromosome 4
- **B.** It is an autosomal recessive condition with incomplete penetrance
- **C.** Primarily a disease affecting the GABA/enkephalin projections from the amygdala to the striatum
- **D.** More common in females than males
- **E.** Has a later onset in successive generations

QUESTIONS 25–32

Directions: The questions below consist of lettered headings followed by a set of numbered items. For each numbered item, select one heading with which it is most closely associated. Each lettered heading may be used once, more than once, or not at all.

- **A.** Trigonocephaly
- **B.** Scaphocephaly
- **C.** Plagiocephaly
- **D.** Brachycephaly
- **E.** Oxycephaly
- **F.** Lacunar skull
- **G.** Kleeblattschädel
- **H.** None of the above

25. Cloverleaf-shaped skull

26. Tower skull

27. Chiari malformation

28. Metopic synostosis

29. Unilaterally flattened head

30. Boat-shaped skull

31. Premature sagittal suture closure

32. Bilaterally flattened head

End of set

33. A 34-year-old male with HIV presents to the emergency room with headaches, confusion, and a right homonymous hemianopia. T1-weighted MRI of the brain with contrast shows a 3- by 4-cm nonenhancing left parieto-occipital lesion, which exhibits increased signal on FLAIR MRI images. What is the most likely etiology of this lesion?

- **A.** A measles infection that disseminated to the brain
- **B.** A monophasic autoimmune attack by T cells against myelin basic protein
- **C.** Perivenular inflammation and demyelination
- **D.** Reactivation of a papovavirus against oligodendrocytes in the subcortical white matter
- **E.** None of the above

34. Patients who undergo rapid correction of hyponatremia are at risk of developing which of the following problems that can lead to seizures, dysarthria, pseudobulbar palsy, coma, and/or death?

- **A.** Marchiafava-Bignami disease
- **B.** Central pontine myelinolysis
- **C.** Acute disseminated leukoencephalopathy
- **D.** Krabbe's disease
- **E.** Alexander's disease

QUESTIONS 35–37

Scenario: A 16-year-old male is trying out for his high school soccer team and noticed severe leg cramps that were relentless in nature. Although he has experienced this problem in the past during exercise, his cramps were never this severe. His neurologic exam was unremarkable, but he was found to have an abnormally deficient level of the enzyme myophosphorylase.

35. What is the likely diagnosis?
- **A.** Von Gierke's disease
- **B.** Pompe's disease
- **C.** McArdle's disease
- **D.** Cori's disease
- **E.** Late-onset Duchenne's dystrophy

36. What is most likely to be seen on urinalysis in this patient?
- **A.** Myoglobinuria
- **B.** Salt wasting
- **C.** Hyperglycemia
- **D.** Hypercalcemia
- **E.** Hyperphosphatemia

37. What is the mode of transmission of this disease process?
- **A.** Autosomal dominant
- **B.** Autosomal recessive
- **C.** X-linked recessive
- **D.** X-linked dominant
- **E.** Polygenetic transmission

End of set

38. All of the following are features of Friedreich's ataxia EXCEPT?
- **A.** It is an autosomal recessive trinucleotide repeat (GAA) disorder involving the frataxin gene
- **B.** Onset of symptoms usually occurs by the age of 10 to 15 years
- **C.** Often results in the degeneration of the posterior columns and spinocerebellar tracts
- **D.** Cerebellar and cerebral cortical ischemic changes can often be associated with concomitant cardiomyopathy
- **E.** With effective treatment, the disease progression associated with neuronal degeneration can be halted about 60% of the time, although heart failure is typically refractory to therapy

39. Lesch-Nyhan syndrome is an X-linked recessive disorder that results from a deficiency of what enzyme?
- **A.** Glucose transporter-1 protein
- **B.** Phenylalanine hydroxylase
- **C.** Hypoxanthine-guanine phosphoribosyltransferase
- **D.** Cystathionine synthase
- **E.** Purine decarboxylase

QUESTIONS 40–47

Directions: The questions below consist of lettered headings followed by a set of numbered items. For each numbered item, select one heading with which it is most closely associated. Each lettered heading may be used once, more than once, or not at all.
- **A.** Scissoring gait
- **B.** Festinating gait
- **C.** Hemiplegic gait
- **D.** Steppage gait
- **E.** Waddling gait
- **F.** Reeling gait
- **G.** Toppling gait
- **H.** None of the above

40. May be secondary to weakness/paralysis of the pretibial and peroneal muscles

41. Parkinson's disease

42. Associated with circumduction of the leg

43. Chronic or progressive Wohlfart-Kugelberg-Welander syndrome

44. May accompany a lesion in the thoracic spine

45. Often seen with foot drop

46. Internal capsule infarct

47. Anterior and lateral borders of shoe sole often worn down

End of set

QUESTIONS 48–51

Scenario: A 34-year-old female suddenly develops a left hemiparesis. She experienced a deep venous thrombosis in her left leg about 4 years earlier.

48. The most likely cause of this patient's deficit is
- **A.** Atrial fibrillation
- **B.** Metastatic brain tumor
- **C.** Multiple sclerosis
- **D.** Lupus anticoagulant
- **E.** Atrial septal defect

49. A nonspecific laboratory feature of this disorder may include which one of the following?

    A. Prolonged PT and PTT that does not reverse when the patient's plasma is mixed with normal plasma
    B. Oligoclonal bands in the CSF
    C. Abnormal dystrophin gene
    D. Elevation of IgE antibodies in the serum
    E. None of the above

50. Which of the following can confirm the diagnosis?

    A. Demonstrating an inhibitor reaction within the clotting system using the thromboplastin inhibition test (TTI) and dilute Russel venom viper assay
    B. Confirming a defect in factor V
    C. Multiple lesions in the deep white matter on magnetic resonance imaging (MRI)
    D. Noting the presence of an atrial septal defect on echocardiography
    E. Excessive bleeding after shaving

51. Optimal therapy for this disease may include

    1. Maintaining an international normalized ratio (INR) of at least 3.0 with warfarin
    2. Corticosteroids
    3. Antiplatelet agents
    4. Plasmapheresis

    A. 1, 2, and 3 are correct
    B. 1 and 3 are correct
    C. 2 and 4 are correct
    D. Only 4 is correct
    E. All of the above

End of set

QUESTIONS 52–54

Scenario: A previously healthy 72-year-old female develops auditory hallucinations and depression. The patient has difficulty providing the details but believes that her son is speaking to her. She is not cooperative during the interview, but the physical examination is unremarkable. She takes multivitamins and an aspirin each day.

52. Which of the following is the most likely diagnosis?

    A. Hyperthyroidism
    B. Complex partial seizures
    C. Alzheimer's disease
    D. Multi-infarct dementia
    E. Hyperparathyroidism

53. The most common way to obtain this diagnosis includes

    A. Obtaining a thyroid-stimulating hormone (TSH) level
    B. Electroencephalography (EEG)
    C. Detailed history and physical examination
    D. Brain biopsy
    E. Obtaining an angiotensin-converting enzyme (ACE) level

54. A treatment regimen for the auditory hallucinations could include

    A. Tacrine
    B. Donepezil
    C. Vitamin E
    D. Haloperidol
    E. All of the above

End of set

55. A 45-year-old lawyer complains of difficulty holding and using his pen. He notes the development of right arm and hand spasms for the past 3 months only when writing. Physical examination is unremarkable. What is the most likely etiology for this patient's signs/symptoms?

    A. Early Parkinson's disease
    B. Athetosis
    C. C7 radiculopathy
    D. Dystonia
    E. Carpal tunnel syndrome

QUESTIONS 56–63

Directions: The questions below consist of lettered headings followed by a set of numbered items. For each item, select one heading with which it is most closely associated. Each lettered heading may be used once, more than once, or not at all.

    A. Anti-Hu antibody
    B. Anti-Ri antibody
    C. Anti-Jo antibody
    D. Anti-Yo antibody
    E. Anti-VGCC antibody
    F. Anti-Tr antibody
    G. Anti-Ta antibody
    H. None of the above

56. Antibody isolated with small cell lung carcinoma; sensory neuropathy, encephalomyelitis

57. Lambert-Eaton myasthenic syndrome

58. Opsoclonus-myoclonus syndrome

59. Reacts with Purkinje cells of the cerebellum

60. Polymyositis

61. Hodgkin disease

62. Antibody primarily found in patients with testicular cancer

63. Retinal degeneration

End of set

64. A mother brings her 4-month-old male infant to your office after witnessing an episode characterized by sudden extensor spasms involving the head, trunk, and limbs. The EEG is most likely to show

    A. 3-Hz spike-wave discharges
    B. Periodic lateralizing epileptiform discharges (PLEDs)
    C. Hypsarrhythmia
    D. Generalized slowing
    E. 4- to 6-Hz spike waves

65. Increased H-reflex latencies in conjunction with normal F wave latencies localize lesions to what location?

    A. Neuromuscular junction
    B. Anterior horn cells of the spinal cord
    C. Dorsal roots
    D. Ventral roots
    E. None of the above

66. All of the following are characteristic of demyelinating neuropathies on motor nerve conduction studies EXCEPT?

    A. Prolonged distal latency
    B. Decreased segmental velocity
    C. Normal or slightly decreased evoked response amplitude
    D. Decreased F wave
    E. Temporal dispersion

67. All of the following are characteristics of normal single-motor-unit potentials on electromyography (EMG) EXCEPT?

    A. Duration of 5–15 ms
    B. Two to four phases
    C. 0.5–3 mV
    D. Fibrillation potentials
    E. Insertional activity

QUESTIONS 68–73

Directions: The questions below consist of lettered headings followed by a set of numbered items. For each numbered item, select one or more than one heading with which it is most closely associated. Each lettered heading may be used once, more than once, or not at all.

    A. Stage 1
    B. Stage 2
    C. Stage 3
    D. Stage 4
    E. Rapid eye movement (REM)
    F. None of the above

68. Sleep spindles and K complexes

69. > 50% delta waves

70. Transition from α waves to slow low-voltage activity

71. Obstructive sleep apnea can be associated with this stage of sleep

72. Night terrors

73. The presence of this stage of sleep during daytime electroencephalography (EEG) suggests sleep deprivation, alcohol withdrawal, or narcolepsy

End of set

74. This electroencephalographic (EEG) finding (Figure 3.74Q) is most consistent with what abnormality?

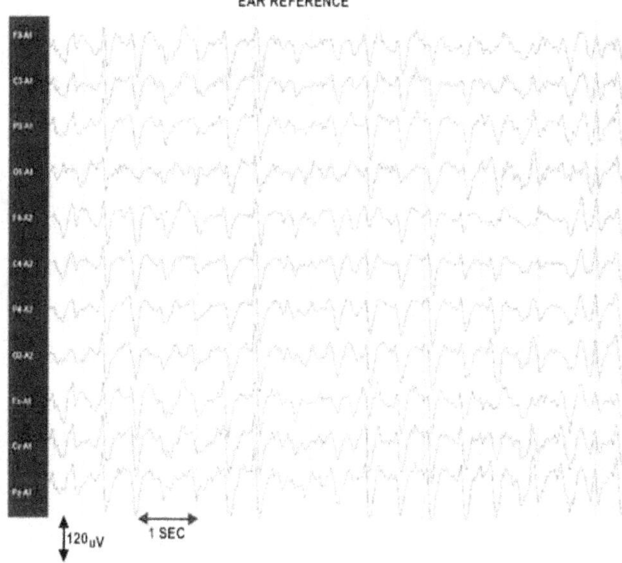

FIGURE 3.74Q

    A. Creutzfeldt-Jakob disease
    B. Hepatic encephalopathy
    C. Massive cerebral infarction
    D. Focal motor seizures
    E. Brain death

75. All of the following are characteristics of narcolepsy EXCEPT?

    A. Associated with excessive daytime sleepiness, sleep paralysis, cataplexy, and hypnagogic hallucinations
    B. Narcoleptics may experience paralysis of voluntary muscles during the initial and terminal periods of the sleep cycle, which often involve the extraocular muscles
    C. Hypnagogic hallucinations often occur at the beginning of the sleep cycle
    D. May exhibit decreased levels of orexin
    E. Associated with the DR2 allele

QUESTIONS 76–78

76. The most likely clinical finding associated with the EEG (Figure 3.76–3.78Q) in this 10-year-old girl would include?

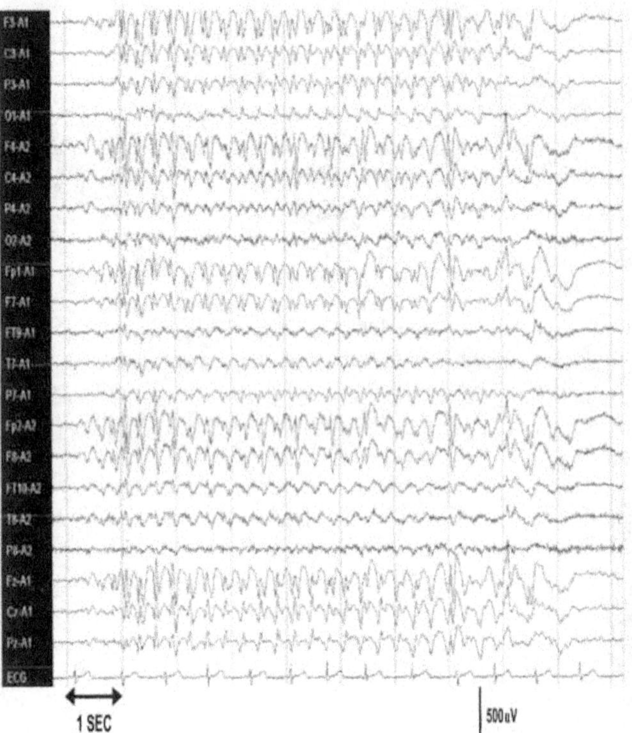

FIGURE 3.76–78Q

A. Drop attacks
B. Infantile spasms
C. Staring spells
D. Oral-alimentary autisms
E. Myoclonic jerks

77. In general, what seizure-activating procedures can be employed to induce seizure activity?

A. Hyperventilation
B. Sleep deprivation
C. Photic stimulation
D. 1 and 3 only
E. All of the above

78. As soon as the seizure stops in this patient, the EEG activity is expected to

A. Return to the interictal state immediately with no postictal depression or slowing
B. Return to the interictal state after a brief period of lateralizing discharges
C. Return to the interictal state after a brief period of paroxysmal bi-occipital activity
D. Resume with normal mu rhythm often seen with this disorder
E. Return to the interictal state with marked depression of background activity in all regions

End of set

QUESTIONS 79–85

Directions: The questions below relate to brain-stem auditory evoked potentials. They consist of lettered headings followed by a set of numbered items. For each numbered item, select one heading with which it is most closely associated. Each lettered heading may be used once, more than once, or not at all.

A. Wave I   E. Wave V
B. Wave II   F. Wave VI
C. Wave III   G. Wave VII
D. Wave IV

79. Inferior colliculus

80. Auditory nerve

81. Medial geniculate body

82. Superior olive

83. Cochlear nucleus

84. Auditory radiation

85. Lateral lemniscus

End of set

86. How can one attempt to normalize the rhythm depicted by this EEG (Figure 3.86Q)?

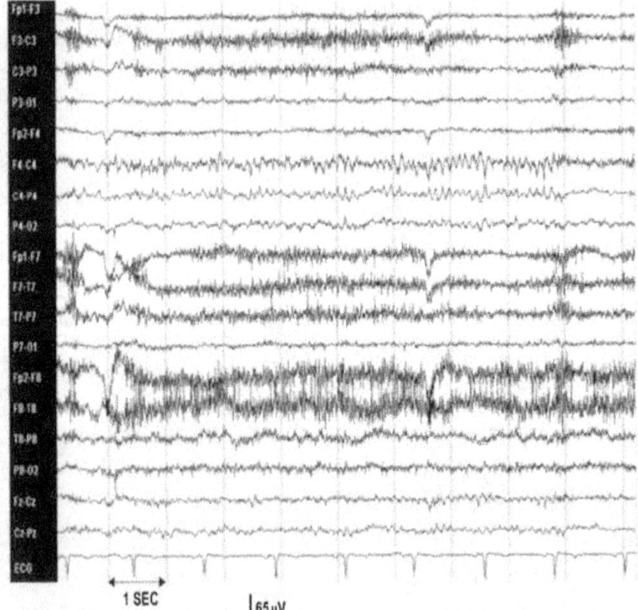

FIGURE 3.86Q

A. Dilantin administration
B. Surgical procedure
C. Phenobarbital administration
D. ACTH administration
E. This rhythm has classically been unresponsive to any medical or surgical intervention

QUESTIONS 87–89

87. The primary center for bladder function that synchronizes bladder contraction with urethral sphincter relaxation is believed to reside in what location?

- **A.** Midbrain tegmentum
- **B.** Hypothalamus
- **C.** Amygdala
- **D.** Pons
- **E.** Thalamus

88. Which of the following bladder abnormalities is most likely to result from acute cauda equina syndrome?

- **A.** Detrusor hyperreflexia
- **B.** Detrusor areflexia
- **C.** Decreased bladder compliance
- **D.** Increased urinary flow rate
- **E.** None of the above

89. All of the following can be used to treat detrusor hyperreflexia EXCEPT?

- **A.** Propantheline (Pro-Banthine)
- **B.** Oxybutynin (Ditropan)
- **C.** Tolterodine (Detrol)
- **D.** Flavoxate (Urispas)
- **E.** Bethanecol (Urecholine)

End of set

90. The components of the somatosensory evoked potential (SSEP) tracing of the median nerve include all of the following EXCEPT?

- **A.** Brachial plexus (Erb's point)
- **B.** Central gray of the spinal cord (N13)
- **C.** Caudal medial lemniscus (P14)
- **D.** Rostral brainstem (N18)
- **E.** Brodmann's areas 5 and 7 (N24)

91. A 52-year-old male with a history of diabetes mellitus and hypertension presents to a local emergency department with left hemiparesis and an evolving infarct involving portions of the right middle cerebral artery (MCA) distribution. A four-vessel angiogram of the brain reveals occlusion of the right MCA proximal to the bifurcation. Data obtained from the National Institute of Neurologic Disorders and Stroke (NINDS) trial showed that administering t-PA within how many hours of stroke resulted in improved functional outcome at 3 months and 1 year?

- **A.** 3 hours
- **B.** 6 hours
- **C.** 8 hours
- **D.** 12 hours
- **E.** 24 hours

92. Since other factors can influence velocities, including blood pressure and overall cerebral blood flow, distinguishing vasospastic from hyperemic increases in MCA blood flow velocities by transcranial Doppler is best achieved by

- **A.** Characterizing all velocities greater than 200 cm/s as the result of vasospasm
- **B.** Repeating the Doppler study within 1 hour to confirm the reading
- **C.** Administer a vasodilating agent in conjunction with the Doppler study to evaluate the percentage change in flow
- **D.** Measuring the "Lindegaard ratio" to help differentiate between vasospastic and hyperemic states
- **E.** Plotting velocity versus vessel diameter on a logarithmic scale

QUESTIONS 93–99

Directions: Match each of the following breathing patterns with the most likely lesion site, using each answer only once.

- **A.** Diencephalon/bilateral cerebral hemispheres
- **B.** Pons
- **C.** High medulla/lower pons
- **D.** Medulla
- **E.** Low midbrain/high pons
- **F.** None of the above

93. Cheyne-Stokes breathing

94. Central neurogenic hyperventilation

95. Cluster breathing

96. Apneustic breathing

97. Ataxic breathing

98. Stertorous breathing

99. Ondine's curse

End of set

100. A poorly controlled hypertensive patient had a sudden onset of hemiplegia and reduced touch and position sense, all of which affected the right side, with bilateral preservation of pain and temperature sensation. There was also weakness on the right side of the tongue and upbeat nystagmus, but no facial droop was noted. An infarct causing this symptomatology would most likely reside in what location?

- **A.** Pontine tegmentum
- **B.** Dorsolateral medulla
- **C.** Midbrain tegmentum
- **D.** Paramedian medulla
- **E.** Posterior limb of the internal capsule

QUESTIONS 101–107

Directions: Match the type of aphasia (numbered items) with the associated clinical findings (lettered options in Table 3.101–3.107Q), using each answer once. (–) indicates abnormality, (+) indicates no abnormality, (+/–) indicates abnormality may be present.

TABLE 3.101–107Q

APHASIA	COMPREHENSION	FLUENCY	NAMING	REPETITION
A	+	–	–	–
B	–	+	–	–
C	+	+	+/–	–
D	+	–	–	+
E	–	+	–	+
F	–	–	–	+
G	–	–	–	–

101. Mixed transcortical

102. Conduction

103. Transcortical motor

104. Global

105. Broca

106. Transcortical sensory

107. Wernicke

End of set

108. Bilateral internuclear ophthalmoplegia can be differentiated from a bilateral medial rectus nuclear lesion by

  A. The presence of normal medial movement with saccades in bilateral INO
  B. The presence of normal medial movement with vestibular stimulation in bilateral INO
  C. The presence of normal convergence in bilateral INO
  D. The presence of normal lateral movement in midline medial recti nuclear lesion
  E. The presence of normal lateral movement in bilateral INO

109. Oculomasticatory myorhythmia is most frequently seen with what abnormality?

  A. Hallervorden-Spatz disease
  B. Progressive supranuclear palsy
  C. Whipple's disease
  D. Arnold-Chiari malformation
  E. Creutzfeldt-Jakob disease

110. What is the best way to differentiate central from peripheral vestibular nystagmus?

  A. The suppression of peripheral nystagmus with fixation
  B. The accentuation of central nystagmus with fixation
  C. The presence of a torsional component with central nystagmus
  D. The presence of increased nystagmus with gaze directed toward the slow phase of nystagmus
  E. The presence of concomitant myoclonic jerks with peripheral nystagmus

111. Amantadine may be classified as what type of medication?

  A. Dopamine receptor agonist
  B. Dopamine receptor antagonist
  C. Muscarinic blocker
  D. Muscarinic activator
  E. None of the above

QUESTIONS 112–117

Directions: Match the following muscles with the associated eye movement, using each answer once, more than once, or not at all.

  A. Superior rectus muscle
  B. Inferior rectus muscle
  C. Lateral rectus muscle
  D. Medial rectus muscle
  E. Superior oblique muscle
  F. Inferior oblique muscle

112. Pure vertical upward movement of the pupil when it is positioned 51 degrees toward the nose (adducted)

113. Pure down movement with the eye abducted 23 degrees

114. Pure down movement with the eye adducted 51 degrees

115. Pure upward movement with the eye abducted 23 degrees

116. Pure intorsion with the eye abducted 39 degrees

117. Pure extorsion with the eye abducted 39 degrees

End of set

118. In a T6 paraplegic (complete cord section), the presence of hypertension, headache, diaphoresis, and bradycardia should be treated with

  A. Propranolol
  B. Bladder catheterization
  C. Arfonad (ganglionic blocker)
  D. 1000 cc bolus of normal saline
  E. Nitroglycerin

119. Small, pinpoint pupils may be seen in all of the following EXCEPT?

A. Pontine tegmental lesions
B. Bilateral diencephalic dysfunction
C. Narcotic intoxication
D. Oculomotor nerve compression
E. Cholinergic drugs

120. Severe shoulder pain followed in several days by proximal arm weakness characterizes the

A. Erb-Duchenne syndrome
B. Parsonage-Turner syndrome
C. Dejerine-Klumpke syndrome
D. Thoracic outlet syndrome
E. None of the above

121. All of the following involve the lower motor CN VII EXCEPT?

A. Ramsay-Hunt syndrome
B. Meige's syndrome
C. Foville's syndrome
D. Benedikt's syndrome
E. Millard-Gubler syndrome

122. Galactorrhea may be due to all of the following EXCEPT?

A. Irritative lesions of the anterior chest wall
B. Levodopa/carbidopa
C. Hypothyroidism
D. Pituitary chromophobe adenomas
E. Contraceptive drugs

123. The "paramedian diencephalic syndrome" includes all of the following EXCEPT ?

A. Hypersomnolence
B. Memory loss
C. Horizontal gaze palsy
D. Apathy
E. Hemiataxia

124. The syndrome of "Dejerine and Roussy" occurs most commonly with lesions of the

A. Ventral lateral (VL) nuclei of the thalamus
B. Ventral posterior (VP) nuclei of the thalamus
C. Intralaminar nuclei of the thalamus
D. Geniculate nuclei
E. Subthalamic nuclei

125. Vitreous hemorrhage associated with subarachnoid hemorrhage is known as

A. Carson syndrome
B. Terson syndrome
C. Collaret syndrome
D. Vicard syndrome
E. Heubner syndrome

QUESTIONS 126–133

Directions: Match the disorder (leukodystrophy) with the enzyme abnormality using each answer once, more than once, or not at all.

A. Krabbe's disease
B. Metachromatic leukodystrophy
C. Adrenoleukodystrophy
D. Pelizaeus-Merzbacher disease
E. Alexander's disease
F. Zellweger's syndrome
G. None of the above

126. Myelin proteolipid

127. Galactocerebrosidase

128. Aryl sulfatase A

129. Arginase

130. Aspartoacylase

131. ATP-binding transporter

132. Long-chain fatty acid metabolism

133. Copper ATPase deficiency

End of set

QUESTIONS 134–142

Directions: Match the disorder (sphingolipidosis) with the associated enzyme abnormality, using each answer once, more than once, or not at all.

A. Tay-Sachs disease (G_{M2} gangliosidosis)
B. Sandhoff's disease
C. Fabry's disease
D. Gaucher's disease
E. Niemann-Pick disease
F. Wolman's disease
G. Batten's disease (neuronal ceroid lipofuscinosis)
H. Cerebrotendinous xanthomatosis
I. G_{M1} gangliosidosis
J. Farber's disease
K. None of the above

134. Sphingomyelinase

135. α-galactosidase A

136. β-glucocerebrosidase

137. β-galactosidase

138. Hexosaminidase A absent; hexosaminidase B increased

139. Hexosaminidase A and B deficient

140. Acid ceramidase

141. Acid lipase

142. Palmitoylprotein thioesterase

End of set

QUESTIONS 143–145

143. What is the inheritance pattern of hereditary hemorrhagic telangiectasia (HHT)?

- **A.** Autosomal recessive
- **B.** Autosomal dominant
- **C.** X-linked
- **D.** Sporadic
- **E.** None of the above

144. HHT is associated with mutations of what gene?

- **A.** EGFR
- **B.** TNF-α
- **C.** TGF-β
- **D.** Superoxide dismutase
- **E.** None of the above

145. Patients with HHT are at high risk for the developing?

- **A.** Brain abscesses
- **B.** Multiple sclerosis
- **C.** Lymphoma
- **D.** Hypoglycemia
- **E.** Myoglobinuria

End of set

146. What is the 1-year stroke risk of asymptomatic 80% carotid artery stenosis?

- **A.** 3%
- **B.** 10%
- **C.** 15%
- **D.** 33%
- **E.** 50%

147. All of the following disorders are associated with defective DNA repair EXCEPT?

- **A.** Xeroderma pigmentosa
- **B.** Fanconi's anemia
- **C.** Bloom's syndrome
- **D.** Ataxia telangiectasia
- **E.** Klinefelter's syndrome

QUESTIONS 148–156

Directions: Match the gene abnormality with the associated syndrome, using each answer once, more than once, or not at all.

- **A.** Trisomy 21
- **B.** Trisomy 18
- **C.** Trisomy 13
- **D.** Trisomy 9
- **E.** Long arm deletion, chromosome 15
- **F.** Short arm deletion, chromosome 4
- **G.** Short arm deletion, chromosome 5
- **H.** Short arm deletion, chromosome 17
- **I.** Decrease in the number of sex chromosomes
- **J.** None of the above

148. Miller-Dieker syndrome

149. Down's syndrome

150. Cri du chat syndrome

151. Patau syndrome

152. Prader-Willi syndrome

153. Edward's syndrome

154. Fragile X syndrome

155. Turner syndrome

156. Associated with Dandy-Walker syndrome in some cases

End of set

157. All of the following disorders are associated with "cherry red" spots EXCEPT?

- **A.** Tay-Sachs disease
- **B.** Sandhoff's disease
- **C.** Sialidosis
- **D.** Niemann Pick disease
- **E.** Galactosemia

158. Increased skin pigmentation is associated with what disorder?

- **A.** Adrenoleukodystrophy
- **B.** Hurler's disease
- **C.** Hunter's disease
- **D.** Cockayne's syndrome
- **E.** Homocystinuria

QUESTIONS 159–164

Directions: Match the clinical feature with the associated disorder, using each answer once, more than once, or not at all.

- **A.** Bulbar palsy
- **B.** Pseudobulbar palsy
- **C.** Both
- **D.** None of the above

159. Atrophic tongue

160. Weak face

161. Absent jaw-jerk reflex

162. Decreased extraocular movements

163. Emotional lability

164. Hyperactive gag

End of set

QUESTIONS 165–170

Directions: Match the virus with the associated genetic content, using each answer once, more than once, or not at all.

  A. DNA virus
  B. RNA virus
  C. Both
  D. None of the above

165. Poliovirus

166. Echovirus

167. Herpes simplex 1 virus

168. Arenavirus

169. Flavivirus

170. Coxsackievirus

End of set

171. What is the normal velocity of a human peripheral nerve when tested by electromyography?

  A. 5–10 meters per second
  B. 10–20 meters per second
  C. 20–30 meters per second
  D. 30–40 meters per second
  E. 40–60 meters per second

QUESTIONS 172–175

Directions: Use the following diagram (Figure 3.172–3.175Q) depicting the basal ganglia circuitry to answer questions 172–175.

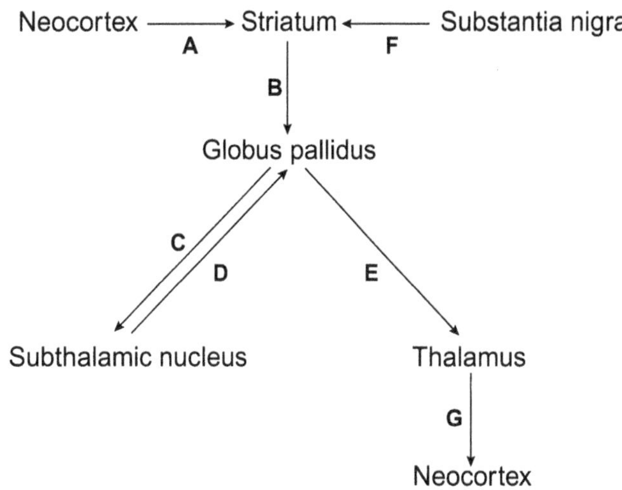

FIGURE 3.172–175Q

172. What is neurotransmitter A?

  A. Glutamate
  B. GABA
  C. Acetylcholine
  D. Dopamine
  E. Substance P

173. What is neurotransmitter C?

  A. Glutamate
  B. GABA
  C. Acetylcholine
  D. Dopamine
  E. Substance P

174. What is neurotransmitter E?

  A. Glutamate
  B. GABA
  C. Acetylcholine
  D. Dopamine
  E. Substance P

175. What is neurotransmitter G?

  A. Glutamate
  B. GABA
  C. Acetylcholine
  D. Dopamine
  E. Substance P

End of set

Neurology Answer Key

1. C	36. A	71. E	106. E	141. F
2. B	37. B	72. C, D	107. B	142. G
3. A	38. E	73. E	108. C	143. B
4. C	39. C	74. B	109. C	144. C
5. B	40. D	75. B	110. A	145. A
6. D	41. B	76. C	111. E	146. A
7. E	42. C	77. E	112. F	147. E
8. E	43. E	78. A	113. B	148. H
9. C	44. A	79. E	114. E	149. A
10. E	45. D	80. A	115. A	150. G
11. E	46. C	81. F	116. E	151. C
12. E	47. C	82. C	117. F	152. E
13. B	48. D	83. B	118. B	153. B
14. C	49. A	84. G	119. D	154. I
15. C	50. A	85. D	120. B	155. I
16. A	51. A	86. B	121. D	156. D
17. B	52. C	87. D	122. B	157. E
18. A	53. C	88. B	123. C	158. A
19. A	54. D	89. E	124. B	159. A
20. E	55. D	90. E	125. B	160. C
21. B	56. A	91. A	126. D	161. A
22. B	57. E	92. D	127. A	162. C
23. E	58. B	93. A	128. B	163. B
24. A	59. F	94. B	129. G	164. B
25. G	60. C	95. C	130. G	165. B
26. E	61. F	96. B	131. C	166. B
27. F	62. G	97. D	132. F	167. A
28. A	63. B	98. F	133. G	168. B
29. C	64. C	99. D	134. E	169. B
30. B	65. C	100. D	135. C	170. B
31. B	66. D	101. F	136. D	171. E
32. D	67. D	102. C	137. I	172. A
33. D	68. B, C	103. D	138. A	173. B
34. B	69. D	104. G	139. B	174. B
35. C	70. A	105. A	140. J	175. A

Neurology Answers

1-C; 2-B; 3-A. Raeder's paratrigeminal neuralgia is often localized adjacent to the trigeminal nerve as it courses through the middle cranial fossa. The cause of this syndrome is often unclear, but it is usually characterized by a partial Horner's syndrome and unilateral trigeminal nerve problems, including tic-like pain, numbness, and/or masseter weakness. Gradenigo's syndrome, also known as apical petrositis, often consists of the classic triad of abducens nerve palsy, retro-orbital pain, and a draining ear. Tolosa-Hunt syndrome is a diagnosis of exclusion; this condition is believed to result from inflammation adjacent to the superior orbital fissure. It is characterized by painful ophthalmoplegia, cranial nerves III, IV, and VI palsies, and recurrent attacks and remissions; it is typically treated with intravenous steroids (Greenberg, pp. 581–582).

4. C. Lesions within the nucleus ambiguus may occur as a result of vascular insults, tumors, syringobulbia, motor neuron disease, and inflammatory disease. Lesions in this location often result in palatal, pharyngeal, and laryngeal paralysis that is often associated with other adjacent cranial nerve and brainstem abnormalities. If the cephalad portion of the nucleus ambiguus is injured, however, laryngeal function is often spared due to the somatotopic organization of this motor nucleus. This is referred to as "palatopharyngeal paralysis of Avellis" (Brazis, pp. 321–322).

5. B. Refer to Table 3-5A. The spinal accessory nerve enters the jugular foramen accompanied by cranial nerves IX and X. Lesions of the jugular foramen including tumors, infections, and fractures can result in Vernet's syndrome, which is characterized by ipsilateral trapezius and sternocleidomastoid muscle weakness, dysphonia and dysphagia, loss of taste over the posterior third of the tongue, and depressed sensation over the pharynx (Brazis, pp. 330–331).

TABLE 3.5A Syndromes involving cranial nerves IX to XII

SYNDROME	NERVES INVOLVED
Collet-Sicard	IX, X, XI, XII
Villaret	IX, X, XI, XII, sympathetic chain, ± VII
Schmidt	X, XI
Tapia	X, XII, ± sympathetic chain, VII
Garcin	All ipsilateral cranial nerves

6. D. An MRI study of the brain in a patient with seizures accompanied by involuntary laughter (gelastic seizures) that alternates with crying or sobbing spells would likely show a lesion in the hypothalamus. A small series of cases have been reported in the literature to date describing this phenomenon; in one report, 4 of 16 patients were found to harbor a hypothalamic hemartoma. Gelastic seizures or laughing fits have been reported to occur in up to 21% of patients with hypothalamic hemartomas. Most patients with this lesion present with isosexual precocious puberty by the age of 3 years, although patients as old as 8 years have been reported. Hypothalamic hemartomas may be associated with midline deformities such as callosal agenesis, optic malformations, and hemispheric dysgenesis (Kaye and Laws, pp. 593–596).

7-E; 8-E; 9-C. In this patient, the multiple motor deficits and signs of anterior horn cell disease unaccompanied by any sensory abnormalities suggest a diagnosis of amyotrophic lateral sclerosis (ALS). Most individuals with ALS die within 5 years of symptom onset, especially if there are both upper and lower motor neuron signs. There is a very high incidence of this disease among the Chamorro Indians of Guam, and there is also an association between ALS and a Parkinson-like dementia complex (Merritt, pp. 710–712).

10. E. Refer to Figure 3.10A. Animal studies and case reports have disclosed two primary lesion sites that may result in akinetic mutism: the mesencephalic-diencephalic reticular activating system including the midbrain reticular formation, thalamus, and hypothalamus, and lesions involving the anterior cingulate gyrus and adjacent mesial frontal lobes. These two major lesion sites occur along the pathways that originate in the mesencephalon and project widely to dopamine receptors located in spinal cord, brainstem, diencephalon, corpus striatum, and mesiofrontal lobes as the ascending dopaminergic activating system. Mutism related to dentate nucleus damage has been shown to occur after removal of cerebellar tumors, especially in children, but this type of mutism is distinct from classic akinetic mutism. (Brazis, p. 566).

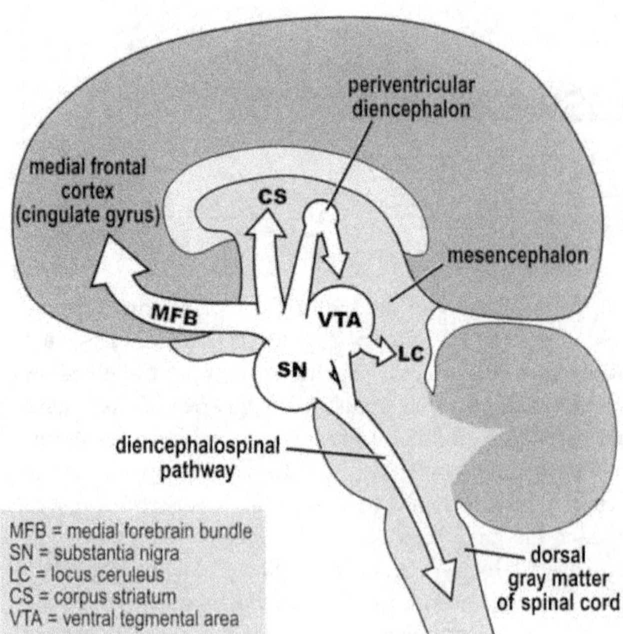

FIGURE 3.10A   Akinetic mutism.

11. E. Tuberculous meningitis is always secondary to an infection elsewhere in the body, especially the lungs. It differs from infections caused by other common bacteria in that the time course is often more protracted, the mortality rate is higher, and the CSF changes may not be very helpful or diagnostic initially. Tuberculous meningitis is also often characterized by marked basal meningitis, as opposed to bacterial meningitis, which tends to produce a meningeal reaction over the convexities of the brain. The diagnosis is often established by isolating the organism from the CSF. CSF findings include slightly increased pressure, moderate pleocytosis of 25 to 500 cells/mm³ with lymphocytic predominance, increased protein content, decreased glucose values in the range of 20 to 40 mg/dL, and the absence of growth on routine CSF culture media. The natural course of the disease is death within 6 to 8 weeks if left untreated. With early diagnosis and treatment, the recovery rate approaches 90%. Treatment is commonly started with four drugs, including isoniazid, rifampin, pyrazinamide, and ethambutol; streptomycin is an alternative in case one of the agents cannot be used. The drug regimen can be modified later, once sensitivities of the mycobacterium are known, but are typically administered for 18 to 24 months (Merritt, pp. 108–111).

12. E. Gerstmann's syndrome can result from injury in the dominant inferior parietal lobule (angular and supramarginal gyri) and is characterized by confusion of the right and left limbs, difficulty in distinguishing the fingers on the hand (finger agnosia), acalculia, and agraphia. Anosognosia, which is characterized by unawareness of the opposite side of the body, often results from lesions in the nondominant parietal lobe and is not a feature of Gerstmann's syndrome (Carpenter, p. 429).

13. B. Refsum disease is an autosomal recessive disease caused by a deficiency of phytanoyl-coenzyme A hydroxylase and accumulation of phytanic acid in the body. This disease is unique among the lipidoses because phytanic acid is not synthesized in the body but is obtained exclusively from the diet. Limiting phytanic acid or its precursor, phytol (dairy products, ruminant fat, and chlorophyl-containing foods), from the diet reduces plasma phytanic acid levels. Plasmapheresis may further help eliminate phytanic acid from the body in severe cases. Symptoms typically begin in childhood but in some patients may be delayed until the fifth decade. Night blindness typically appears first, followed by limb weakness and gait abnormalities. Some patients may develop psychiatric symptoms, peripheral neuropathy, pigmentary retinopathy, deafness, cataracts, bone deformities, or cardiac arrhythmias (Merritt, pp. 514–529, 539–540).

14-C; 15-C; 16-A. The symptoms of acute intermittent porphyria (AIP) are most commonly gastrointestinal, psychiatric, and neurologic. The precise etiology remains uncertain, but large and small nerve fibers, as well as autonomic nerves, have been shown to be affected. Abdominal pain is the most common finding, but often occurs concomitantly with a psychiatric or neurologic disorder. There is usually no abdominal rigidity, but fever, leukocytosis, diarrhea, tachycardia, and hypertension are often evident. Appendicitis or other serious abdominal problems may be difficult to rule out; in fact, some patients have been subjected to laparotomy for abdominal exploration. The most reliable test to confirm AIP is the assay for porphobilinogen deaminase activity in red blood cells, but often a good clinical history and examination can give clues to the diagnosis. The autonomic manifestations, abdominal pain, and anxiety may be reversed with propranolol. Hematin has also been shown to reverse the neuropathy and abdominal pain by suppressing aminolevulinic acid dehydratase levels. This patient's history and multiple clinical findings are not consistent with volume depletion, conversion disorder, appendicitis, or hysteria. Barbiturates, sulfonamides, gabapentin, and hormone replacement therapy may cause or exacerbate AIP (Merritt, pp. 549–551).

17. B. Diphtheria infection produces neuropathy in about 20% of infected patients. *Corynebacterium diphtheriae* is often isolated from the throat and releases an exotoxin (not endotoxin) that can cause myocarditis or symmetric neuropathy. The neuropathy is often characterized by poor visual accommodation, paresis of throat muscles, quadriparesis, and slow nerve conduction velocities secondary to demyelinating neuropathy. This disease can be prevented by immunization and often responds to antibiotics (Merritt, pp. 620–621).

18. A. Although Wernicke's and Korsakoff's syndromes are often described together, these appear to be two distinct entities that result from thiamine deficiency. Wernicke's syndrome consists of mental symptoms (global confusional state), eye movement problems (nystagmus, lateral rectus palsy, and lateral gaze palsy), and gait ataxia, while Korsakoff's syndrome is a purely amnestic syndrome usually associated with lesions in the DM nucleus of the thalamus and mammillary bodies. With treatment (thiamine), ocular abnormalities, nystagmus, and global confusion often improve to varying degrees, leaving Korsakoff's amnesia in about 80% of patients. (Merritt, pp. 924–925).

19. A. Lyme disease is caused by the tick-borne spirochete *Borrelia burgdorferi*. The most common clinical feature is painful sensory radiculitis, which often appears about 3 weeks after the erythema migrans. Other problems include cranial neuropathy (61%), limb weakness (12%), oculomotor paresis, arthralgias, and cardiomyopathy. Peripheral nerve biopsy shows perineurial and epineurial vasculitis and axonal degeneration. The prognosis is good after high-dose antibiotic treatment (usually penicillin) (Merritt, p. 625).

20. E. MELAS, MERFF, LHON, and KSS are a group of disorders related to mitochondrial (mt) DNA abnormalities. Although specific syndromes are often identified by a variety of signs/symptoms, several clinical manifestations seem to be prevalent with mtDNA abnormalities and include short stature, hearing loss, and diabetes mellitus. Lactic acidosis is the most common laboratory finding, while pathologic sectioning reveals enlarged mitochondria in muscle fibers, which forms the basis for ragged red fibers (RRF). Leigh's disease is a disorder of mitochondrial metabolism in which the primary defect involves proteins encoded by nuclear DNA instead of mitochondrial DNA (Ellison, pp. 457–465).

21-B; 22-B; 23-E. Wild, involuntary flinging of an extremity may be secondary to a cerebrovascular accident affecting the subthalamic nucleus and is commonly referred to as hemiballismus. Normally, glutamatergic projections from the subthalamic nucleus to the Gpi and SNr suppress the motor nuclei of the thalamus. After damage to the subthalamic nucleus, the thalamic motor neurons are disinhibited and provide excessive activation of the motor cortex. The dopaminergic projections, however, remain intact, providing a constant and unbalanced activation of motor neurons throughout the basal ganglia. This is the basis for using neuroleptic agents, including dopamine receptor blockers (haloperidol and perphenazine) and presynaptic dopamine depletors (reserpine and tetrabenazine) to treat this disease process (Tarsy, p. 9; Pritchard, pp. 330–331).

24. A. HD is an autosomal dominant condition with complete penetrance that varies in symptom onset from juveniles to late adulthood, with average age onset between 35 and 40 years of age. Sporadic cases of HD are rare. HD, a trinucleotide repeat (CAG) disorder that localizes to chromosome 4, is more common in males than females and exhibits anticipation (earlier onset in successive generations). The abnormal gene product results in protein conformational changes that lead to aggregation in the cytosol and eventually cellular apoptosis. HD primarily affects the GABA/enkephalin projections from the striatum to the external segment of the globus pallidus (indirect pathway), resulting in thalamic facilitation of motor cortical areas and hyperkinesia. Haloperidol may be effective in suppressing abnormal movements early in the disease course, but the disease is inevitably progressive and usually results in death within 20 years from symptom onset (Merritt, pp. 659–664, 696–699).

25-G; 26-E; 27-F; 28-A; 29-C; 30-B; 31-B; 32-D. *Craniosynostosis* refers to the premature closure of cranial sutures. It is more common in males than females, and sagittal synostosis accounts for 50% of all cases of craniosynostosis. Sagittal synostosis is identified in a child with an oblong-shaped skull (scaphocephaly or dolichocephaly), which results in an increased AP skull diameter and a narrowed biparietal diameter. There is usually a palpable "keel" along the course of the sagittal suture. *Trigonocephaly* refers to premature closure of the metopic suture, and results in a wedge-shaped head. Unilateral suture closure (coronal or lambdoid) often results in a misshapen and unilaterally flattened head (plagiocephaly), while premature bilateral coronal or lambdoid suture closure often results in a broad biparietal skull diameter or brachycephaly. Other forms of craniosynostosis can result from premature closure of all the sutures, which can result in a tower-shaped skull (oxycephaly) or a grossly abnormal-appearing skull with a cloverleaf shape (Kleeblattschädel). Lacunar skull can be seen in patients with Chiari II malformation, and does not result from premature closure of the cranial sutures. The indications for surgery with craniosynostosis are usually for intracranial hypertension (VP shunt) and cosmetic deformity (Wilkins, pp. 3673–3679; Merritt, pp. 491–492).

33. D. Progressive multifocal leukoencephalopathy (PML) is a subacute demyelinating disease that results from reactivation of a papovavirus (JC virus) in immunocompromised patients. The reactivated JC virus infects oligodendrocytes, and results in multifocal areas of demyelination predominantly in the subcortical white matter. PML affects 4% of AIDS patients and has been associated with other illnesses characterized by defective cell-mediated immunity, such as lymphomas and leukemias. The lesions of PML are often parieto-occipital, nonenhancing, and exhibit increased signal on T2 and FLAIR MRI with no mass effect. Symptoms of PML depend on the location of lesions and include hemiparesis, visual field cuts, sensory changes, and eventually dementia. The diagnosis of PML is established by biopsy or PCR amplification of JC virus RNA in the CSF. The prognosis of PML is poor, and approximately 80% of patients die within 9 months of symptom onset. Choices A, B, and C are associated with subacute sclerosing panencephalitis (A) and acute disseminated encephalomyelitis (B and C) (Merritt, pp. 151–156).

34. B. Central pontine myelinolysis (CPM) is an acute demyelinating condition that primarily affects the pons, although 10% of cases have concomitant extrapontine myelinolysis. CPM most commonly occurs in alcoholic or malnourished patients who experience rapid correction of chronic hyponatremia. Neurologic symptoms usually occur 2 to 3 days after correction of the hyponatremia and vary extensively. Symptoms include seizures, dysarthria, dysphagia, pseudobulbar palsy, behavioral abnormalities, hyperreflexia, quadriplegia, and coma. Patients may also be completely asymptomatic with CPM. In symptomatic patients, the course is usually rapid and progresses to death within days to weeks of symptom onset. The incidence of CPM is extremely low if the serum sodium is corrected by no more than 12 mmol/L in 24 hours. MRI, brainstem auditory evoked potentials, and CSF studies (increased MBP and protein levels) can all assist in the diagnosis of CPM. Acute disseminated leukoencephalomyelitis, Krabbe's disease, Alexander's disease, and Marchiafava-Bignami disease do not result from rapid correction of hyponatremia (Merritt, pp. 794–796).

35-C; 36-A; 37-B. Glycogen storage diseases are primarily autosomal recessive disorders that result from deficiencies of the enzymes involved with the metabolism of glucose and glycogen. There are more than 12 different types of glycogenoses; they affect different tissues depending on the expression of the defective enzyme. Type I glycogenosis (Von Gierke's disease) is characterized by deficiencies of glucose-6-phosphatase and primarily affects the liver. Patients with Von Gierke's disease present with hepatomegaly and experience severe episodes of hypoglycemia. Type II glycogenosis (Pompe's disease) results from deficiencies of the enzyme acid maltase α–glucosidase and has three different forms. The infantile type of Pompe's disease results in hypotonia, macroglossia, hepatomegaly, cardiomegaly, and death by 2 years of age secondary to cardiac failure. The juvenile and adulthood variants of Pompe's disease are less severe and present with myopathy. Type III glycogenosis (debranching enzyme deficiency or Cori's disease) is rare and results in hepatomegaly, seizures, and growth retardation in children secondary to deficiencies of the debranching enzyme amylo-1,6-glucosidase. Type V glycogenosis (McArdle's disease) is a more benign condition that results in muscle cramps and occasionally myoglobinuria during intense exercise due to deficiencies of the enzyme myophosphorylase. Type VII glycogenosis (Tauri's disease) presents with myalgias, cramps, and early fatigue with exercise (similar to McArdle's disease) in children and is secondary to

deficiencies of the enzyme phosphofructokinase. All of the glycogenoses are autosomal recessive with the exception of type IX and a form of type VIII, which are X-linked recessive (Merritt, pp. 530–531).

38. E. Friedreich's ataxia (FA) is an autosomal recessive trinucleotide repeat (GAA) disorder that involves repeat expansion in the frataxin gene, which encodes a mitochondrial protein and is located on chromosome 9q. The onset of symptoms with FA usually occurs by the age of 10 to 15 years; it is usually fatal by the fifth to sixth decades of life. FA results in degeneration of the posterior columns, spinocerebellar tracts, corticospinal tracts, and Clarke's nucleus in the spinal cord. The medulla (vestibular, cochlear, gracile, and accessory cuneate nuclei), subthalamic nucleus, and pallidum also exhibit evidence of gliosis. Symptoms of FA include ataxic gait, dysarthria, areflexia, lower limb weakness, and loss of vibratory sense and proprioception. Some patients with FA also develop cardiomyopathy, which can lead to cerebellar and cerebral cortical ischemic changes. FA is associated with the development of peripheral neuropathy as well, with concomitant degeneration of the dorsal root ganglia. Orthopedic deformities, such as hammertoes, kyphoscoliosis, and pes cavus are also common. There is no effective treatment for FA (Merritt, pp. 645–646).

39. C. Lesch-Nyhan syndrome (LNS) is an X-linked recessive disorder of purine metabolism that results from deficiencies of the enzyme hypoxanthine-guanine phosphoribosyltransferase (HPRT). Levels of uric acid are increased in LNS secondary to increased purine metabolism, and urate deposition can result in severe nephropathy and gout. Patients with LNS exhibit mental retardation, choreoathetosis, spasticity, self-mutilating behavior, and usually die from renal failure in the second or third decade. Glucose transporter protein syndrome (GTPS) results from deficiencies of the glucose transporter-1 protein (GLUT-1), which is responsible for the facilitative transport of glucose across the blood-brain barrier. Patients with GTPS exhibit decreased CSF glucose levels (hypoglycorrhachia), seizures, developmental delay, microcephaly, ataxia, and hypotonia. Phenylketonuria is an autosomal recessive disorder resulting from phenylalanine hydroxylase deficiency, and cystathionine β-synthase deficiency results in homocystinuria (Merritt, pp. 512–513).

40-D; 41-B; 42-C; 43-E; 44-A; 45-D; 46-C; 47-C. Patients with infarcts or trauma involving the corticospinal tracts on one side often develop a *hemiplegic gait* characterized by a stiff leg that does not freely flex at the hip, knee, or ankle. With movement, the involved leg tends to rotate outward in a semicircle (circumduction), and the toe and outer side of the sole often become worn (less commonly also seen with steppage gait). The arm on the affected side is also usually weak, and is often carried in a flexed position free of any natural movement. *Festinating gait* is a term used to describe the involuntary acceleration or hastening that often accompanies Parkinson's patients. Steppage or equine gait is caused by severe weakness or paralysis of the pretibial or peroneal muscles, with difficulty dorsiflexing and everting the foot. The steps are regular and even, but the advancing foot often hangs with the toes pointing down (footdrop). Walking is accomplished by abnormally high elevation of the involved leg in order for the foot to clear the ground, often producing a characteristic slap as the foot strikes the floor. *Waddling gait* is characteristic of chronic or progressive muscular dystrophy (Wohlfart-Kugelberg-Welander disease) and congenital hip dislocation. *Reeling gait* is a term used to describe the gait of a severely intoxicated patient, which sways in many directions with no attempt to correct the staggering by watching the legs or trunk (as in cerebellar or sensory ataxia). *Toppling gait* may be seen in patients with brainstem lesions, especially in the elderly with a recent stroke, where sudden lurches forward and frequent falls are a prominent feature. It has also been described as a feature of the lateral medullary syndrome (Wallenberg's) and in certain patients with progressive supranuclear palsy and advanced Parkinson's disease. *Scissoring gait* may result from lesions involving the thoracic spine, where abnormal gait may result from the combined effects of weakness and spasticity. The legs are usually maintained in an extended or slightly flexed position at the hips, and knees are often adducted at the hips. With severe spasticity, the legs may cross in front of each other during ambulation, causing a scissoring gait (Merritt, pp. 46–49; Adams, pp. 94–99).

48-D; 49-A; 50-A; 51-A. The lupus inhibitor can be found in up to one-third of systemic lupus erythematosus (SLE) patients. In SLE patients, the associated thrombosis risk can be as high as 10 to 15%, while the risk is less in patients without SLE but still in excess of normal. This disease process is associated with deep venous thrombosis of the legs, ischemic strokes in the brain, and miscarriages (placental dysfunction). Abnormal bleeding does not typically occur, although laboratory findings include prolonged PT and PTT that does not reverse when the patient's plasma is mixed with normal plasma. Diagnosis can be confirmed by the thromboplastin inhibition test (TTI) and antiphospholipid antibody assays. Treatment to prevent thrombosis may include corticosteroids, antiplatelet drugs, and anticoagulation; plasmapheresis is not typically used. Anticoagulation appears to be the best therapy, with a goal of keeping the INR at least 3.0. Atrial fibrillation and atrial-septal defects are common causes of stroke in certain patient populations, but there is no reason to suspect a rhythm or congenital heart problem in this patient. Multiple sclerosis and metastatic brain tumors are not typically associated with deep venous thrombosis unless the patient is immobilized for a prolonged time (Merritt, p. 245).

52-C; 53-C; 54-D. Alzheimer's disease (AD) is a rare cause of new-onset auditory hallucinations in elderly patients. Typically, other forms of cognitive impairment are present, but hallucinations may occasionally precede other manifestations of this disease process. Low doses of haloperidol are often effective in treating the hallucinations, while medications such as tacrine and donepezil may slow the cognitive decline modestly early in the disease course. Several structures in the brain are affected in AD, including the hippocampus (especially CA1), mesial temporal lobe, frontotemporoparietal association areas, and the nucleus basalis of Meynert (n.b.M). The degeneration of cells in the n.b.M (and other basal forebrain nuclei) results in decreased cortical cholinergic input and is associated with decreased levels of ACh and choline acetyltransferase in the hippocampus and neocortex. Patients with AD also exhibit decreased CNS levels of serotonin, norepinephrine, glutamate, and substance P. Ventriculomegaly accompanies the diffuse cerebral neocortical atrophy. Several genes are involved in the pathogenesis of AD including amyloid precursor protein (chromosome 21), presenilin 1 (chromosome 14), and presenilin 2 (chromosome 1). The $\varepsilon 4$ allele of apolipoprotein E (chromosome 19) is associated with an increased risk of developing AD and is associated with 25 to 40% of all cases of AD. In any patient with suspected AD, treatable causes of dementia must be ruled out initially with a good history, physical examination, laboratory data, and imaging studies. Patients with AD are most often diagnosed with a detailed history and physical examination (Merritt, pp. 633–637).

55. D. Writer's cramp is a focal dystonia of unknown etiology. Patients develop sustained muscle contractions that yield abnormal postures or twisting movements when attempting to write. It differs from athetosis by the persistent nature of the abnormal posture or movement. It can be focal (writer's cramp), segmental (e.g., face), or rarely multifocal (e.g., face and leg). Dystonia can also be either primary (inherited) or secondary (stroke, toxin, medication, etc.). The medical treatment is variable, often empiric, and can include local botulinum toxin injections, anticholinergics, benzodiazepines, anticonvulsants, lithium, reserpine, baclofen, and levodopa. Micrographia can be seen with Parkinson's disease but is often accompanied by signs of rigidity, tremor, and bradykinesia. Carpal tunnel syndrome is due to pressure on the median nerve and is associated with numbness, weakness, and pain. A cervical radiculopathy rarely if ever presents with the findings seen in this patient; instead, there is pain, weakness, numbness, and reflex changes in the distribution of the affected nerve (Merritt, pp. 669–677).

56-A; 57-E; 58-B; 59-F; 60-C; 61-F; 62-G; 63-B. Refer to Table 3.56–3.63A (Merritt, pp. 767, 894–895; Rolak, pp. 237–239).

TABLE 3.56–63A   Antibodies and associated disorders

ANTIBODY	CLINICAL SYNDROME	ASSOCIATED DISORDER
Anti-Hu antibody	Encephalomyelitis, sensory neuropathy	Small cell lung cancer
Anti-Ri antibody	Opsoclonus-myoclonus, retinal degeneration	Breast and small cell lung cancer in adults, neuroblastoma in children
Anti-Ta antibody	Limbic and brainstem encephalitis	Brain and testicular tumors
Anti-Tr antibody	Subacute cerebellar disorder with dysarthria, nystagmus (reacts against Purkinje cells)	Hodgkin's disease
Anti-VGCC antibody	Neuromuscular disorder	Lambert-Eaton syndrome
Anti-Ta antibody	Limbic and brainstem encephalitis	Testicular cancer
Anti-Yo syndrome	Cerebellar disorder, brainstem encephalitis	Ovarian, uterine, and breast cancer

TABLE 3.64A   Common epilepsy syndromes and associated clinical and diagnostic findings

SYNDROME	CLINICAL FINDING	EEG ABNORMALITY	MEDICAL TREATMENT
Infantile spasms (West syndrome)	Sudden flexor or extensor spasms of head, trunk, limbs	Hypsarrhythmia	Corticotropin, prednisone, vigabatrin
Juvenile myoclonic epilepsy	Myoclonic jerks usually in the morning; normal intelligence	4- to 6-Hz spike waves and polyspike discharges	Valproate
Petit mal (absence)	Frequent blank staring spells	3-Hz spike-wave discharges	Ethosuximide, valproate
Lennox-Gastaut	Mental retardation, uncontrolled seizures (80% with continued seizures despite therapy)		Valproate, lamotrigine, topiramate
Benign focal epilepsy of childhood	Generalized seizures at night; focal seizures during day; otherwise normal	Di- or triphasic sharp waves over rolandic regions	Appear to be self-limited, but carbamazepine, gabapentin often used
Temporal lobe epilepsy	Most common in adults; involves mesial temporal structures; associated with auras (lip smacking, automatisms)	Focal temporal slowing or epileptiform sharp waves or spikes in anterior temporal lobe region	About 50% have continued attacks despite medication; anterior temporal lobe resection up to 80% effective

64. C. Refer to Table 3.64A (Merritt, pp. 813–836).

65. C. The F wave and H reflex evaluate certain aspects of nerve conduction. Whereas sensory nerve action potentials (SNAP) and compound muscle action potentials (CMAP) are best at evaluating distal nerves, the F wave and H reflex are the two most commonly used methods in evaluating the proximal portions of nerves. The F wave (F response) measures the entire length of the nerve, including the ventral root. It results from supramaximal stimulus of distal motor nerves with impulse propagation in an antidromic direction. The stimulus travels proximally up the motor nerve and stimulates the anterior horn motor neurons. The variable back-firing of nonrefractory anterior horn cells then results in impulse propagation back down the ventral root and motor nerve to the distal electrode. F-wave latencies are most sensitive for disorders causing generalized or multifocal demyelination (GBS or extensive plexopathies). This is because any focal conduction slowing is diluted by the normal conduction velocity over most of the F-wave pathway. The H reflex is the electrical equivalent of the stretch reflex and is obtained with submaximal stimulation of the median and tibial nerves. The H reflex therefore involves an afferent (sensory) limb and an efferent (motor) limb, similar to monosynaptic reflex arcs. The H reflex exhibits increased latency in proximal neuropathies and radiculopathies (i.e., C6, C7, or S1 root lesions). Increased H-reflex latencies in conjunction with normal F-wave latencies localize lesions to the dorsal roots (Adams, pp. 1022–1025; Merritt, pp. 73–76).

66. D. Nerve conduction studies (NCSs) vary in conditions that result in either demyelination or axonal degeneration. Conduction velocity, amplitude of evoked response, latency (latency from the stimulus to recording electrodes), and duration of response all provide information about the integrity of motor and sensory nerves. NCSs of the sensory nerves generate a sensory nerve action potential (SNAP), while NCSs of motor nerves generate a compound muscle action potential (CMAP). Refer to Table 3.66A for summary of electrophysiologic findings with axonal degeneration and demyelinating neuropathies (Merritt, pp. 73–75; Geyer, pp. 226–227; Youmans, pp. 3851–3855).

TABLE 3.66A Electrophysiologic findings with axonal degeneration and demyelination

CHARACTERISTIC	AXONAL DEGENERATION	DEMYELINATION
Motor nerve conduction		
Amplitude	Decreased	Normal/decreased/block
Duration	Normal	Dispersion
Shape	Normal	Normal or multiphasic
Distal latency	Normal or increased	Increased
Velocity	Normal or decreased	Decreased
Sensory nerve conduction		
Amplitude	Decreased or absent	Normal/decreased/absent
Duration	Normal	Increased
Shape	Normal	Sometimes multiphasic
Velocity	Normal or decreased	Decreased
F wave	Increased	Increased
H reflex	Increased	Increased

67. D. Normal muscle potentials appear as waveforms with a duration of 5 to 15 ms, 2 to 4 phases, and an amplitude of 0.5 to 3 mV. Fibrillation potentials are abnormal, involuntary contractions of single muscle fibers that cannot be seen through the skin. They indicate reinnervation of muscle fibers from a variety of causes. Positive sharp waves are similar to fibrillation potentials and appear on EMG as a downward wave after needle insertion, which is indicative of needle irritation of denervated muscle fibers. Insertional activity is the discharge of a single muscle fiber during insertion of the EMG needle and does not necessarily indicate abnormality unless significantly increased activity is seen. Increased insertional activity can also indicate irritable muscle fibers from denervation. Polyphasic units (greater than four phases) are abnormal, and can be seen in both neurogenic and myogenic disorders. In summary, with neurogenic disorders, motor units appear of longer duration and higher amplitude than normal potentials and are usually polypha-

sic. Myopathic potentials are just the opposite, with shorter durations and smaller amplitudes than normal potentials and are also usually polyphasic. Fibrillations, positive sharp waves, and increased insertional activity can be seen with denervated muscle (Merritt, pp. 75–76; Youmans, pp. 3856–3857).

68-B, C; 69-D; 70-A; 71-E; 72-C, D; 73-E. Refer to Table 3.68–3.73A (Merritt, p. 64).

74. B. Triphasic waves are a type of generalized, pseudoperiodic pattern consisting of sharp discharges occurring at typical frequencies of 1 to 2 per second. This is a nonspecific pattern and has to be distinguished from other generalized periodic patterns (CJD, status epilepticus, and hypoxic-ischemic injury). Approximately 50% of patients with triphasic waves have hepatic encephalopathy; the other half have other toxic-metabolic encephalopathies, including

TABLE 3.68–73A Stage of sleep, characteristic EEG findings, and common sleep abnormalities

STAGE OF SLEEP	EEG FINDINGS	ASSOCIATED FINDINGS
Stage 1	Transition from waking to resting state; α-rhythm is replaced by slow, low-voltage activity (2–7 Hz); occipital sharp waves measured at the vertex prominent during this stage, less prominent during stages 2 and 3	
Stage 2	Represents light sleep and consists of sleep spindles (symmetric 12–14 Hz sinusoidal waves) and K complexes (brief high voltage discharges)	
Stage 3	Sleep spindles, K complexes, < 50% delta activity	Somnambulism, night terrors, enuresis
Stage 4	Deep sleep; > 50% delta waves (1–4 Hz)	Somnambulism, night terrors, enuresis
REM	Rapid eye movement (REM) occurs at various intervals throughout night; low-voltage, desynchronized activity; absence of muscle tone; see increases in cerebral blood flow, ICP, and respiratory rate; variable blood pressure and heart rate	Dreaming, obstructive sleep apnea, decline in body temperature, erections, increased during daytime in patients with alcoholism, sleep deprivation, narcolepsy. Accounts for high percentage of sleep in infants

renal failure. Creutzfeldt-Jakob disease is characterized by generalized periodic sharp waves, an acute destructive cerebral lesion (stroke) often results in periodic lateralizing epileptiform discharges (PLEDs) on EEG, and brain death is marked by no activity on EEG (Merritt, pp. 64–65).

75. B. Narcolepsy is a sleep disorder characterized by excessive daytime sleepiness, sleep paralysis, cataplexy, and hypnagogic hallucinations. Narcolepsy affects males and females equally, is associated with the DR2 allele, and usually presents between the ages of 15 and 30 years. Patients with narcolepsy experience increased daytime sleepiness and irresistible sleep attacks during the day that last between 5 and 30 minutes. Patients with narcolepsy sleep more frequently than normal people, but the amount of total sleep is the same in narcoleptics and healthy adults. Narcoleptics also display attacks of cataplexy, which is the abrupt loss of muscle tone and is often precipitated by emotion. Cataplexy reflects REM sleep paralysis during periods of normal wakefulness. REM periods occur early in the sleep cycles of patients with narcolepsy (sleep-onset REM), and this is diagnostic of the condition. Narcoleptics may experience paralysis of voluntary muscles (sleep paralysis) during the initial and terminal periods of the sleep cycle, often with sparing of the extraocular muscles. Hypnagogic hallucinations occur at the beginning of the sleep cycle in narcoleptics; these hallucinations can be auditory or visual. Abnormalities in the hypothalamic projecting system are common in narcolepsy, and patients with this condition exhibit decreased levels of orexin. The treatment of narcolepsy involves adrenergic stimulants, such as methylphenidate (Ritalin), pemoline, and amphetamines. Cataplexy can often be effectively controlled with antidepressants (tricyclics and SSRIs), which suppress REM sleep (Merritt, pp. 843–844).

76-C; 77-E; 78-A. The absence seizure is characterized by a generalized, symmetric, and synchronous 3-Hz spike-slow-wave discharge. This is diagnostic of an absence seizure and is best treated with medications such as ethosuximide (Zarontin) or sodium valproate (Depakote). The common activating procedures usually performed on patients with suspected seizures are hyperventilation, photic stimulation, and sleep. As soon as 3-Hz spike-and-wave bursts stop and the seizure ceases, the EEG returns to its interictal state immediately with no postictal depression or slowing (Merritt, p. 66; Rolak, pp. 365–366).

79-E; 80-A; 81-F; 82-C; 83-B; 84-G; 85-D. Brainstem auditory evoked potentials (BAEPs) are elicited with specific auditory stimuli and result from several important components of the auditory pathway. There are generally seven peaks in the BAEP, which result from the auditory nerve (wave I), cochlear nuclei (wave II), superior olive or trapezoid body (wave III), lateral lemniscus (wave IV), inferior colliculus (wave V), medial geniculate body (wave VI), and auditory

radiations (wave VII). BAEPs are usually preserved with metabolic abnormalities and exhibit prolonged latencies with structural lesions of the brainstem or auditory nerves. BAEPs are abnormal in 90% of patients with acoustic neuromas and usually consist of delayed conduction from CN VIII to the lower pons (prolongation of waves I to III). BAEPs are also abnormal in 33% of multiple sclerosis patients and usually involve increased interpeak latency of waves III to V (Merritt, pp. 68–69).

86. B. A breach rhythm is a rhythmic sharp wave pattern that appears in the region of a skull defect. The skull acts as a "low-pass filter" and screens out high frequencies generated by the cortex. The skull defect allows these higher frequencies to appear. This is the EEG of a man with a history of head trauma and a surgical scar noted within the right frontocentral region (F4, C4) (Rolak, pp. 359–360).

87-D; 88-B; 89-E. There are three major muscle groups that need to be coordinated during micturition: the detrusor muscle, the internal sphincter, and external sphincter. Motor control of the bladder results primarily from parasympathetic function. The detrusor muscle and internal sphincter are heavily influenced by parasympathetic (PNS) fibers with their cell bodies located within the S2, S3, and S4 segments of the spinal cord. Increased PNS activity results in contraction of the detrusor muscle of the bladder and reflex inhibition of the internal sphincter, which aids bladder emptying. The external sphincter, although under voluntary control (pudendal nerve), relaxes in a reflex-type manner after internal sphincter opening and allows for micturition to occur in a synchronous fashion. The sympathetic supply to the bladder originates in cells of the intermediolateral gray column of the upper lumbar cord and passes through spinal nerves to reach the inferior mesenteric ganglia. From there, they travel as postganglionic fibers to the wall of the bladder and internal sphincter. They heavily innervate the bladder neck and trigone (α-adrenergic) and cause bladder neck closure, which aids bladder filling. The primary coordinating center for bladder function is the pontine micturition center, which synchronizes bladder contraction with sphincter relaxation. This center is inhibited by higher cortical levels in adults but not in children. This forms the basis for the uninhibited bladder in children, which contracts when it reaches a critical capacity. This is also seen in adults after severe head injury or the presence of tumors, hydrocephalus, stroke, or other cerebral insults.

Injury to the spinal cord above the sacral voiding center (S2-4) often produces detrusor hyperreflexia (involuntary bladder contractions and smooth sphincter synergy) secondary to preservation of the voiding center (S2-4) and striated or external sphincter dyssynergy due to loss of coordinated sphincter function from the pontine micturition center. Injury below S2 from a cauda equina, conus medullaris, or peripheral nerve lesion produces detrusor areflexia or an atonic bladder, which is characterized by a lack of voluntary bladder contractions and possibly overflow incontinence.

Propantheline, oxybutynin, tolterodine, and flavoxate all have anticholinergic activity and effectively increase the volume at which automatic or reflex contraction occurs in the uninhibited bladder (detrusor hyperreflexia). Bethanechol is a parasympathomimetic agent (primarily muscarinic), which increases detrusor tone and effectively increases bladder emptying. It is often used for patients with detrusor areflexia. α-adrenergic agonists increase bladder filling by contracting the bladder neck, while α-adrenergic antagonists do the opposite. Tamsulosin (Flomax), terazosin (Hytrin), and doxazosin (Cardura) are α-adrenoreceptor antagonists, which have been used in patients with urinary retention (detrusor areflexia) (Greenberg, pp. 112–117; Youmans, pp. 357–383).

90. E. Somatosensory evoked potentials (SSEPs) result from stimulation of peripheral nerves (median and posterior tibial) and are generated by components of the dorsal column sensory pathways. The components of the SSEP tracing of the median nerve include Erb's point (brachial plexus), N13 (central gray of cervical spinal cord), P14 (caudal medial lemniscus), N18 (rostral brainstem), and N20 (primary sensory cortex), but not Brodmann's areas 5 and 7, which are located posterior to the primary sensory cortex. SSEPs are affected by many different pathological conditions that influence the somatosensory system, including strokes, syringomyelia, spondylosis, subacute combined deficiency, and multiple sclerosis. SSEPs are frequently utilized intraoperatively during neurosurgical procedures to monitor the integrity of the spinal cord. Some anesthetics that suppress SSEPs include benzodiazepines, halothane, and thiopental sodium (Pentothal) (Merritt, p. 70).

91. A. The safety and efficacy of thrombolytic therapy has been extensively studied in acute stroke. Data obtained from the National Institute of Neurologic Disorders and Stroke (NINDS) trial showed that administering t-PA within 3 hours of symptom onset resulted in improved functional outcome at 3 months and 1 year. The benefit was seen across all stroke types and was not affected by age, sex, or ethnicity. Although symptomatic intracerebral hemorrhage was higher in the t-PA group, there was no difference in mortality at 3 months. Other trials have assessed the safety of other thrombolytic agents with or without the addition of neuroprotective agents with mixed results. Data from the ATLANTIS trial have provided further information concerning the efficacy and safety of administering t-PA beyond the 3-hour window established by the NINDS trial. Although the drug was not shown to be effective beyond the 3-hour window, the safety profile was similar to that of the NINDS trial. This information provides physicians with some flexibility in administering t-PA beyond the 3-hour window, although

most still advocate its administration in a time frame similar to that established by NINDS (Youmans, pp. 1595–1502).

92. D. Since other factors can influence velocities, including blood pressure and overall cerebral blood flow, distinguishing vasospastic from hyperemic increases in MCA blood flow velocities by transcranial Doppler is best achieved by measuring the cervical carotid artery velocities in addition to the intracranial blood velocities. A "Lindegaard ratio" of V_{MCA}/V_{ICA} greater than 3 is consistent with vasospasm, as hyperemia is associated with increased velocities in both the MCA and ICA, so that the ratio remains the same. Repeating the Doppler study within 1 hour to confirm the reading, administering a vasodilating agent in conjunction with the Doppler study to evaluate the percentage change in flow and plotting the velocity versus vessel diameter on a logarithmic scale will not differentiate between hyperemia and vasospasm (Youmans, pp. 1850–1851).

93-A; 94-B; 95-C; 96-B; 97-D; 98-F; 99-D. Cheyne-Stokes respiration consists of briefs periods of hyperpnea alternating with even shorter periods of apnea and often results from large supratentorial lesions affecting either the cerebral hemispheres or diencephalon. The respiratory drive with this respiratory pattern is highly dependent on the pCO_2 and accumulation causes hyperpnea, which in turn induces a drop in the pCO_2 With this drop in pCO_2, the respiratory stimulus ceases, and a period of apnea ensues. Central neurogenic hyperventilation most often results from pontine lesions in which patients have prolonged and rapid breathing. This breathing pattern can also result from midbrain/high pontine lesions. It may be responsive to morphine or methadone. Apneustic breathing is characterized by a long inspiratory pause, after which the air is retained for several seconds before it is released. It appears to result from lesions of the lateral tegmentum of the pons. Cluster breathing is characterized by a series of breaths following each other in an irregular sequence, which can result from low pontine or high medullary lesions. Ataxic breathing (Biot breathing) has a completely irregular pattern in which breaths with diverse amplitude and length are mixed with periods of apnea, which often follows damage to the dorsomedial medulla. Loss of automatic breathing with preserved voluntary breathing ("Ondine's curse") can also occur with medullary lesions, although they tend to occur in a somewhat lower location than those causing ataxic breathing. Ondine's curse has also been noted to occur after lesions involving the ventrolateral high cervical spinal cord, a location transmitting fibers from the primary medullary respiratory centers. Stertorous breathing is a sign of airway obstruction (Brazis, pp. 568–571; Greenberg, p. 121; Merritt, p. 18).

100. D. The tracts that were most likely affected in this patient run along a paramedian plane in the medulla. In ventrodorsal order they consist of the pyramidal tract, medial lemniscus,

TABLE 3.101–107A   Aphasias and associated clinical findings

APHASIA	COMPREHENSION	FLUENCY	NAMING	REPETITION
Broca's	+	–	–	–
Wernicke's	–	+	–	–
Conduction	+	+	+/–	–
Transcortical motor	+	–	–	+
Transcortical sensory	–	+	–	+
Mixed transcortical	–	–	–	+
Global	–	–	–	–

medial longitudinal fasciculus, and hypoglossal nucleus. This region receives blood from the paramedian branches of the vertebrobasilar system and anterior spinal artery. The face was spared because corticobulbar fibers to the facial nucleus typically depart before reaching the medulla. Pain and temperature were spared because the lateral spinothalamic tracts run in the lateral parts of the medulla, which is supplied by the circumferential arteries. This patient is suffering from medial medullary syndrome (Dejerine's anterior bulbar syndrome) (Carpenter pp. 115–150; Brazis, pp. 345–346).

101-F; 102-C; 103-D; 104-G; 105-A; 106-E; 107-B. Refer to Table 3.101–3.107A. (Merritt, pp. 7–11).

108. C. It is extremely difficult to differentiate between bilateral INO and bilateral medial rectus subnucleus damage unless there is an absence of convergence (as seen with medial rectus subnucleus damage). (Kline, pp. 63–66; Merritt, pp. 215–217).

109. C. *Oculomasticatory myorhythmia* refers to acquired pendular vergence oscillations of the eyes associated with concurrent contraction of the masticatory muscles, which may persist during sleep. This distinct disorder has been recognized only in Whipple's disease (Brazis, p. 231).

110. A. Two main differences that differentiate peripheral from central nystagmus include the effects of fixation on nystagmus as well as the direction of nystagmus. Fixation of the eyes suppresses peripheral but not central nystagmus. Also, peripheral nystagmus, particularly when vertical, usually has a torsional component. Pure vertical and torsional nystagmus are central (Brazis, pp. 223–224).

111. E. Amantadine is an indirect dopaminergic agent that augments dopamine release from storage sites and possibly blocks dopamine reuptake into presynaptic terminals (Merritt, p. 688).

112-F; 113-B; 114-E; 115-A; 116-E; 117-F. The globe of the eye is moved by the action of the superior and inferior oblique muscles as well as the lateral, medial, superior, and inferior recti. The superior rectus muscle elevates the eye when it is

abducted (23 degrees), while the inferior rectus muscle depresses the eye when the globe is abducted (23 degrees). By contrast, when the eye is adducted, the superior rectus muscle intorts the eye (moves it counterclockwise in the case of the left eye), while the inferior rectus muscle extorts the eye (moves the left eye clockwise). The oblique muscles have a similar and complementary action in moving the eyes in a vertical plane. They move the eyeball in a vertical plane when the eye is adducted (51 degrees) and act as rotators (intort, extort) when it is abducted (39 degrees). Unlike the rectus muscles, however, they function as would be expected from their insertional points on the globe. The superior oblique muscle depresses the adducted eye or twists it inwardly when the eye is abducted (counterclockwise in the case of the left eye), and the inferior oblique muscle elevates the adducted eye or extorts it when abducted (moves the left eye clockwise). The action of the lateral and medial rectus muscles causes the eyes to deviate laterally and medially, respectively (Brazis, pp. 156–157).

118. B. Bladder retention and autonomic instability in a T6 paraplegic patient typically resolve with bladder catheterization (Brazis, p. 89; Merritt, p. 422).

119. D. Oculomotor nerve compression typically causes a dilated pupil, whereas a pontine hemorrhage, bilateral diencephalic injury, narcotic administration, and cholinergic drug therapy typically result in small pupils (Merritt, pp. 18–19).

120. B. Neurogenic amyotrophy (Parsonage-Turner syndrome) is characterized by severe, acute pain located in the shoulder and radiating into the arm, neck, and back. To prevent pain, movement of the arm is avoided and the arm is held in a position of flexion at the elbow and adduction at the shoulder (flexion-adduction sign). The muscles innervated by the axillary, suprascapular, and long thoracic nerves are most often affected. The pain usually disappears but is then followed by paresis of the shoulder and proximal musculature (Brazis, p. 57).

121. D. Benedikt's syndrome consists of ipsilateral oculomotor paresis, usually with a dilated pupil, as well as contralateral involuntary movements including intention tremor, hemichorea, or hemiathetosis due to red nucleus damage. Ramsay-Hunt syndrome, Meige's syndrome, Foville's syndrome, and the Millard-Gubler syndrome involve the facial nerve (CN VII) (Brazis, pp. 359–360).

122. B. Levodopa/carbidopa does not typically produce galactorrhea (Merritt, pp. 687–691).

123. C. Infarcts involving the paramedian region of the midbrain and pons may result in decreased level of conciousneness, behavioral changers (agitation, confusion, lack of initiative, apathy), memory loss, vertical gaze and convergence disorders, contralateral hemiataxia, asterixis, motor weakness, and action tremor in the contralateral limbs. Lateral gaze palsies are not typically associated with this syndrome (Brazis, pp. 408–409).

124. B. The syndrome of "Dejerine and Roussy" is characterized by contralateral sensory loss to all modalities, severe dysesthesias of the involved side (thalamic pain), vasomotor disturbances, transient contralateral hemiparesis, and choreoathetoid or ballistic movements. It is most often the result of infarction in the ventral posterior (VP) nuclei of the thalamus, which are supplied by the penetrating branches of the posterior communicating artery (Brazis, p. 548).

125. B. Subarachnoid hemorrhage (or any intracranial hemorrhage) may result in vitreous hemorrhage, also known as Terson's syndrome (Brazis, p. 559).

126-D; 127-A; 128-B; 129-G; 130-G; 131-C; 132-F; 133-G. Refer to Table 3.126–3.133A. Arginase deficiency is associated with urea cycle defects and hyperammonemia, while copper ATPase deficiency results in kinky hair disease (Menke's disease) (Merritt, pp. 521–524, 534–538, 547–548).

134-E; 135-C; 136-D; 137-I; 138-A; 139-B; 140-J; 141-F; 142-G. Refer to Table 3.134–3.142. (Merritt, pp. 518–519).

TABLE 3.126–133A   Leukodystrophies

LEUKODYSTROPHY	INHERITANCE	INVOLVED PROTEIN	HISTOLOGY	CLINICAL FEATURES
Krabbe's disease	AR	Galactocerebrosidase	Globoid macrophages	Spasms, myoclonus, motor loss
Metachromatic	AR	Aryl-sulfatase	PAS + macrophages	Ataxia, motor loss, psychosis
Adrenoleukodystrophy	X-linked	ATP-binding protein	Perivascular inflammation	Seizures, dementia, hypertonia
Pelizaeus-Merzbacher disease	X-linked	Myelin proteolipid	Segmental demyelination	Ataxia, spasticity, nystagmus
Canavan's disease	AR	Aspartoacylase	Spongy white matter	Hypotonia, blindness, myoclonus
Alexander's disease	Sporadic	Unknown	Rosenthal fibers	Seizures, dementia, psychosis

TABLE 3.134–142A   Sphingolipidoses

DISORDER	DEFECTIVE ENZYME	CLINICAL FEATURES
Tay-Sachs disease	Hexosaminidase A absent; Hexosaminidase B increased	Infantile encephalopathy, macular "cherry red" spots, spinal muscular atrophy
G_{M1} gangliosidosis	β-galactosidase	Infantile encephalopathy, organomegaly, macular "cherry red" spot, corneal haze, dementia, seizures, ataxia, dysarthria
Fabry's disease	α-galactosidase	Purple skin lesions, painful hands and feet, renal disease, strokes
Gaucher's disease	β-glucocerebrosidase	Dementia, organomegaly, spasticity, seizures, bony involvement
Niemann-Pick disease	Sphingomyelinase: types A and B Cholesterol esterification gene (NCC1): type C;NPC1 gene: type D	Infantile encephalopathy, organomegaly, "cherry red" spot (30%), lung infiltrates, spasticity, ataxia, seizures
Farber's disease	Acid ceramidase	Swollen joints, subcutaneous nodules, organomegaly, enlarged heart, dysphagia, vomiting
Wolman's disease	Acid lipase	Organomegaly, vomiting, diarrhea, jaundice
Cerebrotendinous xanthomatosis	Unknown	Static encephalopathy, cataracts, ataxia, spasticity, tendon xanthomas
Batten's disease	Palmitoylprotein thioesterase	Visual loss, seizures, ataxia, myoclonic jerks, retinal degeneration, microcephaly

143-B; 144-C; 145-A. HHT or Rendu-Osler-Weber disease, is an autosomal dominant neurocutaneous syndrome that involves mutations in the TGF-β receptor gene. Patients with HHT develop arteriovenous malformations of the liver, lungs, brain, and spine, in descending order of frequency. Patients with HHT also exhibit telangiectasias of the skin and mucosa, and often present with epistaxis. One key distinguishing feature of HHT is the presence of nail bed telangiectasias. The pulmonary shunts that are commonly associated with HHT put patients at significant risk for the development of brain abscesses. Patients with HHT also experience paradoxical cerebral emboli, strokes, and subarachnoid hemorrhage (due to an increased risk of intracranial aneurysms) (Merritt, p. 371; Osborn DN, pp. 106–107).

146. A. Symptomatic carotid artery stenosis and significant asymptomatic carotid artery stenosis are associated with an increased risk of stroke. The North American Symptomatic Carotid Endarterectomy Trial (NASCET) provided strong evidence for the benefit of carotid endarterectomy over maximum medical management of patients with symptomatic ipsilateral carotid artery stenosis between 70 and 99%. In the NASCET study group, patients with mild strokes or ipsilateral hemispheric or retinal TIAs within the past 120 days exhibited a 17% decrease in the rate of all ipsilateral strokes (26% in medical group versus 9% in surgical group), and a 10.6% decrease in major or fatal ipsilateral stroke (13.1% in medical group versus 2.5% in surgical group) at 2 years compared to medical management. Symptomatic patients with less than 50% carotid stenosis should not undergo carotid endarterectomy, and stenosis between 50 and 69% is controversial, with a 6.5% reduction in stroke rate with surgery. Asymptomatic carotid artery stenosis of greater than 75% is associated with a 3.3% risk of stroke per year (2.5% risk of ipsilateral stroke), and stenosis of less than 75% is associated with a 1.3% risk of stroke per year. The Asymptomatic Carotid Atherosclerosis Study (ACAS) concluded that patients with asymptomatic carotid artery stenosis greater than 60% have reduced stroke rates with carotid endarterectomy compared to medical management at 5 years (11.0% stroke rate in medical group versus 5.1% stroke rate in surgical group). However, these results apply to patients in reasonable health and to medical centers that perform carotid endarterectomy with less than 3% perioperative morbidity and mortality (Executive committee for ACAS, pp. 1421–1428; NASCET, pp. 445–453; Merritt, pp. 228, 257).

147. E. Cockayne's syndrome, ataxia telangiectasia, xeroderma pigmentosa, Fanconi's anemia, and Blooms syndrome are associated with defective DNA repair, whereas Klinefelter's syndrome is associated with an increase in the number of sex chromosomes (XXY) (Osborn DN, pp. 11–12).

148-H; 149-A; 150-G; 151-C; 152-E; 153-B; 154-I; 155-I; 156-D. Refer to Table 3.148–3.156A (Osborn DN, pp. 11–12).

TABLE 3.148–156A   Chromosomal disorders

DISORDER	CHROMOSOME ABNORMALITY	ASSOCIATED ABNORMALITIES
Down's syndrome	Trisomy 21	Mental retardation, brain atrophy, Alzheimer's disease, brachycephaly, hypoplastic maxilla, hypotelorism, anomalies of skull base and cervical spine
Edward's syndrome	Trisomy 18	Gyral dysplasia, cerebellar hypoplasia, callosal agenesis, Chiari II, dolichocephaly, low-set ears, hypotelorism, micrognathia
Patau's syndrome	Trisomy 13	Alobar holoprosencephaly, arrhinencephaly, cerebellar dysplasia, ocular anomalies, retinoblastoma development, survival < 9 months
Trisomy 9	Trisomy 9	Dandy-Walker syndrome, subependymal and choroid plexus cysts, progressive hydrocephalus, micrognathia, skeletal and cardiac anomalies
Short arm, chromosome 4 deletion	Short arm, chromosome 4 deletion	Midline defects, cerebellar anomalies, gyral disorders, cardiac defects (CHF)
Cri du chat syndrome	Short arm, chromosome 5 deletion	Severe mental retardation, "cat-like" cry, microcephaly, hypertelorism
Prader-Willi syndrome	Short arm, chromosome 15 deletion	Mental retardation, truncal obesity, short stature, hypogonadism
Miller-Dieker syndrome	Short arm, chromosome 17 deletion	Lissencephaly, hypoplastic corpus callosum, mental retardation, growth deficiency, dysmorphic facies
Fragile X syndrome	Decrease in number of sex chromosomes	Cognitive and behavioral disability, vermian cerebellar hypoplasia, hyperactivity, speech disorder
Turner's syndrome	Decrease in number of sex chromosomes, 45X	Short stature, no major CNS anomalies, webbed neck, coarctation of the aorta, hearing impairment

157. E. Galactosemia is associated with cataracts, not "cherry-red" spots (Geyer, p. 114).

158. A. Increased skin pigmentation is one of the features of adrenoleukodystrophy, while Hurler's syndrome, homocystinuria, and Cockayne's syndrome are associated with corneal clouding (Geyer, pp. 113–114).

159-A; 160-C; 161-A; 162-C; 163-B; 164-B. Patients with bulbar palsy typically have an atrophic tongue with fasciculations, flaccid speech, a weak face, absent jaw-jerk and gag reflexes, and diminished extraocular movements. Patients with pseudobulbar palsy have a normal-sized tongue with spastic speech, a weak face, emotional lability, the presence of jaw-jerk and gag (hyperactive) reflexes, diminished extraocular movements, and the absence of fasciculations (Brazis, p. 321; Merritt, p. 239; Geyer, p. 133).

165-B; 166-B; 167-A; 168-B; 169-B; 170-B. Enteroviruses (poliovirus, coxsackievirus, and echovirus), arboviruses (flaviviruses, bunyaviruses, alphaviruses, rubiviruses), rhabdoviruses (rabies virus), and arenaviruses (lymphocytic choriomeningitis) are RNA viruses, while the herpesviruses (HSV-1, HSV-2, varicella zoster virus, cytomegalovirus, and HHV-6) are DNA viruses. Viral infections of the CNS can result in meningitis, ventriculitis, encephalitis, and myelitis. CSF in patients with viral syndromes of the CNS reveals increased pressure, lymphocytic pleocytosis, mild elevations in protein, and normal glucose levels. Viral (aseptic) meningitis usually peaks in the summer and fall seasons, whereas bacterial meningitis is more common during the winter. The most common causes of viral meningitis are the enteroviruses, but togaviruses are also frequent pathogens. Encephalitis often results from infections with herpes simplex virus, mumps, or arboviruses (Merritt, pp. 134–174).

171. E. The normal conduction velocity of a human peripheral nerve, as tested by electromyography, is approximately 40 to 60 m/s (Adams, p. 1023).

172-A; 173-B; 174-B; 175-A. This is a highly simplified depiction of the basal ganglia circuitry. The neurotransmitters utilized by these neurons are as follows: A, D, and G utilize glutamate; B, C, and E utilize GABA, while F neurons utilize dopamine (Youmans, p. 2684).

Neuropathology Questions

Major Contributor: Kimmo J. Hatanpaa

1. What primary CNS neoplasm is associated with eosinophilic granular bodies?

- **A.** Anaplastic astrocytoma
- **B.** Oligodendroglioma
- **C.** Gemistocytic astrocytoma
- **D.** Pilocytic astrocytoma
- **E.** Germinoma

2. Which of the following is associated with deposition of phosphorylated tau protein?

- **A.** Hirano bodies
- **B.** Neurofibrillary tangles
- **C.** Diffuse amyloid plaques
- **D.** Lewy bodies
- **E.** Granulovacuolar degeneration

3. What neoplasm is depicted in the following photomicrograph (H&E section) (Figure 4.3Q)?

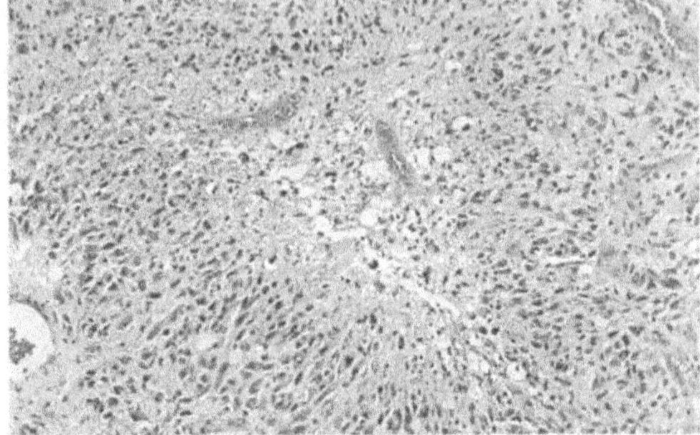

FIGURE 4.3Q

- **A.** Lymphoma
- **B.** Fibrillary astrocytoma
- **C.** Glioblastoma
- **D.** Medulloblastoma
- **E.** Meningioma

4. What chromosome abnormality is associated with neurofibromatosis type 1?

- **A.** 5
- **B.** 7
- **C.** 10
- **D.** 17
- **E.** 20

5. Congenital CMV infection is characterized by all of the following EXCEPT?

- **A.** Periventricular calcifications
- **B.** Microglial nodules
- **C.** Chorioretinitis
- **D.** Megalencephaly
- **E.** Hydrocephalus

6. Which of the following disorders is associated with Opalski cells on microscopic examination?

- **A.** Hallervorden-Spatz disease
- **B.** Werdnig-Hoffman disease
- **C.** Wilson's disease
- **D.** Tay-Sachs disease
- **E.** Gaucher's disease

7. Which of the following proteins compose the Lewy body?

- **A.** Ubiquitin
- **B.** Neurofilaments
- **C.** α–Synuclein
- **D.** Both A and C
- **E.** All of the above

8. Canavan's disease results from deficiencies of which of the following enzymes?

- **A.** Aspartoacylase
- **B.** Aryl sulfatase A
- **C.** Glucocerebrosidase
- **D.** Hexosaminidase A
- **E.** Iduronidase

9. What is depicted in the following photomicrograph (Figure 4.9Q)?

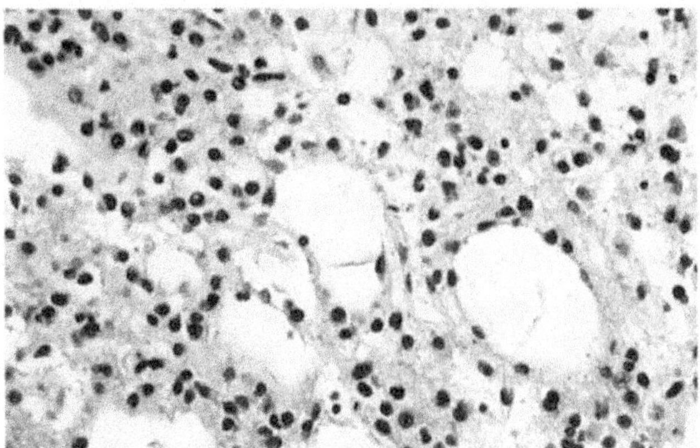

FIGURE 4.9Q

   A. Fibrillary astrocytoma
   B. Reactive astrocytosis
   C. Anaplastic astrocytoma
   D. Clear cell meningioma
   E. Yolk sac tumor

10. Which of the following neoplasms is not associated with neurofibromatosis type 2?

   A. Ependymoma
   B. Schwannoma
   C. Meningioma
   D. Glioma
   E. Plexiform neurofibroma

11. What is the most likely clinical history associated with the following photomicrograph (Figure 4.11Q)?

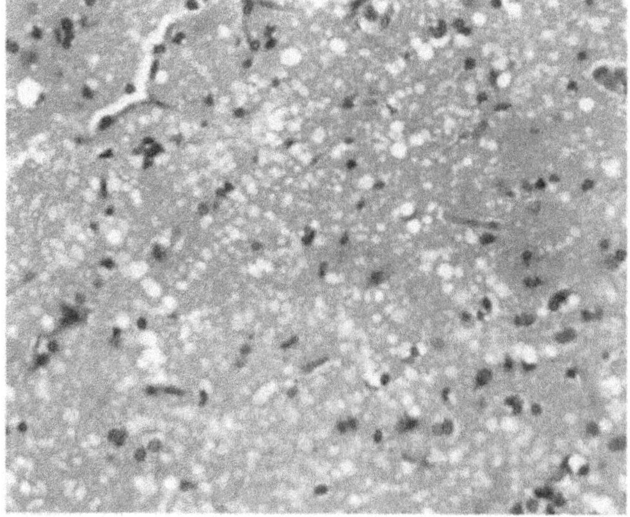

FIGURE 4.11Q

   A. Seizures and progressive hypotonia in infancy
   B. Rapidly progressing dementing illness of an adult
   C. Gradually progressive focal neurologic deficit

   D. Asymptomatic lesion that can often be treated with antibiotics alone
   E. Asymptomatic lesion that typically responds favorably to surgery alone

QUESTIONS 12–16

Directions: Match the following items with their appropriate inclusion body. Some letters may be used more than once.

   A. Actin
   B. Ubiquitin
   C. Polyglucosans
   D. Amyotrophic lateral sclerosis
   E. α–Synuclein

12. Marinesco bodies

13. Lafora bodies

14. Bunina bodies

15. Hirano bodies

16. Pick bodies

End of set

17. What pathologic condition is depicted in the following photomicrograph (Figure 4.17Q)?

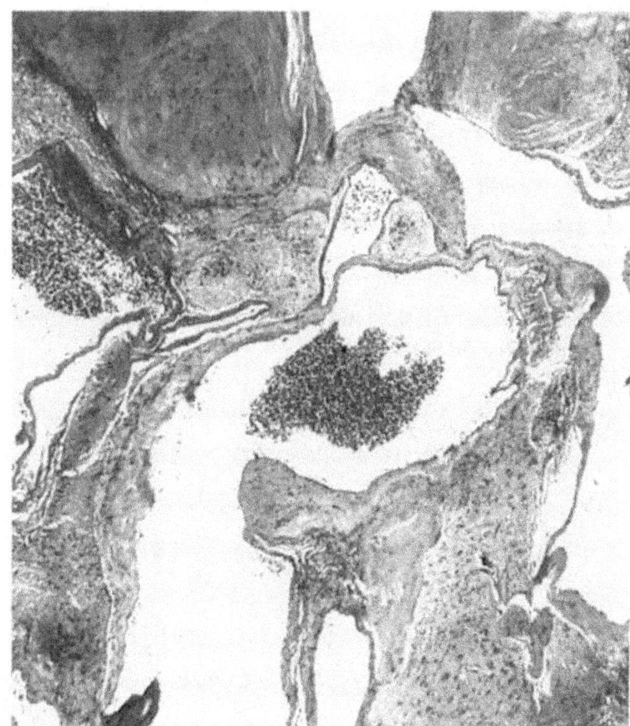

FIGURE 4.17Q

   A. Capillary telangiectasia
   B. Cavernous malformation
   C. Venous angioma
   D. Arteriovenous malformation
   E. Angiomatous meningioma

18. What feature of chronic subdural hematomas is most likely to lead to progressive expansion in size over time?

- **A.** Reinjury of bridging veins
- **B.** Osmotic migration across the dura into the subdural space
- **C.** Hemorrhage in the granulation tissue of the pseudomembrane
- **D.** Breakdown of the blood-brain barrier in adjacent brain parenchyma
- **E.** None of the above

19. What is the most likely etiology of the lesion depicted below in this gross specimen (Figure 4.19Q)?

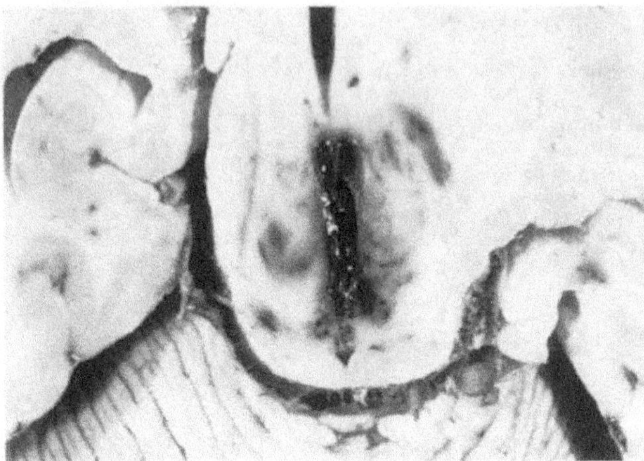

FIGURE 4.19Q

- **A.** Direct contusion
- **B.** Shearing injury
- **C.** Herniation
- **D.** Arterial dissection
- **E.** Arterial rupture

20. What is the most common organism isolated from intracranial abscesses?

- **A.** *Staphylococcus aureus*
- **B.** *Pseudomonas aeruginosa*
- **C.** *Streptococcus pneumoniae*
- **D.** *Streptococcus milleri*
- **E.** *Mycobacterium tuberculosis*

21. What neoplasm is depicted in the following photomicrograph (Figure 4.21Q)?

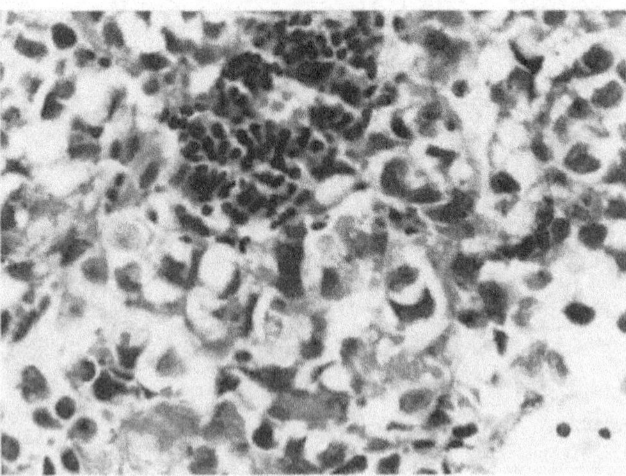

FIGURE 4.21Q

- **A.** Choriocarcinoma
- **B.** Yolk sac tumor
- **C.** Secretory meningoma
- **D.** Germinoma
- **E.** Ependymoma

22. What is the most common cranial nerve affected by neurosarcoidosis?

- **A.** Optic
- **B.** Oculomotor
- **C.** Trigeminal
- **D.** Abducens
- **E.** Facial

23. Which of the following regions of the brain exhibit prominent atrophy with Alzheimer's disease?

1. Hippocampus	**A.** 1, 2, and 3 are correct
2. Occipital lobe	**B.** 1 and 3 are correct
3. Frontal lobe	**C.** 2 and 4 are correct
4. Primary motor cortex	**D.** Only 4 is correct
	E. All of the above are correct

24. Bilirubin deposition in the brain of a neonate with kernicterus is commonly observed in which of the following regions?

1. Subthalamic nucleus	**A.** 1, 2, and 3 are correct
2. Globus pallidus	**B.** 1 and 3 are correct
3. Dentate nucleus	**C.** 2 and 4 are correct
4. Red nucleus	**D.** Only 4 is correct
	E. All of the above are correct

25. A 58-year-old male presents with focal seizures and is found to have a large frontal lobe mass originating from the gray-white junction on MRI. The patient underwent a diagnostic biopsy of this lesion, and the specimen was CD45-negative, vimentin-positive, cytokeratin-AE1/3 positive, and EMA-negative. This is most consistent with which of the following neoplasms?

A. Lymphoma
B. Metastatic carcinoma
C. Glioblastoma
D. Hemangiopericytoma
E. Meningioma

26. Which of the following meningioma variants is depicted in this photomicrograph (Figure 4.26Q)?

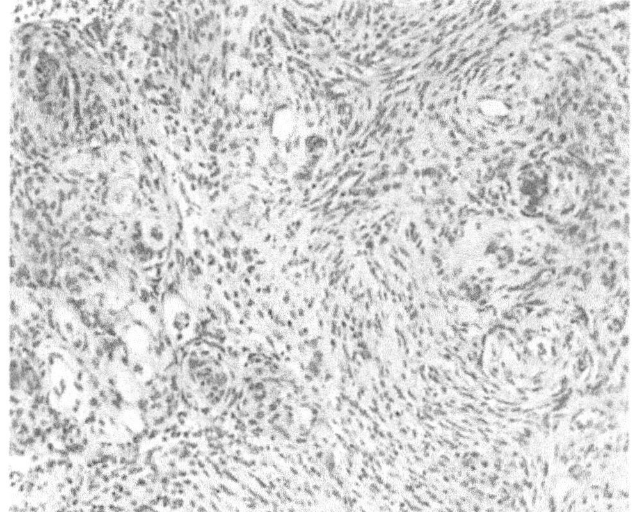

FIGURE 4.26Q

A. Meningothelial
B. Fibrous
C. Transitional
D. Secretory
E. Chordoid

27. Which of the following meningioma variants is associated with more aggressive clinical behavior?

A. Papillary
B. Angiomatous
C. Chordoid
D. Clear cell
E. Metaplastic

28. Which of the following disorders can be inherited in an autosomal dominant fashion via mutations in the superoxide dismutase (SOD1) gene?

A. Refsum's disease
B. Sanfilippo syndrome
C. Zellweger syndrome
D. Amyotrophic lateral sclerosis
E. None of the above

29. Which of the following major histocompatibility complexes is associated with the development of multiple sclerosis?

1. HLA-DR15
2. HLA-DR2
3. HLA-B7
4. HLA-DR4

A. 1, 2, and 3 are correct
B. 1 and 3 are correct
C. 2 and 4 are correct
D. Only 4 is correct
E. All of the above are correct

QUESTIONS 30–34

Directions: Match the following neoplasms with the most common protein/stain using each answer once, more than once, or not at all.

A. Vimentin
B. CD 45
C. CD34
D. S-100
E. Synaptophysin

30. Lymphoma

31. Hemangiopericytoma

32. Sustentacular cell of paraganglioma

33. Meningioma

34. Central neurocytoma

End of set

35. What neoplasm is depicted in the following photomicrograph (Figure 4.35Q)?

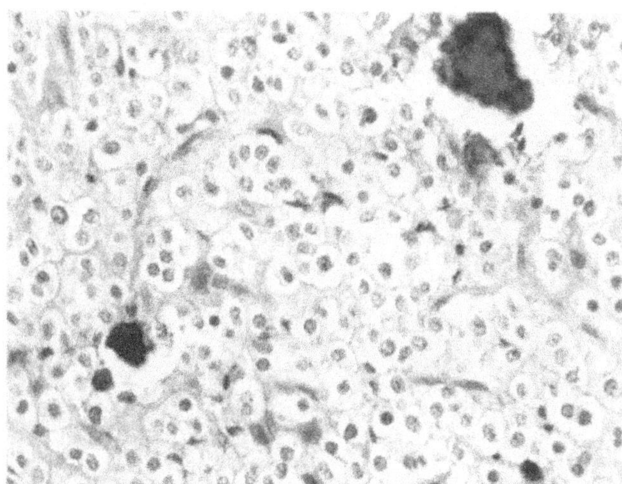

FIGURE 4.35Q

A. Clear cell meningioma
B. Medulloblastoma
C. Fibrillary astrocytoma
D. Oligodendroglioma
E. Hemangiopericytoma

36. What abnormality is depicted in the following photomicrograph (Figure 4.36Q)?

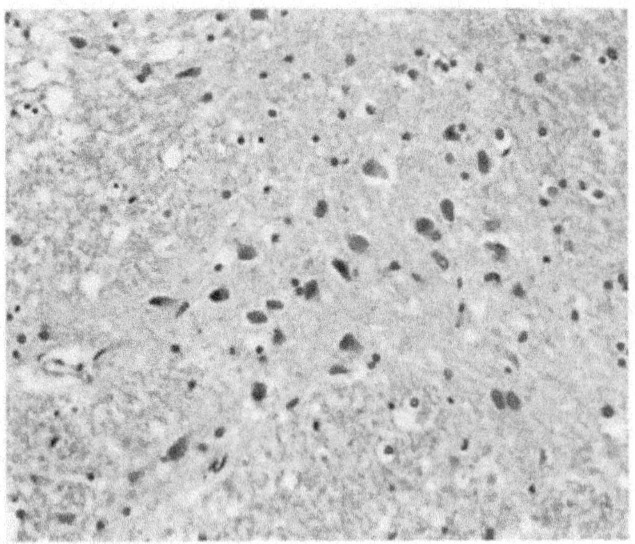

FIGURE 4.36Q

A. Gemistocytic astrocytoma
B. Reactive astrocytosis
C. Acute infarction
D. Viral encephalitis
E. Bacterial meningitis

37. Which of the following is not observed with acute spinal cord injury microscopically?

A. Axonal spheroids
B. Hemorrhagic necrosis
C. Cavitation
D. Inflammatory infiltrates
E. Edema

38. What is the most common chromosomal abnormality associated with meningiomas?

A. Allelic loss of 1p
B. Monosomy 22
C. Allelic loss of 10
D. Allelic loss of 22q
E. Monosomy 2

39. What is the inheritance pattern of Sturge-Weber syndrome?

A. Autosomal recessive
B. Autosomal dominant
C. X-linked recessive
D. Mitochondrial
E. Sporadic

40. Which of the following disorders is associated with the lesion depicted in this photomicrograph (Figure 4.40Q)?

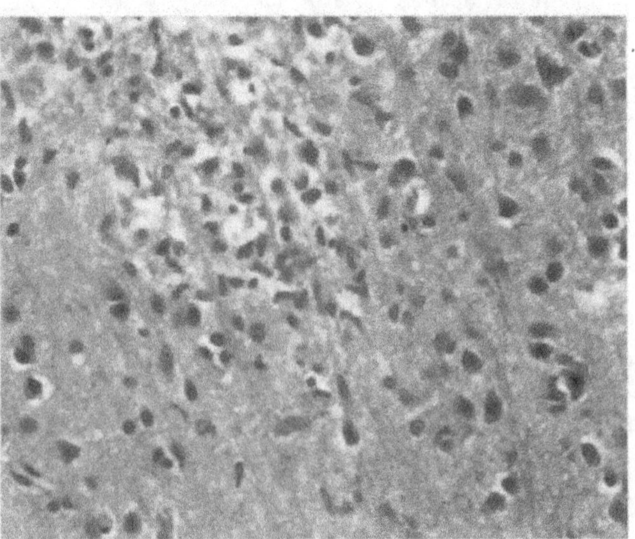

FIGURE 4.40Q

1. HIV encephalitis
2. Toxoplasmosis
3. CMV encephalitis
4. Neurosyphilis

A. 1, 2, and 3 are correct
B. 1 and 3 are correct
C. 2 and 4 are correct
D. Only 4 is correct
E. All of the above are correct

41. Which of the following characteristics is not associated with Hunter syndrome (mucopolysaccharidosis type II)?

A. Lysosomal disorder
B. X-linked recessive inheritance
C. Hepatosplenomegaly
D. Corneal clouding
E. Mental retardation

42. What is depicted in the following photomicrograph (Figure 4.42Q)?

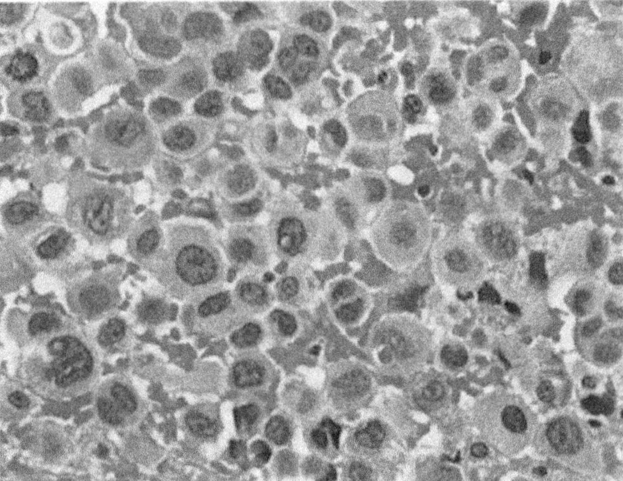

FIGURE 4.42Q

A. Intracranial abscess
B. Intracranial metastases
C. Multiple sclerosis plaque
D. Acute infarction
E. Fungal infection

43. Which of the following disorders is associated with accommodation (ciliary) paralysis, facial paralysis, preservation of extraocular movements, and an ascending sensorimotor polyneuropathy?

A. Neurosarcoidosis
B. Neurosyphilis
C. Diphtheria
D. Lyme disease
E. Guillain-Barré syndrome

QUESTIONS 44–45

The following responses are in reference to questions 44 and 45:

A. Subependymal germinal matrix hemorrhage
B. Choroid plexus hemorrhage
C. Both A and B
D. Neither A nor B

44. The most common cause of intraventricular hemorrhage in term infants

45. The most common cause of intraventricular hemorrhage in premature infants

End of set

46. Which of the following disorders are secondary to defective neuronal migration?

1. Polymicrogyria
2. Schizencephaly
3. Focal nodular heterotopia
4. Holoprosencephaly

A. 1, 2, and 3 are correct
B. 1 and 3 are correct
C. 2 and 4 are correct
D. Only 4 is correct
E. All of the above are correct

QUESTIONS 47–51

Directions: Match the following meningitis-causative organisms with the age group most likely to be afflicted.

A. *Streptococcus pneumoniae*
B. *Haemophilus influenzae*
C. *Listeria monocytogenes*
D. *Proteus mirabilis*
E. *S. epidermidis*

47. Children 1 to 5 years of age

48. Adults

49. Unique to the elderly population

50. Associated with ventriculoperitoneal shunt infections

51. Associated with coexistent cerebral abscesses in neonates

End of set

52. What neoplasm is depicted in the following photomicrograph (Figure 4.52Q)?

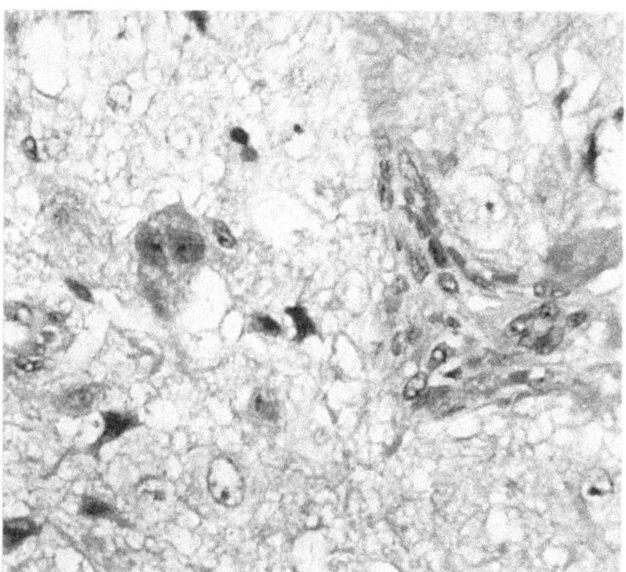

FIGURE 4.52Q

A. Medulloblastoma
B. Ganglion cell tumor
C. Central neurocytoma
D. Ependymoma
E. Anaplastic astrocytoma

53. What neoplasm is depicted in the following photomicrograph (Figure 4.53Q)?

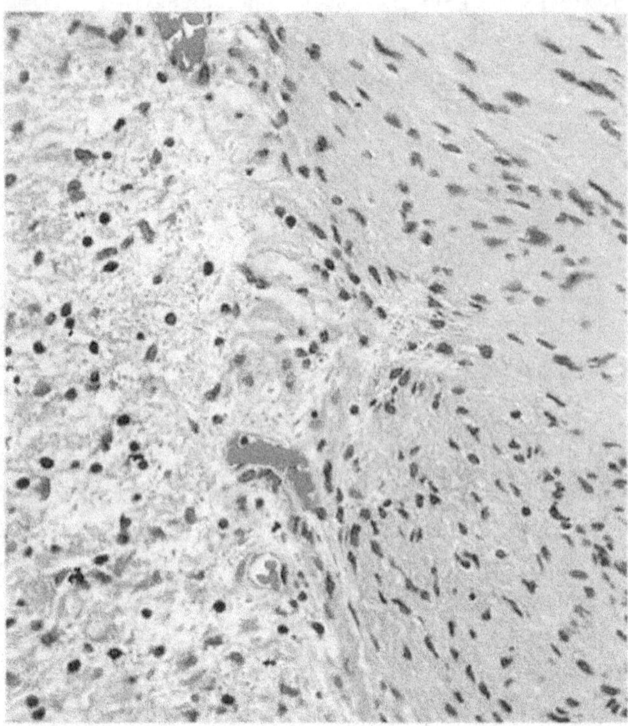

FIGURE 4.53Q

    A. Neurofibroma
    B. Schwannoma
    C. Fibrous meningioma
    D. Malignant nerve sheath tumor
    E. None of the above

54. What neoplasm is depicted in the following photomicrograph (Figure 4.54Q)?

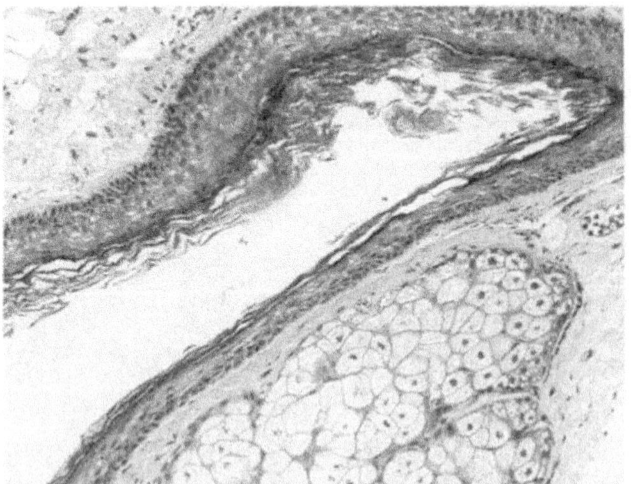

FIGURE 4.54Q

    A. Dermoid cyst (mature teratoma)
    B. Craniopharyngioma
    C. Ependymoma
    D. Yolk sac tumor
    E. None of the above

55. Which of the following conditions is associated with Sprengel's deformity?

    A. Hallervorden-Spatz disease
    B. Leigh's disease
    C. Niemann-Pick disease
    D. Tuberous sclerosis
    E. Klippel-Feil anomaly

56. Which of the following lesions is thought to develop as a consequence of premature disjunction?

    A. Rathke's cleft cyst
    B. Diastematomyelia
    C. Neurenteric cyst
    D. Spinal lipoma
    E. Dandy-Walker malformation

57. Which of the following neoplasms is/are associated with von Hippel-Lindau syndrome?

    1. Pheochromocytomas
    2. Renal cell carcinoma
    3. Cerebellar hemangioblastomas
    4. Endolymphatic sac tumors

    A. 1, 2, and 3 are correct
    B. 1 and 3 are correct
    C. 2 and 4 are correct
    D. Only 4 is correct
    E. All of the above are correct

58. What disorder is associated with the following photomicrograph (Figure 4.58Q)?

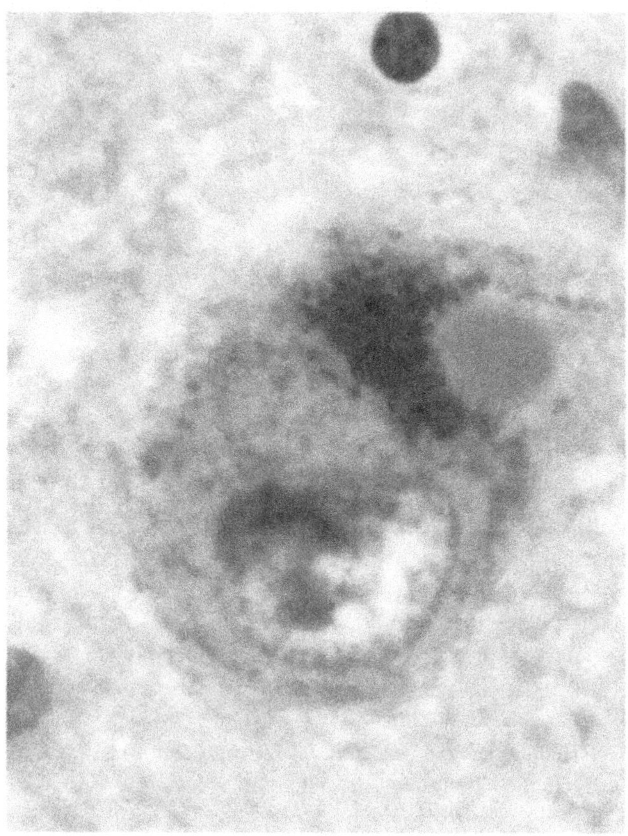

FIGURE 4.58Q

A. Parkinson's disease
B. Corticobasal degeneration
C. Rabies encephalitis
D. Alzheimer's disease
E. None of the above

59. What neoplasm is depicted in the following photomicrograph (Figure 4.59Q)?

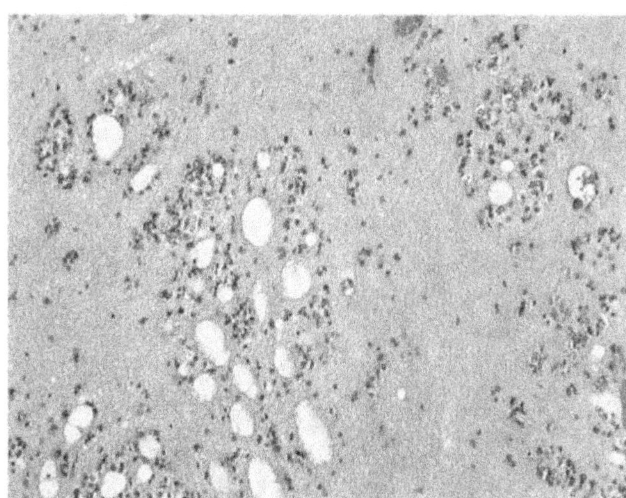

FIGURE 4.59Q

A. Pilocytic astrocytoma
B. Subependymoma
C. Myxopapillary ependymoma
D. Dysembryoplastic neuroepithelial tumor
E. None of the above

60. Which of the following lesions is depicted in these two photomicrographs (two areas of the same lesion) (Figure 4.60Q)?

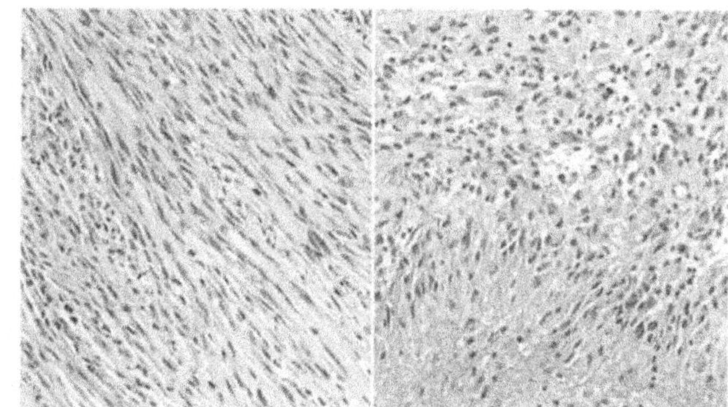

FIGURE 4.60Q

A. Malignant nerve sheath tumor
B. Fibrous meningioma
C. Gliosarcoma
D. Embryonal carcinoma
E. None of the above

61. What is the most likely presentation of the following neoplasm (Figure 4.61Q)?

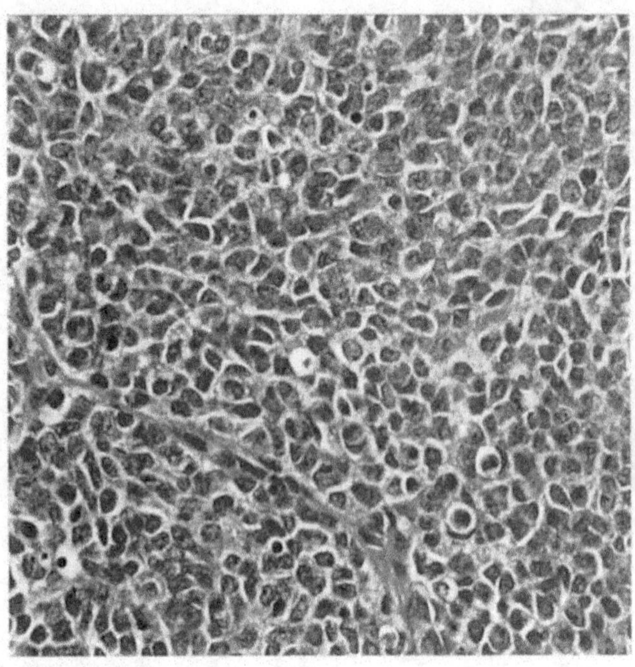

FIGURE 4.61Q

- **A.** Supratentorial mass in a 55-year-old male with a lung mass
- **B.** Complex partial epilepsy in a 12-year-old male
- **C.** Hypopituitarism in a 19-year-old female
- **D.** Nausea, vomiting, and ataxia in a 5-year-old male
- **E.** Hearing loss in a patient with neurofibromatosis type 2

QUESTIONS 62–63

The following answers are in reference to questions 62 and 63.

- **A.** Neurofibromatosis type 1
- **B.** Tuberous sclerosis
- **C.** Both of the above
- **D.** Neither of the above

62. Complete penetrance

63. Incomplete penetrance

End of set

64. Which of the following scenarios is the most likely presentation of the disorder depicted below in this gross specimen (Figure 4.64Q)?

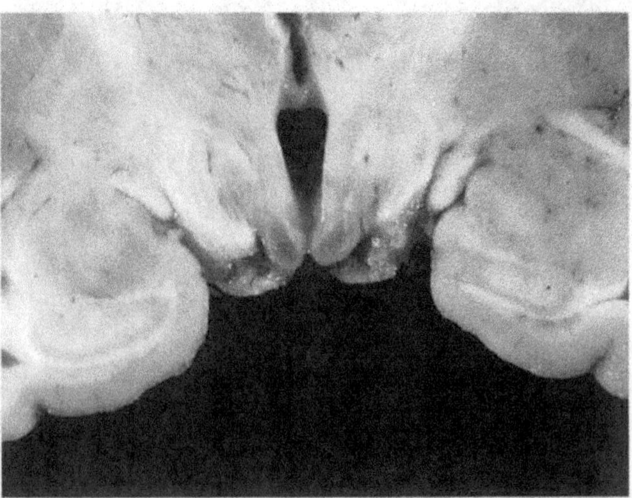

FIGURE 4.64Q

- **A.** Optic neuritis and Uhthoff's sign in a 32-year-old female
- **B.** Ataxia, confusion, and lateral gaze palsy in a 48-year-old male alcoholic
- **C.** Headache, nausea, and vomiting in a 62-year-old female with a systemic malignancy
- **D.** Right hemiparesis in a 75-year-old man with a history of hypertension
- **E.** None of the above

QUESTIONS 65–67

Directions: Match the following questions with the appropriate syndrome using each answer once, more than once, or not at all.

- **A.** Crouzon's disease
- **B.** Apert's syndrome
- **C.** Both of the above
- **D.** Neither of the above

65. Autosomal dominant inheritance

66. Uniformly associated with mental retardation

67. Associated with frontoethmoid synostosis

End of set

68. Craniosynostosis is associated with mutations in which of the following genes?

- **A.** p53
- **B.** Fibroblast growth factor receptor (FGF-R)
- **C.** Interleukin 6 (IL-6)
- **D.** Epidermal growth factor receptor (EGFR)
- **E.** None of the above

69. Which of the following clinical presentations is most consistent with the lesion depicted below in this gross specimen (Figure 4.69Q)?

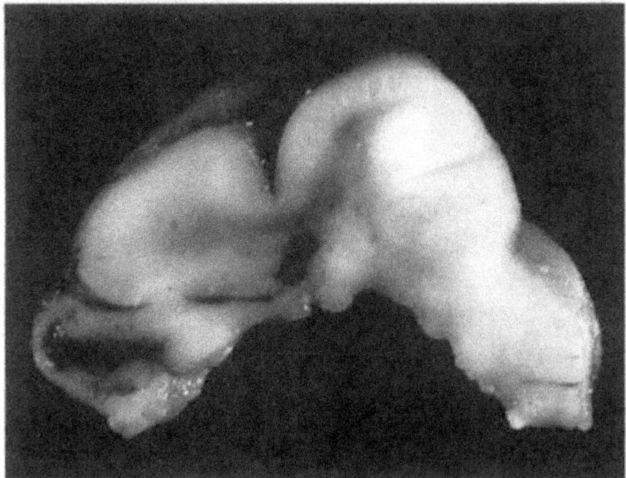

FIGURE 4.69Q

A. Bilateral facial and abducens palsies in the neonate
B. Ipsilateral port wine stain in the distribution of V_1 in a 5-year-old
C. Developmental delay in a 1-year-old
D. Sepsis in the preterm infant
E. Epilepsy in a 6-month-old

70. What is the most likely etiology of the abnormality depicted below (Figure 4.70Q)?

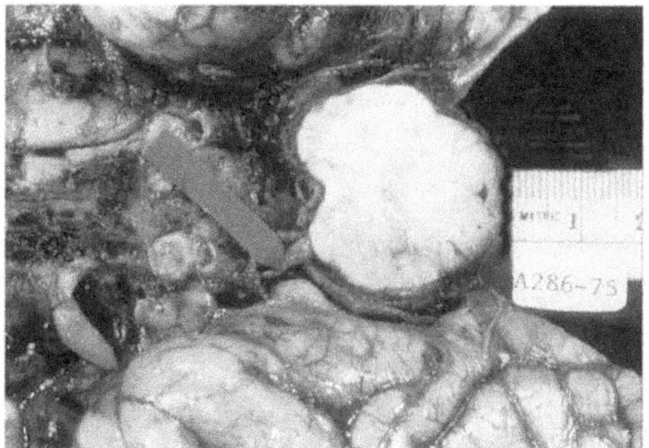

FIGURE 4.70Q

A. Elevated intracranial pressure
B. Atherosclerotic disease
C. CNS infection
D. Neurodegenerative disorder
E. None of the above

71. Which of the following structures are often involved with diffuse axonal injuries?

1. Parasagittal deep white matter
2. Superior cerebellar peduncles
3. Corpus callosum
4. Rostral brainstem

A. 1, 2, and 3 are correct
B. 1 and 3 are correct
C. 2 and 4 are correct
D. Only 4 is correct
E. All of the above are correct

72. What infection is depicted in the following photomicrograph (Figure 4.72Q)?

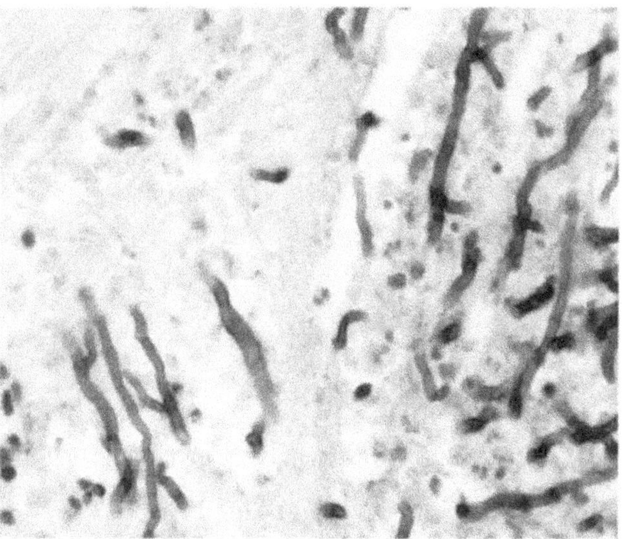

FIGURE 4.72Q

A. Aspergillosis
B. Mucormycosis
C. Cryptococcosis
D. Candidiasis
E. None of the above

73. What disorder is depicted in the following low-power photomicrograph (Figure 4.73Q) of a section stained for myelin?

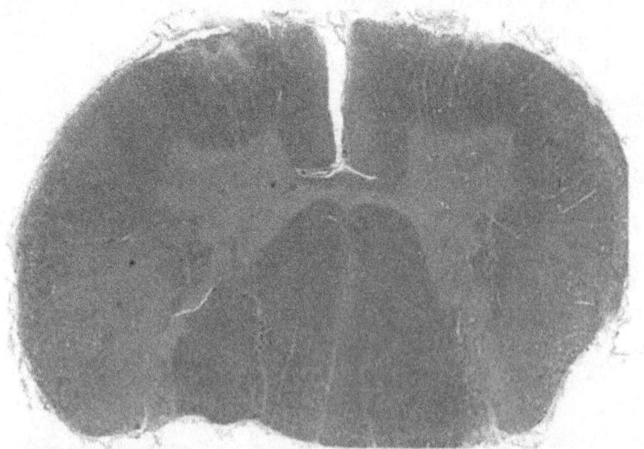

FIGURE 4.73Q

- **A.** Subacute combined degeneration
- **B.** Multiple sclerosis
- **C.** Tabes dorsalis
- **D.** Amyotrophic lateral sclerosis
- **E.** Friedreich's ataxia

QUESTIONS 74–77

Directions: Match the following questions with the appropriate demyelinating disease using each answer either once, more than once, or not at all.

- **A.** Multiple sclerosis
- **B.** Acute disseminated encephalomyelitis
- **C.** Both of the above
- **D.** Neither of the above

74. Monophasic

75. Experimental allergic encephalomyelitis represents the animal model of this disorder

76. Symptoms usually improve with administration of IV steroids

77. Is associated with perivenular inflammation on microscopic examination

End of set

78. What disorder is depicted in the photomicrograph below (Figure 4.78Q)?

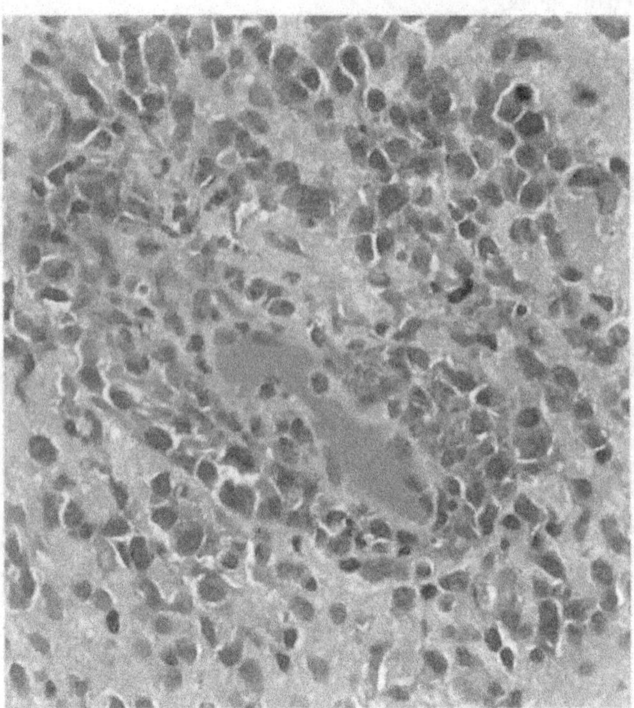

FIGURE 4.78Q

- **A.** Acute disseminated encephalomyelitis
- **B.** CNS lymphoma
- **C.** Viral encephalitis
- **D.** Active MS plaque
- **E.** None of the above

79. What neoplasm is depicted in the following photomicrograph (Figure 4.79Q)?

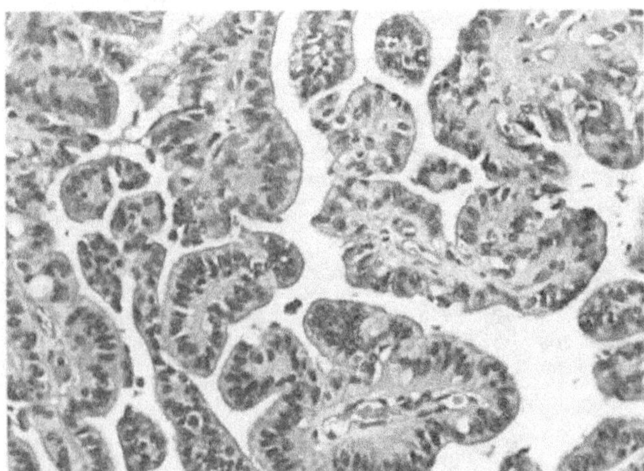

FIGURE 4.79Q

- **A.** Papillary craniopharyngioma
- **B.** Papillary meningioma
- **C.** Colloid cyst
- **D.** Choroid plexus papilloma
- **E.** Pineocytoma

80. All of the following are features of paragangliomas EXCEPT?

- **A.** Contain synaptophysin positive chief cells
- **B.** Contain GFAP positive sustentacular cells
- **C.** Arise from the cauda equina or glomus jugulare
- **D.** WHO grade I lesion
- **E.** Dense core granules on ultrastructural examination

81. What abnormality is depicted in the following gross specimen (Figure 4.81Q)?

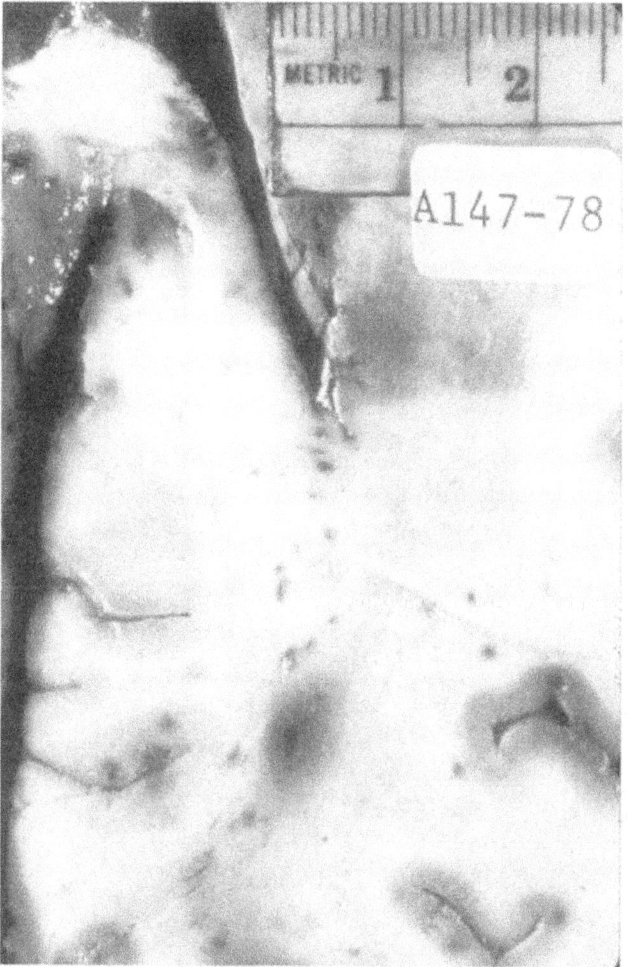

FIGURE 4.81Q

- **A.** Subacute infarct
- **B.** Progressive multifocal leukoencephalopathy
- **C.** Adrenoleukodystrophy
- **D.** Fat embolism
- **E.** Multiple sclerosis plaques

82. Which of the following are useful myelin stains?

1. Weigert
2. Sudan
3. Marchi
4. Phosphotungstic acid/hematoxylin (PTAH)

- **A.** 1, 2, and 3 are correct
- **B.** 1 and 3 are correct
- **C.** 2 and 4 are correct
- **D.** Only 4
- **E.** All of the above

83. What neoplasm is depicted in the following photomicrograph (Figure 4.83Q)?

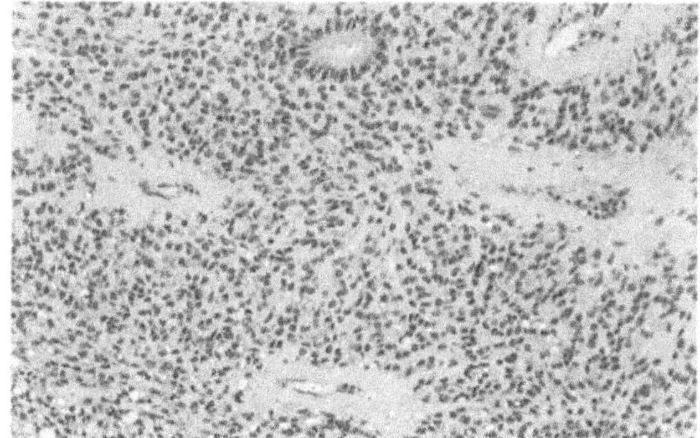

FIGURE 4.83Q

- **A.** Ependymoma
- **B.** Neuroblastoma
- **C.** Central neurocytoma
- **D.** Subependymoma
- **E.** Pilocytic astrocytoma

84. Which of the following CNS neoplasms can exhibit prominent melanin?

1. Schwannomas
2. Embryonal neoplasms
3. Primary malignant melanoma
4. Ependymomas

- **A.** 1, 2, and 3 are correct
- **B.** 1 and 3 are correct
- **C.** 2 and 4 are correct
- **D.** Only 4 is correct
- **E.** All of the above are correct

85. Which of the following disorders is associated with prominent iron deposition within the globus pallidus?

- **A.** Wilson's disease
- **B.** Hallervorden-Spatz disease
- **C.** Wernicke's encephalopathy
- **D.** Pick's disease
- **E.** Ataxia-telangiectasia

86. What abnormality is depicted in the following gross specimen (Figure 4.86Q)?

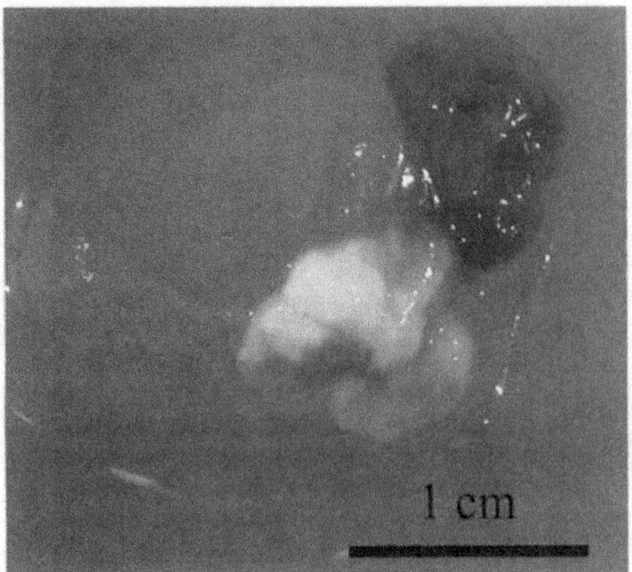

FIGURE 4.86Q

- **A.** Metastatic lesion
- **B.** Intracerebral abscess
- **C.** Cysticercus
- **D.** Arachnoid cyst
- **E.** Cortical tuber

87. Which of the following neurologic complications is associated with Paget's disease?

1. Trigeminal neuralgia
2. Peripheral neuropathy
3. Development of osteogenic sarcoma
4. Hypopituitarism

- **A.** 1, 2, and 3 are correct
- **B.** 1 and 3 are correct
- **C.** 2 and 4 are correct
- **D.** Only 4 is correct
- **E.** All of the above are correct

88. Which of the following disorders exhibits the abnormality depicted in the following photomicrograph (Figure 4.88Q)?

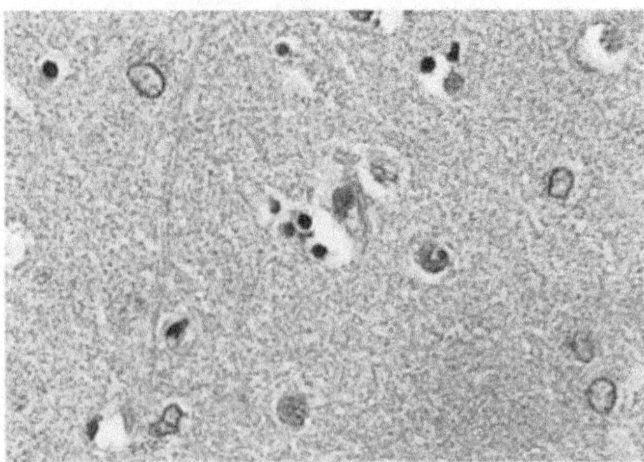

FIGURE 4.88Q

- **A.** Gaucher's disease
- **B.** Niemann-Pick disease
- **C.** Alzheimer's disease
- **D.** Hepatic encephalopathy
- **E.** Pyridoxine deficiency

89. Which of the following infectious disorders is illustrated in the photomicrograph below (Figure 4.89Q)?

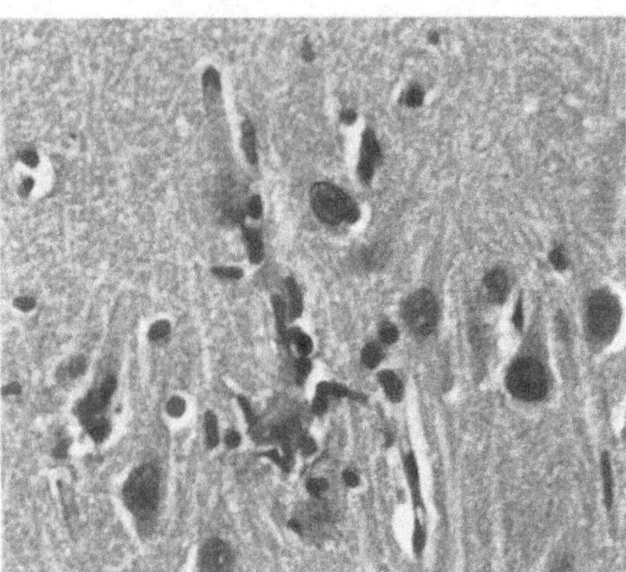

FIGURE 4.89Q

- **A.** Viral encephalitis
- **B.** Creutzfeldt-Jakob disease
- **C.** Bacterial meningitis
- **D.** CNS candidiasis
- **E.** Sarcoidosis

90. What neoplasm is depicted in the following photomicrograph (Figure 4.90Q)?

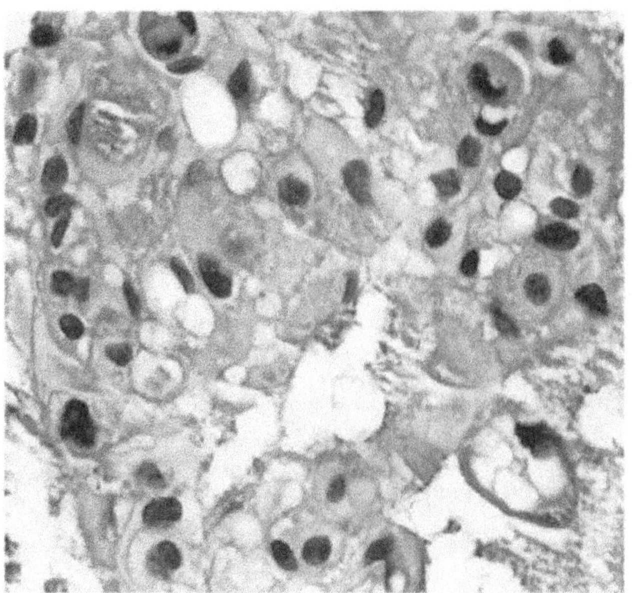

FIGURE 4.90Q

- **A.** Myxopapillary ependymoma
- **B.** Secretory meningioma
- **C.** Hemangiopericytoma
- **D.** Chordoma
- **E.** None of the above

91. Which of the following immunostains is generally not positive with glioblastomas?

- **A.** Vimentin
- **B.** GFAP
- **C.** Keratin AE1/3
- **D.** S-100
- **E.** EMA

92. Which of the following neoplasms is depicted in the following photomicrograph (Figure 4.92Q)?

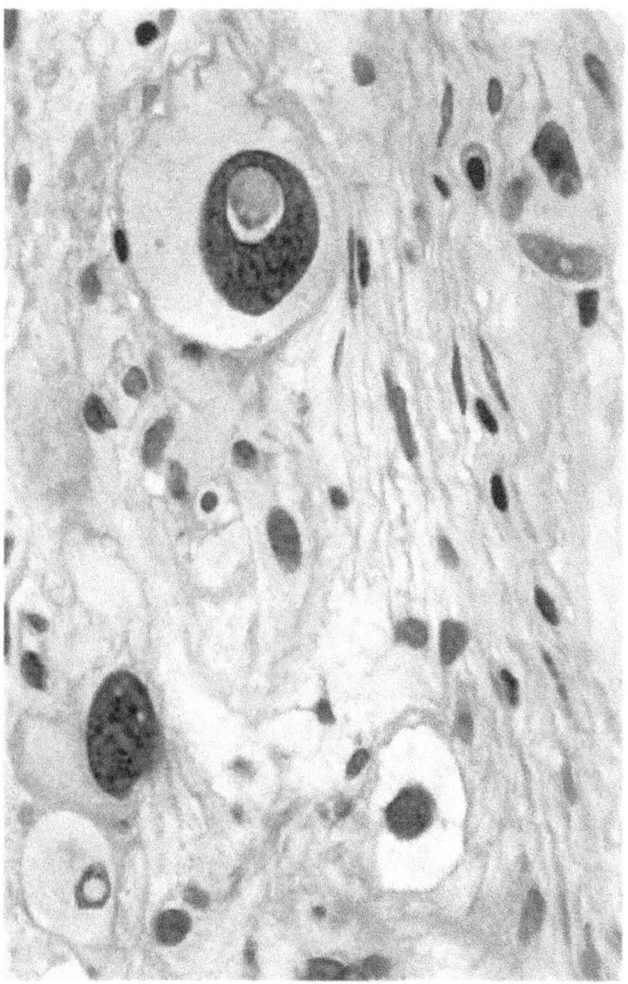

FIGURE 4.92Q

- **A.** Subependymal giant cell astrocytoma
- **B.** Pleomorphic xanthoastrocytoma
- **C.** Glioblastoma multiforme
- **D.** Dysembryoplastic neuroepithelial tumor
- **E.** None of the above

93. What chromosome is associated with Duchenne muscular dystrophy?

- **A.** 1
- **B.** 2
- **C.** 12
- **D.** X
- **E.** 22

94. Which of the following clinical scenarios is most likely associated with the pathologic finding depicted in the photomicrograph below (Figure 4.94Q)?

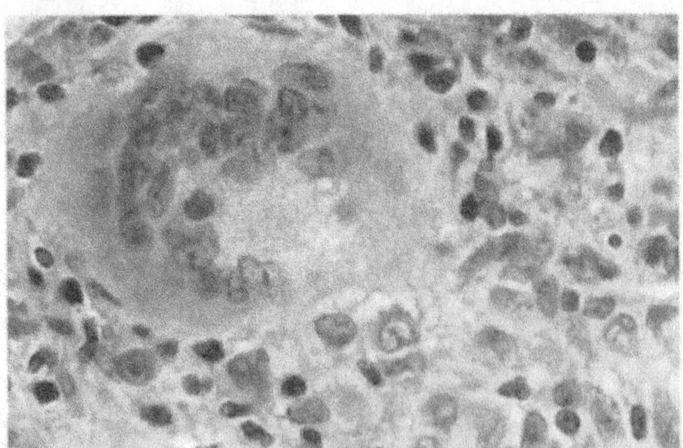

FIGURE 4.94Q

   A. 36-year-old male with fever, nuchal rigidity, and diffuse purpura

   B. Infantile spasms in a 3-week-old neonate

   C. Confusion, lethargy, and gaze palsies in a 42-year-old alcoholic male

   D. Amaurosis fugax in a 68-year-old female

   E. Rapid cognitive decline in a 41-year-old male

95. Which of the following characteristics is not associated with dermatomyositis?

   A. Systemic malignancy

   B. Heliotrope rash

   C. Proximal muscle weakness

   D. Muscle fiber infiltration by T cells

   E. Immunoglobulin deposition that can result in vasculopathy

96. What disorder is depicted in this low-power micrograph (Figure 4.96Q) of the cerebral cortex and underlying white matter, stained for myelin?

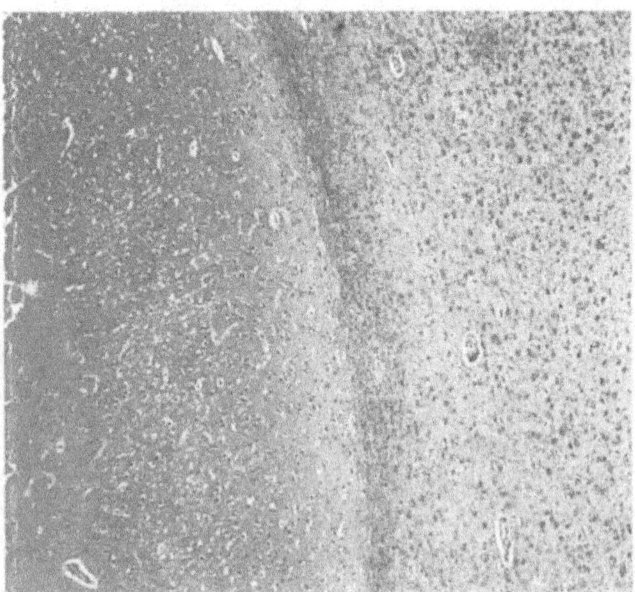

FIGURE 4.96Q

   A. Multiple sclerosis

   B. Cerebral edema

   C. Metachromatic leukodystrophy

   D. Progressive multifocal leukoencephalopathy

   E. Low-grade astrocytoma

97. What neoplasm is depicted in the following photomicrograph (Figure 4.97Q)?

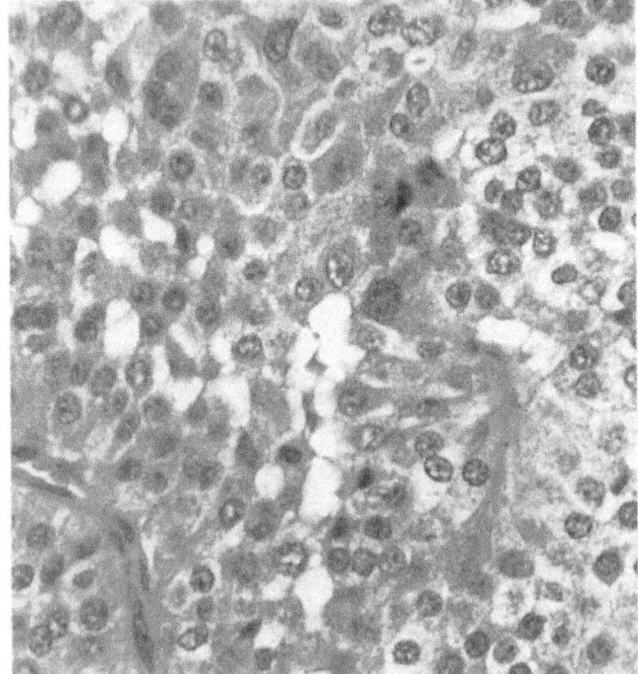

FIGURE 4.97Q

   A. Pituitary adenoma

   B. Metastatic carcinoma

   C. Ganglioglioma

   D. Oligodendroglioma

   E. Pineoblastoma

98. All of the following are associated with Tay-Sachs disease EXCEPT?

- **A.** Autosomal dominant inheritance
- **B.** Results from β-hexosaminidase A deficiency
- **C.** Results in intraneuronal accumulation of G_{M2} gangliosides
- **D.** Associated with blindness in infants
- **E.** Associated with ataxia in young adults

99. Which of the following genetic characteristics is not typically associated with secondary glioblastomas that result from anaplastic progression of low-grade astrocytomas (as opposed to de novo glioblastomas)?

- **A.** Amplification of the epidermal growth factor receptor (EGFR) gene
- **B.** p53 mutations
- **C.** CDK4 gene amplification
- **D.** Loss of heterozygosity of 9p
- **E.** Loss of heterozygosity of 19q

100. What is the most common chromosome involved with cytogenic aberrations in glioblastoma multiforme?

- **A.** Chromosome X
- **B.** Chromosome 11
- **C.** Chromosome 10
- **D.** Chromosome 7
- **E.** Chromosome 22

QUESTIONS 101–102

101. What is depicted in the electron micrograph below (Figure 4.101–4.102Q)?

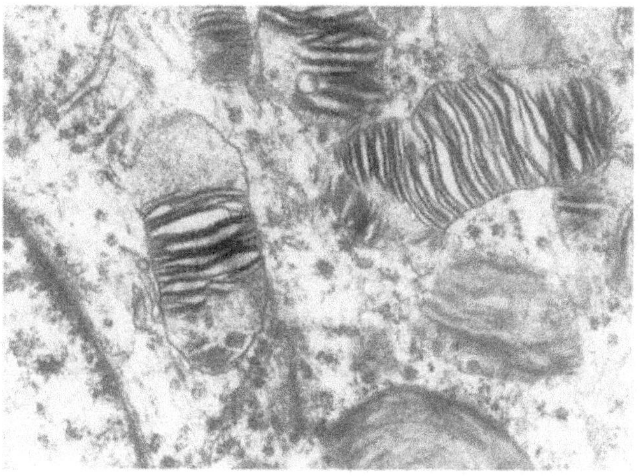

FIGURE 4.101–102Q

- **A.** Ragged red muscle fibers
- **B.** Zebra bodies
- **C.** Bunina body
- **D.** Axonal spheroids
- **E.** Negri body

102. What is the most likely diagnosis?

- **A.** Rabies
- **B.** Pellagra
- **C.** Amyotrophic lateral sclerosis
- **D.** Hurler's syndrome
- **E.** Leber's hereditary optic neuropathy

End of set

103. What is the most likely diagnosis (Figure 4.103Q)?

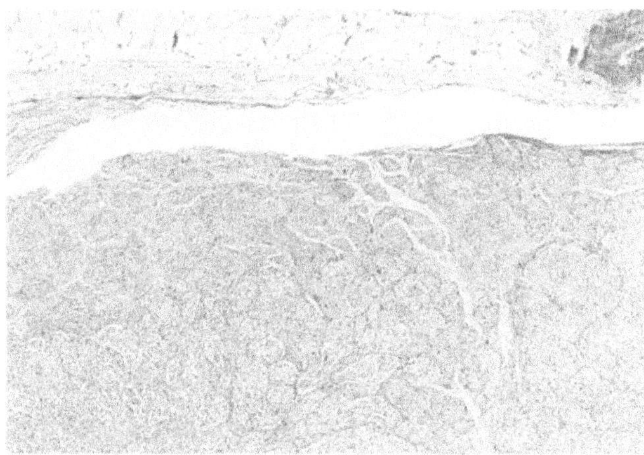

FIGURE 4.103Q

- **A.** Acoustic neuroma
- **B.** Tuberculoma
- **C.** Multiple sclerosis
- **D.** Low-grade astrocytoma
- **E.** Dejerine-Sottas disease

QUESTIONS 104–108

Directions: Match the hormone production (Table 4.104–4.108Q) with the associated germ cell neoplasm (numbered items), using each answer once [(+) = immunoreactive; (–) = not immunoreactive; (+/–) = may be immunoreactive].

TABLE 4.104–108Q

TUMOR	ALPHA FETOPROTEIN (AFP)	BETA SUBUNIT OF HUMAN CHORIONIC GONADOTROPIN (B-HCG)	PLACENTAL ALKALINE PHOSPHATASE
A	–	–	+
B	+/–	+/–	+/–
C	+	+/–	+/–
D	+/–	+	+/–
E	+/–	–	–

104. Teratoma

105. Yolk sac tumor

106. Embryonal carcinoma

107. Germinoma

108. Choriocarcinoma

End of set

109. What is the ultrastructural homologue of the miniature endplate potential?

  A. Vimentin
  B. Synaptic vesicle
  C. Postsynaptic membrane
  D. Gap junctions
  E. Sarcomere

110. What neoplasm is depicted in the photomicrograph below (Figure 4.110Q)?

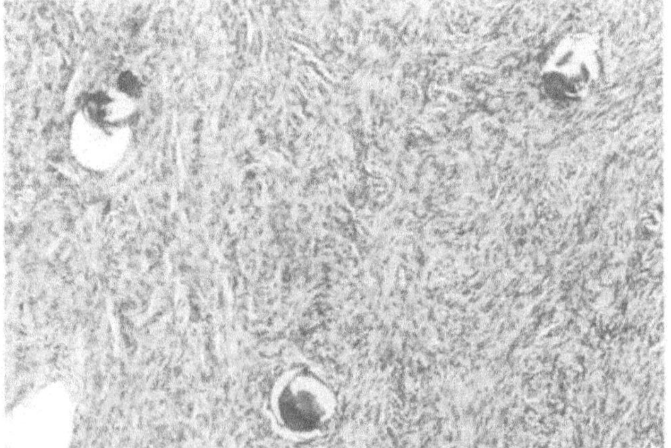

FIGURE 4.110Q

  A. Psammomatous meningioma
  B. Microcystic meningioma
  C. Pilocytic astrocytoma
  D. Craniopharyngioma
  E. Ependymoma

111. What neoplasm is depicted in the photomicrograph below (Figure 4.111Q)?

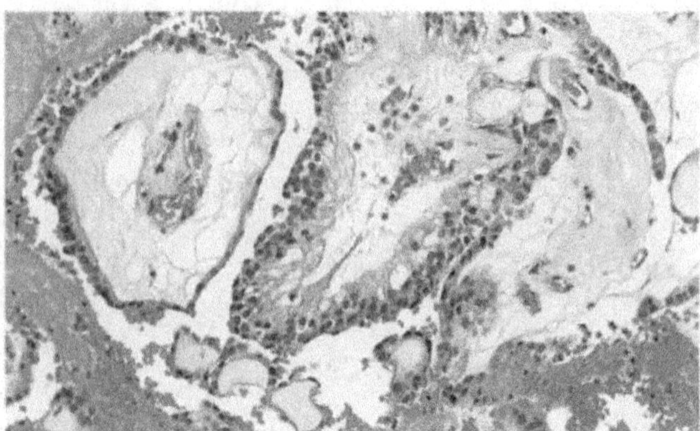

FIGURE 4.111Q

  A. Pleomorphic xanthoastrocytoma
  B. Choroid plexus papilloma
  C. Dermoid tumor
  D. Papillary meningioma
  E. Myxopapillary ependymoma

112. Which of the following meningioma variants is a World Health Organization (WHO) grade II neoplasm?

  A. Psammomatous
  B. Microcystic
  C. Papillary
  D. Secretory
  E. Clear cell

QUESTIONS 113–115

113. Patients with homocystinuria often present with all of the following clinical features EXCEPT?

- **A.** Marfanoid appearance
- **B.** Ectopia lentis
- **C.** Seizures
- **D.** Biconcave (codfish) vertebrae
- **E.** Diabetes insipidus

114. What is the enzyme abnormality of this disorder?

- **A.** Hypoxanthine-guanine phosphoribosyl transferase deficiency
- **B.** Phenylalanine hydroxylase
- **C.** Cystathionine β-synthase deficiency
- **D.** Alpha-ketoacid dehydrogenase deficiency
- **E.** None of the above

115. Treatment of this disease may include all of the following EXCEPT which?

- **A.** Restriction of dietary methionine
- **B.** Pyridoxine supplements
- **C.** Vitamin B_{12} supplements
- **D.** Cysteine supplements
- **E.** L-5-hydroxytryptophan supplements

End of set

116. A photomicrograph from a patient with AIDS is depicted below (Figure 4.116Q). What is the diagnosis?

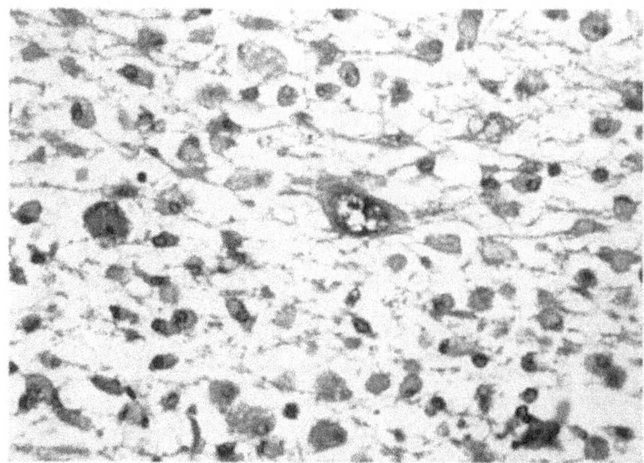

FIGURE 4.116Q

- **A.** Lymphoma
- **B.** Cryptococcal infection
- **C.** HIV encephalopathy
- **D.** Progressive multifocal leukoencephalopathy
- **E.** Toxoplasmosis

117. What is depicted in the photomicrograph below (Figure 4.117Q)?

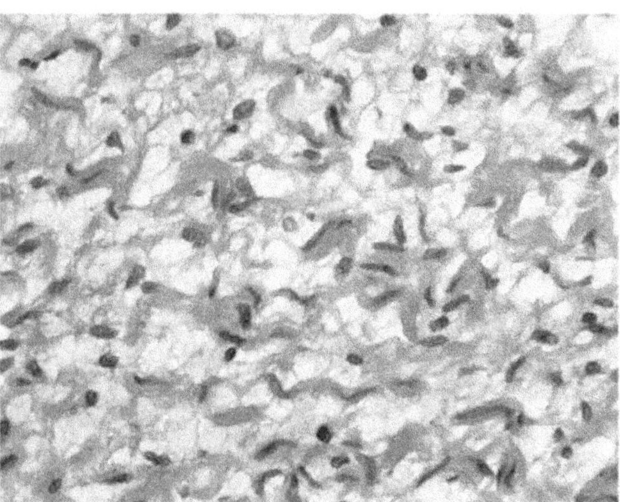

FIGURE 4.117Q

- **A.** Neurofibroma
- **B.** Pilocytic astrocytoma
- **C.** Skeletal muscle
- **D.** Schwannoma
- **E.** Malignant peripheral nerve sheath tumor

QUESTIONS 118–119

118. The neoplasm depicted in the photomicrograph below (Figure 4.118–4.119Q) is typically positive for which immunostains?

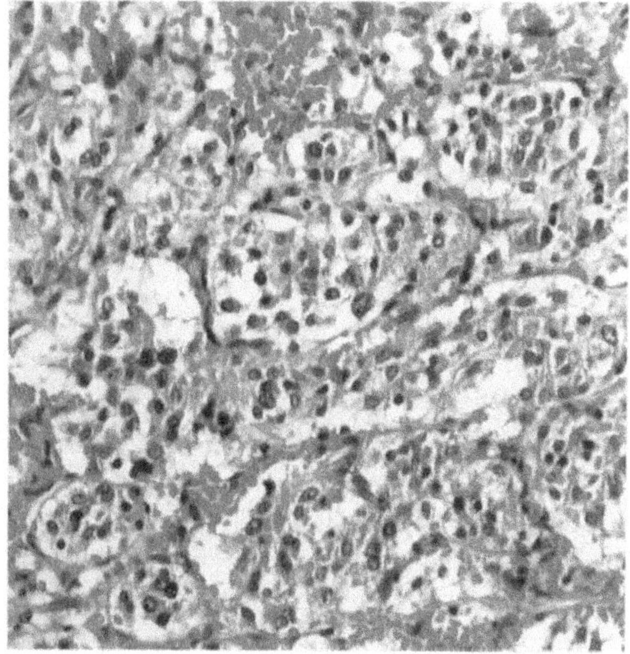

FIGURE 4.118–119Q

1. Synaptophysin	**A.** 1, 2, and 3 are correct
2. S-100	**B.** 1 and 3 are correct
3. Chromogranin	**C.** 2 and 4 are correct
4. GFAP	**D.** Only 4 is correct
	E. All of the above

119. What is the diagnosis?

- **A.** Pituitary adenoma
- **B.** Paraganglioma of the filum terminale
- **C.** Ganglioglioma
- **D.** Germinoma
- **E.** Astrocytoma

End of set

120. What neoplasm is depicted in the photomicrograph below (Figure 4.120Q)?

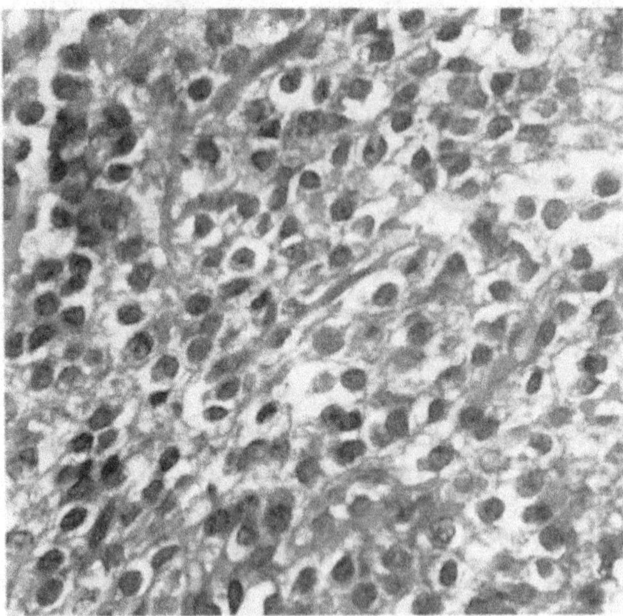

FIGURE 4.120Q

- **A.** Lymphoma
- **B.** Subependymoma
- **C.** Melanoma
- **D.** Medulloblastoma
- **E.** Central neurocytoma

121. Which of the following is correct about a grade II subependymal germinal matrix hemorrhage?

- **A.** Confined to the germinal matrix region
- **B.** Involves the germinal matrix and ventricle without ventricular dilation
- **C.** Involves the germinal matrix, ventricle, and adjacent brain parenchyma
- **D.** Involves the germinal matrix, ventricle, adjacent parenchyma, and basal cisterns
- **E.** Involves the germinal matrix and brain parenchyma only

122. What is depicted by the gross specimen below (Figure 4.122Q)?

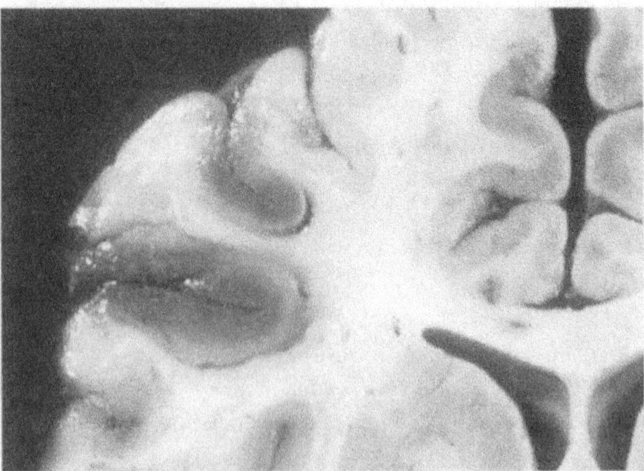

FIGURE 4.122Q

- **A.** Multiple sclerosis
- **B.** Kernicterus
- **C.** Laminar necrosis
- **D.** Heterotopic gray matter
- **E.** Fat emboli

QUESTIONS 123–124

123. What is depicted by the gross specimen below (Figure 4.123–4.124Q)?

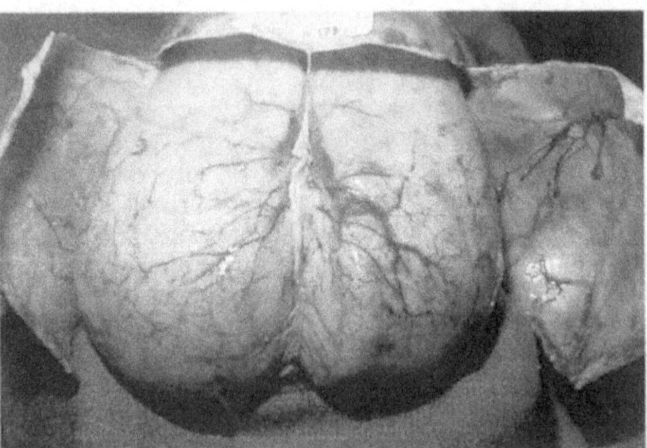

FIGURE 4.123–124Q

- **A.** Tuberous sclerosis
- **B.** Sturge-Weber syndrome
- **C.** Occipital encephalocele
- **D.** Agyria
- **E.** Subdural empyema

124. This abnormality often results from faulty

- **A.** Primary neurulation
- **B.** Secondary neurulation
- **C.** Diverticulation and cleavage
- **D.** Cellular migration
- **E.** Myelination

End of set

QUESTIONS 125–126

125. What is depicted in the photomicrograph below (Figure 4.125–4.126Q)?

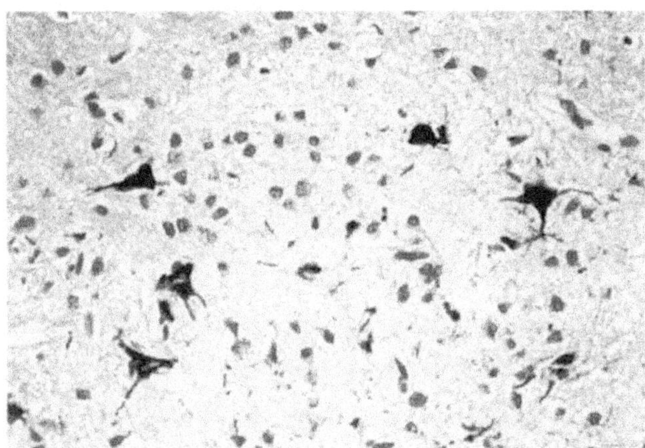

FIGURE 4.125–126Q

- **A.** Pick bodies
- **B.** Chronic multiple sclerosis plaque
- **C.** Cortical dysplasia
- **D.** Siderocalcinosis
- **E.** Neurofibrillary tangles

126. The finding in this photomicrograph may have resulted from what pathologic event?

- **A.** An autoimmune disorder
- **B.** Neurodegeneration
- **C.** Viral infection
- **D.** Developmental anomaly
- **E.** Chronic infarct

End of set

127. What is depicted in the photomicrograph below (Figure 4.127)?

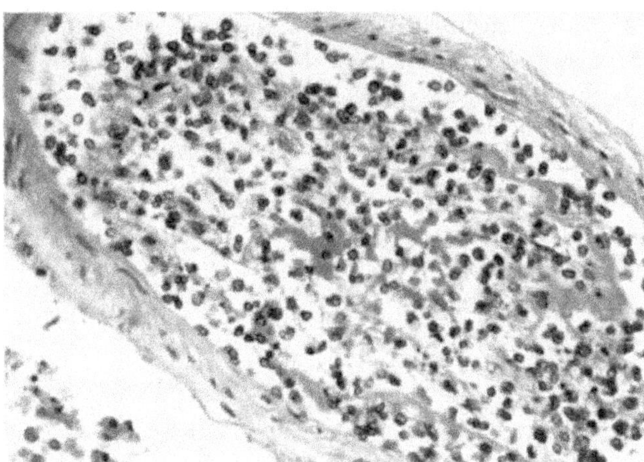

FIGURE 4.127Q

- **A.** Bacterial meningitis
- **B.** Ependymoma
- **C.** Anaplastic astrocytoma
- **D.** Amyloid angiopathy
- **E.** None of the above

QUESTIONS 128–130

128. What infectious process is depicted in the photomicrograph below (Figure 4.128–4.130Q)?

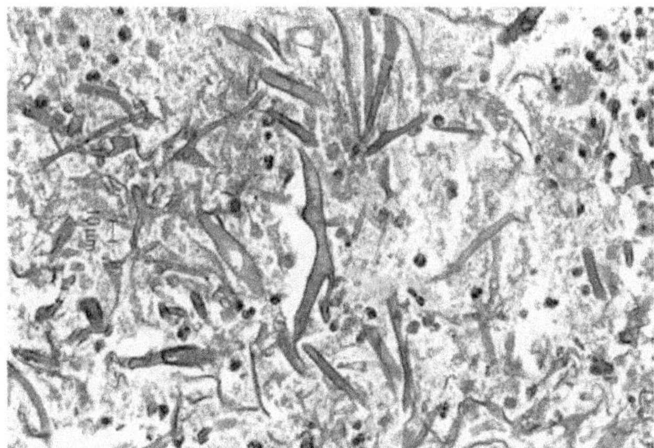

FIGURE 4.128–130Q

- **A.** Aspergillosis
- **B.** Mucormycosis
- **C.** Rabies
- **D.** Histoplasmosis
- **E.** Toxoplasmosis

129. This infection most commonly spreads to the brain by what route?

    A. Hematogenous spread from the lungs
    B. Through the trigeminal nerve from the skin
    C. Through the cribriform plate from the nasal mucosa
    D. From the facial vein secondary to a tooth abscess
    E. From the middle ear canal

130. What patients have an increased risk of acquiring this infection?

    A. Those with HIV
    B. Pregnant patients
    C. Diabetic patients with ketoacidosis
    D. Coal miners
    E. Veterinarians

End of set

QUESTIONS 131–132

131. What neoplasm is depicted in the photomicrograph below (Figure 4.131–4.132Q)?

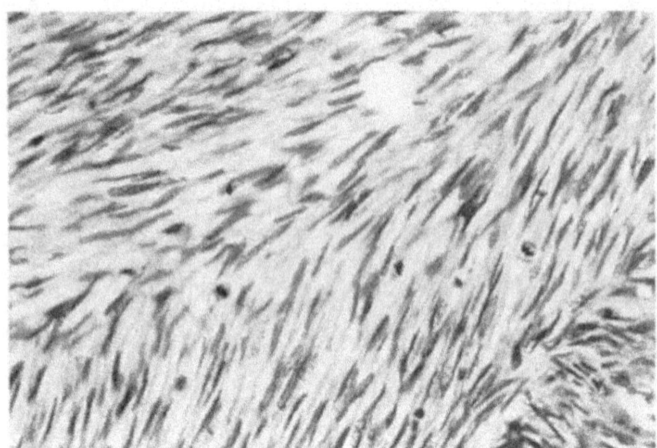

FIGURE 4.131–132Q

    A. Pilocytic astrocytoma
    B. Transitional meningioma
    C. Malignant nerve sheath tumor
    D. Acoustic neuroma
    E. Pituitary adenoma

132. This neoplasm most often involves which cranial nerve?

    A. Oculomotor (CN III)
    B. Trigeminal nerve (CN V)
    C. Facial nerve (CN VII)
    D. Vestibulocochlear nerve (CN VIII)
    E. Spinal accessory nerve (XI)

End of set

QUESTIONS 133–135

Directions: Match the metastatic neoplasm with the corresponding photomicrograph (Figures 4.133–4.135Q a, b, c) depicted below, using each answer once.

(a)

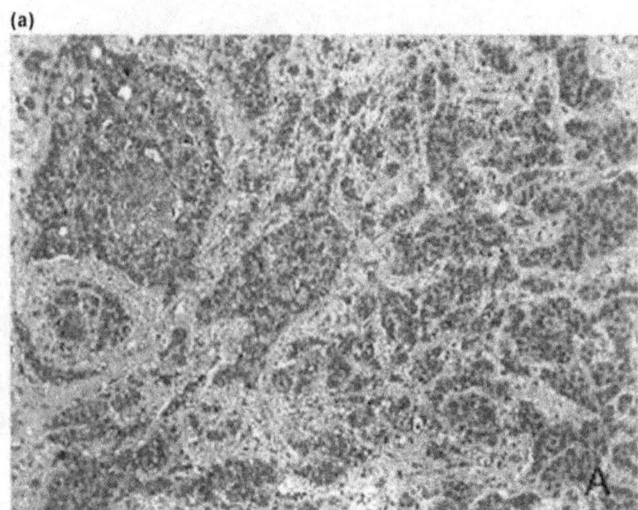

(b)

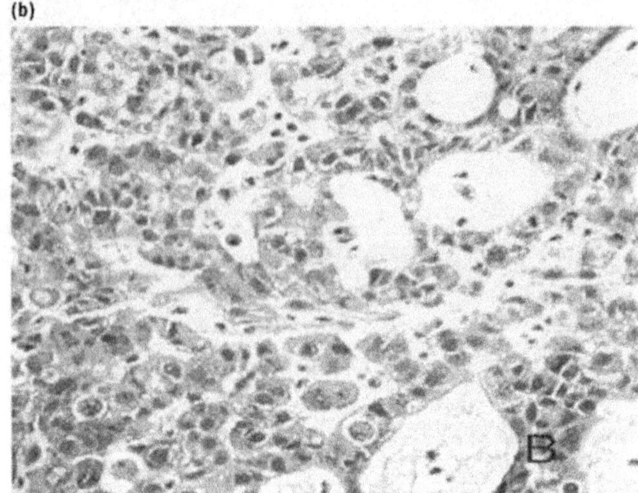

(c)

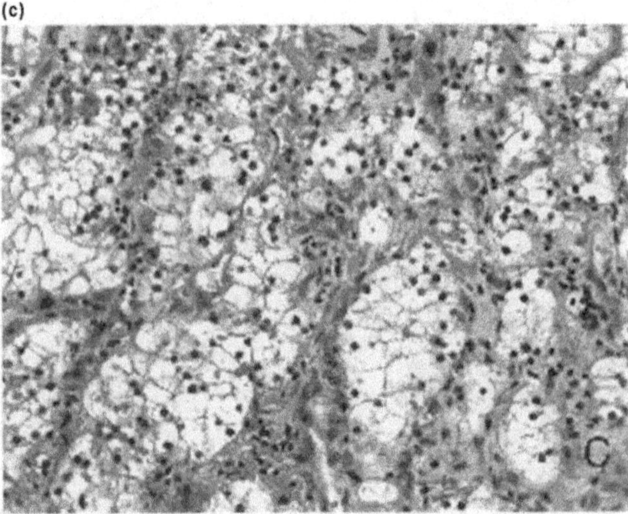

FIGURE 4.133–135Q

133. Renal cell carcinoma

134. Breast cancer

135. Lung adenocarcinoma

End of set

136. What is depicted in the photomicrograph below (Figure 4.136Q)?

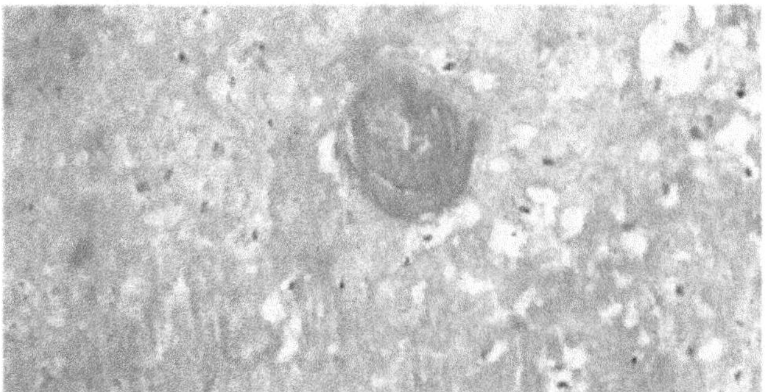

FIGURE 4.136Q

  A. Central pontine myelinosis
  B. Low-grade astrocytoma
  C. Subependymoma
  D. Radiation necrosis
  E. Microglial nodule

137. What is depicted on this gross section (Figure 4.137Q)?

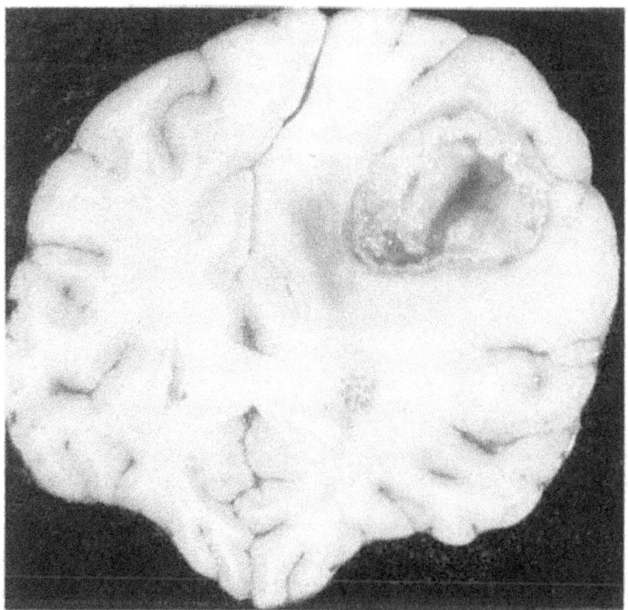

FIGURE 4.137Q

  A. Multiple sclerosis plaque
  B. Pilocytic astrocytoma
  C. Lymphoma
  D. Cerebral abscess
  E. Embolic infarct

QUESTIONS 138–139

138. What is depicted in the photomicrograph below (Figure 4.138–4.139Q)?

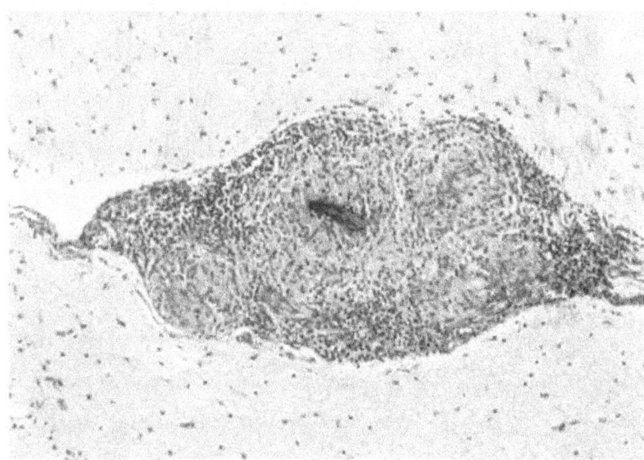

FIGURE 4.138–139Q

  A. Amputation neuroma
  B. Noncaseating granuloma
  C. Acoustic neuroma
  D. Paraganglioma
  E. Chronic multiple sclerosis plaque

139. This finding would be most consistent with what diagnosis?

  A. Acoustic neuroma
  B. Trauma
  C. Neurosarcoidosis
  D. Tuberculosis
  E. Leigh's disease

End of set

QUESTIONS 140–149

Directions: Match the following questions with the type of neuropathy produced using each answer once, more than once, or not at all.

  A. Axonal
  B. Demyelinating
  C. Both
  D. None of the above

140. Thallium

141. Thiamine

142. Colchicine

143. Nitrous oxide

144. HIV

145. Chloramphenicol

146. Phenytoin

147. AIDS

148. Gold

149. Diphtheria

End of set

150. What is depicted in the photomicrograph below (Figure 4.150Q)?

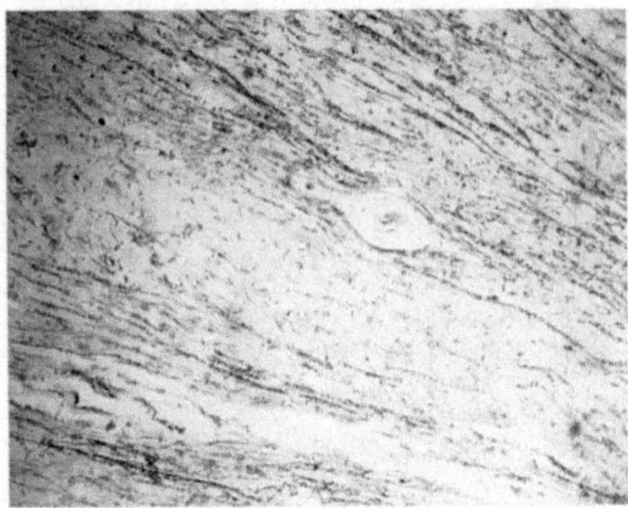

FIGURE 4.150Q

A. Acute infarct
B. Chronic infarct
C. Progressive multifocal leukoencephalopathy
D. Amyloid angiopathy
E. Neurofibrillary tangles

QUESTIONS 151–156

Directions: Match the inclusion body with the associated photomicrograph (Figures 4.151–4.156Q a, b, c, d, e, f) using each answer once.

(a)

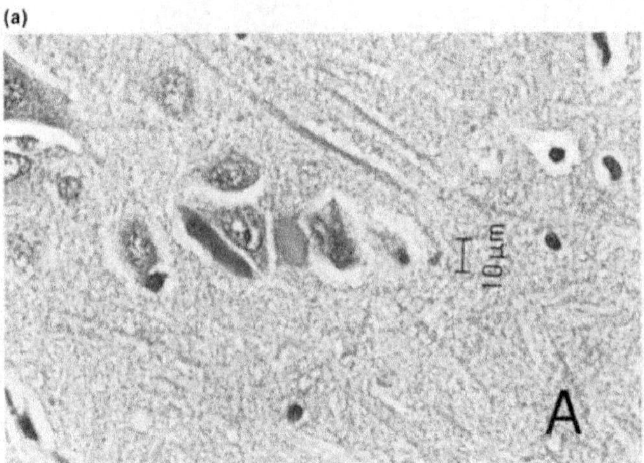

(b)

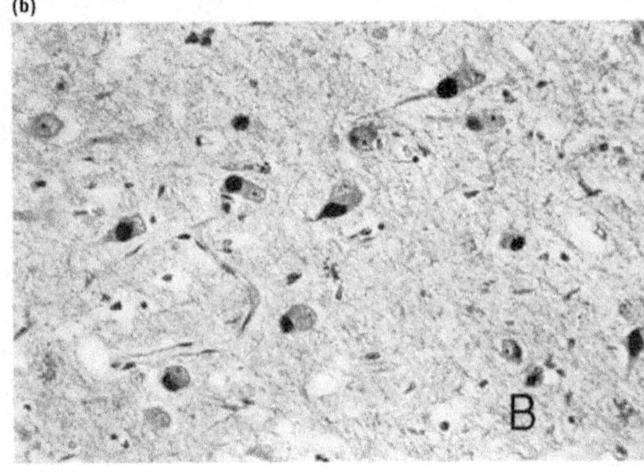

(c)

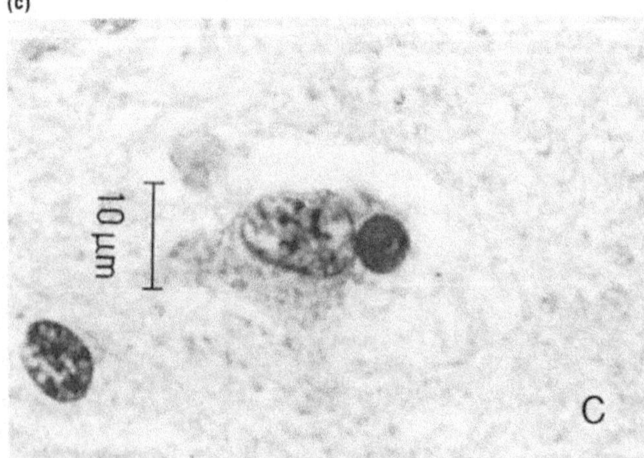

FIGURE 4.151–156Q

(d)

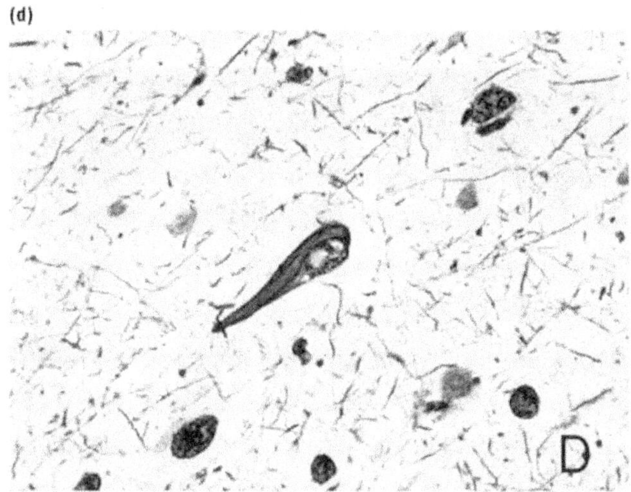

(e)

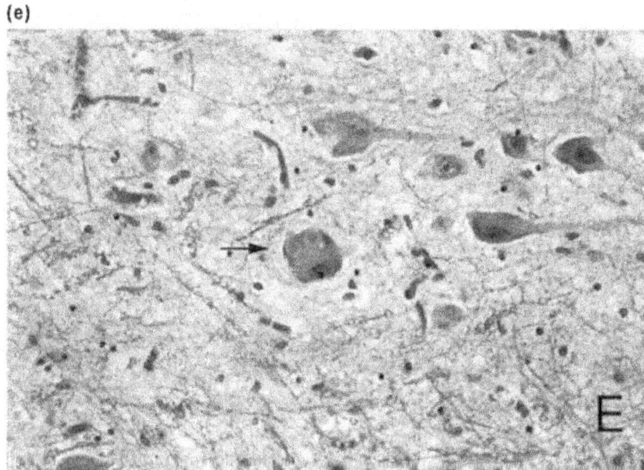

(f)

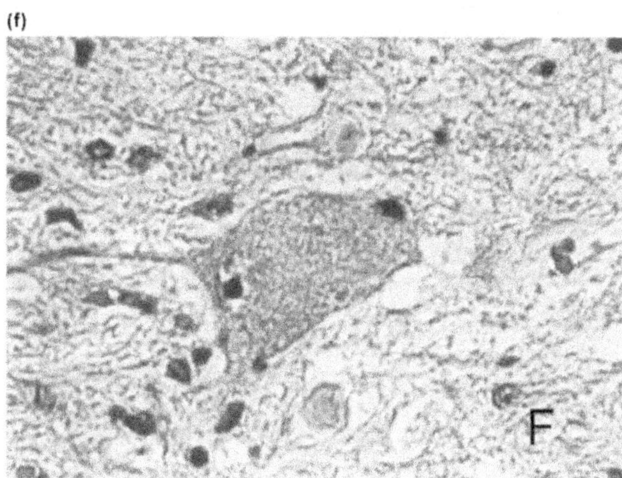

FIGURE 4.151–4.156Q Continued

151. Negri body

152. Hirano body

153. Lewy body

154. Pick body

155. Neurofibrillary body

156. Bunina body

End of set

QUESTIONS 157–159

157. What neoplasm is associated with opsoclonus, my-oclonus, and encephalopathy?

- **A.** Astroblastoma
- **B.** Teratoma
- **C.** Neuroblastoma
- **D.** Rhabdoid tumor
- **E.** Pilocytic astrocytoma

158. This neoplasm most commonly originates from the

- **A.** Sympathetic chain
- **B.** Adrenal glands
- **C.** Ependymal cells
- **D.** Pineal gland
- **E.** Optic nerve

159. What gene is most frequently amplified in patients harboring this lesion?

- **A.** N-*myc*
- **B.** *Ras*
- **C.** *RB1*
- **D.** *MEN1*
- **E.** *p53*

End of set

QUESTIONS 160–168

Directions: Match the medication with the associated complication, using each answer once, more than once, or not at all.

- **A.** Isotretinoin
- **B.** Tamoxifen
- **C.** Interleukin-2
- **D.** Cyclosporine
- **E.** Anti-CD3
- **F.** Vinblastine
- **G.** Vincristine
- **H.** Carboplatin
- **I.** None of the above

160. Muscle pain

161. Pseudotumor cerebri

162. Decreased visual acuity

163. Peripheral neuropathy, hearing loss, cortical blindness

164. Hypertrichosis

165. Tremor

166. Parkinsonism

167. Decreased ADH secretion

168. Primary CNS lymphoma

End of set

169. Hypertrophied nerves often accompany all of the following conditions EXCEPT?

A. Amyloidosis
B. Refsum's disease
C. Leprosy
D. Acromegaly
E. Alcoholism

170. What is depicted in this gross specimen (Figure 4.170Q)?

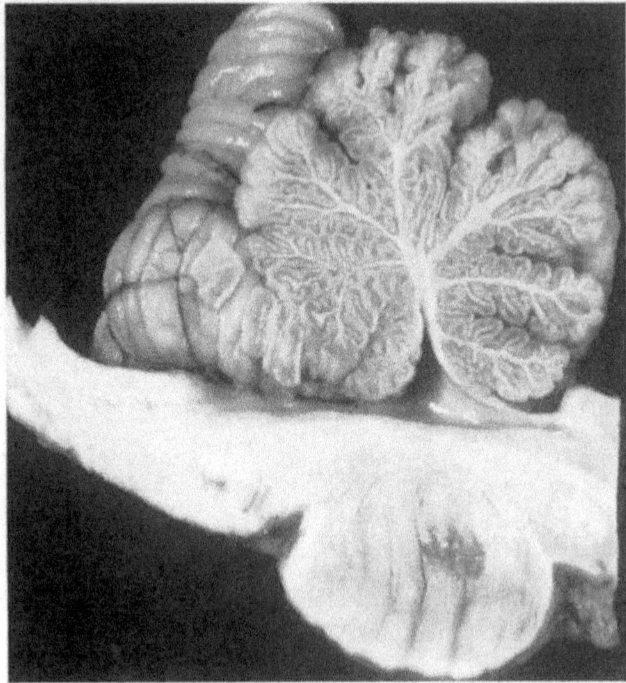

FIGURE 4.170Q

A. Alcoholic cerebellar degeneration
B. Metastatic tumor
C. Multiple sclerosis
D. Chiari malformation
E. Aqueductal stenosis

171. What is depicted in this gross specimen (Figure 4.71Q)?

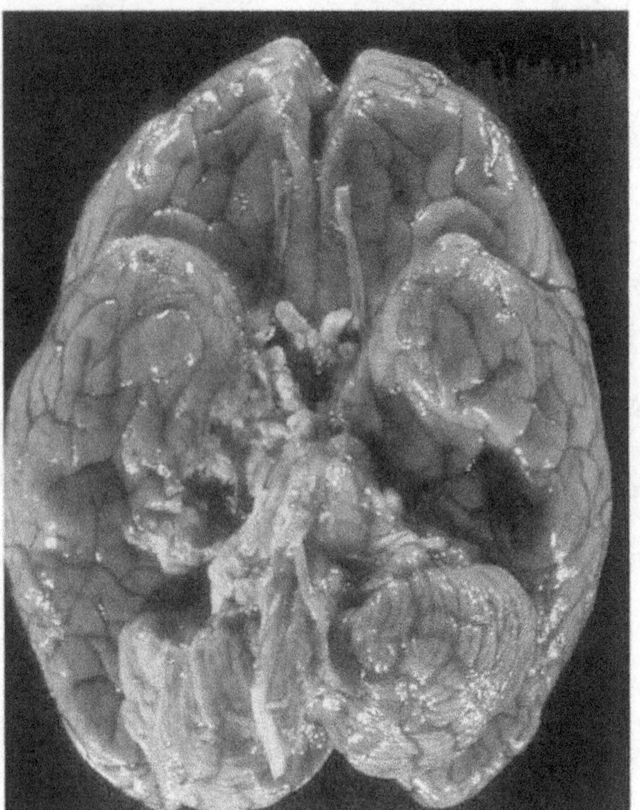

FIGURE 4.171Q

A. Acoustic neuroma
B. Tuberculosis
C. Epidermoid tumor
D. Basilar apex aneurysm
E. Optic nerve glioma

172. What is depicted in the photomicrograph below (Figure 4.172Q)?

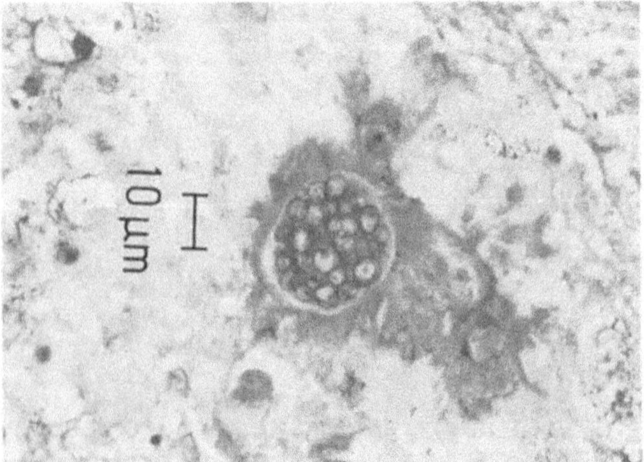

FIGURE 4.172Q

A. Coccidioidomycosis
B. Histoplasmosis
C. Toxoplasmosis
D. Cryptococcal meningitis
E. Mucormycosis

173. What is depicted in this gross specimen (Figure 4.173Q)?

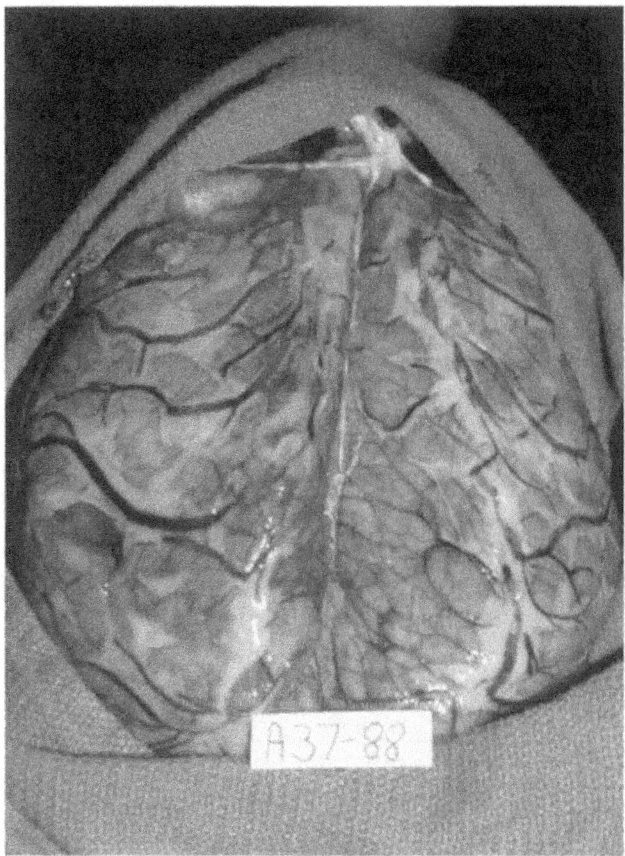

FIGURE 4.173Q

A. Purulent meningitis
B. Traumatic brain injury
C. Embolic stroke
D. Watershed infarct
E. None of the above

174. What fungal species is characterized by nonseptate hyphae?

A. *Candida*
B. *Cryptococcus*
C. *Blastomyces*
D. *Mucor*
E. *Cladosporium*

175. What is depicted in the photomicrograph below (Figure 4.175Q)?

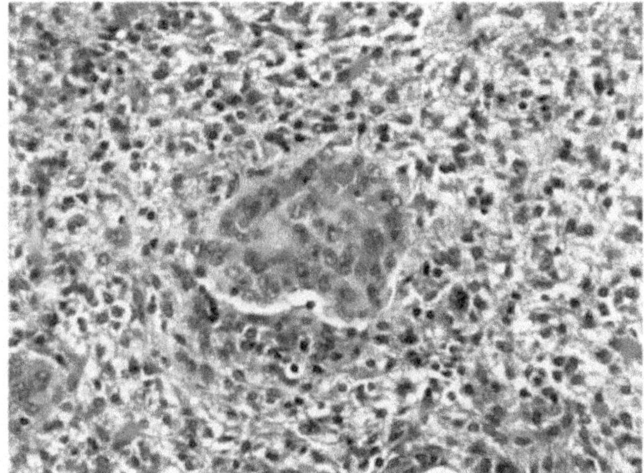

FIGURE 4.175Q

A. Glomeruloid vascular proliferation of a glioblastoma
B. Homer-Wright rosette of a pinealcytoma
C. Microglial nodule
D. Angiomatous meningioma
E. Neuronophagia

Neuropathology Answer Key

1. D	36. C	71. E	106. B	141. A
2. B	37. C	72. A	107. A	142. A
3. C	38. B	73. D	108. D	143. A
4. D	39. E	74. B	109. B	144. B
5. D	40. E	75. B	110. A	145. A
6. C	41. D	76. C	111. E	146. A
7. E	42. B	77. B	112. E	147. A
8. A	43. C	78. B	113. E	148. A
9. A	44. B	79. D	114. C	149. B
10. E	45. A	80. B	115. E	150. B
11. B	46. B	81. D	116. D	151. C
12. B	47. B	82. A	117. A	152. A
13. C	48. A	83. A	118. A	153. E
14. D	49. C	84. E	119. B	154. B
15. A	50. E	85. B	120. E	155. D
16. B	51. D	86. C	121. B	156. F
17. D	52. B	87. E	122. C	157. C
18. C	53. B	88. D	123. D	158. B
19. C	54. A	89. A	124. D	159. A
20. D	55. E	90. D	125. D	160. F
21. D	56. D	91. E	126. E	161. A
22. E	57. E	92. B	127. A	162. B
23. B	58. A	93. D	128. B	163. H
24. A	59. B	94. D	129. C	164. D
25. C	60. C	95. D	130. C	165. D
26. C	61. D	96. C	131. C	166. C
27. A	62. A	97. A	132. B	167. G
28. D	63. B	98. A	133. C	168. D
29. A	64. B	99. A	134. A	169. E
30. B	65. C	100. D	135. B	170. A
31. C	66. B	101. B	136. D	171. C
32. D	67. C	102. D	137. D	172. A
33. A	68. B	103. E	138. B	173. A
34. E	69. E	104. E	139. C	174. D
35. D	70. A	105. C	140. A	175. A

Neuropathology Answers

1. D. Pilocytic astrocytomas typically have a biphasic appearance. They usually consist of regions of elongated cells arranged in compact fascicles intermixed with regions of stellate cells that encompass microcysts. Pilocytic astrocytomas can exhibit some nuclear pleomorphism and hyperchromasia, but mitoses and necrosis are absent. These tumors are classically associated with Rosenthal fibers and intracellular eosinophilic globules (granular bodies). Intracellular eosinophilic conglomerations can also be observed in pleomorphic xanthoastrocytoma but not anaplastic astrocytoma or oligodendroglioma. Gemistocytic astrocytoma is characterized by large, plump astrocytes with diffuse, glassy cytoplasm (Ellison, pp. 630–634; WHO, pp. 25, 45–54, 56–64).

2. B. Neurofibrillary tangles (NFTs) are cytoplasmic, basophilic structures that are prevalent in neurons in patients with Alzheimer's disease (AD). NFTs contain large amounts of paired helical filament protein, which largely consists of hyperphosphorylated tau. Tau protein is also phosphorylated in normal brain; however, these phosphate groups are easily removed by phosphatases. The hyperphosphorylated tau of NFTs is largely resistant to phosphatases, which may be a key feature in its deposition in AD. Other key features of AD include Hirano bodies (which are composed of actin), amyloid plaques, and granulovacuolar degeneration (which primarily affects hippocampal neurons). Amyloid plaques are extracellular deposits of amyloid and preamyloid material, which are easily demonstrated with silver stains and immunohistochemical stains for Aβ peptide. Diffuse plaques contain normal neuronal processes and lack tau protein. Classic (mature) plaques often consist of dense core regions with a peripheral halo and may stain positive for tau protein (Ellison, pp. 550–565).

3. C. Glioblastoma multiforme (GBM) is characterized by cellular pleomorphism and a diversity of histologic appearances. Regardless of the predominant histologic pattern of a particular GBM, cytologic pleomorphism, nuclear hyperchromasia, and frequent mitoses are often observed. By definition, tumor necrosis and/or microvascular proliferation is present. Pseudopalisading of neoplastic cells around a central necrotic region (pseudopalisading necrosis), as depicted here, is characteristic of GBMs. These features easily distinguish GBM from low-grade astrocytomas; medulloblastomas exhibit a more homogenous population of small blue cells that lack pseudopalisading necrosis. Lymphomas are characterized by sheets of neoplastic lymphocytes that often surround blood vessels and occasionally exhibit necrosis (Ellison, pp. 628–630; WHO, pp. 27–28, 29–39, 129–132, 199–201).

4. D. Neurofibromatosis type 1 is associated with abnormalities of the neurofibromin gene, which is located on chromosome 17q11. NF1 exhibits autosomal inheritance with almost complete penetrance; however, approximately 50% of all cases are secondary to spontaneous mutations. Neurofibromin is a guanosine triphosphatase–activating protein that is important for cell proliferation and differentiation (Ellison, pp. 695–696; WHO, pp. 216–218).

5. D. Congenital CMV infection represents the most common intrauterine viral infection, affecting 0.5 to 2.0% of all births. Macroscopically, CMV infection is characterized by microcephaly, periventricular and basal ganglial calcifications, and hydrocephalus. Microscopically, CMV infections exhibit microglial nodules, cytomegalic inclusion cells, ventriculoencephalitis, and gliosis. Infants with congenital CMV infections can also exhibit mental retardation, seizures, chorioretinitis, optic atrophy, sensorineural hearing loss, and death in 30% of acute infections (Ellison, pp. 284–286).

6. C. Opalski cells are round, with a small central nucleus and prominent granular eosinophilic cytoplasm. These cells are most commonly observed in the globus pallidus in patients with Wilson's disease (hepatolenticular degeneration) and acquired hepatic encephalopathy (Ellison, pp. 429–432).

7. E. Lewy bodies are associated with Parkinson's disease and are composed of neurofilament proteins (form the cytoskeleton of the inclusion), ubiquitin (involved in cytosolic proteolysis), αB crystallin (neurofilament chaperone protein), and α–synuclein (catalyze phosphorylation of neurofilaments). Immunohistochemical stains for ubiquitin are among the most sensitive methods of identifying Lewy bodies (Ellison, pp. 511–513).

8. A. Canavan's disease (spongiform leukodystrophy) is an autosomal recessive disorder characterized by extensive vacuolation of the white matter due to the widespread loss of myelin at the gray-white junction. Although cortical neurons are normal, there are numerous Alzheimer type II astrocytes within the gray matter. Cortical changes include enlarged pale astrocytes in the deeper cortical layers that contain abnormally long mitochondria with ladder-like cristae, an abnormality unique to Canavan's disease. Canavan's disease does not spare the subcortical U fibers and is a result of deficiencies of the enzyme aspartoacylase (Ellison, pp. 121–122, 125).

9. A. Fibrillary astrocytoma is characterized by atypical astrocytes in a loose fibrillary matrix. The neoplastic cells lack visible cytoplasm and show features of mild nuclear atypia, such as hyperchromasia, elongation, or angulation. As in this case, microcysts are often prominent. Mitoses, necrosis, and endothelial proliferation are not observed. Reactive astrocytosis can occasionally be confused with a fibrillary astrocytoma; however, astrocytosis is characterized by an even distribution of slightly enlarged astrocytic nuclei with abundant cytoplasm and long, tapering processes. There is usually no significant hypercellularity in reactive astrocytosis. Microcysts are also not observed with reactive astrocytosis (Ellison, pp. 623–628; WHO, pp. 24–25).

10. E. NF-2 is an autosomal dominant condition that is most commonly associated with bilateral schwannomas of the eighth cranial nerve and multiple intracranial meningiomas. NF-2 is also associated with schwannomas of other cranial nerves, spinal meningiomas, astrocytomas (spinal, brainstem, and cerebellar), and spinal ependymomas. Spinal schwannomas are occasionally observed with NF-2, although spinal neurofibromas and plexiform neurofibromas are not (WHO, pp. 219–222; Ellison, pp. 696–699; Kaye and Laws, pp. 71–76).

11. B. The photomicrograph illustrates the classic spongiform change that is associated with Creutzfeldt-Jakob disease (CJD). CJD usually affects adults in the sixth to eighth decades of life. Approximately 85% of all cases of CJD are sporadic and 10% are familial. Microscopically, CJD is characterized by neuronal loss, astrocytosis, spongiform change (fine vacuolation of the neuropil), and a lack of inflammation. Clinically, CJD is characterized initially by subtle motor signs and ataxia, followed by a rapidly progressive dementing illness that culminates in severe myoclonus, akinetic mutism, and death within 1 year from initial symptom onset. The prion diseases, including CJD, Gerstmann-Straussler-Scheinker disease, fatal familial insomnia, and kuru, are believed to have a common molecular pathology that involves the conversion of a normal cellular protein (encoded on human chromosome 20), called prion protein (PrP), into an abnormal isoform that is resistant to protease degradation (PrP^{res}). This abnormal isoform is believed to accumulate within cells, and also outside of cells in the form of amyloid. Although immunostaining for PrP^{res} is diagnostic for CJD, the CSF immunoassay for protein 14-3-3 has 96%

sensitivity and specificity for detecting CJD among patients with dementia. The characteristic EEG findings include bilateral, symmetric, and periodic bi- or triphasic synchronous sharp-wave complexes (periodic spikes, 0.5 to 2/s), which have 70% sensitivity and 86% specificity for CJD. Fully effective and recommended operating room procedures for instrument sterilization includes steam autoclaving for 1 hour at 132°C or immersion in 1N sodium hydroxide (NaOH) for 1 hour at room temperature. Partially effective procedures include steam autoclaving at either 121 or 132°C for 15 to 30 minutes, immersion in 1N NaOH for 15 minutes, or immersion in sodium hypochlorite (household bleach) undiluted or up to 1:10 dilution (0.5%) for 1 hour. Ineffective sterilization procedures include boiling, UV light, ionizing radiation, ethylene oxide, ethanol, formalin, beta-propiolactone, ammonium compounds, iodine, or acetone (Ellison, pp. 585–598; Greenberg, pp. 228–231).

12-B; 13-C; 14-D; 15-A; 16-B. Marinesco bodies are small eosinophilic intranuclear inclusions that are prominent in neurons of the substantia nigra and are composed largely of ubiquitin and intermediate filaments. Lafora bodies are composed of polysaccharide polymers (polyglucosans) and have a round core that is strongly PAS-positive. Bunina bodies are small eosinophilic inclusions that are observed in motor neuron diseases such as amyotrophic lateral sclerosis. Hirano bodies are brightly eosinophilic cytoplasmic inclusions that are prominent in hippocampal neurons in Alzheimer's disease. Hirano bodies are composed of actin and actin-associated proteins. Pick bodies are slightly basophilic neuronal cytoplasmic inclusions that are observed in all layers of the cerebral cortex and some subcortical nuclei in patients with Pick's disease. Pick bodies consist of ubiquitin, tubulin, tau, and chromogranin-A (Ellison, pp. 7–10, 504–505, 552, 566–567, 570–572).

17. D. Arteriovenous malformations (AVMs) are characterized by clusters of dilated vessels of varying diameters with abnormally thick or thin walls and occasional intervening brain parenchyma. AVMs often contain calcification, and the surrounding brain parenchyma may exhibit prominent astrocytosis. Capillary telangiectasias consist of much smaller, uniformly thin-walled vascular channels without evidence of hemorrhage or surrounding astrocytosis. Cavernous malformations are characterized by tightly packed hyalinized vascular channels without elastic tissue. There is usually no intervening brain parenchyma. Venous angiomas are composed of thin-walled, dilated vascular channels interspersed among normal brain parenchyma (Ellison, pp. 226–233).

18. C. Chronic subdural hematomas (SDH) are usually initiated from the tearing of bridging veins, which can often be precipitated by minimal trauma in patients with significant cerebral atrophy. After the initial hemorrhagic event, a pseudomembrane organizes immediately beneath the fibrous dura along the surface of the hematoma. This pseudomembrane develops dense granulation tissue with prominent neovascularization. Large-caliber vessels in this granulation tissue are initially unstable and tend to bleed spontaneously, which leads to progressive, stepwise enlargement of the SDH (Ellison, pp. 210–211).

19. C. This specimen exhibits a prominent pontine hemorrhage, known as a Duret hemorrhage. Duret hemorrhages occur when internal herniation (usually transtentorial herniation) results in compression or stretching of pontine perforating vessels. This leads to ischemic damage in the pons, which then undergoes secondary hemorrhagic conversion. This type of hemorrhage is not a direct result of trauma and occurs only after prolonged elevations in intracranial pressure with concomitant herniation (Ellison, pp. 257–259).

20. D. *Streptococcus milleri* is the most common isolate from intracranial abscesses. Many intracranial abscesses are polymicrobial, however. Infants are particularly susceptible to developing abscesses in association with the development of meningitis from infections by *Citrobacter diversus* or *Proteus mirabilis*. Brain abscesses often result from hematogenous seeding in a septic patient (25%), or direct spread from infections of the middle ear, paranasal sinuses, or dental roots (50%) (Ellison, pp. 330–335; Greenberg, p. 218).

21. D. Germinomas are characterized by groups of round neoplastic cells that contain clear cytoplasm with interspersed regions of lymphocytic infiltrates. It is the presence of chronic inflammation in this specimen that distinguishes this tumor from the other choices and is characteristic of germinomas. Choriocarcinoma exhibits a bilaminar pattern of syncytiotrophoblastic giant cells interspersed among smaller neoplastic cells, which is often associated with necrosis and hemorrhage. Yolk sac tumor is characterized by a loose arrangement of clear cells and occasional Schiller-Duval bodies. Secretory meningiomas exhibit typical meningothelial or transitional patterns with occasional intracellular eosinophilic globules. Ependymomas are characterized by uniform neoplastic cells with higher nuclear-cytoplasmic ratios arranged in pseudorosettes, with the rare observance of true rosettes (Ellison, pp. 645–647, 667–670, 680–683, 710; WHO, pp. 72–77, 129–137, 179, 208–214).

22. E. The facial nerve is by far the most commonly involved cranial nerve with neurosarcoidosis. In fact, the most common clinical presentation of neurosarcoidosis is unilateral facial nerve palsy. Other neurologic manifestations may include deafness, vertigo, aseptic meningitis, hydrocephalus, diabetes insipidus, or hypothyroidism. Intracranial disease is quite commonly associated with peripheral nervous system and muscle involvement (Ellison, pp. 346–348; Greenberg, pp. 79–80).

23. B. The gross brain of patients with Alzheimer's disease usually exhibits prominent atrophy of the medial temporal lobes, anterior frontal lobes, and the parietal lobes. The hippocampus is particularly affected, whereas the motor cortex and occipital lobes are usually spared (Ellison, pp. 550–565).

24. A. Bilirubin deposition with kernicterus is evidenced by yellow staining of several deep gray structures in the gross specimen. The most commonly involved regions include the lateral thalamus, globus pallidus, and subthalamic nucleus. The hippocampus, colliculi, substantia nigra pars reticulata, dentate nucleus, inferior olives, brainstem reticular formation, and cranial nerve nuclei are also affected. It is the unconjugated form of bilirubin that is toxic, and its accumulation leads to neuronal necrosis with subsequent gliosis (Ellison, pp. 50–52).

25. C. Glioblastoma multiforme exhibits staining for both vimentin and S-100. GBMs are usually focally positive for GFAP as well. With small tissue biopsies, it can be difficult to distinguish GBM from metastatic carcinoma and lymphoma. Metastatic carcinoma exhibits staining for epithelial membrane antigen (EMA) and cytokeratins, while lymphoma is CD45-positive, which distinguishes these neoplasms from GBM. GBM, however, occasionally exhibits cross reactivity with some keratin stains (e.g., AE1/3). Hemangiopericytoma is vimentin-positive and EMA-negative; however, it does not exhibit AE1/3 cross-reactivity (Ellison, pp. 628–632, 689–694, 732–735, 745–750; WHO, pp. 29–39, 190, 198–203, 250–253).

26. C. Meningothelial meningiomas exhibit sheets or lobules of cells with oval nuclei and indistinct cell borders. Rudimentary whorls are often present. Fibrous meningiomas exhibit streaming of elongated (spindle-shaped) nuclei with prominent surrounding collagen deposition. Transitional meningiomas contain elements of both meningothelial and fibrous variants. Transitional variants exhibit whorls or lobules as well as a fascicular (streaming) pattern of neoplastic cells, as depicted here. Secretory meningiomas can exhibit a transitional or meningothelial pattern; however, many cells contain prominent eosinophilic (PAS-positive) globules. Chordoid meningiomas exhibit columns of cells surrounded by a mucoid matrix, thus resembling a chordoma (WHO, pp. 176–184; Ellison, pp. 703–716).

27. A. Papillary meningiomas are unique variants that exhibit a high nuclear-cytoplasmic ratio, prominent mitoses, metastasis throughout the CNS via CSF pathways, and occasional metastasis outside the CNS. Other meningioma variants are considered atypical if they exhibit prominent mitoses, increased cellularity, sheet-like growth patterns, and necrosis. Anaplastic meningiomas are frankly malignant lesions that exhibit prominent cellular pleomorphism and necrosis. Atypical and anaplastic meningiomas are more likely to exhibit local invasion and recur after resection; however, distant metastasis is usually confined to papillary meningiomas (Ellison, pp. 711–715; WHO, pp. 179–180).

28. D. Amyotrophic lateral sclerosis (ALS) is a neurodegenerative disorder that results in the loss of upper and lower motor neurons. Although the cause of ALS is unknown, 5 to 10% of all cases of ALS are inherited in an autosomal dominant fashion. Approximately 25% of these familial cases of ALS are secondary to mutations of the copper/zinc superoxide dismutase (SOD1) gene located on chromosome 21q. Refsum's disease results from deficiencies of the enzyme phytanoyl CoA hydroxylase, which results in the accumulation of phytanic acid. Clinical manifestations of Refsum's disease include ataxia, peripheral neuropathy, and retinitis pigmentosa. Sanfilippo syndrome is one of the mucopolysaccharidoses and results from defective glycosaminoglycan (heparan sulfate) metabolism. Zellweger syndrome is a peroxisomal disorder that is associated with pachygyria, polymicrogyria, and various heterotopias (Ellison, pp. 93, 445–447, 452–454, 501–507; Merritt, pp. 539–540).

29. A. Multiple sclerosis (MS) is classically associated with the HLA-DR2 allele, and HLA-DR15 is common in Northern Europeans with MS. The HLA alleles A3, B7, and DR3 are also overrepresented in the MS population. The incidence and prevalence of MS vary with latitude, increasing with greater distance from the equator. If, however, an individual migrates to a higher-risk latitude after the teen years, that individual's risk of developing MS is no greater than the risk associated with the original region (Ellison, pp. 389–404).

30-B; 31-C; 32-D; 33-A; 34-E. Hemangiopericytoma is vimentin-positive, with focal reactivity to CD34 as well. The sustentacular cell of paragangliomas exhibits immunoreactivity for S-100, while chief cells exhibit chromogranin-A and synaptophysin positivity. Meningiomas are vimentin-positive, with occasional focal reactivity for EMA, S-100, and cytokeratins. Notably, meningiomas are GFAP-negative. Central neurocytoma exhibits immunoreactivity for synaptophysin, GFAP, and neurofilament proteins. Primary CNS T-cell lymphomas are CD 45– and CD 3–positive, while B-cell lymphomas usually show immunoreactivity to CD 79a and CD 20 (Ellison, pp. 656–659, 691–692, 703–716, 732–735).

35. D. Oligodendrogliomas are characterized by uniform cells, arranged back to back, and interspersed prominent branching capillaries ("chicken-wire" vasculature). Artifactual clearing of the cytoplasm ("fried-egg" appearance), as depicted here, results from delayed formalin fixation and is not always observed. The neoplastic cells of oligodendrogliomas contain monomorphic round nuclei. Oligodendrogliomas frequently exhibit loss of heterozygosity on chromosome 1p and 19q and rarely contain *p53* mutations. Very few cells in these neoplasms exhibit immunoreactivity for GFAP. Clear cell meningiomas resemble oligodendrogliomas microscopically, but like other meningiomas, clear cell meningiomas contain bands of collagen. They also lack the chicken-wire vasculature of oligodendrogliomas (Ellison, pp. 641–644; WHO, pp. 56–64).

36. C. Microscopically, acute cerebral infarcts (after 8 to 12 hours) exhibit neuronal eosinophilia, pyknosis, and vacuolation of the neuropil. Subacute infarcts (2 to 4 days) also exhibit neuronal eosinophilia; however, they may also contain neutrophil infiltrates, occasional necrotic microvessels, and scattered foamy histiocytes. Chronic infarcts exhibit foamy macrophages, reactive astrocytosis, thin-walled blood vessels (neovascularization), and ferrugination of residual neurons surrounding a cystic (acellular) cavity. Gemistocytic astrocytomas exhibit large plump eosinophilic cells with glassy cytoplasm and are hypercellular. Viral encephalitis can exhibit neuronal eosinophilia, especially in the early stages; however, inclusion bodies are usually observed in conjunction with prominent lymphocytic infiltrates. Bacterial meningitis exhibits prominent infiltrates of neutrophils and lymphocytes, often with infiltration of leptomeningeal and cortical vessels. The above photomicrograph illustrates neuronal eosinophilia and pyknosis with vacuolation of the surrounding neuropil and a paucity of inflammation. This is most consistent with an acute cerebral infarction (Ellison, pp. 197–203, 627; WHO, p. 25).

37. C. Acute spinal cord injury is characterized by axonal swellings (spheroids), hemorrhagic necrosis of gray and white matter, and variable amounts of surrounding edema. Over the following weeks there is infiltration of macrophages and a gradual removal of myelin and neuronal debris. Posttraumatic syrinx formation, or cavitation, is a relatively late feature of spinal cord injury, often occurring months to years after the original injury. The gray matter often shows prominent fibroblastic proliferation and associated collagenous fibrosis, as well as hyaline thickening of small blood vessels (Ellison, pp. 262–269).

38. B. Monosomy 22 is by far the most common cytogenetic abnormality of meningiomas, and greater than 75% of all meningiomas exhibit loss of heterozygosity for chromosome 22q markers. Allelic losses of chromosomes 1p, 10, and 14q are associated with progression to more aggressive meningiomas (atypical and anaplastic). Despite the occurrence of (multiple) meningiomas with NF-2, which also localizes to chromosome 22, the tumor suppressor gene that is responsible for tumorigenesis with meningiomas in patients without neurofibromatosis is separate from the NF-2 gene locus (Ellison, p. 715; Kaye and Laws, p. 78).

39. E. Sturge-Weber syndrome (encephalotrigeminal angiomatosis) is a neurocutaneous disorder that occurs sporadically. The disorder is characterized by port wine stains in the distribution of the sensory fibers of the trigeminal nerve, with associated ocular angiomas and leptomeningeal venous angiomas of the ipsilateral cerebral hemisphere. Occasionally the cerebral hemispheres are involved bilaterally. Most patients with Sturge-Weber syndrome develop epilepsy over time, and many exhibit progressive neurologic deficits such as hemiparesis, hemisensory loss, and homonymous hemianopsia. On microscopic analysis, there is widespread gliosis and dystrophic calcification of the involved brain parenchyma, with iron and calcium deposition in large, tortuous meningeal vessels. The treatment of this disorder is largely symptomatic (Ellison, pp. 107–108).

40. E. This photomicrograph depicts a microglial nodule. Microglia typically have rod-shaped nuclei and are CD68-positive. Microglia proliferate in many chronic CNS infections and viral encephalitides. Microglial nodules sometimes contain neurons with viral inclusion bodies, and they are commonly observed with neurosyphilis, toxoplasmosis, and many different viral infections of the CNS (e.g., CMV, HIV, arboviruses, polioviruses). The aggregation of microglia and macrophages around dying neurons is called "neuronophagia" (Ellison, pp. 273–275, 277, 303–304, 319, 324).

41. D. Hunter syndrome is a lysosomal disorder that results from deficiencies of the enzyme iduronate sulfatase. It is inherited in an X-linked recessive fashion and usually presents in the first 2 to 4 years of life. Clinical findings of Hunter syndrome include delayed growth (short stature), coarse facial features, joint stiffness, macrocephaly, progressive hearing loss, hepatosplenomegaly, and various degrees of mental retardation. Hurler syndrome (MPS I), not Hunter syndrome, is associated with corneal clouding (Ellison, pp. 445–446).

42. B. CNS metastatic lesions can occur anywhere but are typically located at the gray-white junction of the cerebral hemispheres. This H&E photomicrograph depicts a malignant metastatic melanoma characterized by areas of hemorrhage, prominent nucleoli (dark spot inside nucleus), and some tumor cells containing melanin pigment (brown). Grossly, metastases can be firm, or they can exhibit a soft, necrotic central region. Hemorrhage is often associated with metastatic melanoma, renal cell carcinoma, or choriocarcinoma. Metastases rarely involve the brainstem or spinal cord. Intracranial abscesses can also occur at the gray-white junction as a result of hematogenous spread, and they usually occur in the MCA distribution. Grossly, abscesses usually exhibit a well-defined capsule that is thicker toward the cortical surface and thinner toward the deep surface. The center of a brain abscess contains purulent, necrotic debris. MS plaques are well-demarcated gray areas of discoloration that commonly occur at the lateral angles of the lateral ventricles. Foci of cavitation are rare with MS plaques but can be observed with fulminant, acute plaques. Acute infarcts exhibit only slight blurring of the gray-white junction with dusky discoloration, often in major vascular territories (Ellison, pp. 197–202, 327–334, 389–398, 743–750).

43. C. Diphtheria infections can result in paralysis of accommodation (ciliary ganglion), followed by facial and oropharyngeal paralysis with preservation of extraocular movements. The fifth to eighth week of the illness is associated with an ascending sensorimotor polyneuropathy in approximately 20% of all cases; this results in a mild to severe paralysis. The disease course is shortened by early treatment with antitoxin and antibiotics, and the majority of patients eventually make a full recovery. Symptoms of neurosarcoidosis include cranial nerve palsies (facial weakness, hearing loss, vertigo, optic atrophy), hypopituitarism, hydrocephalus, and ataxia. Neurosyphilis is associated with cranial nerve palsies, hydrocephalus, arteritis, seizures, and eventually psychosis and cognitive decline. Lyme disease results in an enlarging maculopapular rash with central clearing (erythema chronicum migrans), followed by the development of axonal neuropathies, lymphocytic meningitis, encephalopathy, polyradiculitis, and cranial nerve palsies. Lyme disease can also affect the joints and cardiovascular system. Guillain-Barré syndrome (GBS) is an acute ascending monophasic motor polyneuropathy that can involve the face, limbs, and even respiratory musculature. GBS is not typically associated with any sensory loss or ciliary paralysis, however (Ellison, pp. 342–349; Merritt, pp. 613–615).

44-B; 45-A. Subependymal germinal matrix hemorrhage is usually observed in low-birth-weight premature infants and can result in intraventricular hemorrhage. The microcirculation of the periventricular matrix zone is extremely fragile and persists in the neonate until 34 weeks of gestation. This microcirculation is prone to hemorrhage, with hypoxia and secondary failures of autoregulation. Choroid plexus hemorrhage is the most common cause of intraventricular hemorrhage in the term infant and can result in anything from minimal (asymptomatic) hemorrhage to massive intraventricular hemorrhage (Ellison, pp. 34–37).

46. B. Disorders of abnormal neuronal migration include agyria, pachygyria, polymicrogyria, cortical dysplasia, and focal and diffuse heterotopias. Schizencephaly and porencephaly are fetal hypoxic-ischemic lesions, and holoprosencephaly results from a failure of the normal growth and cleavage of the prosencephalic vesicles (Ellison, pp. 29–32, 62–68, 71–80, 82–85, 87–89).

47-B; 48-A; 49-C; 50-E; 51-D. Pediatric patients with bacterial meningitis are usually due to infection by *Streptococcus pneumoniae*, *Neisseria meningitidis*, or *Haemophilus influenzae*. The incidence of *H. influenzae* meningitis in the pediatric population has decreased significantly in the past decade because of the widespread use of the *H. influenzae* B vaccination. Bacterial meningitis in the adult population is usually secondary to infection by *S. pneumoniae* or *N. meningitidis*. Meningitis in the elderly commonly results from *S. pneumoniae* and gram-negative rods. *Listeria monocytogenes* can also afflict this older population. Neonatal bacterial meningitis is usually a result of infection by group B streptococci and *Escherichia coli*; however, *Citrobacter diversus* and *Proteus mirabilis*-related meningitis are associated with the development of concomitant cerebral abscesses in this population (Ellison, pp. 327–330; Merritt, pp. 103–107).

52. B. Ganglion cell tumors (gangliocytomas and gangliogliomas) are characterized by neoplastic ganglion cells, with or without a component of neoplastic glial tissue (usually with an astrocytic morphology). Neoplastic ganglion cells resemble normal neurons but are abnormally large and round, arranged in clusters, and contain an eccentric nucleus with a prominent nucleolus. The classic finding is binucleation, seen in one of the ganglion cells here, which never occurs in normal neurons. Gangliogliomas occasionally exhibit nuclear pleomorphism, but mitoses are absent. Ganglion cells exhibit immunoreactivity for synaptophysin and neurofilaments. Medulloblastomas are characterized by a uniform population of small blue cells with hyperchromatic nuclei, minimal cytoplasm, mitoses, and occasional foci of necrosis. Central neurocytoma consists of uniform round cells with few mitoses. Ependymomas also contain uniform cells with round nuclei that often form pseudorosettes and rarely form true (ependymal) rosettes (Ellison, pp. 645–647, 653–657, 667–672; WHO, pp. 72–77, 96–98, 129–137).

53. B. Schwannomas are characterized by compact arrangements of interwoven fascicles of cells (Antoni A areas) and spindle-shaped cells arranged in a loose myxoid stroma (Antoni B areas). The Antoni A areas often exhibit sequential palisading nuclei (Verocay bodies), shown here. Thickened blood vessels with hyaline walls may be seen. Neurofibromas are characterized by spindle-shaped cells with wavy nuclei arranged haphazardly within a mucoid matrix with interspersed bundles of collagen ("shredded carrots" appearance). Fibrous meningiomas consist of spindle-shaped cells with intermixed collagen and lack a mucoid matrix and Verocay bodies. Malignant nerve sheath tumors can also exhibit a fascicular pattern; however, this tumor is highly cellular and contains frequent mitoses and necrosis. The presence of Verocay bodies in this specimen is consistent with a schwannoma (Ellison, pp. 695–702, 707, 715; WHO, pp. 164–166, 172–174, 176–184).

54. D. Mature teratomas, the most common of which is the dermoid cyst depicted here, exhibit a mixture of ectodermal, mesodermal, and endodermal components. These neoplasms are well circumscribed and rarely associated with malignant transformation into carcinomas or sarcomas. Dermoid cysts are lined by squamous epithelium and contain adnexal structures such as sebaceous glands (shown in this example). Craniopharyngiomas (adamantinomatous) are characterized by collections of squamous cells with intermingled clusters of keratinized ghost cells, calcification, and cholesterol clefts (Ellison, pp. 683–684, 724–727, 737–739).

55. E. Klippel-Feil anomaly results from the failure of cervical vertebral (somite) segmentation. Klippel-Feil anomaly is classically associated with the triad of short neck, low posterior hairline, and limited cervical motion. Approximately one-third of all Klippel-Feil cases are associated with congenital elevation of the scapula, which is known as Sprengel's deformity. Klippel-Feil is also associated with diastematomyelia, Chiari I malformations, basilar impression, and genitourinary abnormalities (Merritt, p. 490).

56. D. *Disjunction* refers to the separation of superficial ectoderm from neural ectoderm during development. It is thought that premature disjunction allows cells of mesodermal origin to migrate between these two layers of ectoderm, which can lead to the formation of lipomas (Wilkins, pp. 3497–3499).

57. E. Von Hippel-Lindau syndrome (VHL) is an autosomal dominant neurocutaneous disorder that is associated with chromosome 3p. VHL patients develop hemangioblastomas of the brainstem, cerebellum, and spinal cord. VHL is also associated with the development of retinal angiomas, paragangliomas, endolymphatic sac tumors, pheochromocytoma, epididymal cystadenoma, renal and pancreatic cysts, and renal cell carcinoma. The production of erythropoietin by hemangioblastomas can occur with VHL and result in polycythemia (Ellison, pp. 736–738; WHO, pp. 223–226; Kaye and Laws, pp. 75–76).

58. A. The Lewy body is an intracellular neuronal inclusion characterized by the presence of a hyaline eosinophilic core and a pale halo. Lewy bodies are observed within the substantia nigra in Parkinson's disease and within the cerebral cortex in certain forms of dementia (e.g., "dementia with Lewy bodies"). Rabies encephalitis is characterized by the presence of Negri bodies, which are intracellular inclusions resembling red blood cells, and Babès' nodules, which are clusters of microglia. Corticobasal degeneration is characterized by the presence of swollen cortical neurons (ballooned neurons), gliosis, and microvacuolation (Ellison, pp. 287–289, 512–514).

59. B. Subependymomas are characterized by the presence of clusters of cells with round nuclei and interspersed regions of very low cellularity ("islands of blue in a sea of pink"). Subependymomas often exhibit microcysts; however, nuclear pleomorphism and mitoses are universally absent. Myxopapillary ependymomas classically exhibit collars of epithelioid cells surrounding pools of mucin with central blood vessels. Dysembryoplastic neuroepithelial tumor (DNET) is a supratentorial cortical neoplasm of children and young adults that is usually located in the temporal lobe and presents with seizures. Microscopically, DNETs exhibit nodules of oligodendrocyte-like cells, mucinous cysts, and neurons that appear to "float" in the mucinous cysts (Ellison, pp. 651, 659–661; WHO, pp. 78–81, 103–106).

60. C. Gliosarcoma is a variant of glioblastoma multiforme. The presenting features, demographic characteristics, cytogenetic changes, and prognosis of the gliosarcoma (Feigin tumor) are all similar to that of the glioblastoma. Microscopically, the gliosarcoma consists of two distinct cell populations: sarcomatous areas containing spindle-shaped cells arranged in a streaming fashion (left photomicrograph) and areas of conventional glioblastoma (right photomicrograph). Malignant nerve sheath tumors also contain spindle-shaped neoplastic cells; however, areas of conventional glioblastoma are not observed. Embryonal carcinoma exhibits large cells with slight pleomorphism arranged in solid, glandular, papillary, or cribriform patterns. Spindle-shaped cells are absent in embryonal carcinoma (Ellison, pp. 628–632, 682, 700–702; WHO, pp. 42–44).

61. D. This photomicrograph illustrates a medulloblastoma, which is characterized by a population of undifferentiated cells with hyperchromatic nuclei and minimal cytoplasm. Medulloblastomas exhibit prominent mitoses, with focal regions of necrosis and apoptosis. Occasionally cells may form rosettes that lack a central canal or blood vessel (Homer-Wright rosettes). Medulloblastomas often spread throughout the CNS via CSF pathways. Approximately 50% of all medulloblastomas present in children less than 10 years of age; they are usually located in the cerebellar vermis in children. Therefore this tumor could lead to ataxia and hydrocephalus, which is consistent with answer D (Ellison, pp. 667–672; WHO, pp. 129–137).

62-A; 63-B. Neurofibromatosis type 1 (NF-1) is an autosomal dominant neurocutaneous disorder that localizes to chromosome 17. The NF-1 gene is very large and associated with a high spontaneous mutation rate. Approximately 50% of all NF-1 cases are secondary to spontaneous mutations. NF-1 is associated with 100% penetrance and variable expressivity. Tuberous sclerosis (TS) is also an autosomal dominant neurocutaneous disorder that is associated with a high spontaneous mutation rate. TS can result from mutations at two different loci, one located on chromosome 9 and the other on chromosome 11. Tuberous sclerosis is associated with approximately 80% penetrance and variable expressivity (Kaye and Laws, pp. 69–72, 75; WHO, pp. 216–222; Ellison, pp. 695–697).

64. B. This gross specimen exhibits bilateral petechial hemorrhages within the mamillary bodies, which is associ-

ated with Wernicke's encephalopathy. Wernicke's encephalopathy is associated with thiamine deficiency and is commonly observed in chronic alcoholics and some patients with gastrointestinal disorders. Patients with Wernicke's encephalopathy exhibit ataxia, gaze palsies, confusion, and apathy, which is often reversible with the administration of thiamine. The chronic form of the disease is known as Korsakoff's psychosis and is associated with retrograde and anterograde amnesia, with concomitant confabulation, usually irreversible (Ellison, pp. 415–418).

65-C; 66-B; 67-C. Crouzon's disease is an autosomal dominant condition that results in bilateral coronal, frontosphenoid, and frontoethmoid synostosis. Patients with Crouzon's disease have a high incidence of hydrocephalus; however, the vast majority achieve normal IQ's with adequate treatment of the hydrocephalus. Facial features of Crouzon's disease include proptosis, maxillary hypoplasia, and a "parrot's beak" nose. Apert's syndrome is an autosomal dominant condition that involves premature closure of all cranial sutures. These patients have facies that resemble those of Crouzon's disease and also have a high incidence of hydrocephalus. Apert's syndrome is associated with syndactyly, short thumbs, and a uniformly decreased IQ even with adequate treatment of the hydrocephalus (Wilkins, pp. 3693–3694).

68. B. *Craniosynostosis* refers to the premature closure of cranial sutures; this condition is often associated with Crouzon's disease and Apert's syndrome, although many cases are isolated and sporadic as well. Many cases of craniosynostosis are associated with mutations of the fibroblast growth factor receptor gene. Craniosynostosis is more common in males, and isolated sagittal synostosis (scaphocephaly) accounts for approximately 50% of all cases (most common type of synostosis) (Wilkins, pp. 3673–3676).

69. E. Tuberous sclerosis (TS) often presents in children between the ages of 1 and 6 months with seizures, which usually consists of infantile spasms. Approximately 90% of all patients with TS experience seizures, and the vast majority also exhibit various degrees of mental retardation. TS is associated with the development of cortical tubers, which are firm, pale nodules that project from the cortical surface, as depicted in this gross specimen. TS is also associated with subependymal nodules and the development of subependymal giant cell astrocytoma (Ellison, pp. 108–110; WHO, pp. 227–230).

70. A. Prolonged elevations in intracranial pressure can result in various herniation syndromes. Transtentorial herniation of the uncus through the tentorial incisura can result in compression of the ipsilateral oculomotor nerve, midbrain, and ipsilateral posterior cerebral artery, with subsequent infarction. Prolonged herniation can result in the development of hemorrhagic necrosis within the pons and midbrain (Duret hemorrhages) as a consequence of penetrating arteriolar compression and ischemia. This gross specimen illustrates transtentorial herniation of the uncus, with notable indentation of the surrounding cerebrum by the tentorium cerebelli (Ellison, pp. 257–259).

71. E. Diffuse axonal injury (DAI) results from acceleration/deceleration injuries of the brain. DAI can exhibit prominent petechial hemorrhages within the corpus callosum, interventricular septum, dorsolateral brainstem, superior cerebellar peduncles, and parasagittal deep white matter on gross specimens. Microscopically, DAI specimens exhibit prominent axonal spheroids, especially with silver stains. DAI varies in severity from minimal disturbances in level of consciousness to vegetative states with subsequent death (Ellison, pp. 249–253).

72. A. Cerebral aspergillosis is usually secondary to hematogenous dissemination from the lungs or local spread from the paranasal sinuses of *Aspergillus fumigatus* or *Aspergillus flavus*. Symptoms of cerebral aspergillosis are variable and include headache, seizures, cranial nerve palsies, hemiparesis, and elevated intracranial pressure. *Aspergillus* has a tendency to exhibit prominent vascular invasion, with subsequent vascular thrombosis, infarction, and hemorrhage. *Aspergillus* is characterized by septate hyphae that are readily demonstrated on silver stains. In contrast, mucormycosis exhibits broad nonseptate hyphae, candidiasis exhibits budding yeasts and pseudohyphae, and cryptococcosis exhibits only a yeast form with CNS infections (Ellison, pp. 351–355, 357–362).

73. D. Amyotrophic lateral sclerosis (ALS) affects primarily the anterior and lateral corticospinal tracts of the spinal cord, as evidenced by the loss of myelinated axons (as depicted in the specimen). Subacute combined degeneration (SACD) results from vitamin B_{12} (cobalamin) deficiency and exhibits symmetric demyelination in the posterior and lateral columns of the spinal cord. In severe cases of SACD, the anterior columns can also be involved. Tabes dorsalis results from chronic inflammation of the dorsal roots and dorsal root ganglia and is usually observed 15 to 20 years after initial infection with syphilis. The posterior columns are primarily affected in tabes dorsalis. Friedreich's ataxia (FA) is an autosomal recessive disorder that localizes to chromosome 9 and results in deterioration of the posterior columns, spinocerebellar tracts, Clarke's nucleus, and distal (thoracolumbar) corticospinal tracts (Ellison, pp. 344–345, 417–420, 501–508, 533–534).

74-B; 75-B; 76-C; 77-B. Acute disseminated encephalomyelitis (ADEM), also known as postinfectious encephalomyelitis, is a monophasic demyelinating disorder that usually follows a viral infection or vaccination (especially rabies vaccine). ADEM results from T-cell autoimmune attacks against myelin basic protein and usually presents with fever, headache, nuchal rigidity, and focal neurologic deficits. ADEM is characterized by perivenular inflammation and demyelination on microscopic analysis. Patients with ADEM usually exhibit a full recovery (10 to 20% have permanent neurologic deficits), and the disease course is generally shorter with the administration of IV steroids. Experimental allergic encephalomyelitis (EAE) is a monophasic autoimmune response that occurs in genetically susceptible animals after immunization with myelin basic protein. EAE is actually the animal model of ADEM, although there is a chronic relapsing form of the disease that resembles MS and has provided much of the immunologic information that there is about MS in humans. MS is typically a chronic relapsing/remitting demyelinating disorder that affects adults between the third to fifth decades of life and is more common in women than men. Approximately 85% of acute MS exacerbations improve with the administration of IV methylprednisolone. Acute MS plaques can exhibit perivascular inflammation; however, arterioles are involved (as well as venules). Interferon β-1b Betaserone), interferon β-1a (Avonex), and Copaxone are generally utilized to decrease the frequency of MS attacks (Ellison, pp. 389–404, 405–407; Merritt, pp. 151–153, 773–791; Greenberg, pp. 69–71).

78. B. CNS lymphoma is characterized by numerous malignant lymphocytes that tend to invade the walls of blood vessels. Lymphoma cells are prominent in the perivascular spaces, and they diffusely invade brain parenchyma toward the periphery of the lesion. More than 80% of these tumors are diffuse large B-cell lymphomas. The surrounding brain often exhibits reactive astrocytosis, which can resemble other inflammatory disorders. Interspersed small reactive (nonneoplastic) lymphocytes are usually observed as well and provide contrast to the larger, polymorphous malignant lymphocytes, which facilitates distinguishing lymphoma from other inflammatory conditions. B-cell lymphomas are positive for CD20 (Ellison, pp. 689–694; WHO, pp. 198–203).

79. D. Choroid plexus papillomas (CPPs) exhibit a columnar epithelium with an underlying fibrovascular network and prominent papillary projections. CPPs exhibit slight nuclear crowding and loss of the normal "cobblestone" surface, which differentiates them from normal choroid plexus. CPPs are generally positive for S-100, transthyretin, and cytokeratin. Papillary meningiomas are aggressive tumors that exhibit prominent mitoses, a high nuclear-cytoplasmic ratio, and poorly defined papillary structures. Papillary craniopharyngiomas are composed of papillae of squamous cells without fibrovascular cores. Colloid cysts are lined by a single layer of columnar cells. Many of the cells of a colloid cyst wall are ciliated, and mucin-containing goblet cells may also be located within the epithelial layer (WHO, pp. 84–86, 180, 244–246; Ellison, pp. 685–688, 713, 724–727, 738–740).

80. B. Paragangliomas usually arise from the cauda equina or jugular bulb (glomus jugulare tumors) and consist of lobules of chief cells (Zellballen) surrounded by a single layer of sustentacular cells. Chief cells are labeled with synaptophysin, neurofilament, and chromogranin immunostains. Sustentacular cells are S-100–positive. Myxopapillary ependymomas can also originate from the cauda equina region; however, they are GFAP-positive, whereas paragangliomas are GFAP-negative. Paragangliomas are WHO grade I lesions (Ellison, pp. 651, 658–659; WHO, pp. 78–79, 112–114).

81. D. Fat embolism is usually observed in trauma patients with multisystem injuries and is often associated with long bone fractures. Grossly, fat embolism is characterized by multiple petechial hemorrhages that affect both the gray and white matter of the cerebral hemispheres diffusely, with concomitant regions of perivascular (gray) discoloration. Microscopically, fat embolism exhibits hemorrhagic lesions surrounding capillaries with signs of fibrinoid necrosis. Lipid globules can be demonstrated in necrotic regions with oil red O stains. Progressive multifocal leukoencephalopathy (PML) results from JC virus (polyomavirus) reactivation in the CNS of immunocompromised patients. PML exhibits foci of gray discoloration with regions of necrosis and cavitation, primarily in the deep white matter. Adrenoleukodystrophy is characterized by extensive white matter demyelination with sparing of the subcortical U fibers, and involves the parieto-occipital regions more extensively than the frontotemporal region. This specimen exhibits multiple petechial hemorrhages in both the cortical gray and deep white matter, which is most consistent with fat embolism (Ellison, pp. 254–256, 298–300, 454–456).

82. A. PTAH stains for collagen, while the Sudan, Weigert, and Marchi are useful myelin stains (Wheater, pp. 102, 149, 309).

83. A. Ependymomas are characterized by the presence of uniform cells with round nuclei, mild nuclear pleomorphism, and indistinct cytoplasmic borders. Pseudorosettes (with a central blood vessel) are commonly observed in ependymomas; however, true rosettes with a central lumen (shown in the mid-upper portion of the picture) are less frequent. Some ependymomas exhibit epithelial differentiation and the presence of true gland-like canals. Ependymomas are GFAP-positive. The presence of numerous perivascular pseudorosettes in the above specimen is most consistent with an ependymoma (Ellison, pp. 645–651; WHO, pp. 72–77).

84. E. Melanocytes are present within the leptomeninges of the CNS and can lead to the formation of malignant melanoma, diffuse melanosis, and melanocytomas. All of these neoplasms exhibit prominent melanin. Occasionally, schwannomas, ependymomas, pineal neoplasms, and embryonal neoplasms can also exhibit prominent melanin (Ellison, pp. 734–737).

85. B. Hallervorden-Spatz disease (HSD) is an autosomal recessive disorder that presents with progressive gait disturbance, dystonia, dysarthria, and choreoathetosis in children and young adults. An adult variant of HSD presents with progressive cognitive decline and extrapyramidal signs. T2-weighted MRI exhibits prominent hypointensity within the globus pallidus in patients with HSD ("eye of the tiger" sign), which is secondary to the accumulation of iron pigment. Microscopically, HSD is characterized by the presence of gliosis, axonal spheroids, and occasional Lewy bodies and neurofibrillary tangles within the globus pallidus and substantia nigra (pars reticulata). Wilson's disease (hepatolenticular degeneration) is also characterized by abnormalities of the pallidum; however, prominent iron deposition is not observed (Ellison, pp. 134–136, 603–605).

86. C. Neurocysticercosis results from ingestion of the larval form of *Taenia solium*. These larvae migrate throughout the body and can involve the eyes, liver, brain, lung, and skeletal muscle. Grossly, neurocysticercosis exhibits the presence of a variable number of cysts that usually involve the cortical gray matter. Viable cysts are often 1 to 2 cm in diameter; they become fibrotic and calcified with degeneration. Occasionally a prominent scolex is observed within the viable cysts (Ellison, pp. 377–381).

87. E. Paget's disease is characterized by initial excessive bone resorption by osteoclasts, followed by the progressive deposition of disorganized vascular bone. Paget's disease can involve any bone in the body and can exhibit neurologic symptoms by neural compression, fracture/dislocations, hemorrhage, vascular insufficiency ("steal" phenomena), and malignant degeneration into osteogenic sarcoma or fibrosarcoma with local invasion. Common neurologic symptoms associated with Paget's disease include cranial nerve palsies (optic atrophy, trigeminal neuralgia, facial paralysis, hearing loss), entrapment neuropathies, hypopituitarism, myeloradiculopathy, and brainstem compression (Wilkins, pp. 3887–3889).

88. D. Alzheimer type II astrocytes exhibit an enlarged vesicular nucleus with peripheral chromatin and minimal cytoplasm. Alzheimer type II astrocytes can be observed in the caudate, putamen, thalamus, hypothalamus, and brainstem of patients with Wilson's disease and acquired hepatic encephalopathy (Ellison, pp. 430–432).

89. A. Neuronophagia (the aggregation of macrophages and microglia around dying neurons) is classically associated with poliovirus infections of the CNS; however, it can also be observed with other CNS viral infections (Ellison, pp. 274–276).

90. D. Chordomas usually arise within the sacrum or clivus and are characterized microscopically by the presence of cells with prominent vacuolated cytoplasm (physaliphorous cells) surrounded by a mucinous matrix (Ellison, p. 746).

91. E. Glioblastomas generally exhibit widespread reactivity for vimentin and focal reactivity for GFAP and S-100; they are not reactive with cytokeratin markers such as epithelial membrane antigen (EMA). An exception to this is cytokeratin AE1/3, which is occasionally cross-reactive with glioblastomas (WHO; pp. 29–39, Ellison, pp. 628–632).

92. B. Pleomorphic xanthoastrocytoma (PXA) is a WHO grade II lesion that is usually located superficially in the cerebrum of children and young adults. It has variable biologic behavior. Some may progress to become aggressive neoplasms, which behave like glioblastomas, whereas others have a more favorable prognosis, carrying a 70% 10-year survival rate. PXAs exhibits prominent cytologic pleomorphism, with occasional nuclear hyperchromasia and atypical nuclei. Many of the neoplastic cells with PXA contain prominent eosinophilic cytoplasm, but groups of undifferentiated cells may also be found. Cytoplasmic lipid accumulation is found with variable frequency in some cells, which often appear xanthomatous or vacuolated. Unlike most gliomas, they are often surrounded by dense pericellular reticulin. Mitoses and necrosis are rarely observed, and PXA is generally GFAP- and S-100–positive. PXA can be differentiated from a glioblastoma by the presence of extensive reticulin deposition, intracellular eosinophilic accumulations, and the lack of mitotic figures, neovascularization, and necrosis (Ellison, pp. 634–637; WHO, pp. 52–54).

93. D. Duchenne muscular dystrophy results from the complete absence of the protein dystrophin, which is encoded by a gene located on chromosome Xp21. Duchenne muscular dystrophy exhibits X-linked recessive inheritance (Merritt, p. 737).

94. D. Giant cell arteritis (GCA) occurs almost exclusively in the elderly and is associated with polymyalgia rheumatica, fever, malaise, weakness, and visual loss. The ESR is elevated in approximately 95% of all cases of GCA. Temporal artery biopsy is often diagnostic for GCA; however, skip lesions can occur with involved arteries, which can lead to false-negative biopsies. Microscopically, GCA is characterized by prominent granulomatous inflammation of arterial walls, marked intimal hyperplasia, and frequent multinucleated giant cells, as depicted in this example (Ellison, pp. 182–183).

95. D. Dermatomyositis is an inflammatory disorder of the muscles and skin that has been associated with infections, vaccinations, hypothyroidism, sarcoidosis, and systemic malignancy (10% of all cases). Dermatomyositis results primarily from B-cell infiltration of the perimysium and blood vessels, with concomitant immunoglobulin deposition that can result in vasculitis. Muscle fiber degeneration occurs in a perifascicular pattern with dermatomyositis; cutaneous findings include scaly macules of the extensor surfaces of the fingers (Gottron sign) and a rash of the eyelids (heliotrope), nose, and cheeks. T-cell infiltration of muscle fibers with subsequent muscle fiber necrosis is a characteristic of polymyositis (Merritt, pp. 763–768).

96. C. The white matter exhibits prominent demyelination with relative sparing of the subcortical U fibers, which is characteristic of several leukodystrophies, including metachromatic leukodystrophy (Ellison, pp. 451–456).

97. A. Pituitary adenomas usually consist of minimally atypical monomorphic cells, which can be arranged in sheets as well as in acinar, papillary, or trabecular patterns. The cells occasionally form perivascular pseudorosettes. Cytologic pleomorphism and mitoses are infrequently observed in pituitary adenomas (Ellison, pp. 717–724).

98. A. Tay-Sachs disease is a metabolic disorder that results from a deficiency (or absence) of the lysosomal enzyme β-hexosaminidase A, which is encoded by a gene on chromosome 15. This enzyme normally degrades the lipid G_{M2} ganglioside, and its absence results in intracellular accumulation of this compound, which is toxic to neurons. Tay-Sachs disease is inherited in an autosomal recessive pattern, and the defective allele has an increased incidence in Jews of eastern European (Ashkenazi) descent, Cajuns of southern Louisiana, and French Canadians of parts of Quebec. There are both infantile and juvenile forms of the disease, depending on the amount of residual functional enzyme that is present within the neuron. Infantile forms of the disease are severe and result in blindness, deafness, dysphagia, paralysis, and eventually death (usually by 5 years of age). Juvenile forms of the disease are more indolent and are associated with dementia, ataxia, psychosis, and a gradually progressive neurologic deterioration. Tay-Sachs disease often produces a "cherry red spot" on the retina on funduscopic evaluation (Ellison, pp. 437–438).

99. A. Glioblastoma multiforme (GBM) can occur de novo without any prior evidence of neoplasia or secondarily as a result of anaplastic progression from low-grade astrocytomas. There are many cytogenetic differences between primary (de novo) and secondary GBMs. Secondary GBMs are associated with *p53* gene mutations (chromosome 17), *CDK4* gene amplification, and loss of heterozygosity (LOH) of chromosomes 13q (Rb), 9p, and 19q. Epidermal growth factor receptor (EGFR) and MDM2 gene amplifications are more commonly associated with de novo GBMs. The most frequent abnormality associated with the progression of malignant astrocytomas overall is LOH on chromosome 10 (Ellison, pp. 623–624; WHO, pp. 36–39).

100. D. Approximately 80% of all glioblastomas exhibit gains of part or all of chromosome 7. Other common nonrandom cytogenetic aberrations of glioblastoma multiforme include the loss of chromosome 10 (60%), deletion or rearrangements of chromosome 9p (35%), and the acquisition of double minute chromosomes (33%). LOH involving various alleles on chromosome 17 (22%), chromosome 22 (19%), and chromosome 13 (14%) has also been observed regularly in glioblastoma karyotypes (Kaye and Laws, p. 77).

101-B; 102-D. Note the stacked lamellar membranes or stored gangliosides ("zebra bodies") on this electron micrograph in a patient with Hurler's syndrome (Ellison, pp. 445–447).

103. E. Note the prominent "onion bulb" formations in this peripheral nerve, which has undergone marked demyelination and subsequent remyelination in a patient with Dejerine-Sottas disease (Merritt, pp. 608–609).

104-E; 105-C; 106-B; 107-A; 108-D. Refer to Table 4.104–4.108A. (Ellison, p. 683; Kaye and Laws, pp. 778–786).

109. B. The ultrastructural homologue of the miniature endplate potential (MEPP) is the synaptic vesicle, which produces a MEPP after being released from the presynaptic terminal (Kandel, pp. 258–262).

110. A. Note the presence of psammoma bodies intermingled with whorling meningothelial cells in this photomicrograph, depicting a psammomatous meningioma (Ellison, pp. 708–709).

111. E. This photomicrograph depicts a myxopapillary ependymoma with markedly thickened blood vessel walls and cells with a delicate fibrillary cytoplasm surrounding mucin-rich areas (Ellison, pp. 646–651).

112. E. Anaplastic, rhabdoid, and papillary meningiomas are WHO grade III neoplasms and carry the worst prognosis, while atypical, chordoid, and clear cell meningiomas are WHO grade II variants. The best prognosis is seen with WHO grade I meningiomas, which include the psammomatous, angiomatous, microcystic, secretory, metaplastic, and lymphoplasmacytic variants (Ellison, pp. 709–712).

113-E; 114-C; 115-E. Patients with homocystinuria (autosomal recessive, chromosome 21) have a variable onset and may present with a marfanoid habitus, codfish vertebrae (biconcave), eye anomalies (ectopia lentis, myopia, glaucoma, optic atrophy), mental retardation, seizures, behavioral disorders, and strokes (beginning at age 5 to 9 months). The pathophysiology includes intimal thickening and fibrosis of blood vessels, which may lead to arterial and venous thrombosis. It is the result of cystathionine β-synthase deficiency, which leads to the accumulation of homocysteine and methionine. There is also impaired methylation of homocysteine to methionine from enzyme deficiency or cofactor B_{12} deficiency. Treatment may include restriction of dietary methionine as well as pyridoxine, vitamin B_{12}, and cysteine supplements. Hypoxanthine-guanine phosphoribosyl transferase deficiency results in Lesch-Nyhan syndrome, phenylalanine hydroxylase deficiency results in phenylketonuria, and alpha-ketoacid dehydrogenase deficiency can produce maple syrup urine disease (Merritt, p. 256; Geyer, pp. 102–106).

116. D. Note the prominent pleomorphic astrocyte and oligodendrocytes with viral inclusions in this immunocompromised patient with PML. Patients with this disease present with focal neurologic deficits including dysarthria, limb weakness, visual disturbances, ataxia, personality changes, and occasionally seizures. PML usually progresses rapidly over the course of weeks to months, resulting in increasing neurologic impairment, coma, and death. Treatment of the underlying immunocompromised state can lead to remission (Ellison, pp. 298–300).

117. A. Note the haphazardly arranged spindle cells with wavy nuclei and a prominent matrix of mucin and collagen in this photomicrograph depicting a neurofibroma (Ellison, pp. 699–701).

118-A; 119-B. Note the nests of chief cells (Zellballen) surrounded by a fibrovascular stroma and sustentacular cells

TABLE 4.104–108A

TUMOR	ALPHA FETOPROTEIN (AFP)	BETA SUBUNIT OF HUMAN CHORIONIC GONADOTROPIN (β-HCG)	PLACENTAL ALKALINE PHOSPHATASE
Germinoma	–	–	+
Embryonal carcinoma	+/–	+/–	+/–
Yolk sac tumor	+	+/–	+/–
Choriocarcinoma	+/–	+	+/–
Teratoma	+/–	–	–

in this photomicrograph depicting a paraganglioma of the filum terminale. These neoplasms show immunoreactivity to synaptophysin and chromogranin; ultrastructural examination reveals dense-core granules. Sustentacular cells are immunoreactive to S-100 protein (Ellison, pp. 658–659).

120. E. Note the sheets of cells with uniform round nuclei, which is characteristic of central neurocytomas. These neoplasms most often show synaptophysin immunoreactivity, although a small astrocytic component is often present that is GFAP-positive. Ultrastructural features include dense-core and clear vesicles, microtubules, and intermediate filaments (Ellison, pp. 656–658; WHO, pp. 107–109).

121. B. Subependymal germinal matrix hemorrhage (SEH) usually occurs in premature infants (less than 34 weeks' gestation) with low birth weight and is usually located adjacent to the head of the caudate nucleus or thalamus. SEH is the most common cause of intraventricular hemorrhage (IVH) in premature infants. Grade I SEH is confined to the germinal matrix, grade 2 extends into the lateral ventricle from the germinal matrix, grade 3 consists of IVH with hydrocephalus, and grade IV involves extension into the brain parenchyma (Ellison, pp. 34–37).

122. C. Laminar necrosis can be related to intrapartum difficulties, congenital heart disease, and vascular collapse in an infant. It often involves the depths of the sulci (as depicted here), and the necrosis can be in a laminar or pseudolaminar pattern (Ellison, pp. 37–43).

123-D; 124-D. Note the absence of sulci and gyri along the cerebral convexities of this specimen depicting agyria, which results from abnormal cellular migration during embryologic development (Ellison, pp. 71–76).

125-D; 126-E. Note the prominent calcifications of residual neurons adjacent to a chronic infarct in this photomicrograph depicting siderocalcinosis (Ellison, pp. 190–191).

127. A. Note the presence of a prominent inflammatory infiltrate within the lumen of this blood vessel with concomitant vascular thrombosis in this photomicrograph depicting bacterial meningitis (Ellison, pp. 327–331).

128-B; 129-C; 130-C. Note the presence of broad, nonseptate hyphae in this photomicrograph depicting mucormycosis, a fungal infection most often seen in diabetic patients with ketoacidosis. It most commonly enters the cranial cavity from the nasal mucosa via the cribriform plate. Mucormycosis is often fatal within a few days unless surgical debridement and antifungal therapy is initiated early (Ellison, pp. 353–355).

131-C; 132-B. Note the fascicular arrangement of these neoplastic cells that exhibit a high nuclear-cytoplasmic ratio

and prominent mitosis in this photomicrograph depicting a malignant nerve sheath tumor (MNST). This neoplasm usually involves the trigeminal nerve intracranially but most often originates from the cervical or brachial plexi. MNST carries a poor prognosis, and approximately 50% of patients harboring this lesion have NF1 (Ellison, pp. 700–702).

133-C; 134-A; 135-B. The most common metastatic brain tumors originate from the lung, breast, skin, and kidney. Photomicrograph A depicts a lesion with an area of necrosis and branching as well as sharply angulated lobules, which is most consistent with metastatic breast carcinoma. Photomicrograph B depicts metastatic lung adenocarcinoma, which is thyroid transcription factor-1 (TTF-1) positive, and thyroglobulin negative. Photomicrograph C shows a hypervascular tumor with lobules of clear cells, which is most consistent with renal cell carcinoma [EMA (+), CAM 5.2 (+), CD 10 (+)] (Ellison, pp. 743–749; WHO, pp. 250–253).

136. D. Note the areas of necrosis without intact cells or nuclei and the hyalinized, necrotic vessel in this photomicrograph depicting radiation necrosis (Ellison, p. 632; Berger, pp. 471–474; Greenberg, pp. 507–515).

137. D. Note the prominent capsule and central purulent region in this gross section depicting a brain abscess. The central area of necrosis and surrounding capsule formation are characteristic features of the fourth stage of abscess formation (capsular stage). Refer to Table 5.97–5.100A for a summary of the stages of abscess formation (Ellison, pp. 330–336).

138-B; 139-C. Note the noncaseating sarcoid granuloma containing prominent epithelioid cells and multinucleated giant cells. Tuberculosis is associated with caseating granulomas, whereas MS plaques, paragangliomas, amputation neuromas, and acoustic neuromas are not associated with granuloma formation (Ellison, pp. 346–348).

140-A; 141-A; 142-A; 143-A; 144-B; 145-A; 146-A; 147-A; 148-A; 149-B. Patients with axonal neuropathies (most common) usually have symmetric distal sensory loss with weakness, atrophy, and loss of ankle jerks. Nerve conduction velocity (NCV) studies show mild slowing without conduction block or temporal dispersion as well as decreased amplitudes of compound motor action potentials (CMAP) and sensory nerve action potentials (SNAP). EMG studies show evidence of distal denervation. Demyelinating neuropathies typically present with sensory loss of larger fibers more than smaller fibers, and usually motor more than sensory involvement. NCV studies can show marked slowing, conduction block, temporal dispersion, prolonged F waves, and prolonged distal latencies with demyelinating diseases. EMG studies show denervation, based on chronicity. Of note, HIV-positive patients with neuropathy typically have a demyelinating process, whereas patients with AIDS rarely present with a demyelinating neuropathy but instead with an axonal neuropathy (Merritt, pp. 620–624; Geyer, p. 164).

150. B. Note the presence of hypocellularity, gliosis, demyelination, and a lack of inflammation in this photomicrograph depicting a chronic infarct (Ellison, pp. 197–201).

151-C; 152-A; 153-E; 154-B; 155-D; 156-F. Lewy bodies (E), the hallmark of Parkinson's disease, are intracellular cytoplasmic inclusions containing an eosinophilic core surrounded by a pale halo. They are predominantly found in the substantia nigra and consist of ubiquitin, neurofilaments, α–synuclein, and αβ crystallin. Bunina bodies (F) are small eosinophilic cytoplasmic inclusions that are observed in patients with ALS. They can be demonstrated with H&E stains; however, they are best identified with ubiquitin staining techniques. Hirano bodies (A) are eosinophilic cytoplasmic inclusions composed of actin and actin-associated proteins; they are particularly prominent in the CA1 sector of the hippocampus in patients with Alzheimer's disease (AD) and Pick's disease. Neurofibrillary tangles (D) are intraneuronal inclusions composed of phosphorylated tau, which is a microtubule-associated cytoskeletal protein. Phosphorylated tau forms helical filaments, which can be found within the neocortex and pyramidal cells of the hippocampus in patients with AD. The microscopic hallmark of Pick's disease is the Pick body (B), which is a spherical cytoplasmic inclusion (composed of phosphorylated tau) that is mildly basophilic and contains a well-demarcated margin. Negri bodies (C) are oval or round cytoplasmic inclusions that can be found throughout the CNS but are most prominent in Purkinje cells. The appearance of Negri bodies is similar to that of red blood cells (Ellison, pp. 288–289, 504, 513–514, 552, 556–559, 570–572).

157-C; 158-B; 159-A. Neuroblastoma most commonly occurs in the first decade of life and can present with opsoclonus, myoclonus, and encephalopathy. This lesion most commonly originates from the adrenal glands (40% of neuroblastic tumors), followed by the abdominal (25%), thoracic (15%), cervical (5%), and pelvic sympathetic ganglia (5%); it is associated with amplification of the N-*myc* gene. The cerebral form tends to favor the frontoparietal lobes, although it is rare. Treatment typically includes surgical resection and radiation therapy to the tumor bed. Recurrence is frequent after excision (WHO, pp. 153–161; Merritt, p. 330; Geyer, p. 146).

160-F; 161-A; 162-B; 163-H; 164-D; 165-D; 166-C; 167-G; 168-D. Refer to Table 4.160–4.168A. (Kaye and Laws, pp. 378–385; Geyer, pp. 154–155).

169. E. Hypertrophied nerves may occur with neurofibromatosis, Refsum's disease, leprosy, hereditary sensory motor neuropathy (HSMN) III > II > I, acromegaly, neurofibromatosis, and amyloidosis. Hypertrophied nerves are not typically seen in patients with alcoholism (Merritt, p. 605).

170. A. Note the prominent atrophy of the cerebellar vermis in this gross specimen depicting alcoholic cerebellar degeneration (Ellison, pp. 488–489).

171. C. Note the prominent epidermoid within the right cerebellopontine angle cistern in this gross specimen (Ellison, pp. 737–739).

172. A. Note the prominent spherules containing endospores in this photomicrograph depicting coccidioidomycosis. The spherules and enclosed endospores usually appear basophilic when stained with H&E but are better demonstrated by methenamine silver impregnation. Pulmonary infection can occur in the absence of underlying disease and

TABLE 4.160–168A   Chemotherapeutic agents and potential side effects

CHEMOTHERAPY	SIDE EFFECTS
Cyclosporin	Hypertrichosis, anorexia, nausea, vomiting, confusion, psychosis, tremor, primary CNS system lymphoma
Isotretinoin	Pseudotumor cerebri, headache, dry skin, hepatotoxicity, and rarely pancreatitis
Vincristine	Peripheral axonal neuropathy, autonomic neuropathy, decreased ADH secretion, bone marrow sparing
Interleukin-2	Parkinsonism, brachial plexopathy
Cisplatin	Peripheral neuropathy, high-frequency hearing loss, myelosuppression, nephrotoxicity
Carboplatin	Peripheral neuropathy, hearing loss, transient cortical blindness, less renal toxicity than cisplatin
Paclitaxel (Taxol)	Peripheral neuropathy
Tamoxifen	Decreased visual acuity
Vinblastine	Peripheral neuropathy, muscle pain
Nitrosourea (BCNU)	Myelosuppression, nausea, vomiting, pulmonary fibrosis, encephalopathy

is generally self-limiting, although there may be residual fibrosis and calcification. Coccidioidomycosis is most often associated with occupations involving exposures to large amounts of dust. Hematogenous spread is rare and is most often seen in patients with diabetes, immunosuppression, or pregnancy. CNS involvement is usually a late, terminal event (Ellison, pp. 362–363).

173. A. This gross section depicts prominent exudates along the cerebral convexities as well as focal areas of hemorrhage and thrombosed veins; these are characteristic of purulent meningitis (Ellison, pp. 328–330).

174. D. Forms of fungi in CNS infection include yeasts (*Blastomycosis, Candida, Coccidioides, Cryptococcus, Histoplasma, Paracoccidioides, Sporotrichum,* and *Torulopsis*) as well as branching septate (*Aspergillus, Cladosporium, Fusarium*) and nonseptate hyphae (*Mucor*) and pseudohyphae, which are larger than yeasts but smaller than true hyphae (some *Candida* species) (Ellison, pp. 351–354).

175. A. Note the glomeruloid vascular proliferation in this photomicrograph depicting a glioblastoma (Ellison, p. 631).

Neuroradiology Questions

1. What tumor commonly exhibits high signal intensity on T2-weighted images, low signal intensity on T1-weighted images, and high signal intensity (restricted diffusion) on diffusion MR images?

- **A.** Pineoblastoma
- **B.** Glioblastoma
- **C.** Arachnoid cyst
- **D.** Epidermoid
- **E.** Meningioma

2. A 12-year-old male presented with symptoms of ataxia and diplopia and exhibited facial weakness, hemiparesis, and internuclear ophthalmoplegia on neurologic examination. His T2-weighted MRI (Figure 5.2Q) illustrates which of the following tumors?

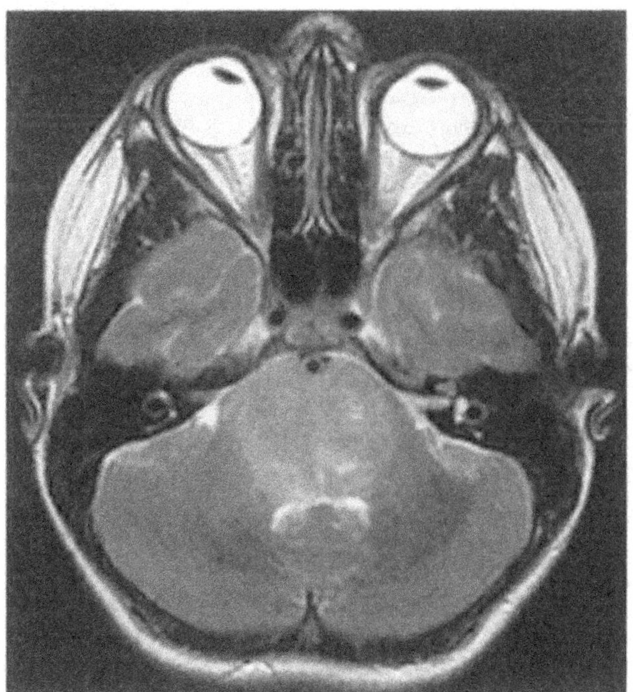

FIGURE 5.2Q

- **A.** Lymphoma
- **B.** Choriocarcinoma
- **C.** Yolk sac tumor
- **D.** Ependymoma
- **E.** Infiltrating astrocytoma

3. What MR sequence is the most sensitive in identifying intracerebral cavernous malformations?

- **A.** T1-weighted
- **B.** T2-weighted
- **C.** Gradient echo
- **D.** Fast spin echo
- **E.** Diffusion

4. What is the most common intracranial tumor associated with neurofibromatosis type 1?

- **A.** Optic nerve glioma
- **B.** Ependymoma
- **C.** Neurofibroma
- **D.** Meningioma
- **E.** Medulloblastoma

5. What surgical approach would be most suitable for a patient with mild tinnitus and the lesion depicted in the following enhanced T1-weighted MRI (Figure 5.5Q)?

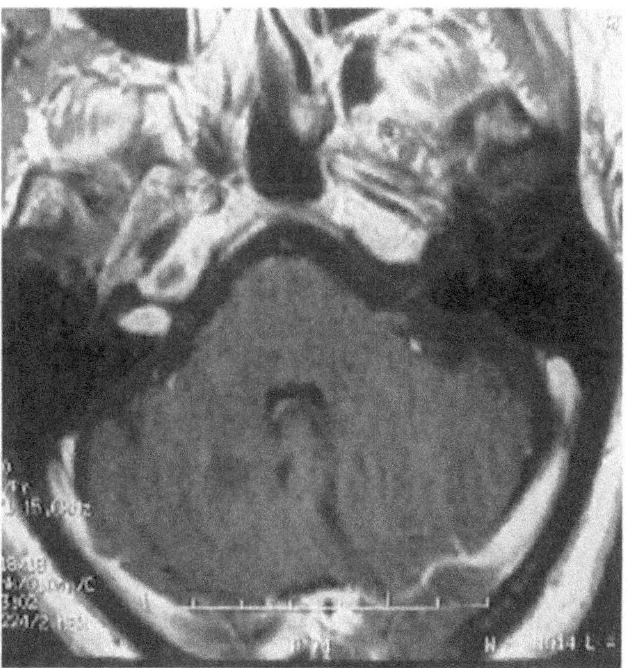

FIGURE 5.5Q

- **A.** Retrosigmoid
- **B.** Translabyrinthine
- **C.** Middle fossa
- **D.** Transpetrosal infratemporal fossa
- **E.** Transcochlear

6. This lateral internal carotid angiogram (Figure 5.6Q) illustrates what persistent fetal circulation?

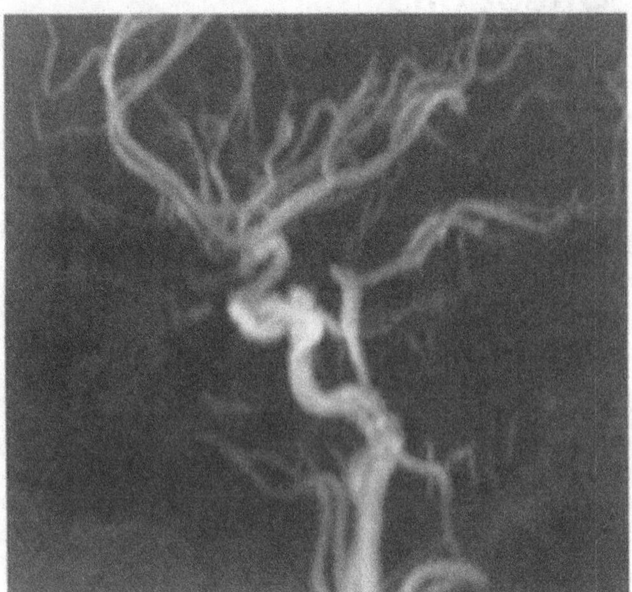

FIGURE 5.6Q

    A. Primitive trigeminal artery
    B. Persistent otic artery
    C. Persistent hypoglossal artery
    D. Proatlantal intersegmental artery
    E. None of the above

7. Which of the following ratios is typically decreased with primary CNS neoplasms on MR spectroscopy?

    A. Myoinositol:total creatine
    B. Choline:N-acetyl aspartate
    C. Choline:total creatine
    D. N-acetyl aspartate:total creatine
    E. Myoinositol:N-acetyl aspartate

8. An 8-year-old female presented with symptoms of persistent headaches, nausea, and emesis for 1 week. The patient was somewhat lethargic and was noted to have a mild left hemiparesis on examination. Axial contrasted T1-weighted MRI (Figure 5.8Q) illustrates what abnormality?

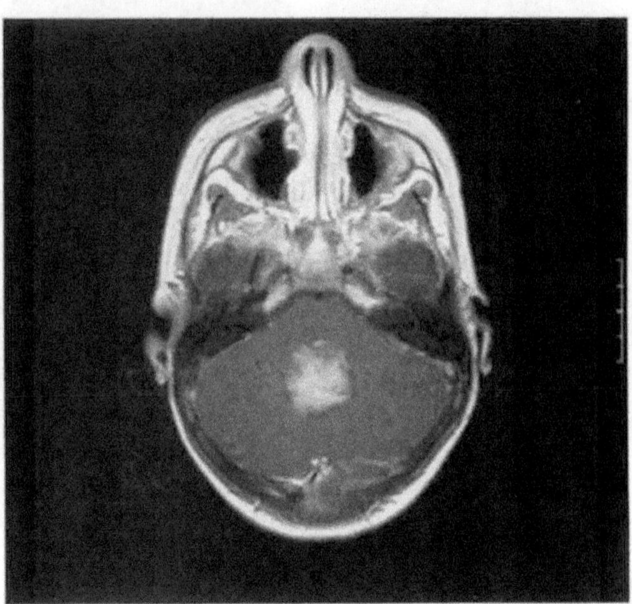

FIGURE 5.8Q

    A. Pilocytic astrocytoma
    B. Subependymoma
    C. Choroid plexus papilloma
    D. Hemangioblastoma
    E. Medulloblastoma

9. Which of the following features is usually NOT observed with oligodendrogliomas on MRI?

    A. Calcification
    B. Hemorrhage
    C. Cystic
    D. Heterogenous signal on T1-weighted images
    E. Intense homogenous enhancement

10. Which of the following characteristics is NOT observed in tuberous sclerosis (Bourneville disease)?

    A. Autosomal recessive inheritance pattern
    B. Cortical hamartomas
    C. Subependymal giant cell astrocytoma
    D. Cardiac rhabdomyomas
    E. Mental retardation

11. What is the appropriate management of the lesion depicted in this lateral internal carotid angiogram (Figure 5.11Q)?

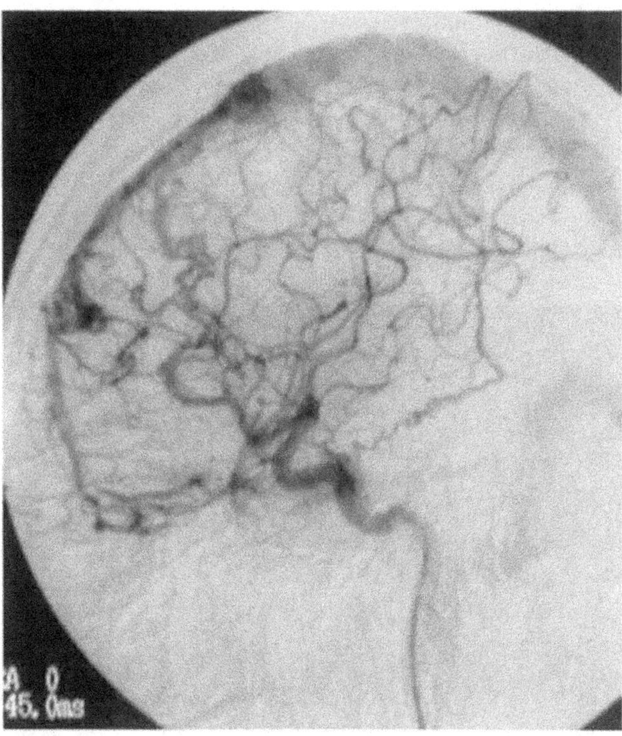

FIGURE 5.11Q

A. Repeat angiography in 6 to 12 months
B. Oral anticoagulation
C. No further treatment is required
D. Urgent surgical treatment
E. Follow up MRA in 6 to 12 months

12. Which of the following locations is typically NOT involved with diffuse axonal injuries?

A. Brainstem
B. Deep white matter
C. Cerebellum
D. Corpus callosum
E. Thalamus

13. A 12-year-old male presented with partial complex seizures. The patient was neurologically intact. MRI revealed a cystic right mesial temporal lobe lesion that is hypointense to brain on T1-weighted images and hyperintense on T2-weighted images, with mild rim enhancement. The most likely diagnosis is which of the following?

A. Ganglioglioma
B. Pleomorphic xanthoastrocytoma
C. Pilocytic astrocytoma
D. Germinoma
E. Glioblastoma

QUESTIONS 14–20

Directions: Match the following MR imaging characteristics with the appropriate intracranial hematoma. Some letters may be used once, more than once, or not at all.

A. Hyperacute (up to 4 to 6 hours)
B. Acute (7 to 72 hours)
C. Early subacute (4–7 days)
D. Late subacute (1 to 4 weeks)
E. Early chronic (weeks to months)
F. Late chronic (months to years)

14. Extracellular methemoglobin

15. Oxyhemoglobin

16. Isointense on T1, hypointense on T2

17. Deoxyhemoglobin, echinocytes

18. Hyperintense on T1, hypointense on T2

19. Isointense on T1, hyperintense on T2

20. Intracellular methemoglobin

End of set

21. A 38-year-old male presented with a 2-day history of severe headache, photophobia, and emesis. On examination, the patient was neurologically intact. The patient's CT scan is pictured below (Figure 5.21Q). Which of the following is NOT necessary in the management of this entity?

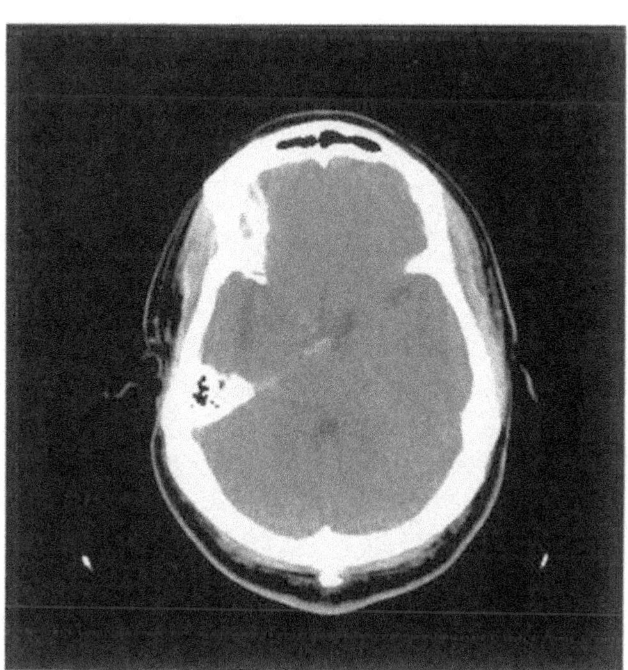

FIGURE 5.21Q

A. Angiography
B. Cardiac monitoring
C. Monitoring of electrolytes
D. Hyperdynamic therapy
E. Monitoring for hydrocephalus

22. What abnormality is depicted in this axial T2-weighted MRI (Figure 5.22Q)?

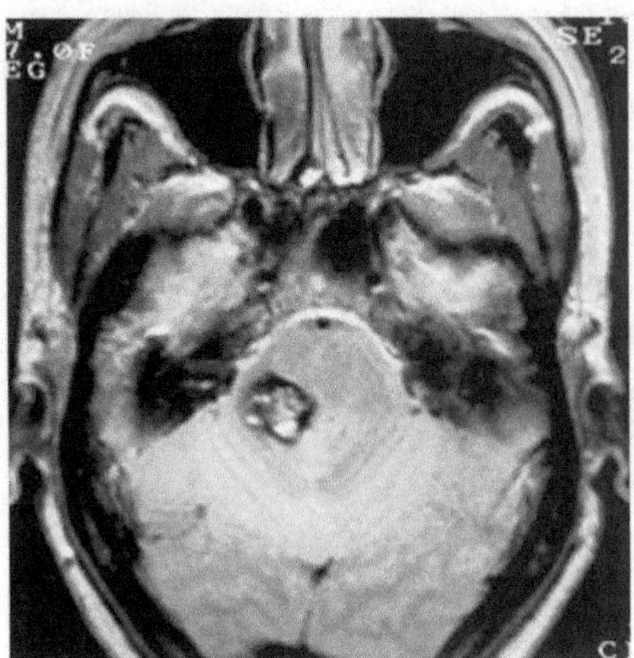

FIGURE 5.22Q

- **A.** Oligodendroglioma
- **B.** Capillary telangiectasia
- **C.** Cavernous malformation
- **D.** Venous angioma
- **E.** Choriocarcinoma

23. A 44-year-old male presented with a cutaneous melanoma. After local resection and radiation therapy, the patient underwent a CT scan of the chest/abdomen/pelvis, nuclear bone scan, and lumbar puncture for systemic staging. The patient had no evidence of systemic metastases and his CSF cytology was negative. The patient presented 2 weeks later with new-onset frontal headaches that were exacerbated with ambulation. The patient underwent an MRI of the brain; a contrasted axial T1-weighted image is illustrated below (Figure 5.23Q). What would be the most appropriate next step in management of this disorder?

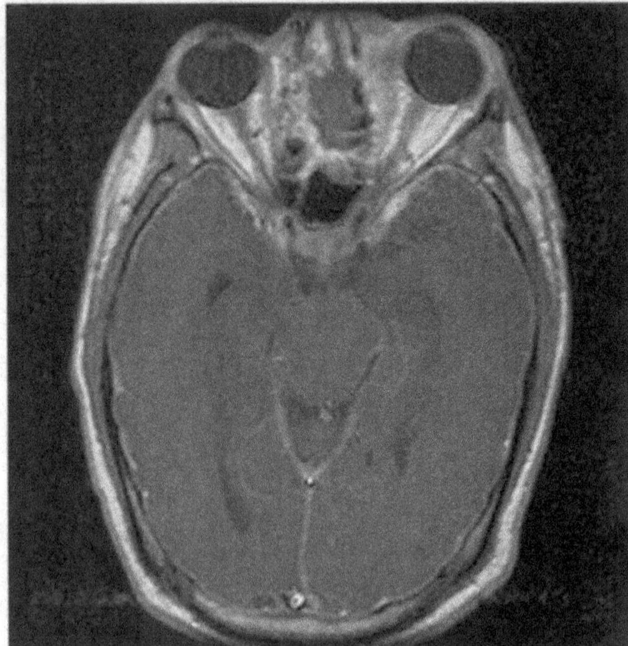

FIGURE 5.23Q

- **A.** Meningeal biopsy
- **B.** Repeat lumbar puncture
- **C.** Epidural blood patch
- **D.** Cerebral angiography
- **E.** None of the above

24. What is the vessel (arrow) on this lateral internal carotid angiogram (Figure 5.24Q) commonly associated with?

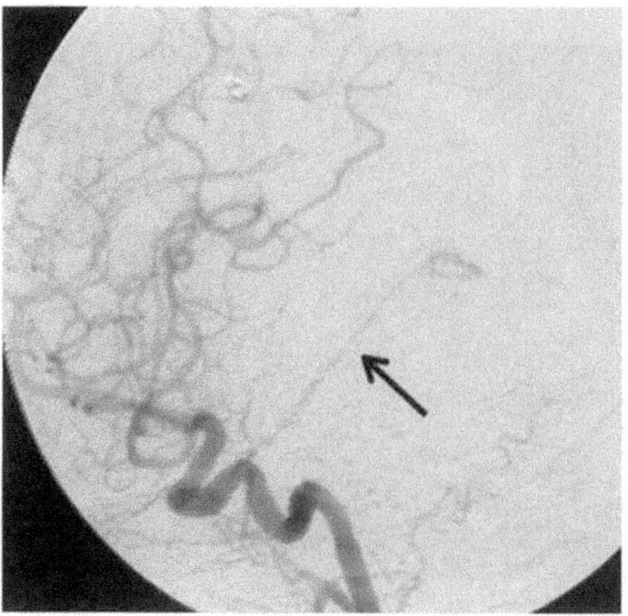

FIGURE 5.24Q

1. Tentorial meningioma
2. Venous angioma
3. Dural arteriovenous fistula
4. Choroid plexus papilloma

A. 1, 2, and 3 are correct
B. 1 and 3 are correct
C. 2 and 4 are correct
D. Only 4 is correct
E. All of the above are correct

25. What abnormality is depicted on this axial T2-weighted MR scan (Figure 5.25Q)?

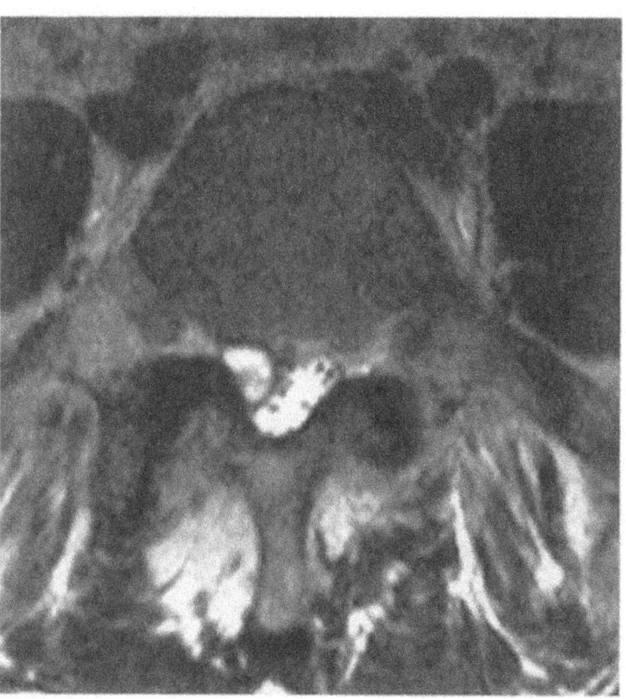

FIGURE 5.25Q

A. Herniated disc fragment
B. Neurofibroma
C. Synovial cyst
D. Osteochondroma
E. Neurenteric cyst

26. Which of the following characteristics is NOT associated with the disorder illustrated in this sagittal T2-weighted MRI (Figure 5.26Q)?

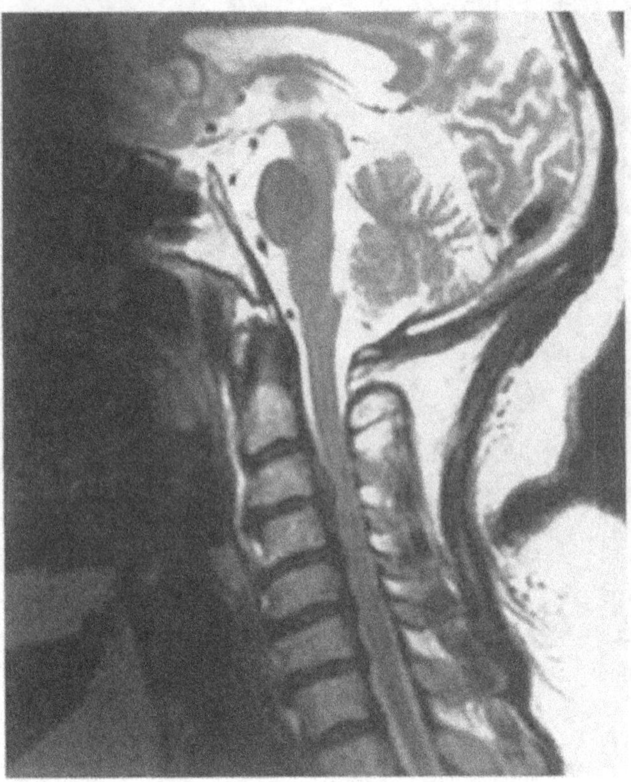

FIGURE 5.26Q

    A. Highest prevalence in the Japanese population
    B. 70% of all cases involve the cervical spine
    C. Commonly presents with progressive myelopathy
    D. C5 radiculopathy is a common complication of anterior surgical approaches
    E. Commonly identified on plain spinal x-rays

27. A 55-year-old female presented with the acute onset of a mild right hemiparesis. What neoplasm is depicted in the following enhanced T1-weighted MRI (Figure 5.27Q)?

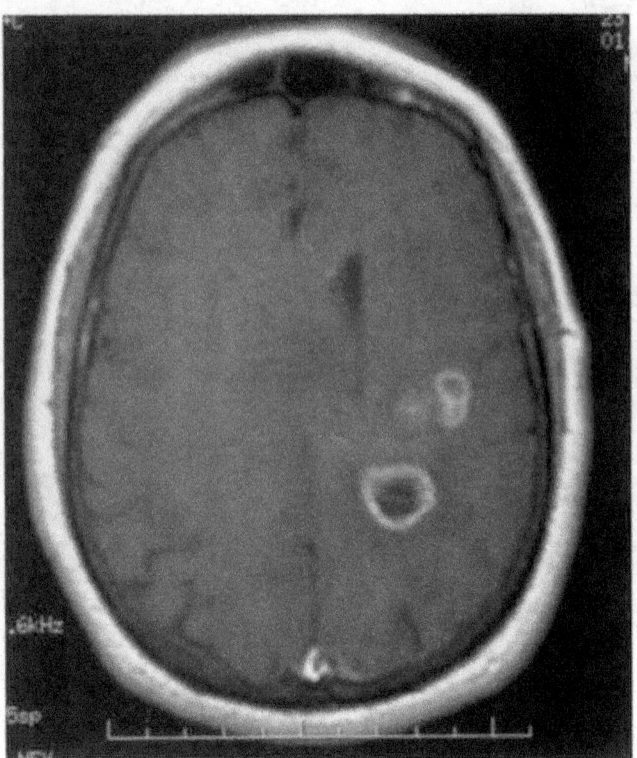

FIGURE 5.27Q

    A. CNS lymphoma
    B. Teratoma
    C. Oligodendroglioma
    D. Glioblastoma multiforme
    E. Melanoma

28. Which of the following characteristics is NOT associated with the abnormality depicted in the following CT scan (Figure 5.28Q)?

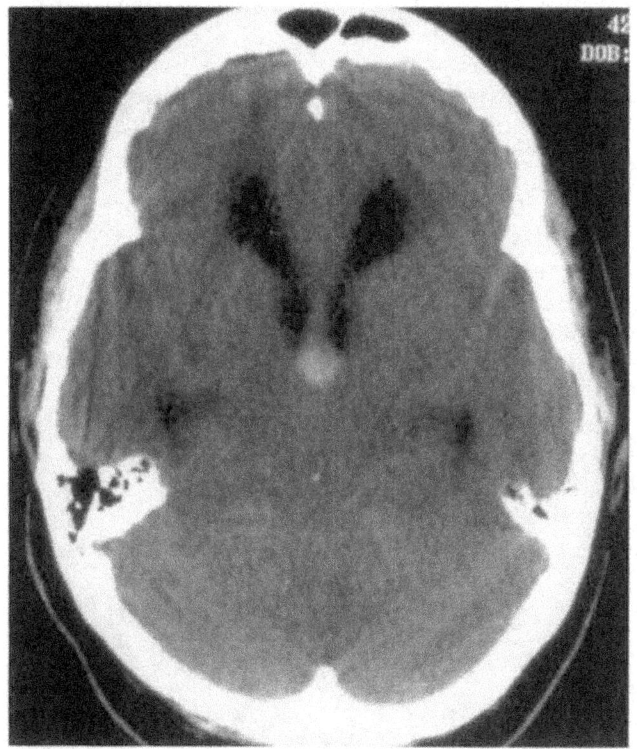

FIGURE 5.28Q

- **A.** Most commonly presents with headaches
- **B.** Most commonly hyperdense on CT scan
- **C.** Most commonly hyperintense to cortex on T1-weighted MRI
- **D.** Derived from ectoderm
- **E.** Does not exhibit malignant degeneration

29. What abnormality is depicted in the following enhanced T1-weighted MRI (Figure 5.29Q)?

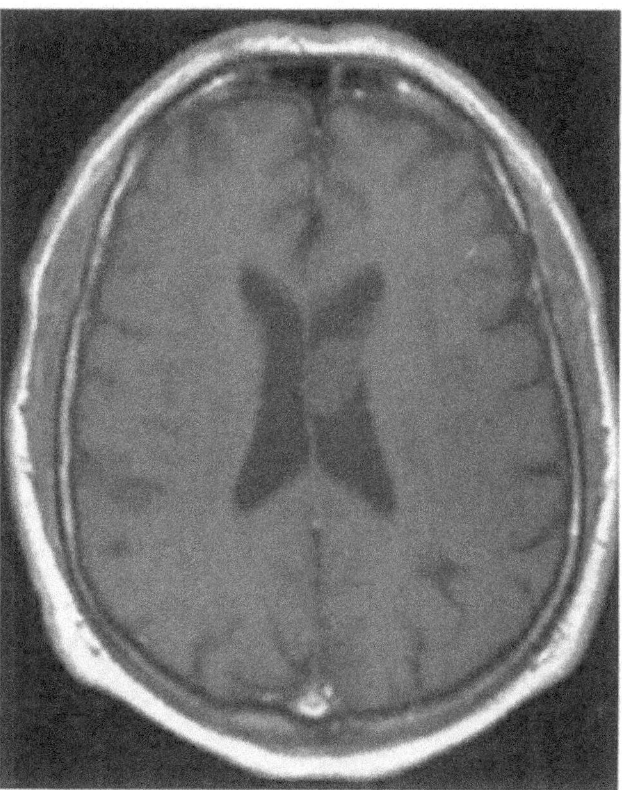

FIGURE 5.29Q

- **A.** Ependymoma
- **B.** Meningioma
- **C.** Pilocytic astrocytoma
- **D.** Central neurocytoma
- **E.** Choroid plexus papilloma

30. An 18-year-old male presented with a 6-month history of progressive occipital headaches and local scalp tenderness and edema. What abnormality is depicted in this patient's unenhanced axial CT scan (Figure 5.30Q)?

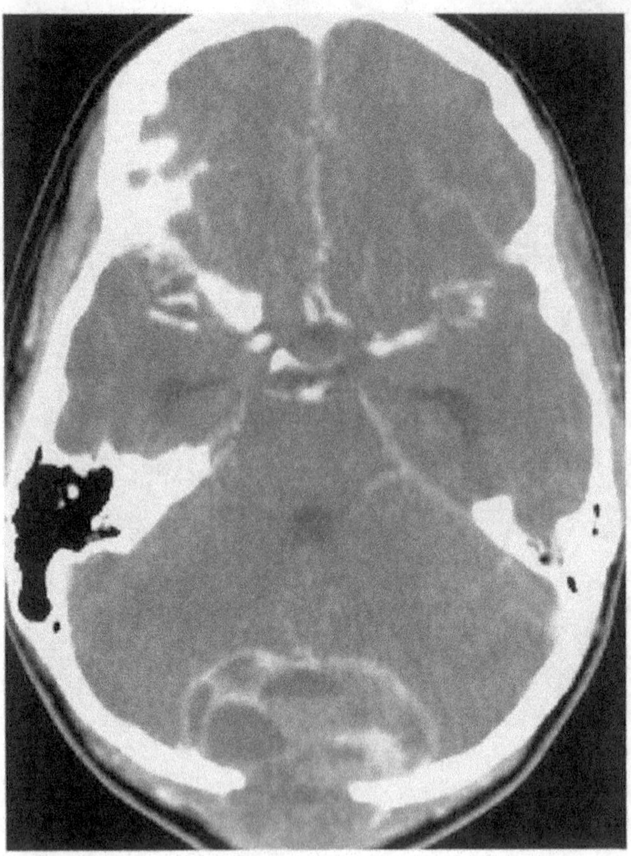

FIGURE 5.30Q

- **A.** Giant cell tumor
- **B.** Osteoid osteoma
- **C.** Eosinophilic granuloma
- **D.** Aneurysmal bone cyst
- **E.** Osteosarcoma

QUESTIONS 31–34

Directions: Match the labeled region on the following axial T2-weighted MRI (Figure 5.31–5.34Q) with the corresponding cortical structure. Letters may be used more than once or not at all.

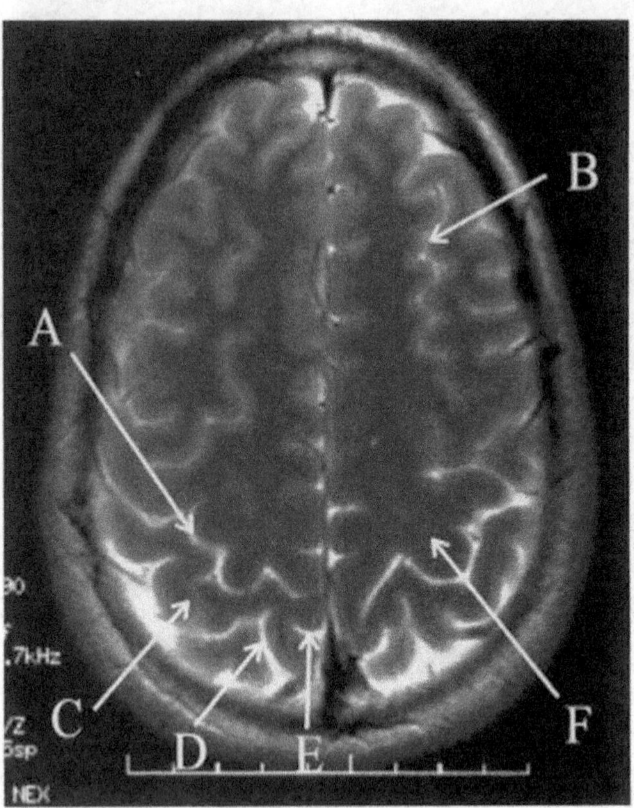

FIGURE 5.31–34Q

31. Primary motor cortex

32. Postcentral sulcus

33. Central sulcus

34. Superior frontal sulcus

End of set

35. Which of the following disorders is exhibited in this axial contrasted T1-weighted MRI (Figure 5.35Q)?

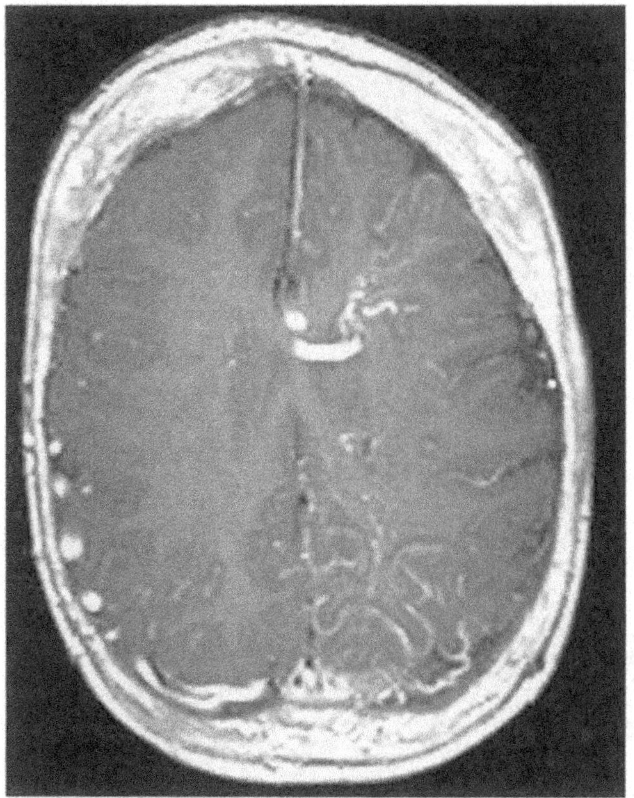

FIGURE 5.35Q

A. Sturge-Weber syndrome
B. Tuberous sclerosis
C. Wyburn-Mason syndrome
D. Laurence-Moon-Biedl syndrome
E. Neurofibromatosis type 1

36. Which of the following abnormalities is depicted in this left carotid artery AP angiogram (Figure 5.36Q)?

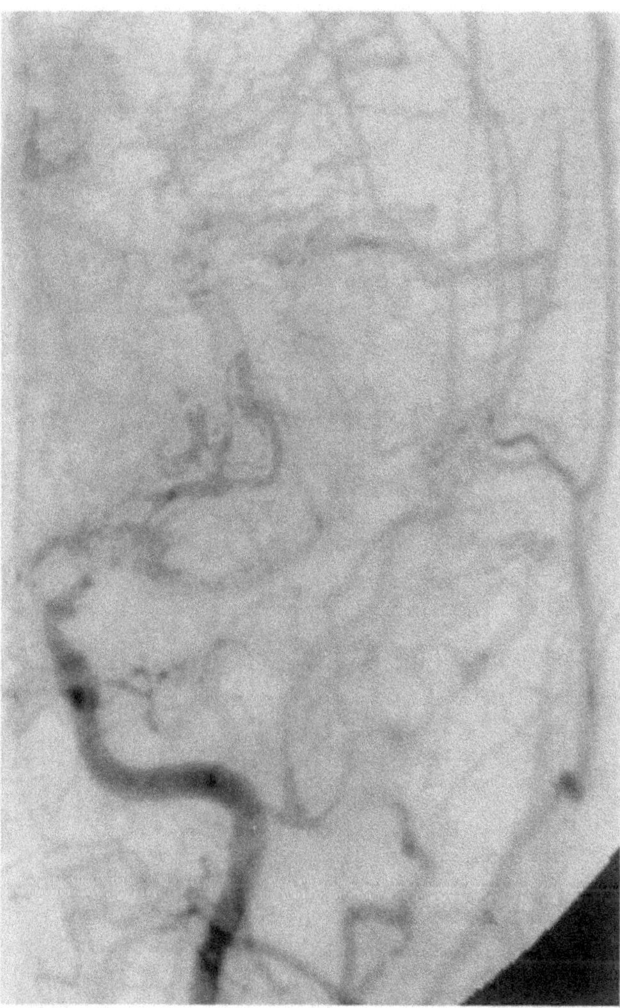

FIGURE 5.36Q

A. Acute embolic occlusion
B. Arterial dissection
C. Dural arteriovenous malformation
D. Moyamoya
E. Vasculitis

37. Which of the following conditions is NOT associated with regional hypometabolism with fluorine-18 deoxyglucose (FDG) positron emissions tomography (PET) imaging?

A. Epileptic foci
B. Radiation necrosis
C. Glioblastoma multiforme
D. Fibrillary astrocytoma
E. None of the above

38. A premature infant exhibited infantile spasms shortly after admission to the neonatal intensive care unit. The patient's T2-weighted MRI (Figure 5.38Q) depicts what abnormality?

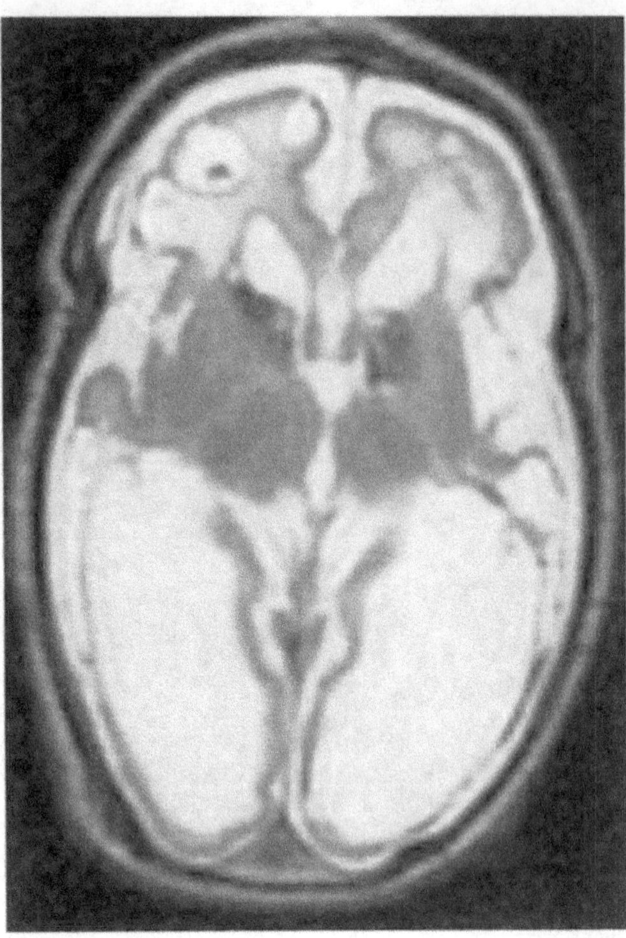

FIGURE 5.38Q

   A. Cortical dysplasia
   B. Bilateral porencephaly
   C. Holoprosencephaly
   D. Congenital cytomegalovirus infection
   E. Hydranencephaly

39. What is the approximate age of the hematoma depicted below on this nonenhanced axial T1-weighted MRI?

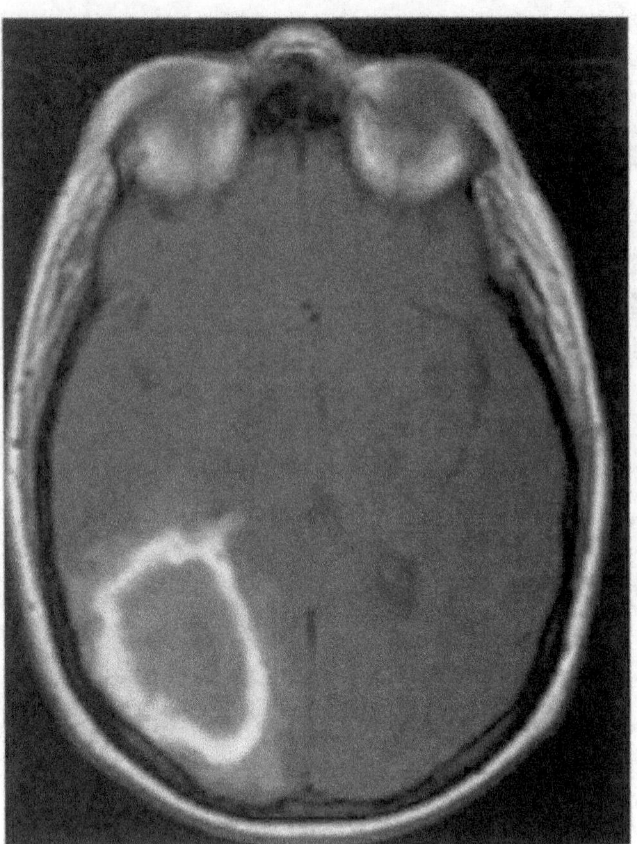

FIGURE 5.39Q

   A. Hyperacute
   B. Acute
   C. Early subacute
   D. Late subacute
   E. Chronic

40. A 15-year-old male presented with headaches and polyuria. Contrasted sagittal T1-weighted MRI (Figure 5.40Q) depicts what disorder?

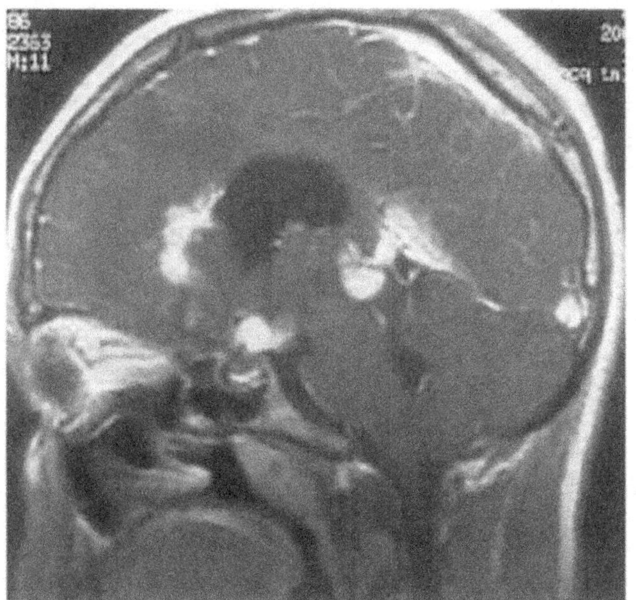

FIGURE 5.40Q

A. Histiocytosis X

B. Lipoma

C. Germinoma

D. Hypothalamic glioma

E. Pineoblastoma

41. What abnormality is depicted on the following lateral internal carotid artery angiogram (Figure 5.41Q)?

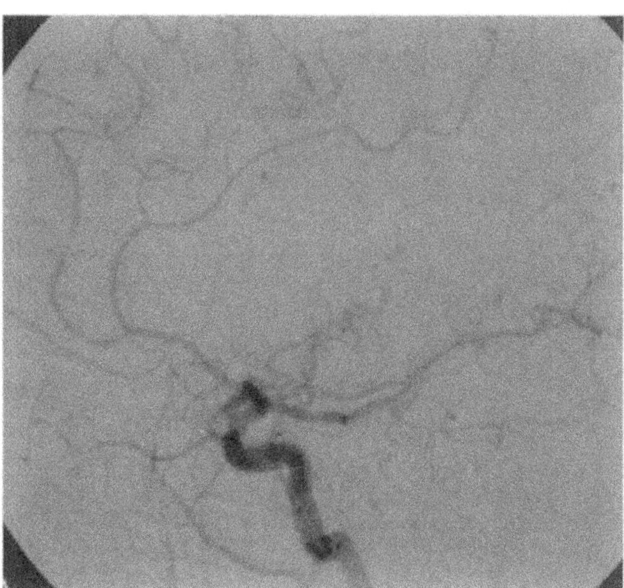

FIGURE 5.41Q

A. Arteriovenous malformation

B. Primary angiitis of the CNS

C. Cavernous malformation

D. Embolic stroke

E. Moyamoya

42. A 35-year-old male with a history of AIDS presented with altered mental status and low-grade fever. Contrasted axial T1-weighted MRI (Figure 5.42Q) depicts what abnormality?

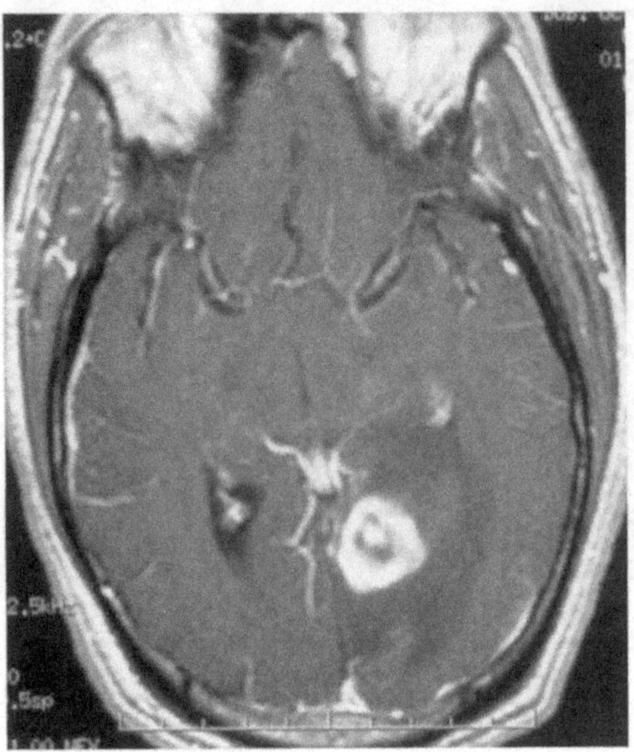

FIGURE 5.42Q

    A. CNS lymphoma
    B. Progressive multifocal leukoencephalopathy
    C. Cryptococcoma
    D. Tuberculoma
    E. Toxoplasmosis

43. A 4-month-old neonate presented with macrocephaly. Axial unenhanced CT scan (Figure 5.43Q) depicts what abnormality?

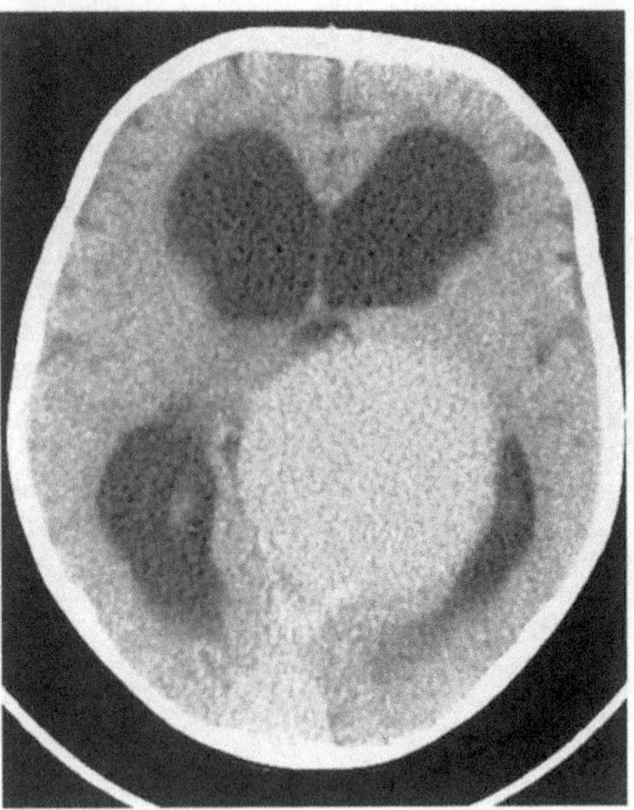

FIGURE 5.43Q

    A. Pineoblastoma
    B. Vein of Galen malformation
    C. Sinus pericranii
    D. Cavernous malformation
    E. Teratoma

44. What abnormality is depicted on the following unenhanced sagittal T1-weighted MRI (Figure 5.44Q)?

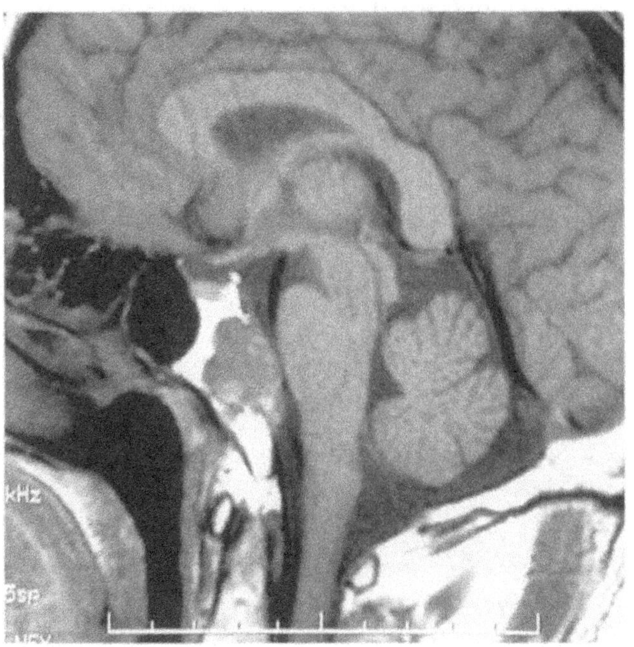

FIGURE 5.44Q

A. Pituitary adenoma
B. Rathke's cleft cyst
C. Meningioma
D. Chordoma
E. Fibrous dysplasia

45. An 8-week-old infant presented with a palpable scalp mass. What lesion is depicted in the following plain skull film (Figure 5.45Q)?

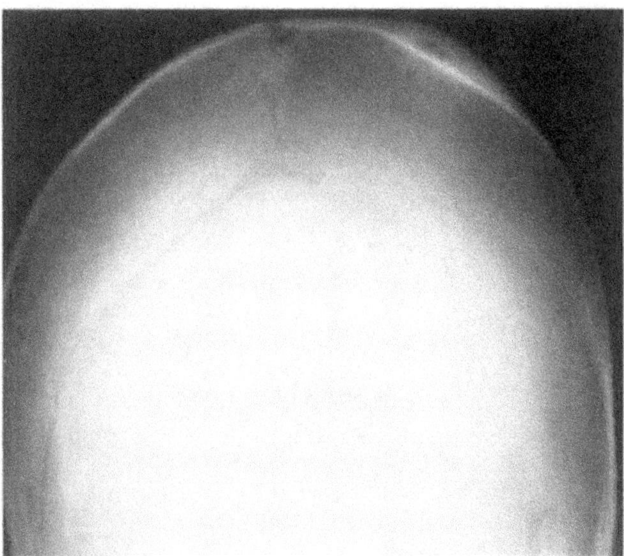

FIGURE 5.45Q

A. Cephalhematoma
B. Dermoid
C. Eosinophilic granuloma
D. Osteochondroma
E. Aneurysmal bone cyst

46. The following axial contrasted T1-weighted MRI is located at the L3-4 disc space (Figure 5.46Q). What structure is most likely to be affected by the abnormality depicted in this MRI?

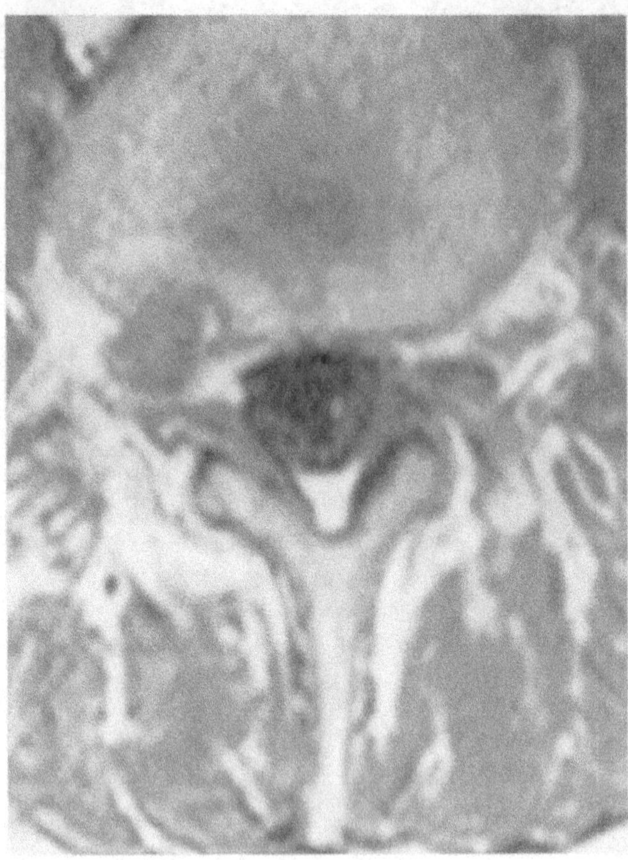

FIGURE 5.46Q

   A. L3 nerve root
   B. L4 nerve root
   C. Both of the above
   D. Neither of the above

QUESTIONS 47–51

Directions: Match the following locations and demographic information with the most likely involved primary CNS neoplasm. Letters may be used more than once or not at all.

   A. Pilocytic astrocytoma   **E.** Meningioma
   B. Schwannoma   **F.** Choroid plexus papilloma
   C. Pineoblastoma   **G.** Medulloblastoma
   D. Germinoma   **H.** Hemangioblastoma
                           I. None of the above

47. Pineal region, 15-year-old male

48. Cerebellum, 58-year-old female

49. Cerebellopontine angle, 42-year-old female

50. Posterior fossa, 12-year-old male

51. Atrium, 8-year-old male

End of set

52. What is the approximate age of the following hematoma on this noncontrasted axial CT scan (Figure 5.52Q)?

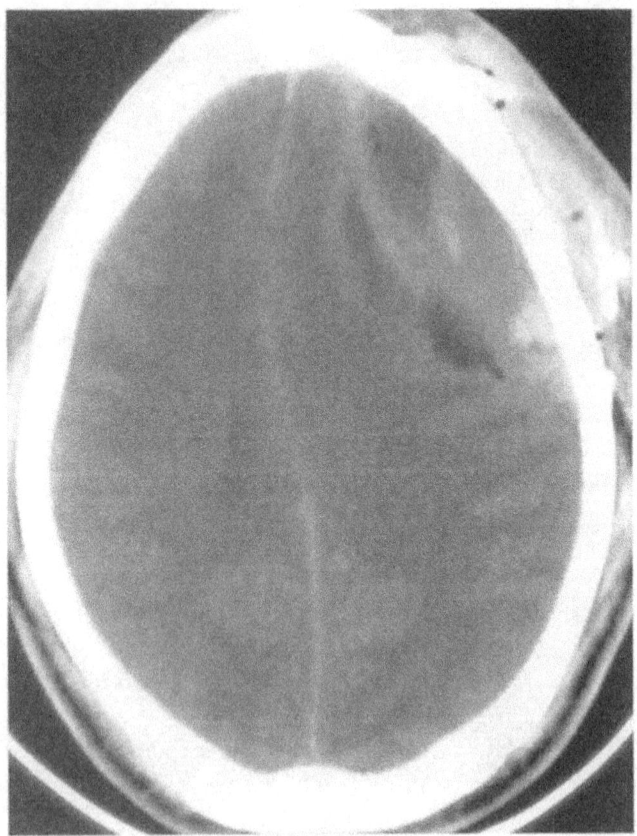

FIGURE 5.52Q

   A. Hyperacute
   B. Acute
   C. Early subacute
   D. Late subacute
   E. Chronic

53. Which of the following characteristics is NOT associated with the disorder depicted in this lateral thoracic spine radiograph (Figure 5.53Q)?

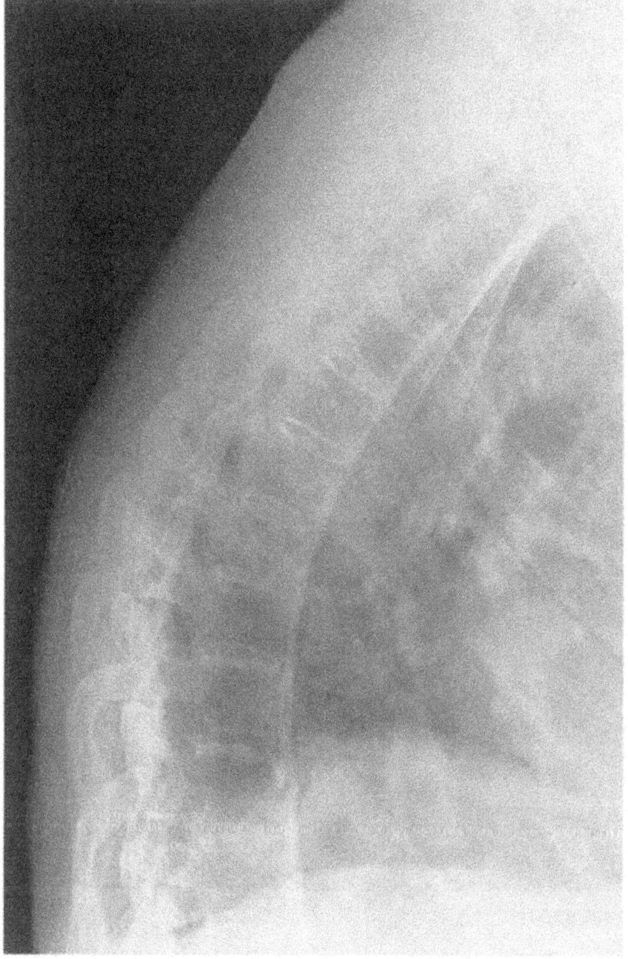

FIGURE 5.53Q

  A. Craniocervical instability
  B. More common in young males
  C. Pathologic fractures
  D. HLA D15
  E. Sacroiliitis

54. What is the most likely histologic appearance of the neoplasm depicted in the following sagittal T2-weighted MRI (Figure 5.54Q)?

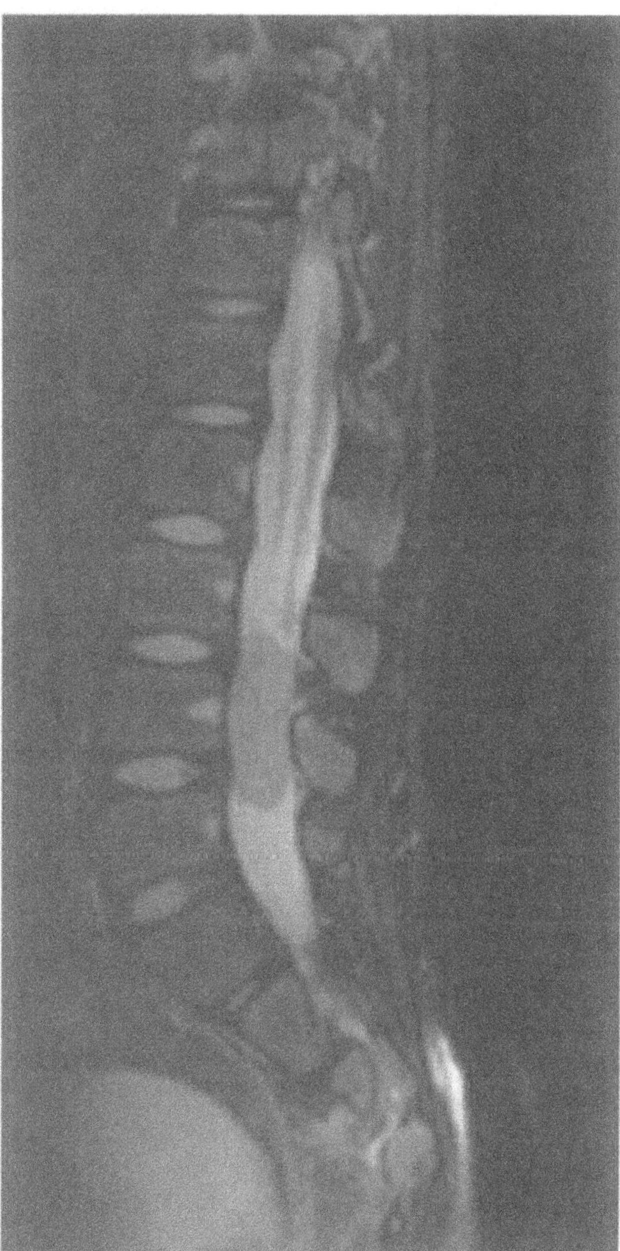

FIGURE 5.54Q

  A. Small blue cells with prominent mitoses and necrosis
  B. Whorls of cells with intermingled fascicular arrangements
  C. Elongated cells with prominent cytoplasmic processes and minimal pleomorphism
  D. Clusters of cuboidal cells separated by a prominent mucoid matrix
  E. Lipid-containing cells within a dense network of vascular channels

55. What is depicted in this noncontrasted axial T1-weighted MRI (Figure 5.55Q)? The lesion did not exhibit enhancement with the administration of gadolinium.

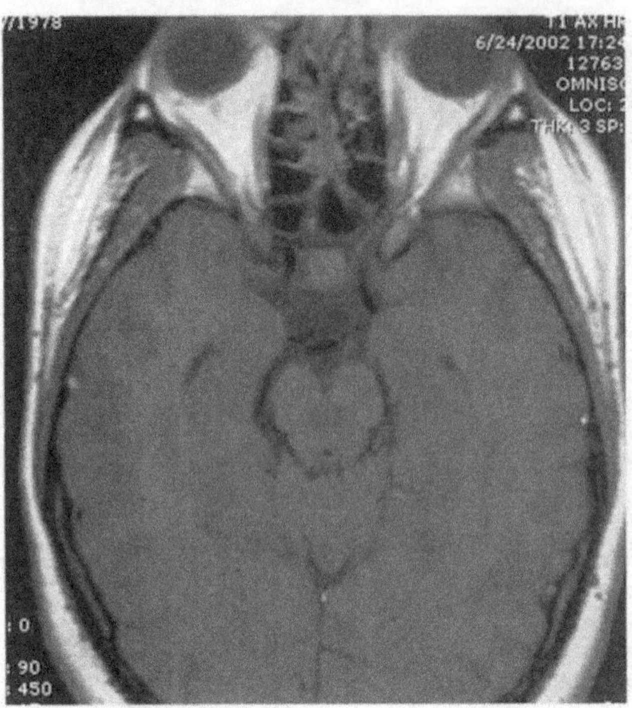

FIGURE 5.55Q

    A. Pituitary adenoma
    B. Craniopharyngioma
    C. Lipoma
    D. Rathke's cleft cyst
    E. Histiocytosis X

56. What abnormality is depicted on the following axial T2-weighted MRI (Figure 5.56Q)?

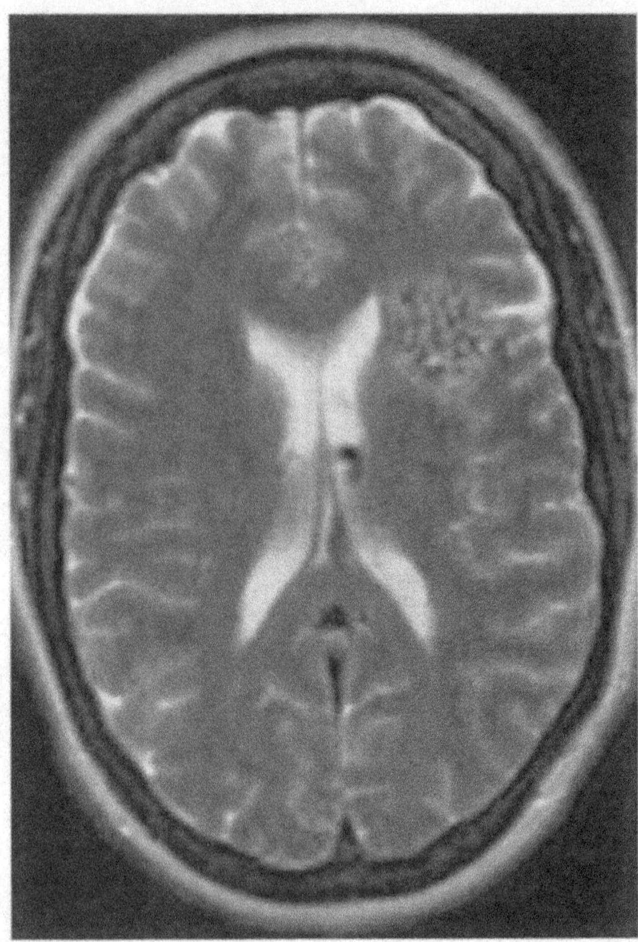

FIGURE 5.56Q

    A. Arteriovenous malformation
    B. Oligodendroglioma
    C. Cavernous malformation
    D. Multiple sclerosis plaque
    E. Hemangioblastoma

57. A 48-year-old female presented with headaches, nausea, and ataxia. The contrasted axial T1-weighted MRI below (Figure 5.57Q) depicts what abnormality?

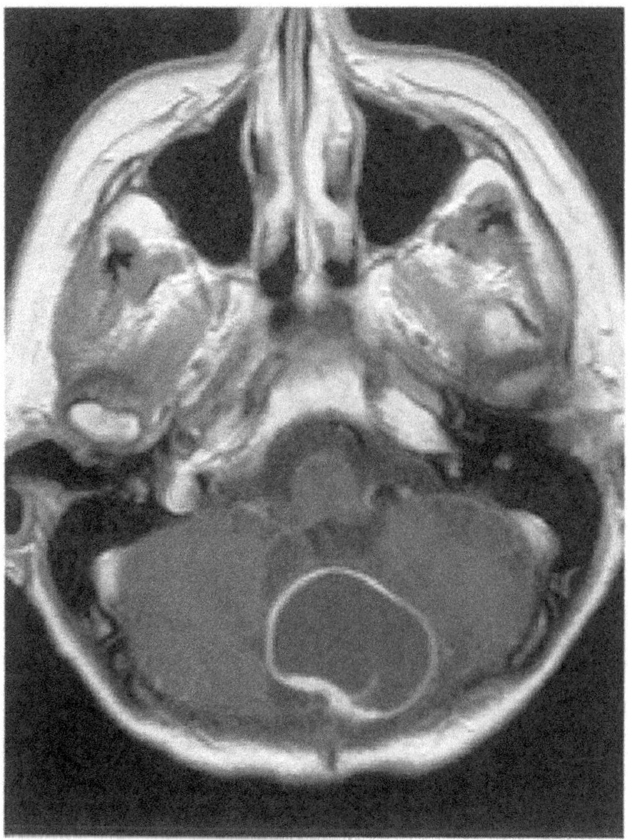

FIGURE 5.57Q

A. Pilocytic astrocytoma
B. Choroid plexus papilloma
C. Hemangioblastoma
D. Metastatic lesion
E. Ganglioglioma

58. What lesion is depicted in the following AP cervical spine radiograph (Figure 5.58Q)?

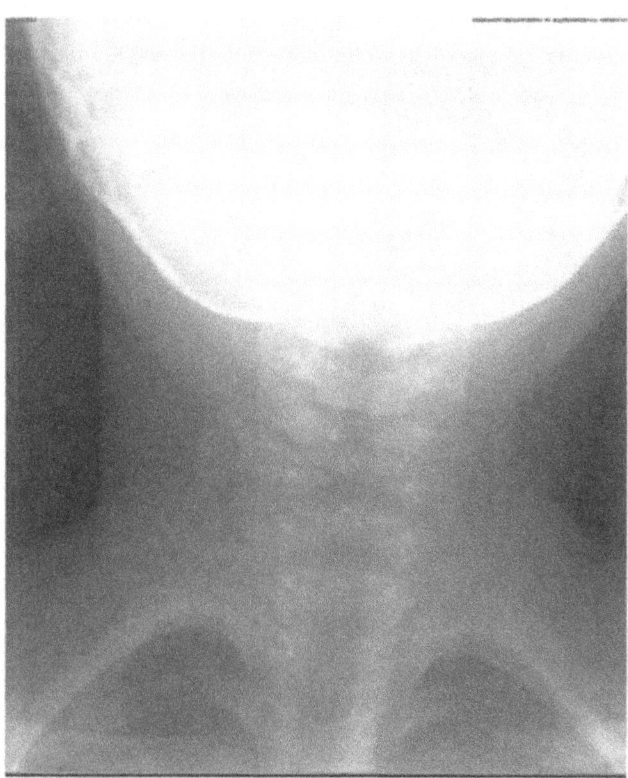

FIGURE 5.58Q

A. Eosinophilic granuloma
B. Osteoblastoma
C. Osteoid osteoma
D. Osteosarcoma
E. Osteochondroma

59. A 5-year-old male presented with generalized seizures and developmental delay. What abnormality is depicted on the patient's axial T2-weighted MRI (Figure 5.59Q)?

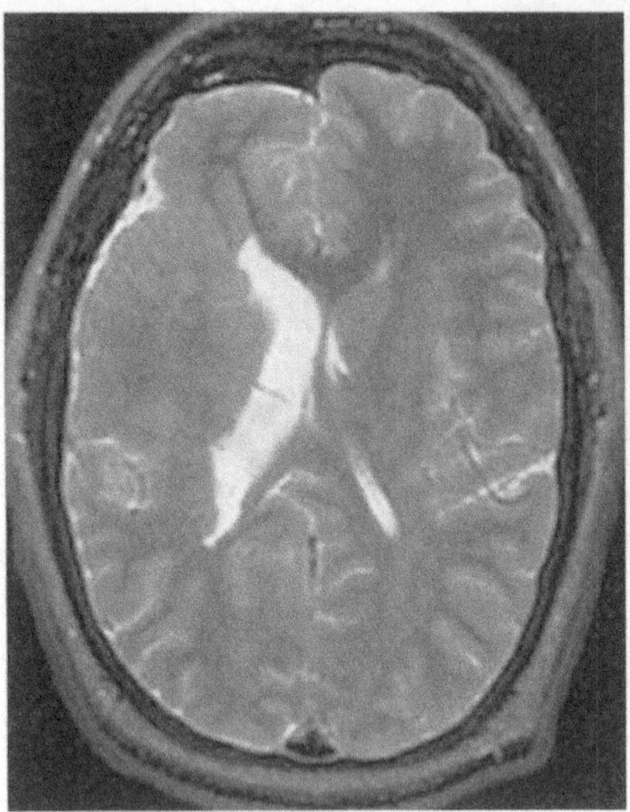

FIGURE 5.59Q

- **A.** Pachygyria
- **B.** Lobar holoprosencephaly
- **C.** Tuberous sclerosis
- **D.** Nodular heterotopia
- **E.** Septo-optic dysplasia

60. Which of the following imaging abnormalities is NOT associated with neurofibromatosis type 1?

- **A.** Optic nerve gliomas
- **B.** Basal ganglia hamartomas
- **C.** Thoracic meningoceles
- **D.** Spinal schwannomas
- **E.** Posterior vertebral body scalloping

61. A 21-year-old female with a prior 2-week history of nasal congestion and frontal headaches presents with fever, leukocytosis, and confusion. Based on the patient's axial contrasted T1-weighted MRI (Figure 5.61Q), what is the appropriate next step in the management of this condition?

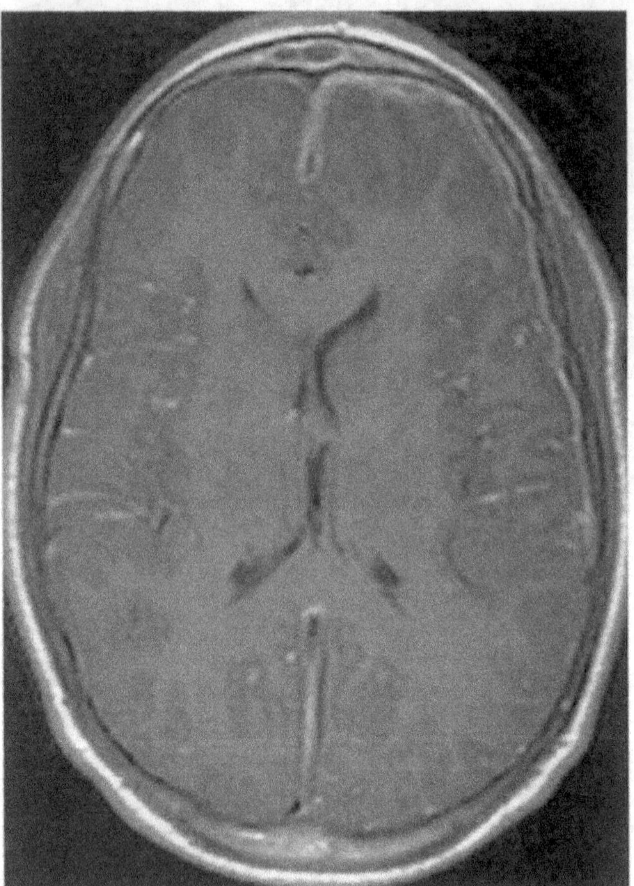

FIGURE 5.61Q

- **A.** Administration of broad-spectrum IV antibiotics
- **B.** Administration of IV steroids
- **C.** Lumbar puncture
- **D.** Emergent surgical evacuation
- **E.** ICU observation with repeat CT scan in 24 hours

62. Which of the following disorders is associated with multiple intracranial arteriovenous malformations, often involving the visual pathways and the mesencephalon?

- **A.** Wyburn-Mason syndrome
- **B.** Meningioangiomatosis
- **C.** Blue rubber bleb nevus syndrome
- **D.** Sturge-Weber syndrome
- **E.** None of the above

63. Which of the following characteristics is NOT associated with the disorder depicted in the following CT myelogram (Figure 5.63Q)?

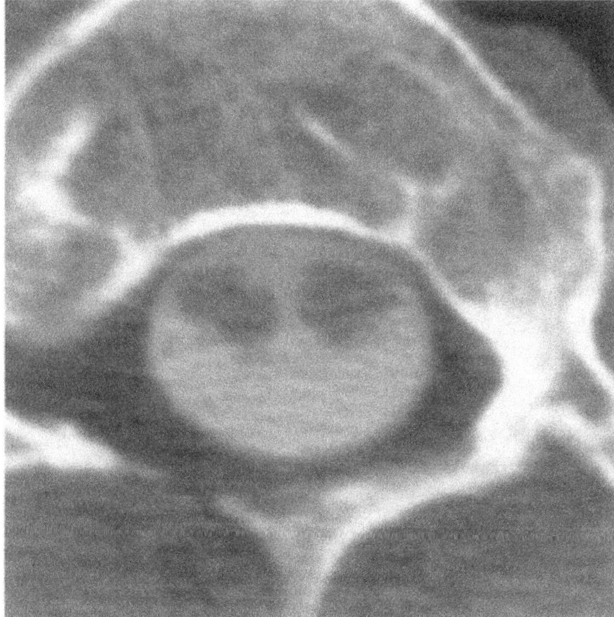

FIGURE 5.63Q

- **A.** Tethered cord
- **B.** Klippel-Feil syndrome
- **C.** Chiari I malformation
- **D.** Scoliosis
- **E.** Spina bifida

64. Which of the following neurologic symptoms would a patient with the following noncontrasted CT scan (Figure 5.64Q) be most likely to exhibit?

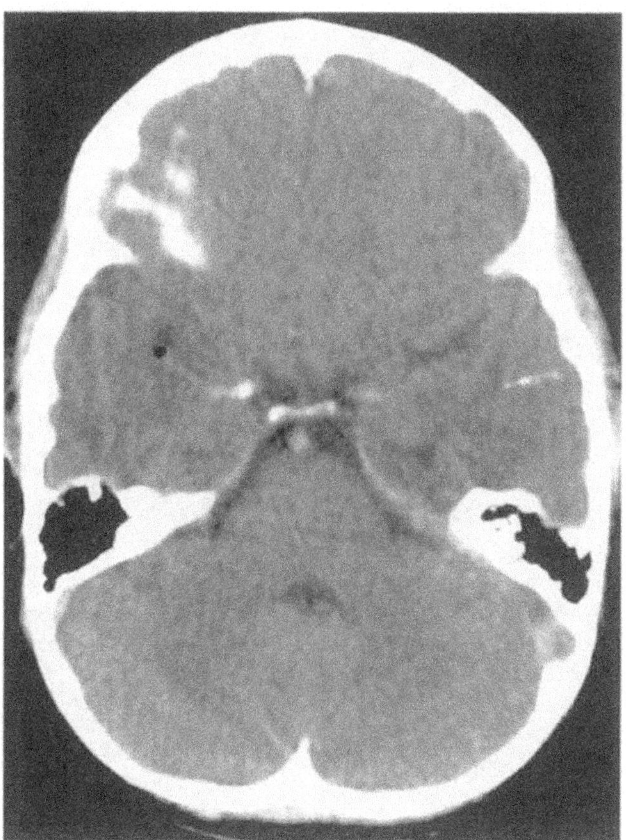

FIGURE 5.64Q

- **A.** Confusion and lethargy
- **B.** Left hemiparesis
- **C.** Right homonymous hemianopsia
- **D.** Bilateral temporal hemianopsia
- **E.** Receptive aphasia

65. What is the most likely etiology of the lesion demonstrated in the following lateral internal carotid angiogram (midarterial phase) (Figure 5.65Q)?

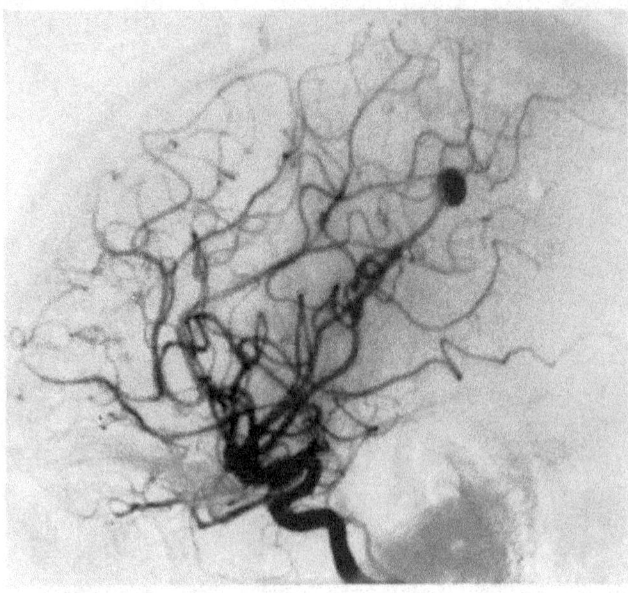

FIGURE 5.65Q

A. Trauma
B. Congenital
C. Infection
D. Dissection
E. Atherosclerosis

66. Which of the following disorders is NOT typically associated with agenesis of the corpus callosum?

A. Holoprosencephaly
B. Aicardi syndrome
C. Dandy-Walker malformation
D. Klippel-Feil syndrome
E. Trisomy 13

67. Which of the following characteristics is commonly observed on plain skull films in patients with Sturge-Weber syndrome?

1. Thickened calvarium
2. Enlarged frontal sinus
3. "Tram-track" calcifications
4. Elevation of the petrous temporal bone

A. 1, 2, and 3 are correct
B. 1 and 3 are correct
C. 2 and 4 are correct
D. Only 4 is correct
E. All of the above are correct

68. All of the following are true about basilar impression (BI) EXCEPT?

A. Most common acquired anomaly of the craniocervical junction
B. Often accompanied by Down's syndrome, Klippel-Feil syndrome, and Chiari malformation
C. Characterized by upward displacement of foramen magnum margins (occipital bone) and cervical spine (odontoid process) into the posterior fossa
D. McRae's line can help make the diagnosis
E. May be seen after trauma

69. Which of the following spinal neoplasms is typically found in an intradural-extramedullary location?

1. Neurofibroma
2. Ganglioneuroma
3. Schwannoma
4. Ependymoma

A. 1, 2, and 3 are correct
B. 1 and 3 are correct
C. 2 and 4 are correct
D. Only 4 is correct
E. All of the above are correct

QUESTIONS 70–74

Directions: Match the sellar lesion with the appropriate imaging characteristic using each answer either once, more than once, or not at all.

A. Pituitary macroadenoma
B. Rathke's cleft cyst
C. Both of the above
D. None of the above

70. Hypointense on T1-weighted images

71. Enhances with administration of gadolinium

72. Hyperintense on T2-weighted images

73. Exhibits calcification

74. Primarily intrasellar location

End of set

75. What is the mechanism of injury in the following spine fracture (axial CT scan) (Figure 5.75Q)?

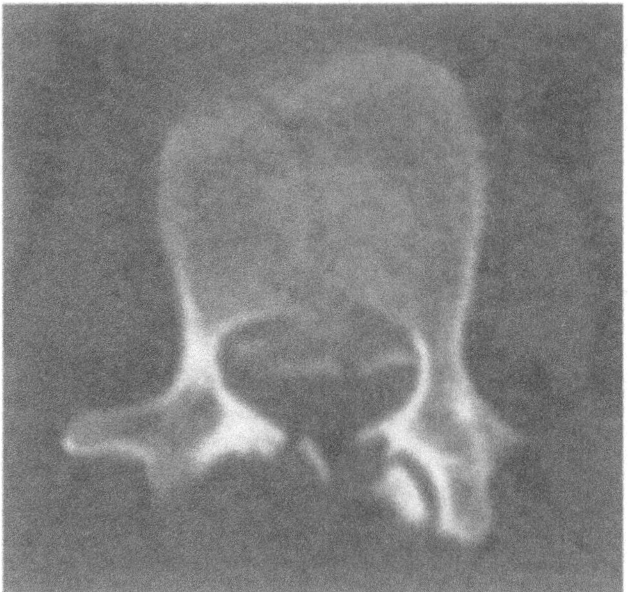

FIGURE 5.75Q

- **A.** Fracture-dislocation
- **B.** Axial compression
- **C.** Flexion-distraction
- **D.** Hyperextension
- **E.** None of the above

76. What is the most likely etiology for the abnormality depicted in the following axial FLAIR MRI (Figure 5.76Q)?

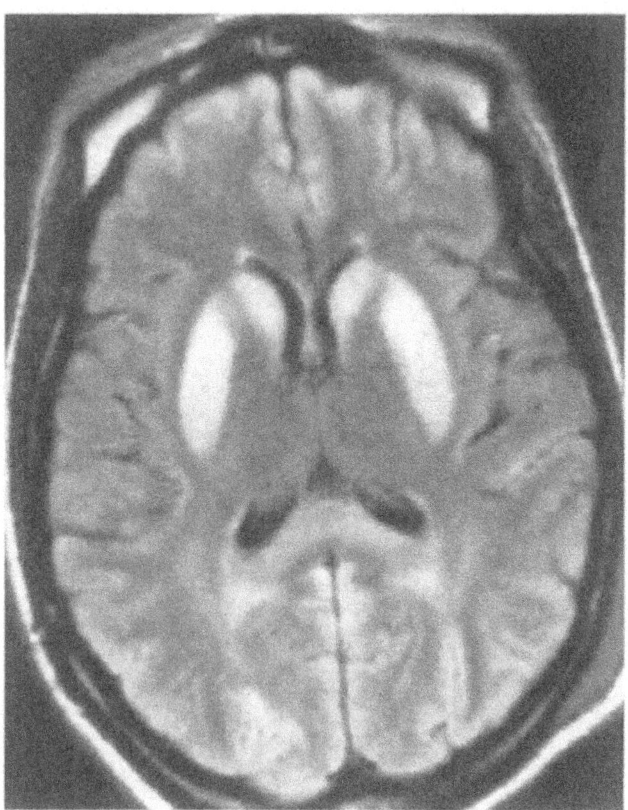

FIGURE 5.76Q

- **A.** Embolic
- **B.** Metabolic
- **C.** Congenital
- **D.** Hypoxic
- **E.** Infectious

77. What intramedullary neoplasm is illustrated in this early arterial phase vertebral artery angiogram (Figure 5.77Q)?

78. What neoplasm is depicted on this external carotid angiogram (midarterial phase) (Figure 5.78Q)?

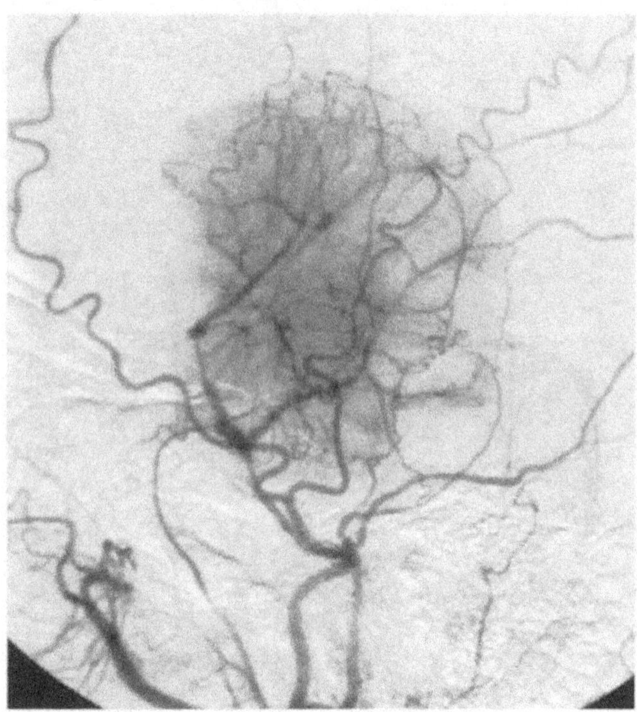

FIGURE 5.78Q

    A. Astrocytoma
    B. Choroid plexus papilloma
    C. Hemangioblastoma
    D. Meningioma
    E. Central neurocytoma

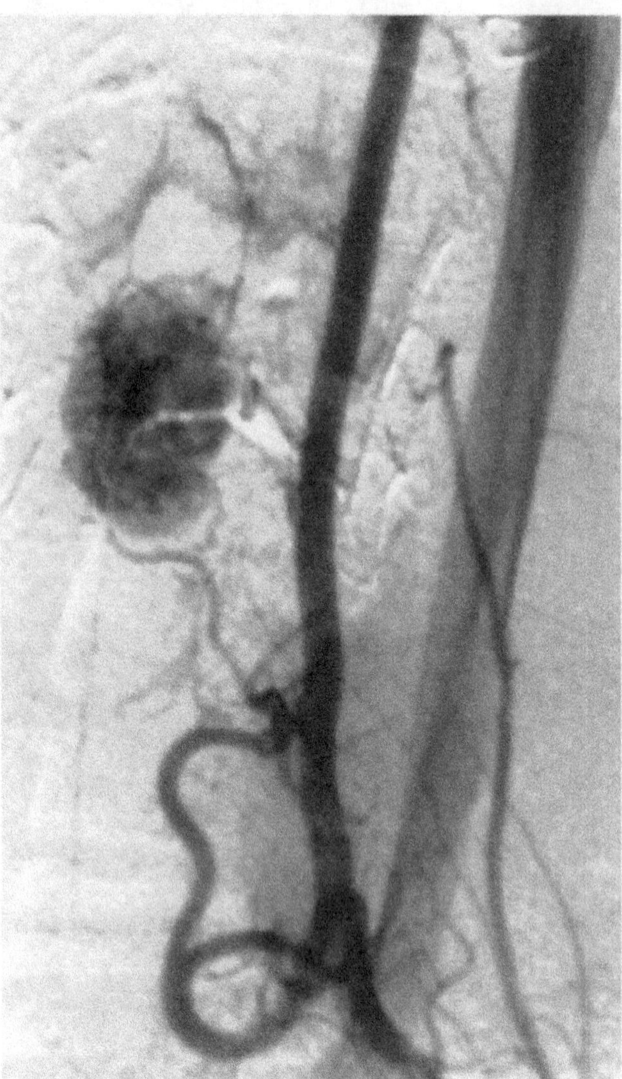

FIGURE 5.77Q

    A. Astrocytoma
    B. Ependymoma
    C. Hemangioblastoma
    D. Meningioma
    E. None of the above

79. Which of the following characteristics is NOT associated with the disorder depicted in this lateral skull radiograph (Figure 5.79Q)?

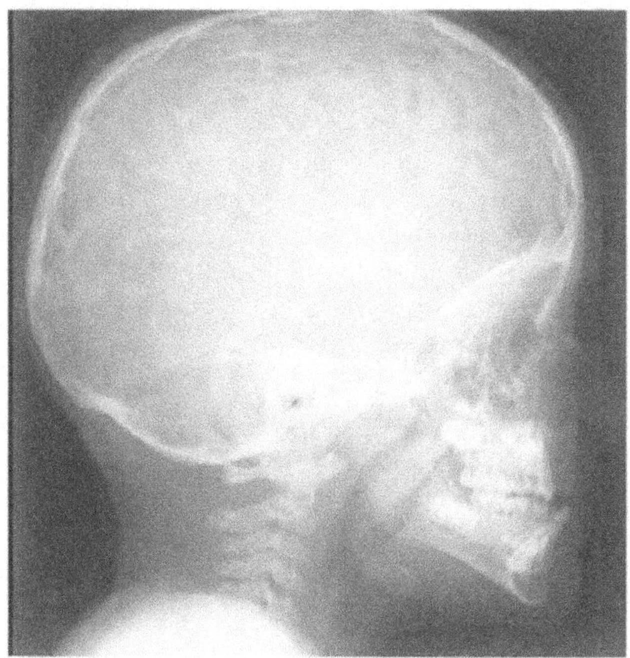

FIGURE 5.79Q

A. Craniosynostosis
B. Syndactyly
C. Mental retardation
D. Autosomal dominant inheritance pattern
E. Ptosis

80. Which of the following imaging characteristics is/are associated with multiple sclerosis?

1. Periventricular hyperintense lesions on T2-weighted images
2. Basal ganglia hypointense lesions on T2-weighted images
3. Callososeptal lesions with extension into deep white matter
4. No enhancement with administration of gadolinium

A. 1, 2, and 3 are correct
B. 1 and 3 are correct
C. 2 and 4 are correct
D. Only 4 is correct
E. All of the above are correct

81. What is the most common management of the lesion depicted in the following 3D CT reconstruction (Figure 5.81Q)?

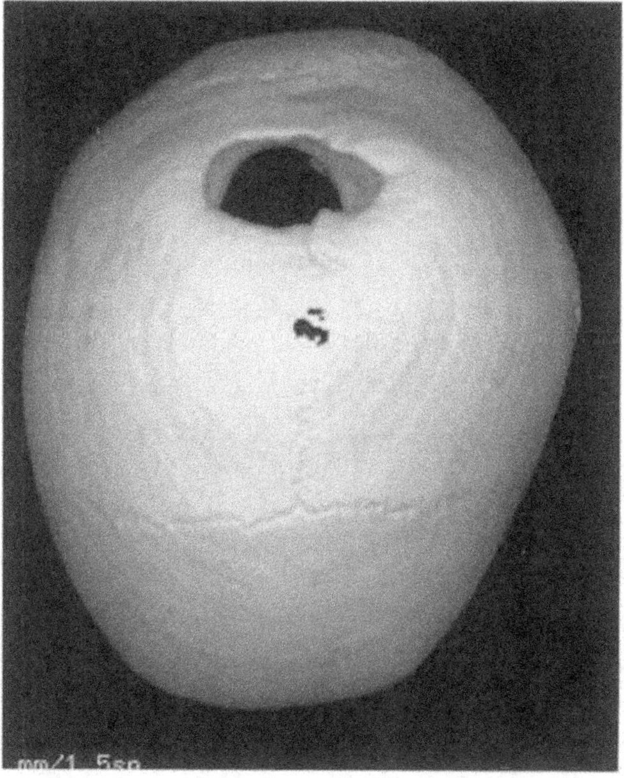

FIGURE 5.81Q

A. Surgical resection
B. Focused radiation
C. Chemotherapy
D. IV steroids
E. Observation

82. What abnormality is depicted in the following lateral carotid angiogram (midarterial phase) (Figure 5.82Q)?

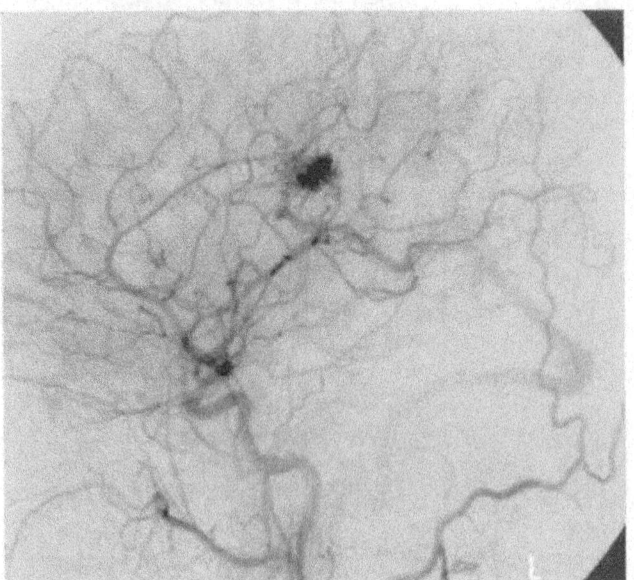

FIGURE 5.82Q

    A. High-grade astrocytoma
    B. Hemangioblastoma
    C. Arteriovenous malformation
    D. Cavernous malformation
    E. Venous angioma

83. A 72-year-old man presented with bitemporal hemianopsia. The following contrasted T1-weighted MRI exhibits what abnormality (Figure 5.83Q)?

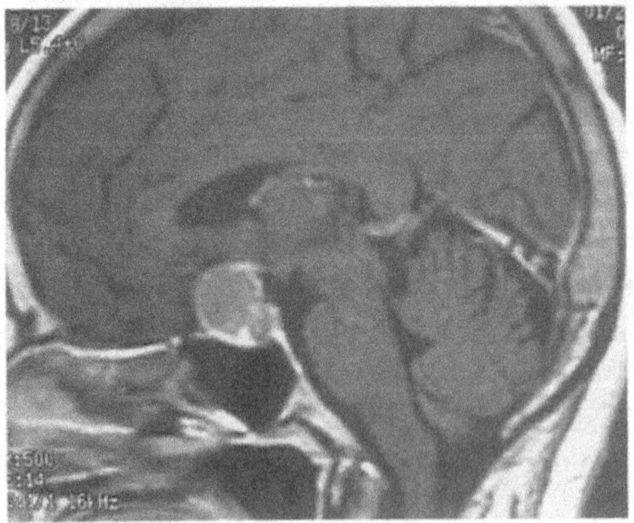

FIGURE 5.83Q

    A. Pituitary adenoma
    B. Craniopharyngioma
    C. Rathke's cleft cyst
    D. Pilocytic astrocytoma
    E. Metastatic tumor

84. What is the inheritance pattern of the disorder depicted in the following nonenhanced axial T1-weighted MRI (Figure 5.84Q)?

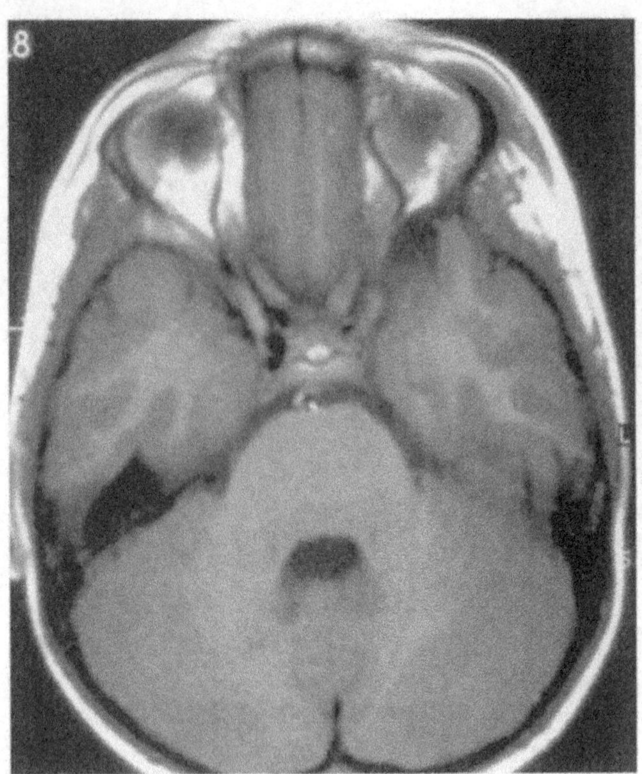

FIGURE 5.84Q

    A. Autosomal dominant
    B. Autosomal recessive
    C. X-linked
    D. Sporadic
    E. Mitochondrial

85. What abnormality is depicted on this cervical internal carotid angiogram (Figure 5.85Q)?

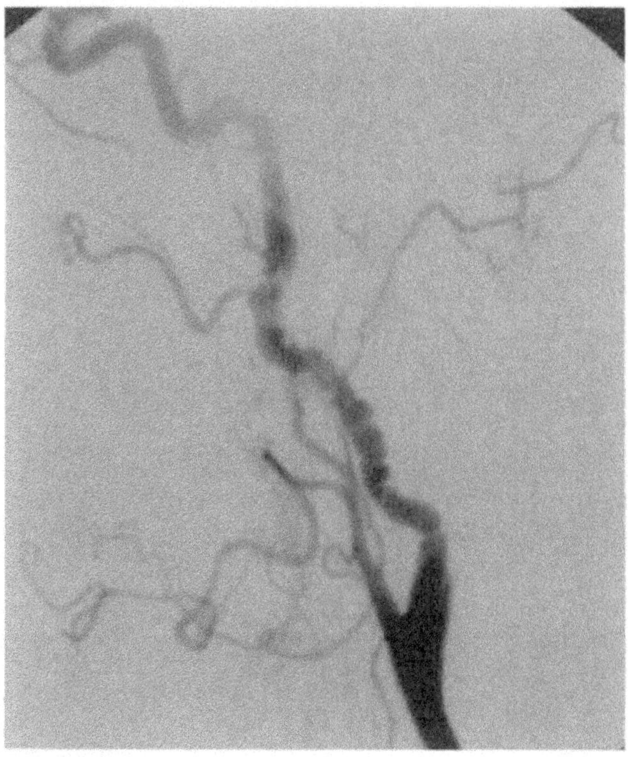

FIGURE 5.85Q

A. Arterial dissection
B. Takayasu's arteritis
C. Marfan's syndrome
D. Fibromuscular dysplasia
E. None of the above

86. What is the most common T2-weighted image appearance and location, respectively, of an arachnoid cyst?

A. Hyperintense, suprasellar cistern
B. Hyperintense, middle cranial fossa
C. Hypointense, suprasellar cistern
D. Hypointense, middle cranial fossa
E. Isointense, cerebellopontine angle

87. What neoplasm is depicted on the following contrasted T1-weighted MRI in an asymptomatic adult male (Figure 5.87Q)?

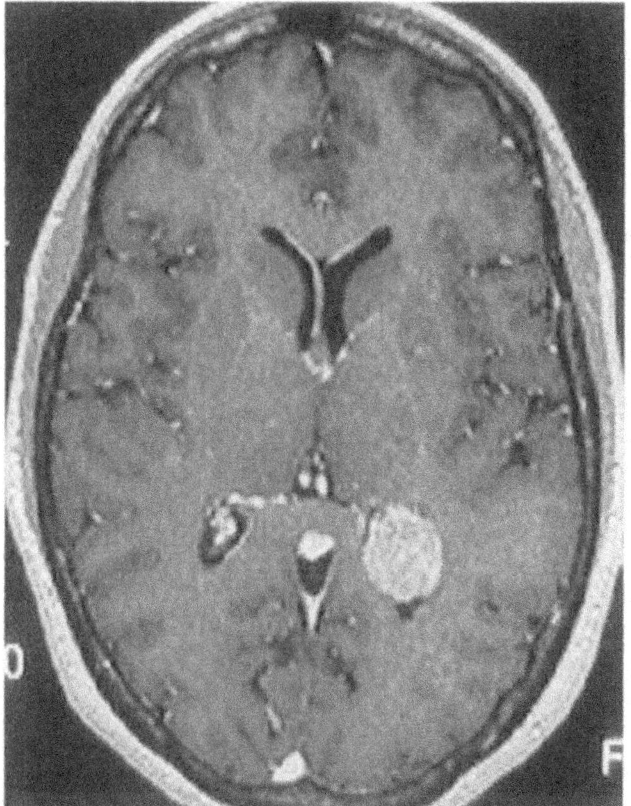

FIGURE 5.87Q

A. Choroid plexus papilloma
B. Ependymoma
C. Subependymoma
D. Astrocytoma
E. Meningioma

88. What abnormality is depicted on the following noncontrasted T1-weighted MRI (Figure 5.88Q)?

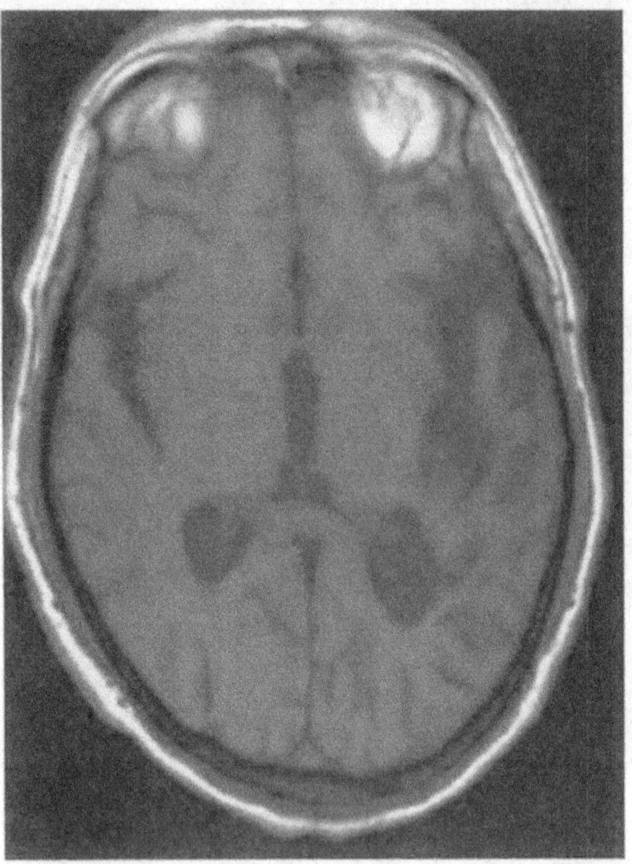

FIGURE 5.88Q

A. Multiple sclerosis plaque
B. Acute infarct
C. Chronic infarct
D. Astrocytoma
E. None of the above

89. Which of the following imaging characteristics is NOT associated with fibrous dysplasia?

A. Sclerotic bone on CT scan
B. Hypointense signal of bony lesions on T1-weighted imaging
C. Hyperintense signal of bony lesions on T2-weighted imaging
D. Variable enhancement patterns
E. Cystic components

90. Which of the following imaging characteristics is NOT typically associated with primary CNS lymphoma?

A. Isodense on unenhanced CT scans
B. Prominent enhancement
C. Slightly hyperintense on T2-weighted imaging
D. Multifocal
E. Often involves the basal ganglia

91. What is the mechanism of injury for the condition depicted in this axial CT scan (Figure 5.91Q)?

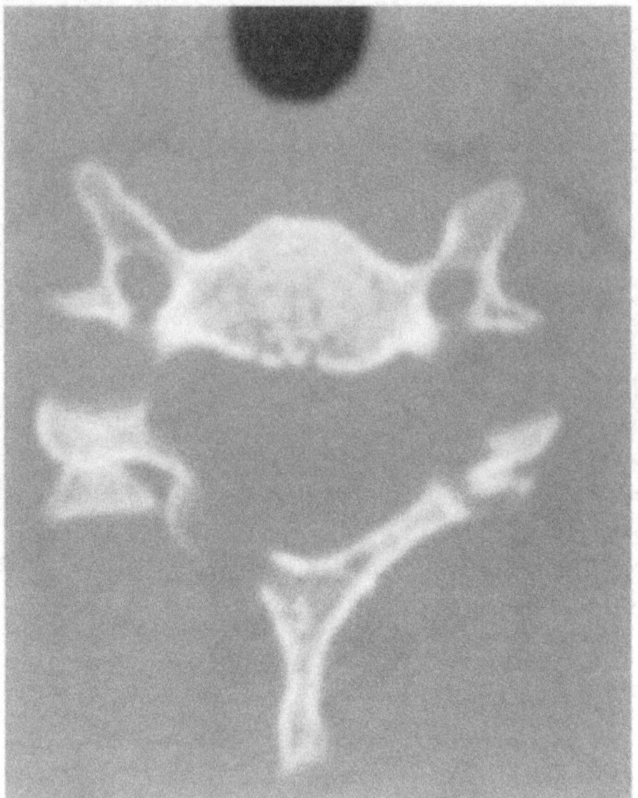

FIGURE 5.91Q

A. Hyperflexion
B. Hyperextension
C. Axial loading
D. Flexion/rotation
E. Distraction

92. Which of the following neoplasms are generally hypointense on T1-weighted images and hyperintense on T2-weighted images with variable enhancement patterns?

1. Pilocytic astrocytoma
2. Pleomorphic xanthoastrocytoma
3. Ganglioglioma
4. Dysembryoplastic neuroepithelial tumor

A. 1, 2, and 3 are correct
B. 1 and 3 are correct
C. 2 and 4 are correct
D. Only 4 is correct
E. All of the above are correct

93. Which of the following characteristics is NOT observed with acoustic neuromas on MRI?

A. Hypointense to brain on T1-weighted images
B. Hypointense to brain on T2-weighted images
C. Variable enhancement patterns
D. Cystic degeneration
E. Hemorrhage

94. A 54-year-old male with diabetes mellitus presented with complaints of progressive lower back pain. The patient's neurologic exam was normal, and his sagittal T2-weighted MRI is depicted below. What is the most likely etiology of this patient's kyphotic deformity (Figure 5.94Q)?

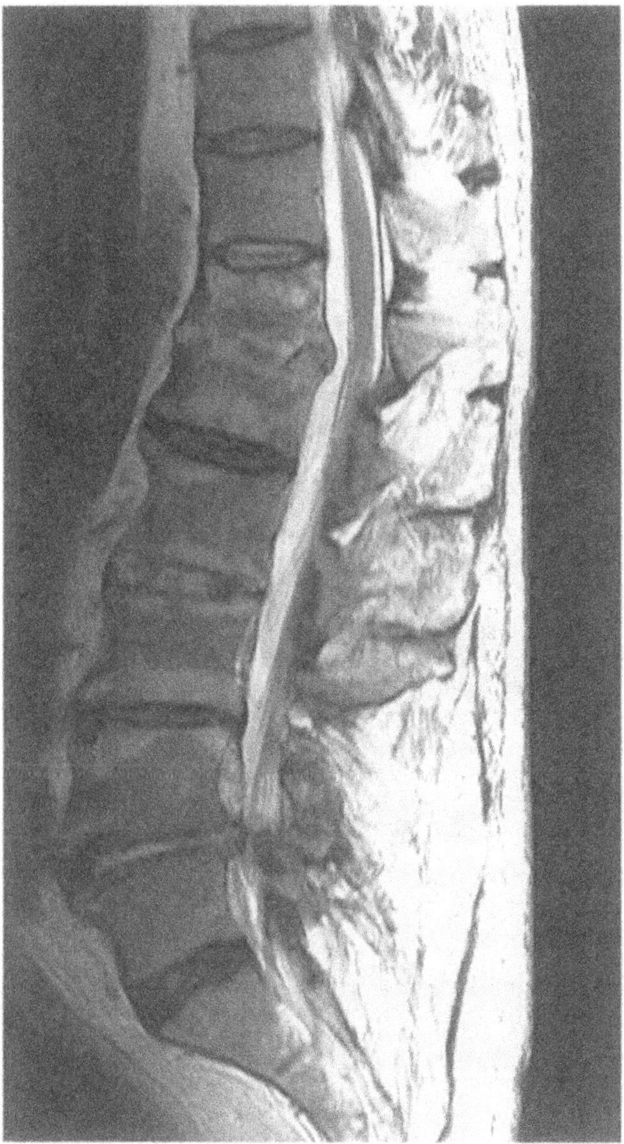

FIGURE 5.94Q

A. Isthmic spondylolisthesis
B. Discitis/osteomyelitis
C. Rheumatoid arthritis
D. Intervertebral disc herniation
E. None of the above

95. A 38-year-old male experienced transient left upper extremity sensory changes after a motor vehicle collision. A CT scan of the head was unremarkable. The patient's right internal carotid angiogram (AP view) is exhibited below (Figure 5.95Q). What is the appropriate next step in management?

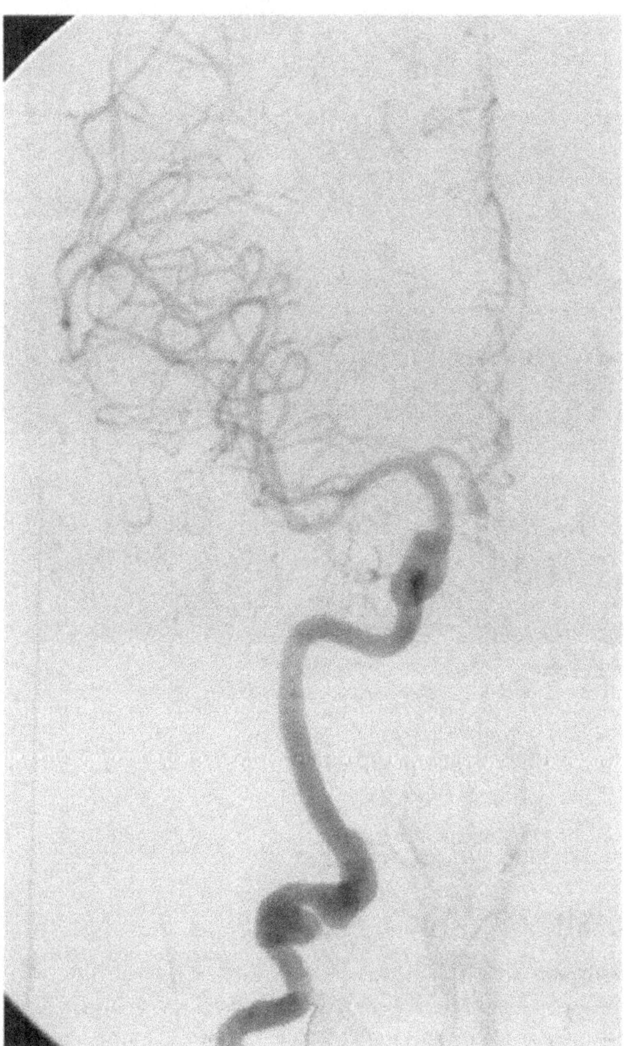

FIGURE 5.95Q

A. Endovascular treatment
B. Anticoagulation
C. Antiplatelet agents
D. Surgical intervention
E. Repeat angiography in 2 to 3 months

96. A 47-year-old female presents to your office with the MRI (axial view) exhibited below (Figure 5.96Q). What is the likely diagnosis?

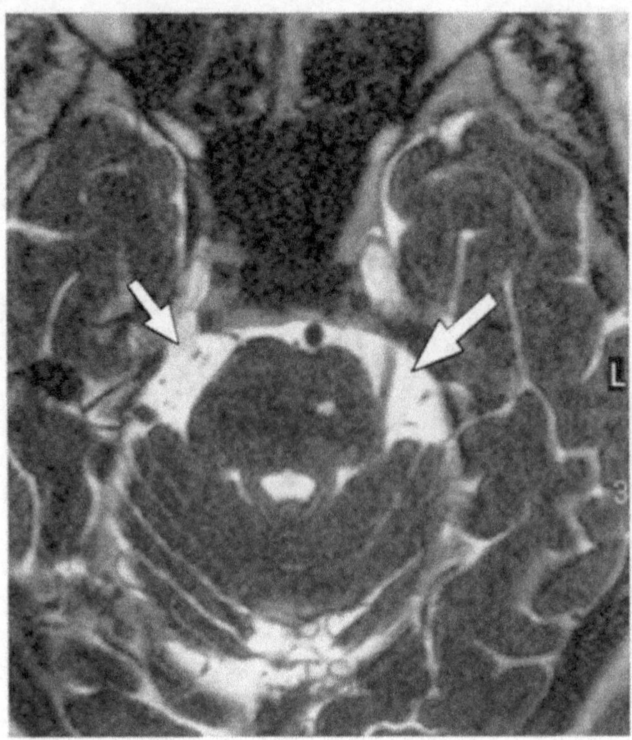

FIGURE 5.96Q

    A. Posterior fossa arachnoid cyst
    B. Arterial-venous malformation
    C. Trigeminal neuralgia
    D. Hemifacial spasm
    E. Multiple sclerosis

QUESTIONS 97–100

Directions: Match each of the following stages of abscess formation with the appropriate imaging and/or histologic characteristics, using each answer once, more than once, or not at all.

    A. Early cerebritis
    B. Late cerebritis
    C. Early capsule
    D. Late capsule
    E. None of the above

97. Well-formed collagen capsule and gliotic layer around abscess

98. Ring enhancement usually appears by this stage

99. Inflammatory response poorly demarcated, toxic changes in neurons, perivascular infiltrates

100. Neovascularity, necrotic center, reticular matrix, and capsule less well developed alongside ventricle

End of set

QUESTIONS 101–105

Directions: Figure 5.101–5.105Q is a coronal CT scan through the right orbit. Match the anatomic structures with the corresponding letterhead using each answer once.

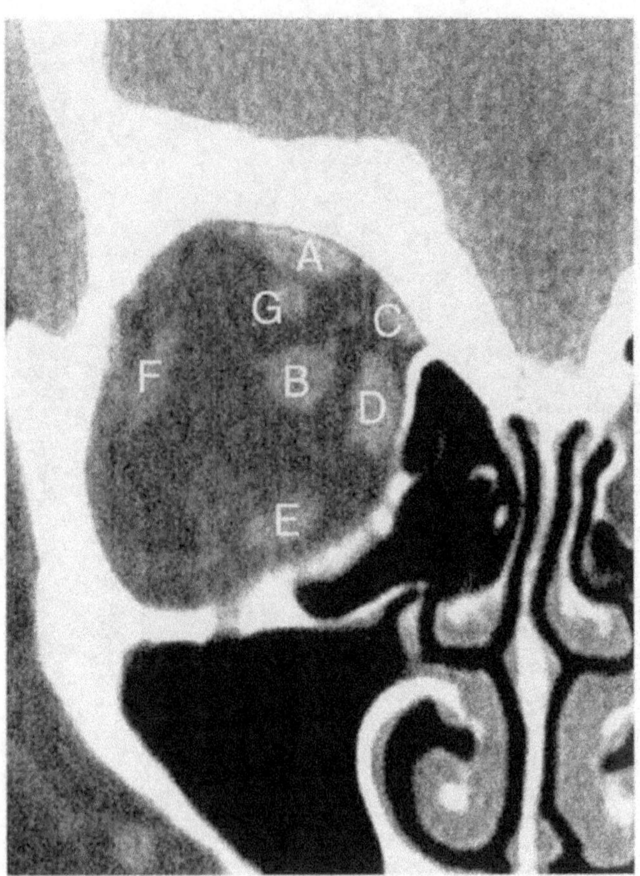

FIGURE 5.101–105Q

101. Optic nerve

102. Levator palpebrae superioris muscle

103. Superior oblique muscle

104. Inferior rectus muscle

105. Superior rectus muscle

End of set

QUESTIONS 106–107

106. A 42-year-old HIV-positive male presented to the emergency department with a 3-week history of headaches and confusion. His postcontrast MRI scan is depicted below (Figure 5.106–5.107Q). What is the most likely diagnosis?

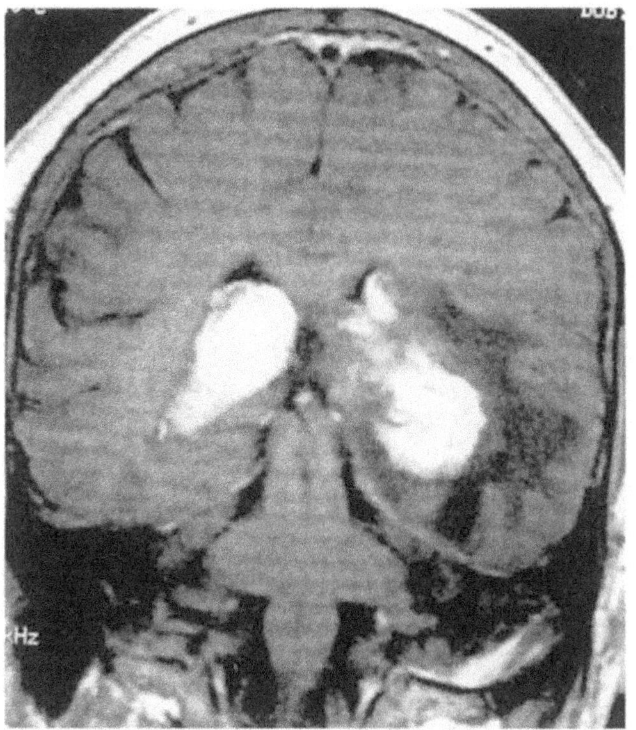

FIGURE 5.106–107Q

- A. Cryptococcal abscess
- B. Toxoplasmosis
- C. Lymphoma
- D. Progressive multifocal leukoencephalopathy (PML)
- E. HIV encephalopathy

107. What microbial agent is most often associated with this lesion?

- A. Herpes simplex virus
- B. JC virus
- C. Epstein-Barr virus
- D. *Treponema pallidum*
- E. *Toxoplasma gondii*

End of set

QUESTIONS 108–111

108. A 34-year-old male presents with increasing neck and back pain, quadriparesis, and bowel and bladder incontinence. His MRI is depicted below (Figure 5.108–5.111Q). These lesions most likely represent

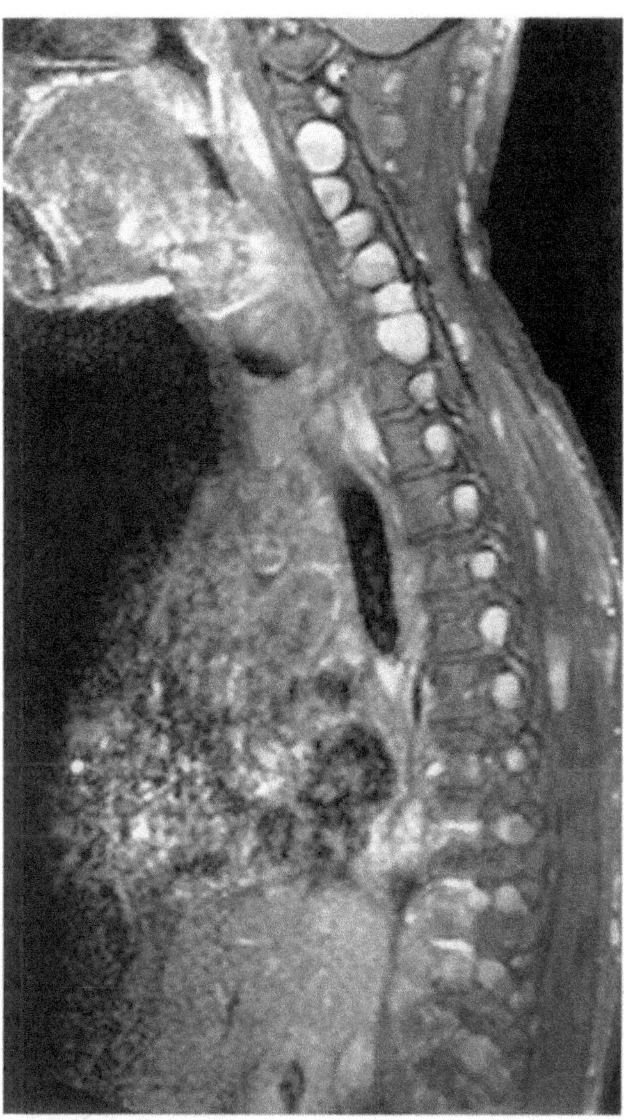

FIGURE 5.108–111Q

- A. Spinal ependymomas
- B. Spinal schwannomas
- C. Spinal neurofibromas
- D. Spinal meningiomas
- E. Metastatic disease

109. What is the diagnosis?

- A. Sturge-Weber syndrome
- B. Neurofibromatosis type I (NF-1)
- C. Neurofibromatosis type II (NF-2)
- D. Metastatic prostate cancer
- E. Disseminated medulloblastoma

110. Diagnostic criteria for this condition may include all of the following EXCEPT?

   A. Six or more café-au-lait spots each > 5 mm in greatest diameter in prepubertal individuals, or > 15 mm in greatest diameter in postpubertal patients

   B. Two or more Lisch nodules

   C. Two or more neurofibromas of any type or one plexiform neurofibroma

   D. Sphenoid dysplasia

   E. Bilateral acoustic neuromas

111. What is the inheritance pattern?

   A. Autosomal recessive

   B. Autosomal dominant

   C. X-linked recessive

   D. X-linked dominant

   E. Pleiotropic mitochondrial disorder

End of set

QUESTIONS 112–114

112. What is depicted on the gradient echo MRI sequence below (Figure 5.112–5.114Q)?

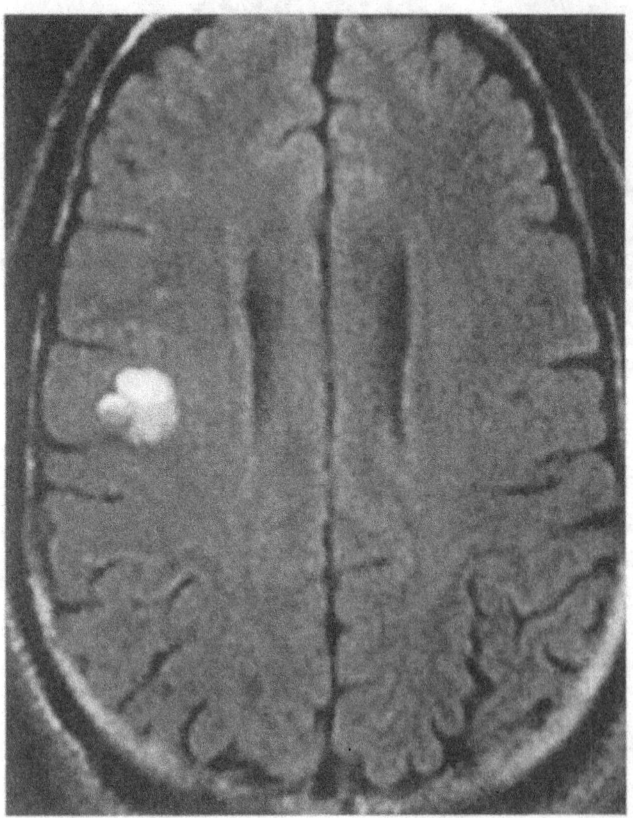

FIGURE 5.112–114Q

   A. Amyloid hemorrhage

   B. Cavernous malformation

   C. Capillary telangiectasia

   D. Metastatic tumor with hemorrhage

   E. Hemangioblastoma

113. This lesion may be associated with all of the following EXCEPT which?

   A. Venous malformation

   B. 0.5% incidence

   C. Multiplicity

   D. Mutation in a gene on chromosome 7q

   E. Erythropoietin secretion

114. Angiographic findings may include

   A. Vascular blush

   B. Associated aneurysm

   C. External carotid artery collaterals supplying this lesion

   D. An early draining vein

   E. All of the above

End of set

115. What is depicted on the lateral angiogram below (Figure 5.115Q)?

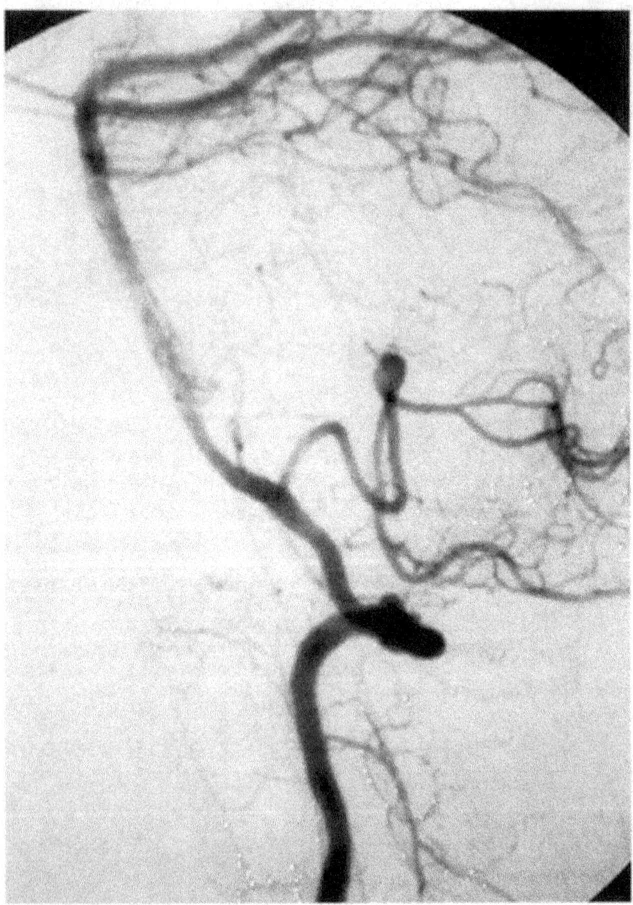

FIGURE 5.115Q

   A. Aneurysm

   B. Dural arterial-venous fistula

   C. Cavernous malformation

   D. Persistent hypoglossal artery

   E. Proatlantal intersegmental artery

116. All of the following may accompany the finding depicted on the MRI below (Figure 5.116Q) EXCEPT?

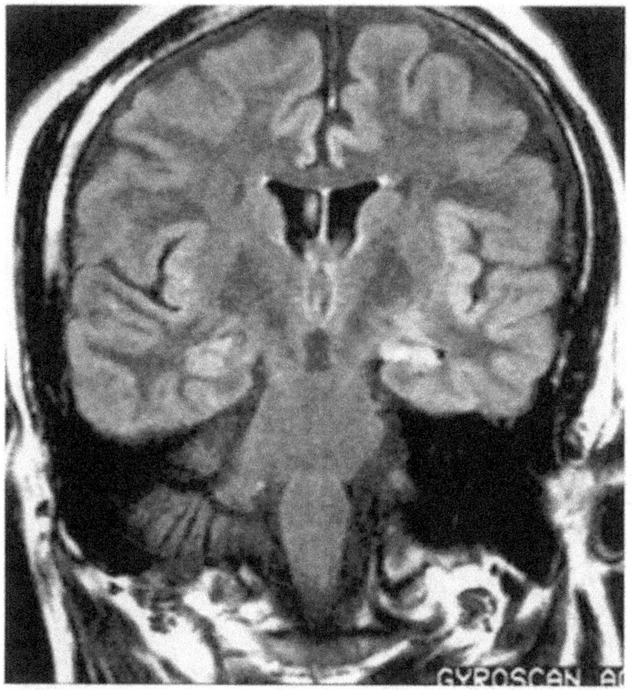

FIGURE 5.116Q

A. Oroalimentary automatisms

B. Epigastric aura

C. Hypermetabolism of the affected temporal lobe on interictal fluorodeoxyglucose PET scanning

D. Posturing of the contralateral arm

E. History of complicated febrile seizures

117. A type II split-cord malformation, which consists of two hemicords separated by a nonrigid fibrous septum, results from faulty development during what embryologic stage?

A. Primary neurulation

B. Secondary neurulation

C. Ventral induction

D. Cellular migration

E. Myelination

118. The finding on this CT scan (Figure 5.118Q) is most consistent with

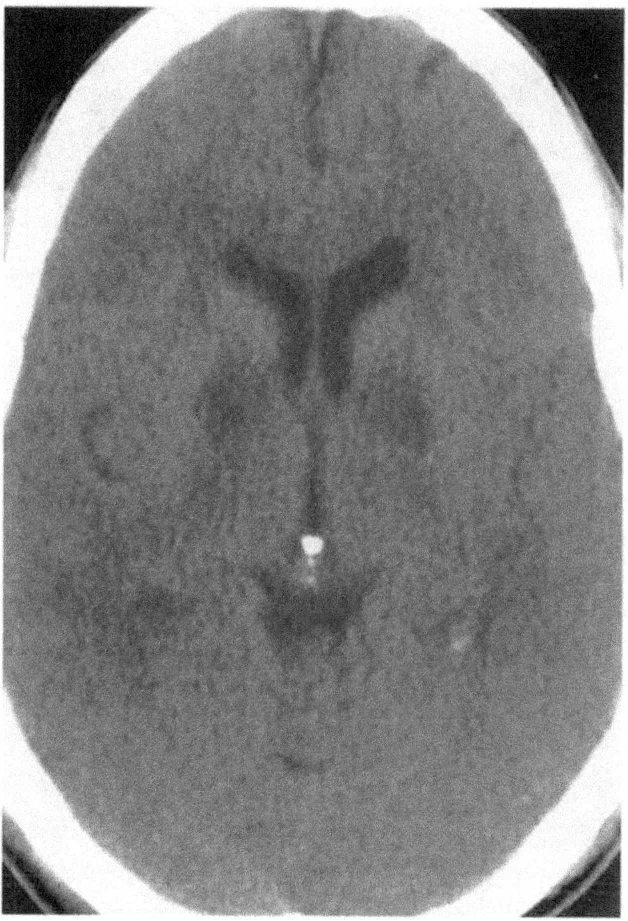

FIGURE 5.118Q

A. Severe closed head injury

B. Neurocysticercosis

C. Child abuse

D. Carbon monoxide poisoning

E. Cryptococcal infection

QUESTIONS 119–120

119. What is the most likely diagnosis depicted on the diffusion-weighted MRI scan below (Figure 5.119–5.120Q)?

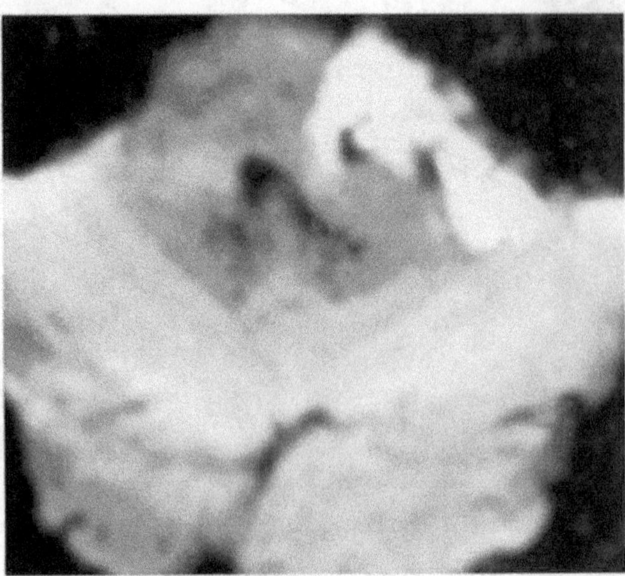

FIGURE 5.119–120Q

   A. Aneurysm
   B. Acoustic neuroma
   C. Meningioma
   D. Epidermoid tumor
   E. Arachnoid cyst

120. How would the application of a fat-saturation pulse during MRI alter the signal characteristics of this lesion?

   A. The signal would suppress
   B. The signal would remain the same
   C. The lesion would show similar characteristics to CSF
   D. It would produce increased signal intensity
   E. It would result in a chemical shift artifact

End of set

121. What is depicted in the following contrasted axial T1-weighted MRI (Figure 5.121Q)?

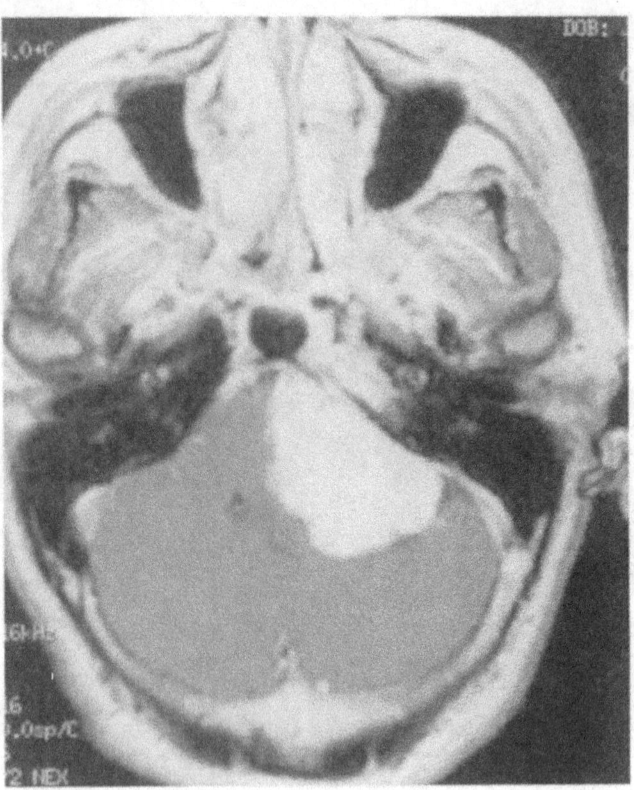

FIGURE 5.121Q

   A. Vestibular schwannoma
   B. Dural metastasis
   C. Hemangiopericytoma
   D. Meningioma
   E. Astrocytoma

QUESTIONS 122–124

122. Refer to Figure 5.122–5.124Q. What is the diagnosis?

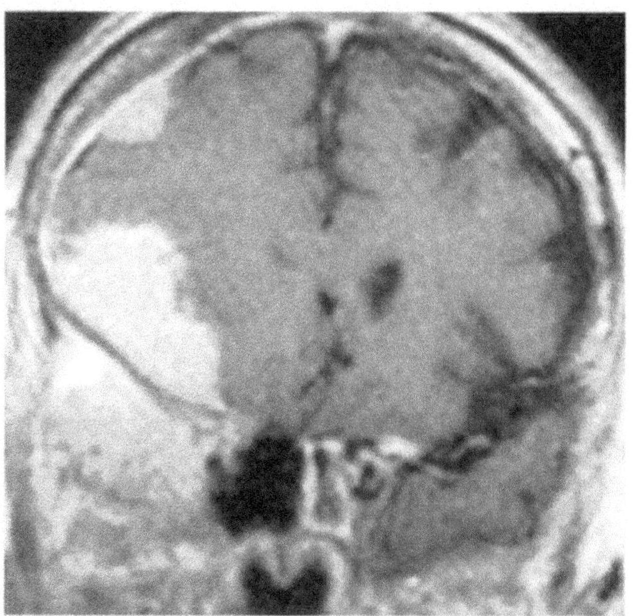

FIGURE 5.122–124Q

- **A.** Neurofibromatosis type 1 (NF-1)
- **B.** Neurofibromatosis type II (NF-II)
- **C.** Tuberous sclerosis
- **D.** Sturge-Weber syndrome
- **E.** Wyburn-Mason syndrome

123. This disorder most commonly occurs with mutations of what chromosome?

- **A.** Chromosome 3
- **B.** Chromosome 9
- **C.** Chromosome 16
- **D.** Chromosome 17
- **E.** Chromosome 22

124. What is the incidence of this condition?

- **A.** 1 per 3000
- **B.** 1 per 10,000
- **C.** 1 per 20,000 to 50,000
- **D.** 1 per 80,000
- **E.** 1 per 100,000

End of set

QUESTIONS 125–126

125. Refer to Figure 5.125–5.126Q. What is the diagnosis?

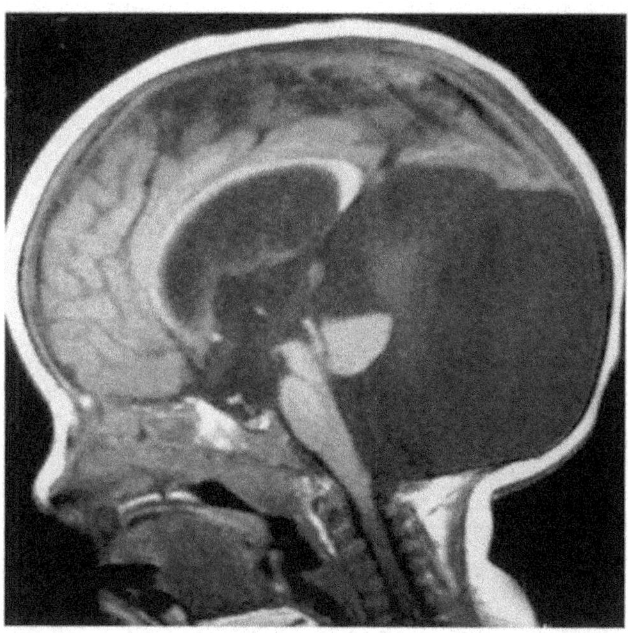

FIGURE 5.125–126Q

- **A.** Retrocerebellar arachnoid cyst
- **B.** Porencephaly
- **C.** Dandy-Walker malformation
- **D.** Mega cisterna magna
- **E.** Chiari III malformation

126. The most common anomalies outside of the CNS occur in what system?

- **A.** Renal
- **B.** Pulmonary
- **C.** Gastrointestinal
- **D.** Endocrine
- **E.** Cardiac

End of set

QUESTIONS 127–128

127. A 28-year-old male presents with right leg weakness and the sagittal MRI depicted below (Figure 5.127–5.128Q). What should be the next diagnostic test performed?

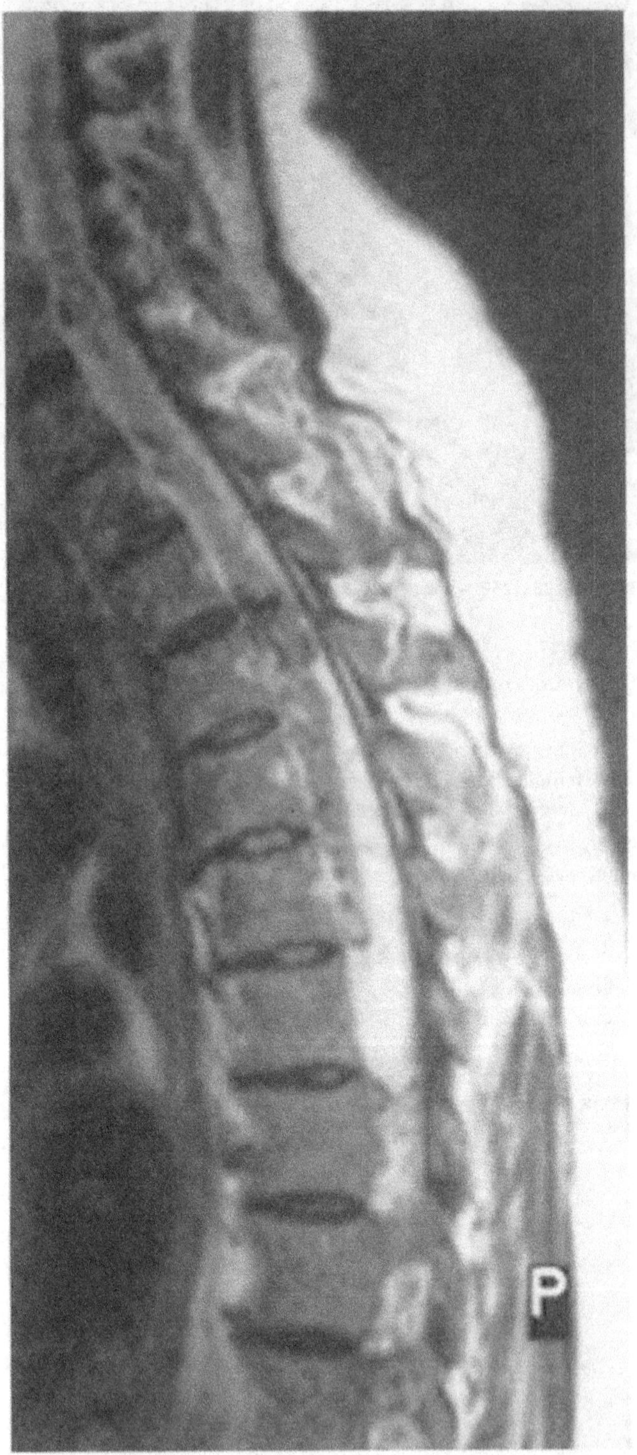

FIGURE 5.127–128Q

A. Computed tomography (CT)
B. Magnetic resonance angiography (MRA)
C. Myelography
D. Angiography
E. Electromyography

128. What is the most likely diagnosis?

A. Paraganglioma
B. Ependymoma
C. Cavernoma
D. Arteriovenous malformation
E. Hemangioblastoma

End of set

129. Refer to Figure 5.129Q. What is the diagnosis?

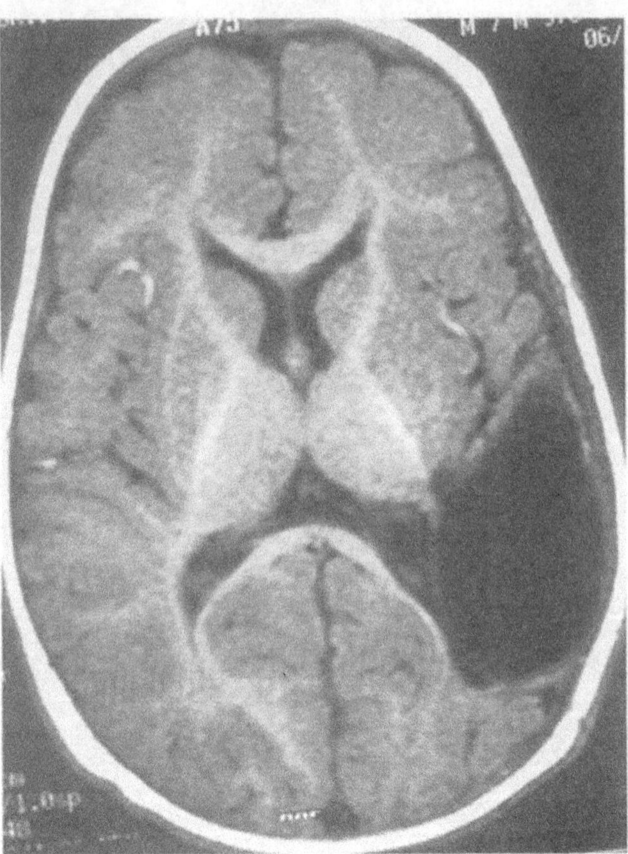

FIGURE 5.129Q

A. Schizencephaly
B. Wyburn-Mason syndrome
C. Arachnoid cyst
D. Left parietal astrocytoma
E. Porencephaly

130. Refer to Figure 5.130Q. What is the diagnosis?

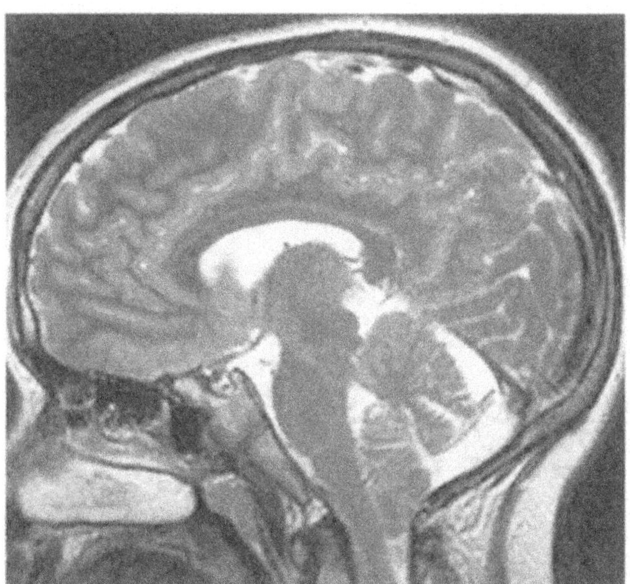

FIGURE 5.130Q

A. Chiari I malformation
B. Chiari II malformation
C. Basilar invagination
D. Tuberous sclerosis
E. Pachygyria

131. Refer to Figure 5.131Q. What is the most likely diagnosis (coronal contrasted T1-weighted MRI)?

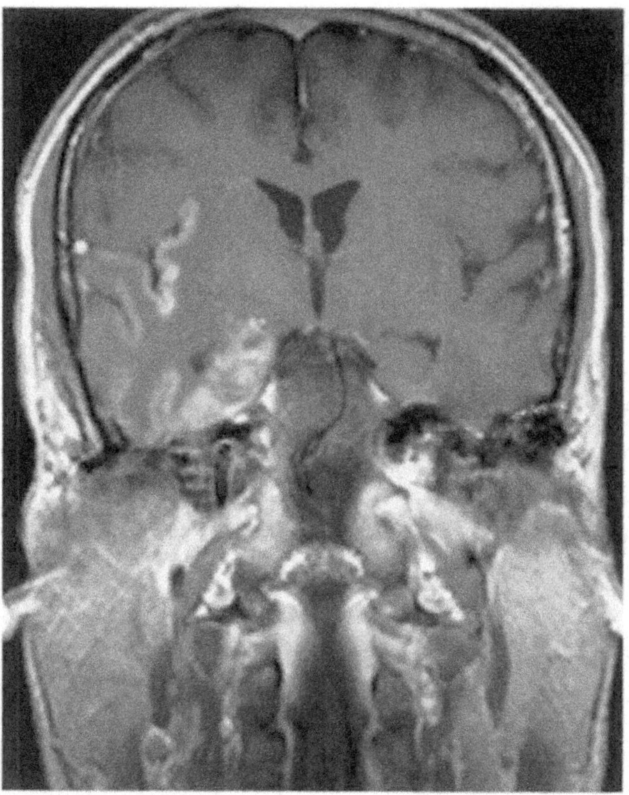

FIGURE 5.131Q

A. Herpes simplex encephalitis
B. Bacterial meningitis
C. Malignant glioma
D. Coccidioidomycosis
E. Lymphoma

132. Refer to Figure 5.132Q. What is the most likely diagnosis?

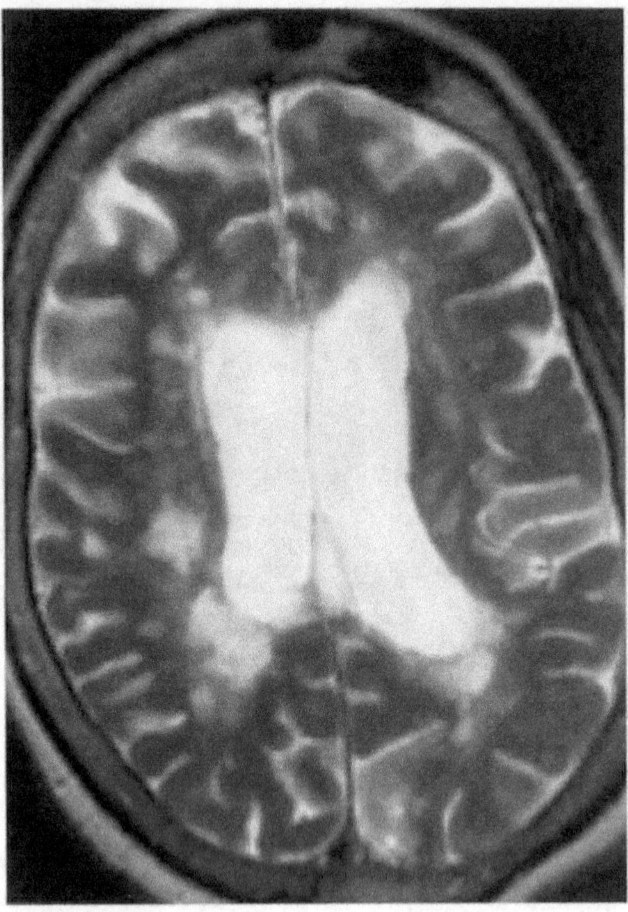

FIGURE 5.132Q

A. Metastatic disease
B. Multiple sclerosis
C. Multiple lacunar infarcts
D. Canavan's disease
E. Alexander's disease

133. Refer to Figure 5.133Q. What is the most likely diagnosis?

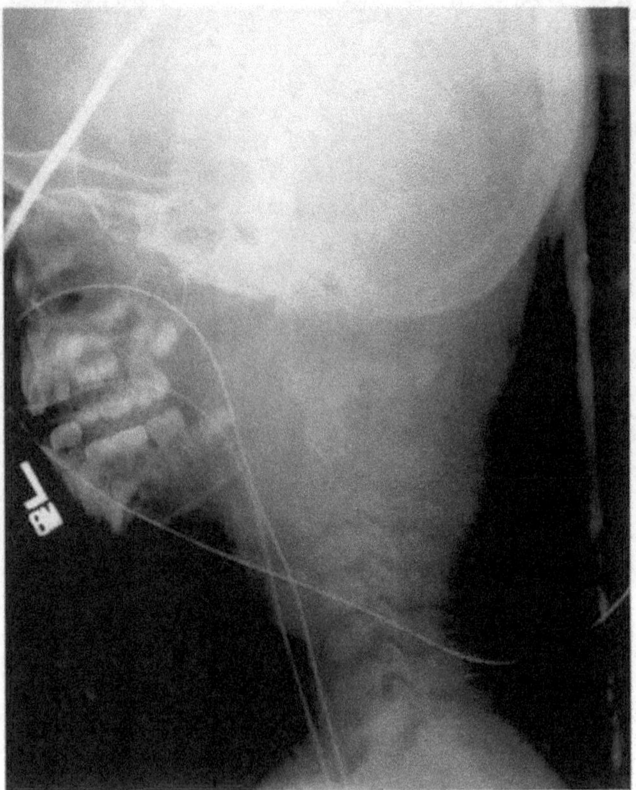

FIGURE 5.133Q

A. Odontoid fracture
B. Atlanto-occipital dissociation
C. Hangman's fracture
D. Condylar fracture
E. Transverse ligament disruption

134. The atlantodental interval (ADI) does not usually exceed what length in an adult?

A. 2 mm
B. 3 mm
C. 4 mm
D. 5 mm
E. 6 mm

QUESTIONS 135–136

135. Refer to Figure 5.135–5.136Q. What is the diagnosis?

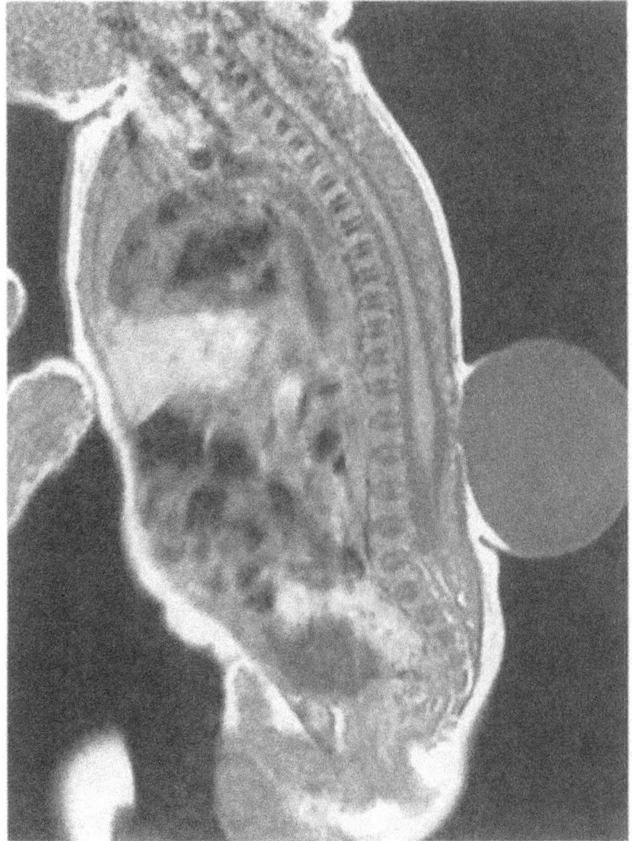

FIGURE 5.135–136Q

   A. Sacral lipoma
   B. Meningocele
   C. Myelomeningocele
   D. Lipomyelomeningocele
   E. Myelocystocele

136. This disorder often develops during faulty development of what embryologic stage?

   A. Secondary neurulation
   B. Disjunction
   C. Ventral induction
   D. Neuronal proliferation
   E. Cellular migration

End of set

QUESTIONS 137–139

137. Refer to Figure 5.137–5.139Q. What is the diagnosis (axial FLAIR MRI)?

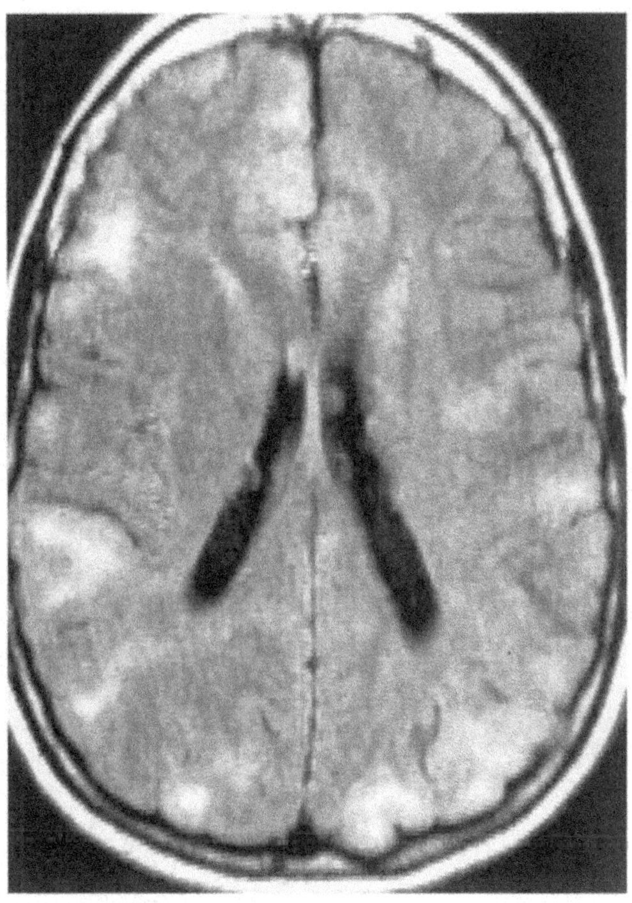

FIGURE 5.137–139Q

   A. Von Hippel-Lindau disease
   B. Tuberous sclerosis
   C. Sturge-Weber syndrome
   D. Multiple metastatic tumors
   E. Rendu-Osler-Weber disease

138. What is the inheritance pattern of this disease?

   A. Autosomal dominant
   B. Autosomal recessive
   C. X-linked
   D. Sporadic
   E. Pleiotropic

139. What is the most common neoplasm associated with this disorder?

   A. Subependymal giant cell astrocytoma
   B. Pilocytic astrocytoma of the optic nerve
   C. Meningioma
   D. Neurofibroma
   E. Cutaneous melanoma

End of set

QUESTIONS 140–141

140. What is depicted on this lateral angiogram (Figure 5.140–5.141Q)?

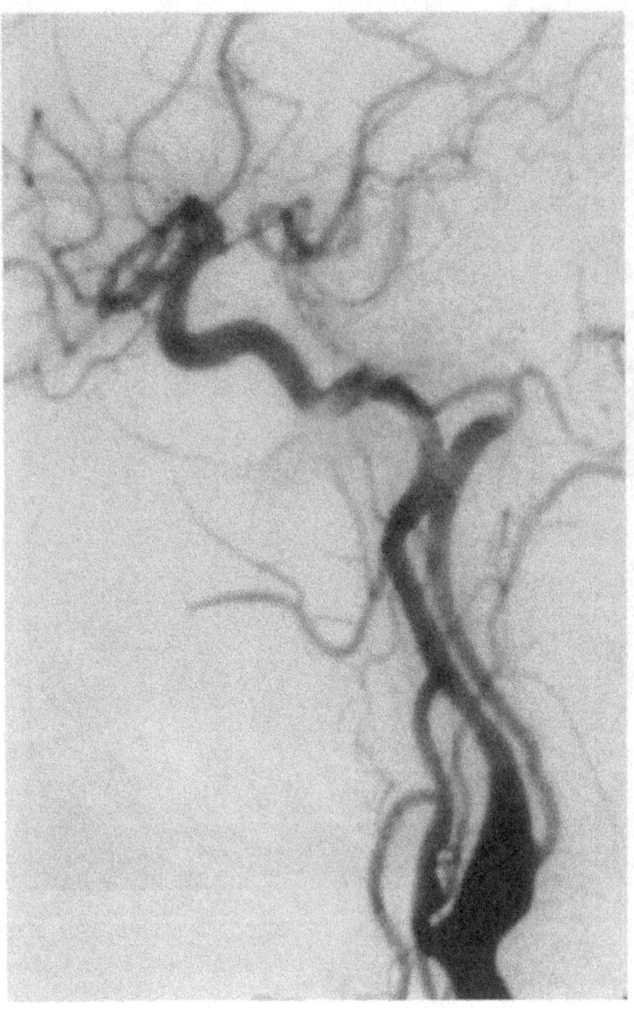

FIGURE 5.140–141Q

- **A.** Atherosclerotic changes
- **B.** Developmental anomaly
- **C.** Traumatic injury
- **D.** Neoplastic process
- **E.** Iatrogenic process

141. What should be the next course of treatment?

- **A.** Aspirin therapy and repeat angiogram in 3 months
- **B.** Warfarin therapy with a goal of keeping the INR > 2.0
- **C.** Carotid endarterectomy
- **D.** Carotid stent placement and anticoagulation
- **E.** No treatment

End of set

QUESTIONS 142–143

142. Refer to Figure 5.142–5.143Q. What is the diagnosis?

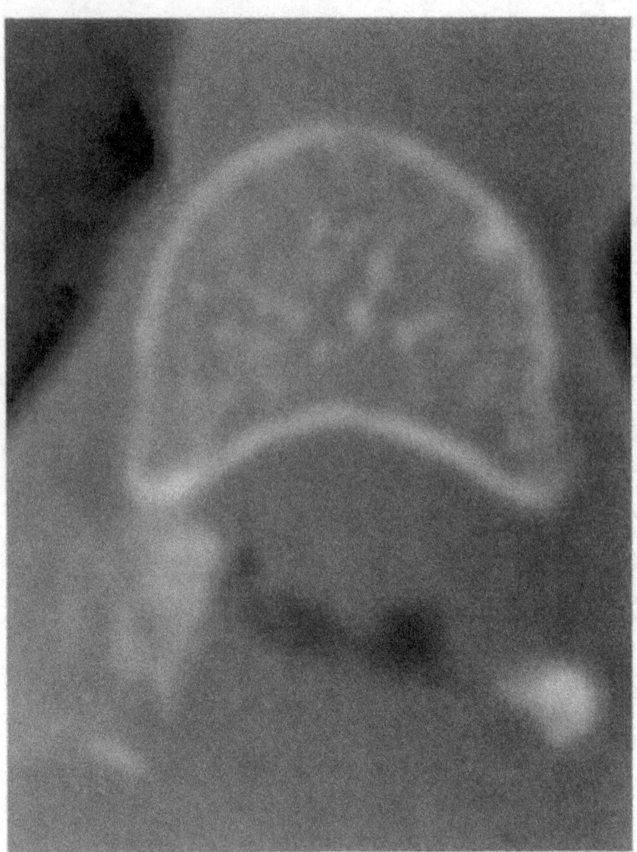

FIGURE 5.142–143Q

- **A.** Osteomyelitis
- **B.** Hemangioma
- **C.** Eosinophilic granuloma
- **D.** Osteoid osteoma
- **E.** Metastatic disease

143. The next course of management should include

- **A.** A serum white blood cell count, sedimentation rate, and MRI
- **B.** A spinal angiogram
- **C.** CT-guided biopsy
- **D.** Flexion-extension views of spine
- **E.** No further intervention is necessary

End of set

144. What is the appearance of an acute intracerebral hematoma on a T2-weighted MRI?

- **A.** Hyperintense
- **B.** Isointense
- **C.** Similar to the appearance of CSF
- **D.** Markedly hypointense to surrounding brain
- **E.** Hyperintense to isointense

145. What is the most common location for choroid plexus papillomas in adults?

- **A.** Third ventricle
- **B.** Lateral ventricle
- **C.** Fourth ventricle
- **D.** Cerebellopontine angle
- **E.** Sylvian fissure

146. All of the following are common causes of a regionally thickened skull on imaging studies EXCEPT?

- **A.** Paget's disease
- **B.** Meningioma
- **C.** Fibrous dysplasia
- **D.** Hyperostosis frontalis interna
- **E.** Shunted hydrocephalus

147. What is the most likely diagnosis in a patient with a long history of complicated asthma and the unenhanced sagittal T1-weighted MRI depicted below (Figure 5.147Q)?

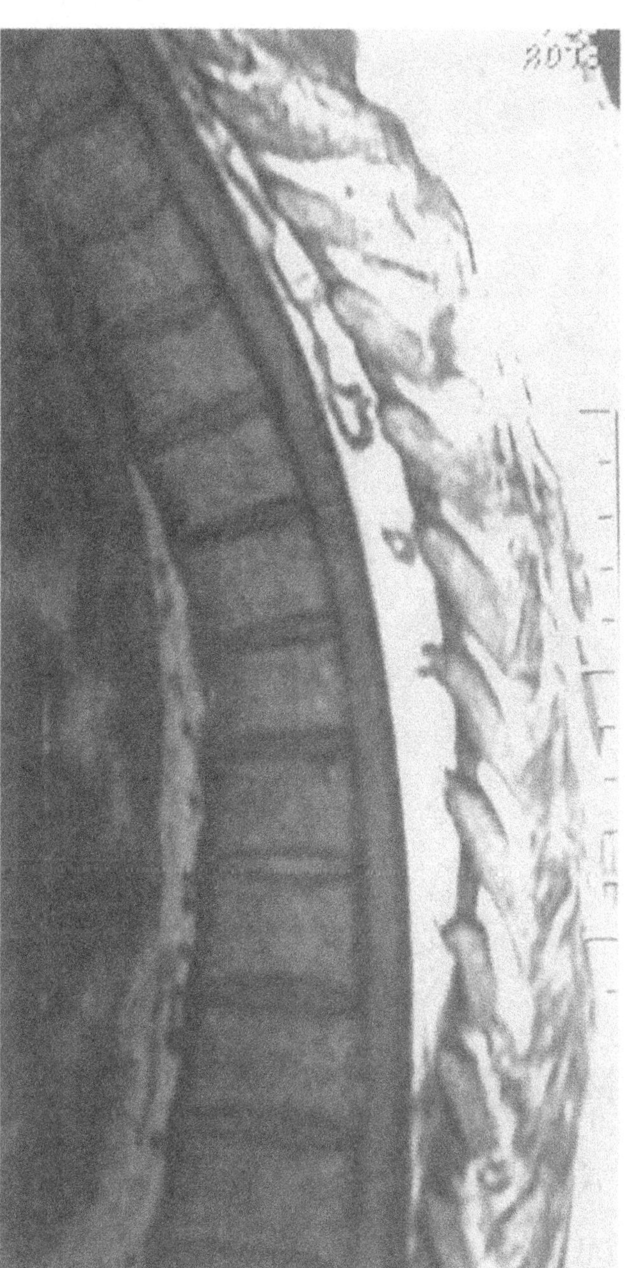

FIGURE 5.147Q

- **A.** Eosinophilic granuloma
- **B.** Burst fracture
- **C.** Epidural hematoma
- **D.** Spinal lipomatosis
- **E.** Osteomyelitis

QUESTIONS 148–149

148. Refer to Figure 5.148–5.149Q. What is the most likely diagnosis in an 8-year-old male without a history of trauma?

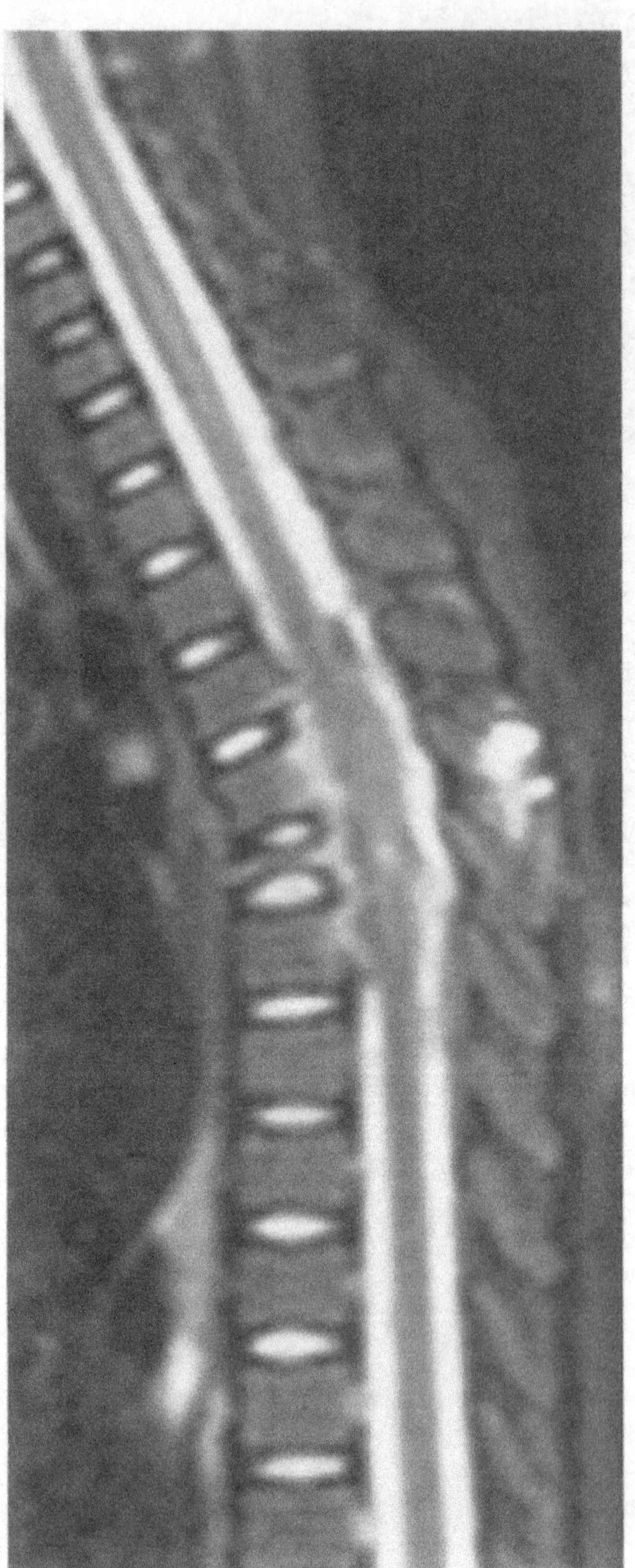

A. Hemangioma
B. Osteomyelitis
C. Eosinophilic granuloma
D. Giant cell tumor
E. Osteosarcoma

149. What would be the most likely appearance of this lesion on an axial CT scan?

A. A lytic lesion without surrounding sclerosis
B. A lytic lesion with surrounding sclerosis
C. An osteolytic lesion surrounded by expanded, thinned, eggshell-like cortical bone
D. A lytic area surrounding a central area of sclerosis
E. None of the above

End of set

150. What is the most likely diagnosis (Figure 5.150Q)?

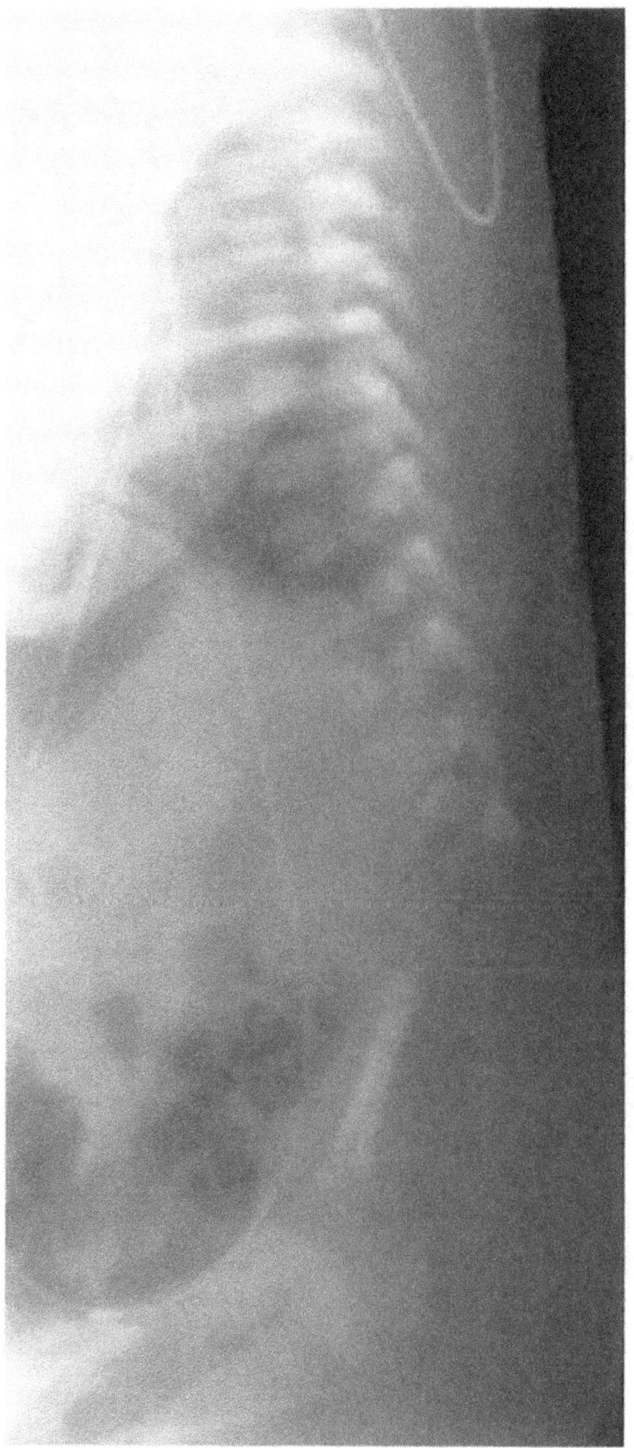

FIGURE 5.150Q

- **A.** Myelomeningocele
- **B.** Caudal regression syndrome
- **C.** Diastomyelia
- **D.** Spondylosis
- **E.** Spondylolisthesis

QUESTIONS 151–152

151. Refer to Figure 5.151–5.152Q. What is typically the initial treatment for this abnormality?

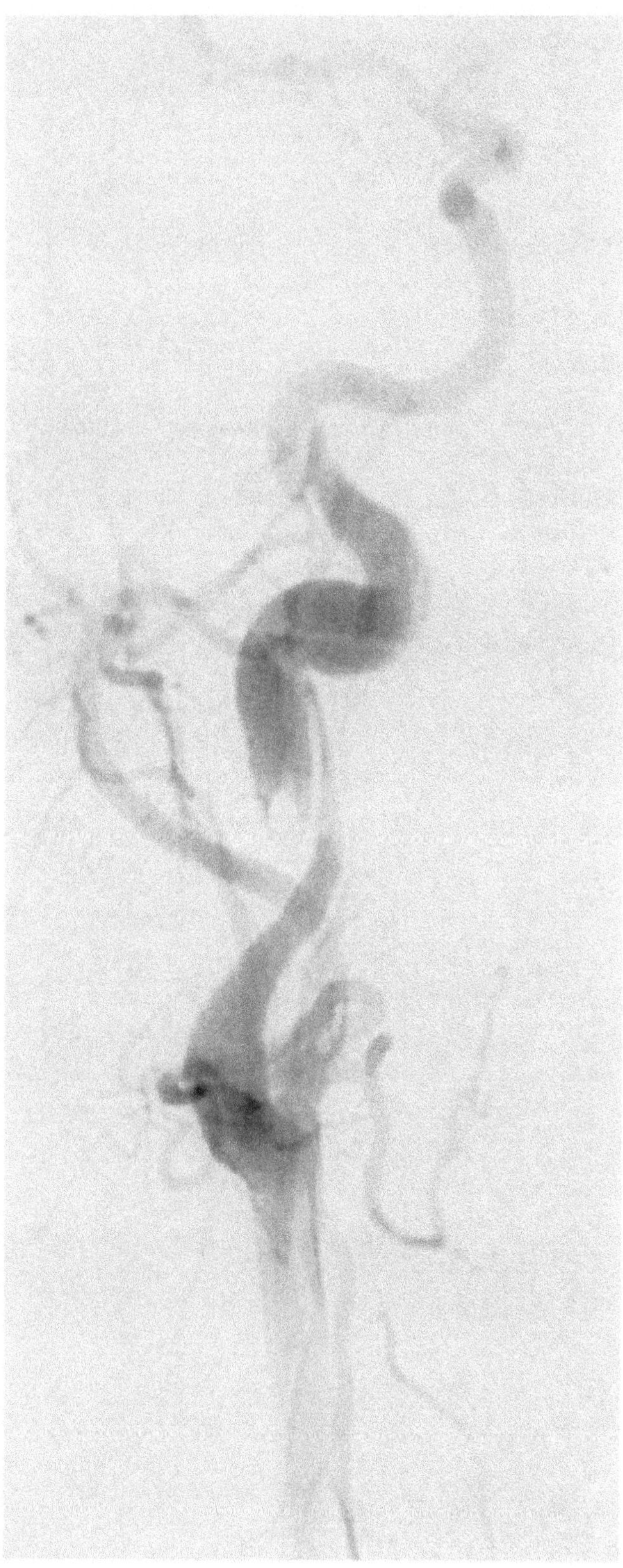

FIGURE 5.151–152Q

A. Anticoagulation
B. Superficial temporal artery to middle cerebral artery bypass
C. High-flow saphenous vein bypass
D. Carotid stenting
E. Carotid endarterectomy

152. What is the diagnosis?

A. Fibromuscular dysplasia
B. Carotid artery dissection and pseudoaneurysm formation
C. Tumor encasement of the internal carotid artery
D. Atherosclerotic carotid artery disease
E. None of the above

End of set

153. What tumor is least likely to metastasize to the brain?

A. Breast
B. Lung
C. Melanoma
D. Prostate
E. Renal

QUESTIONS 154–156

154. What abnormality is depicted on the sagittal MRI below (Figure 5.154–5.156Q)?

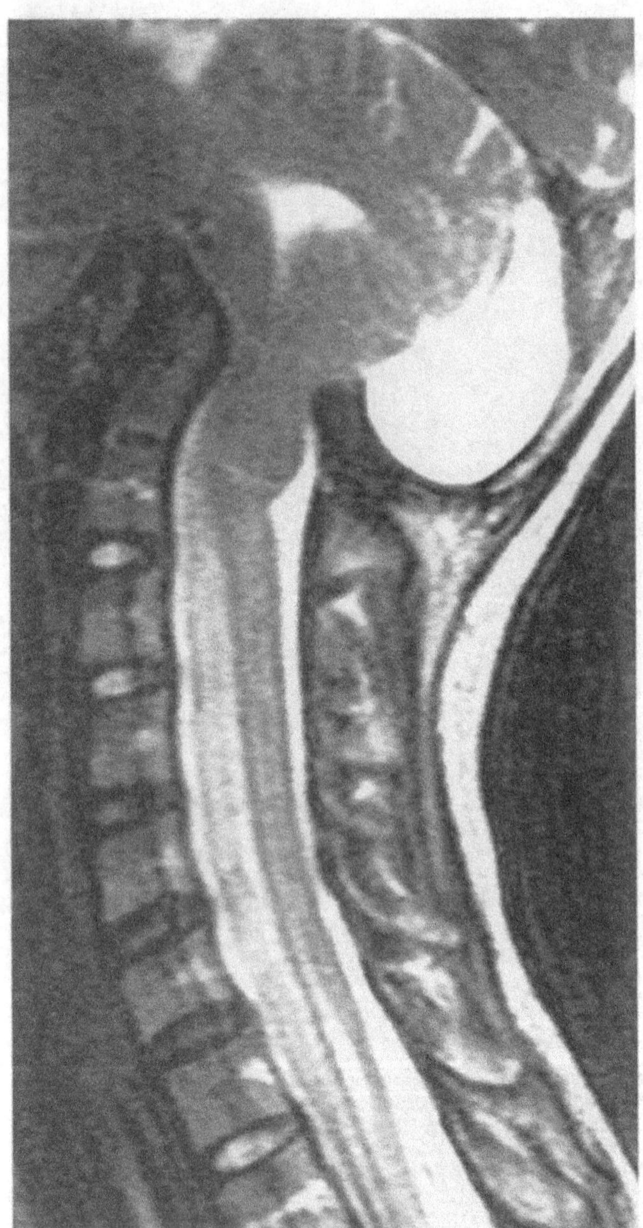

FIGURE 5.154–156Q

A. Klippel-Feil syndrome
B. Histiocytosis X
C. Basilar invagination
D. Os odontoideum
E. None of the above

155. This abnormality is often associated with all of the following conditions EXCEPT?

- **A.** Rheumatoid arthritis
- **B.** Chiari malformations
- **C.** Klippel-Feil syndrome
- **D.** Down's syndrome
- **E.** Dandy-Walker malformation

156. Reference lines used to evaluate this condition may include

1. McRae's line
2. Chamberlain's line
3. McGregor's line
4. Wackenheim's clivus-canal line

- **A.** 1, 2, and 3 are correct
- **B.** 1 and 3 are correct
- **C.** 2 and 4 are correct
- **D.** Only 4 is correct
- **E.** All of the above

End of set

157. A 53-year-old male underwent an uncomplicated right L4-5 microdiscectomy for an L5 radiculopathy. Approximately 5 weeks later the patient again developed right leg pain and weakness in a similar distribution to his preoperative symptoms. Pre- and post-contrasted T1-weighted MRI scans revealed a large soft tissue mass in the vertebral canal posterior to the L5 vertebral body. There was compression of the thecal sac and nearly complete obliteration of the epidural fat at that level. On the postcontrast image, a well-defined rim of enhancement was seen outlining the soft tissue mass. What is the most likely diagnosis?

- **A.** Arachnoiditis
- **B.** Postoperative scar formation
- **C.** Recurrent herniated disc fragment
- **D.** Synovial cyst
- **E.** Epidural venous plexus

158. A 58-year-old male presents with a severe headache and left-sided hemiparesis. His CT scan is depicted below (Figure 5.158Q). What is the most likely diagnosis?

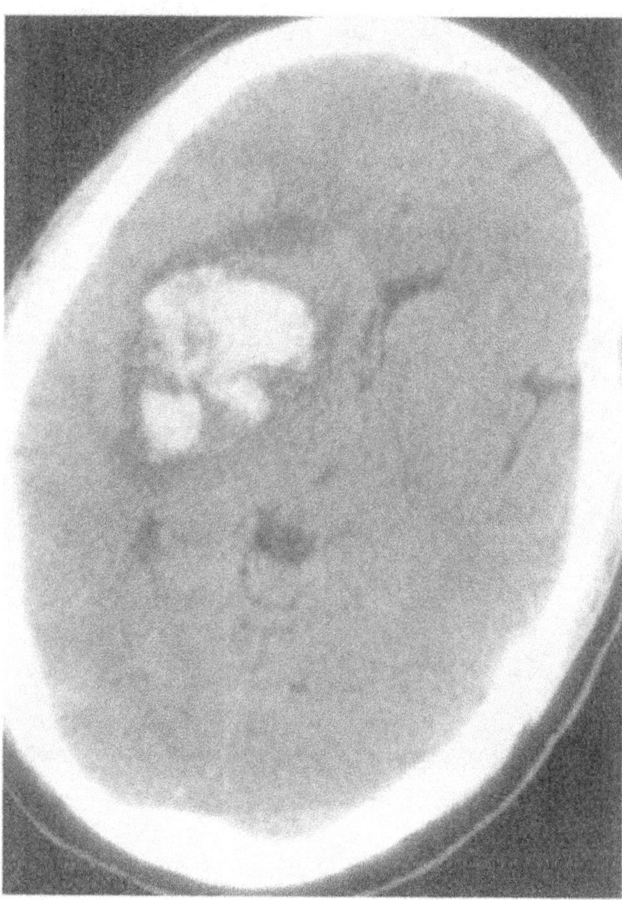

FIGURE 5.158Q

- **A.** Hypertensive hemorrhage
- **B.** Ruptured middle cerebral artery aneurysm
- **C.** Amyloid angiopathy
- **D.** Vasculitis
- **E.** Ruptured arterial-venous malformation

159. Refer to Figure 5.159Q. What is the diagnosis?

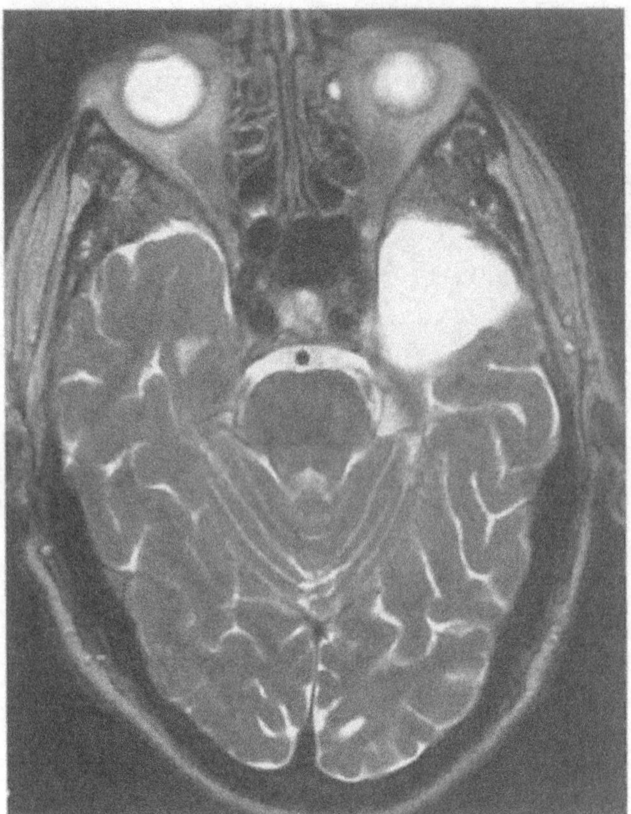

FIGURE 5.159Q

- **A.** Enterogenous cyst
- **B.** Schizencephaly
- **C.** Arachnoid cyst
- **D.** Pilocytic astrocytoma
- **E.** Epidermoid tumor

160. Refer to Figure 5.160Q. What is the diagnosis?

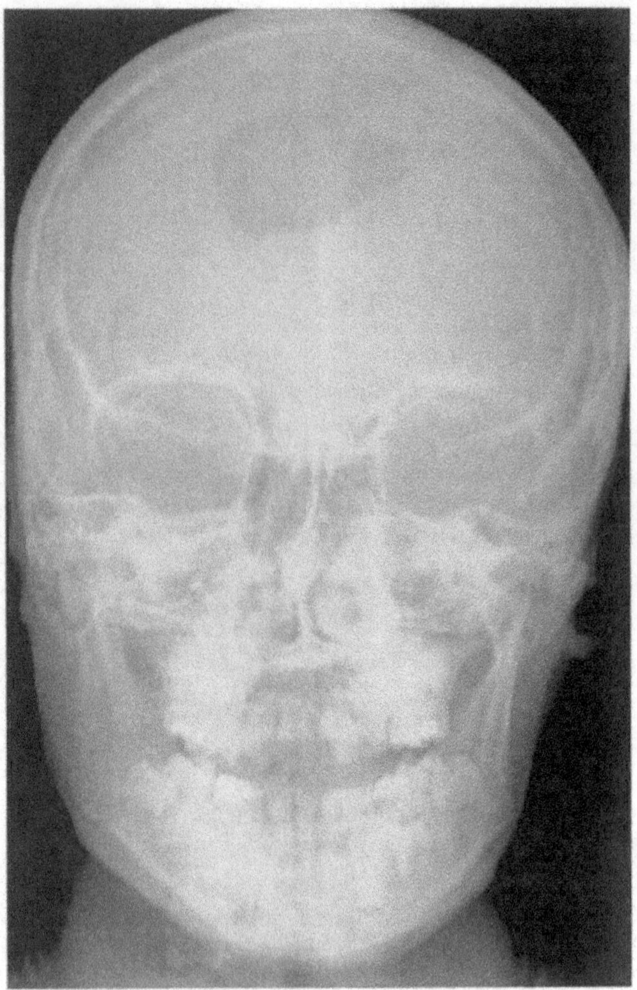

FIGURE 5.160Q

- **A.** Eosinophilic granuloma
- **B.** Giant cell tumor
- **C.** Hemangioma
- **D.** Parietal foramen
- **E.** Osteosarcoma

QUESTIONS 161–162

161. What is depicted on the angiogram below (Figure 5.161–5.162Q)?

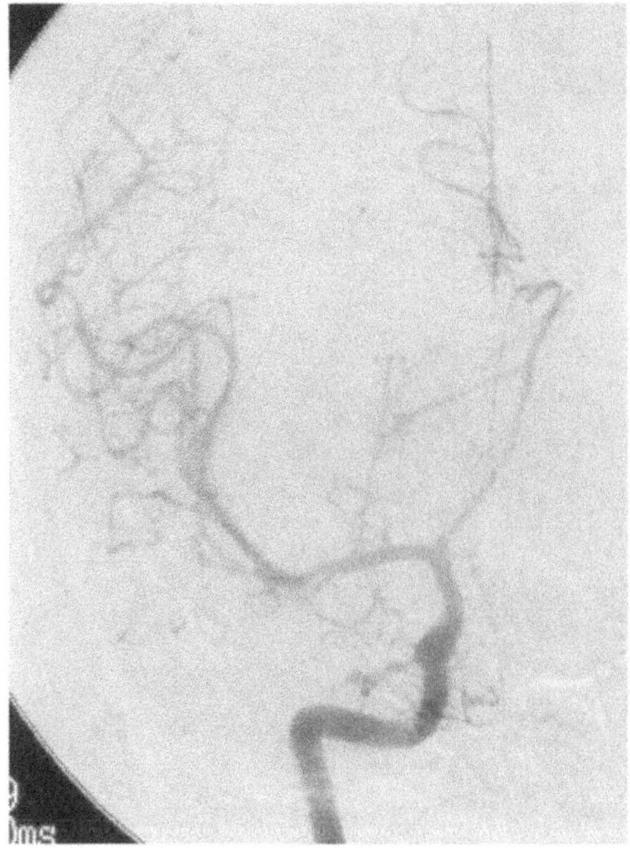

FIGURE 5.161–162Q

A. Transtentorial herniation
B. Transalar herniation
C. Subfalcine herniation
D. Arterial-venous fistula
E. Persistent trigeminal artery

162. Where is the lesion responsible for this finding most likely located?

A. Parietal lobe
B. Frontal lobe
C. Occipital lobe
D. Lateral ventricle
E. Temporal lobe

End of set

QUESTIONS 163–169

Directions: Match each of the following HIV opportunistic infections and neoplasms with the most likely imaging characteristic, using each answer either once, more than once, or not at all.

A. HIV encephalopathy
B. Toxoplasmosis
C. Progressive multifocal encephalopathy
D. Primary CNS lymphoma
E. Cryptococcal disease
F. Cytomegalovirus
G. None of the above

163. Lacunar infarctions resulting from "gelatinous pseudocysts"

164. Asymmetric, multifocal areas of T1 and T2 prolongation in the periventricular and/or peripheral white matter without sparing of subcortical U fibers

165. Parieto-occipital involvement classically described, but lesions can also affect the basal ganglia, brainstem, and cerebellum

166. Symmetric patchy or confluent areas of high signal intensity on T2-weighted images involving the centrum semiovale; frontal predominance

167. "Eccentric target sign"

168. Characteristic rim of generalized periventricular hyperintensity on proton density-weighted images or fluid-attenuated Inversion recovery (FLAIR)

169. Ependymal enhancement often nodular and irregular

End of set

QUESTIONS 170–171

170. Refer to Figure 5.170–5.171Q. What is the diagnosis?

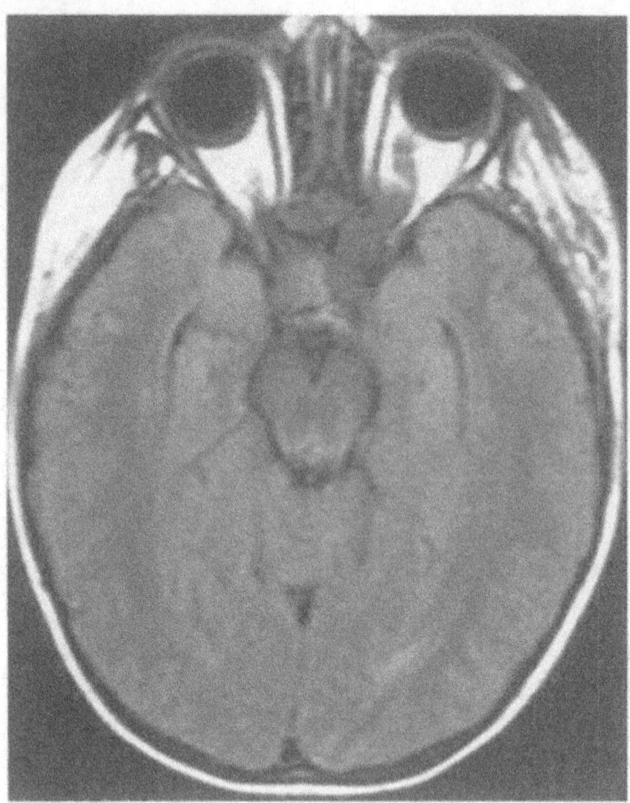

FIGURE 5.170–171Q

   A. Sphenoid wing meningioma
   B. Optic nerve glioma
   C. Hypothalamic hemartoma
   D. Capillary telangiectasia
   E. Ophthalmic artery aneurysm

171. This lesion is most often associated with

   A. Neurofibromatosis type 1
   B. Monosomy 22
   C. Tuberous sclerosis
   D. 1 to 3% risk of rupture per year
   E. None of the above

End of set

172. What is the most likely etiology of the findings depicted on the CT scan below (Figure 5.172Q)?

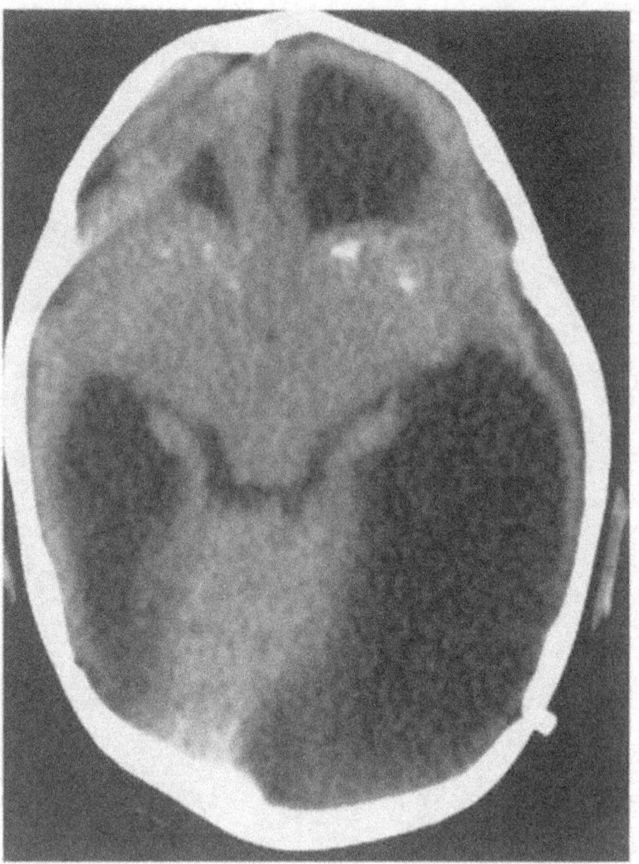

FIGURE 5.172Q

   A. Hemosiderosis
   B. Intrauterine infection
   C. Aqueductal stenosis
   D. Severe closed head injury
   E. Fahr's disease

QUESTIONS 173–174

173. What disorder is characterized by fused thalami, a monoventricle, a peripheral rim of undifferentiated cerebral tissue, severe craniofacial abnormalities, polydactyly, and trisomy 13?

   A. Semilobar holoprosencephaly
   B. Lobar holoprosencephaly
   C. Alobar holoprosencephaly
   D. Septo-optic dysplasia
   E. Arhinencephaly

174. This disorder results from failure of what embryologic stage?

   A. Cellular migration
   B. Diverticulation and cleavage
   C. Cellular differentiation
   D. Myelination
   E. Induction

End of set

175. What is the most common location for spinal cellular ependymomas?

   A. Cervical spine
   B. Thoracic spine
   C. Lumbar spine
   D. Cauda equina
   E. Conus medullaris

Neuroradiology Answer Key

1. D	36. D	71. A	106. C	141. E
2. E	37. C	72. B	107. C	142. B
3. C	38. D	73. D	108. C	143. E
4. A	39. C	74. C	109. B	144. D
5. C	40. C	75. B	110. E	145. C
6. A	41. D	76. D	111. B	146. E
7. D	42. E	77. C	112. B	147. D
8. E	43. B	78. D	113. E	148. C
9. E	44. D	79. C	114. A	149. A
10. A	45. A	80. A	115. A	150. B
11. D	46. A	81. E	116. C	151. A
12. C	47. D	82. C	117. B	152. B
13. A	48. H	83. A	118. D	153. C
14. D	49. B	84. A	119. D	154. D
15. A	50. A	85. D	120. B	155. E
16. B	51. F	86. B	121. D	156. E
17. B	52. A	87. E	122. B	157. C
18. C	53. D	88. C	123. E	158. A
19. A	54. D	89. C	124. C	159. C
20. C	55. D	90. A	125. C	160. D
21. D	56. A	91. A	126. E	161. C
22. C	57. C	92. E	127. D	162. E
23. C	58. E	93. B	128. D	163. E
24. B	59. D	94. B	129. E	164. C
25. C	60. D	95. B	130. A	165. C
26. E	61. D	96. C	131. A	166. A
27. D	62. A	97. D	132. B	167. B
28. D	63. C	98. B	133. B	168. F
29. D	64. B	99. A	134. B	169. D
30. D	65. C	100. C	135. B	170. B
31. F	66. D	101. B	136. A	171. A
32. D	67. E	102. A	137. B	172. B
33. A	68. A	103. C	138. A	173. A
34. B	69. A	104. E	139. A	174. B
35. A	70. D	105. G	140. B	175. A

Neuroradiology Answers

1. D. Epidermoids are usually located off of the midline along the basilar cisterns. These tumors often resemble CSF, and thus arachnoid cysts, on T1- and T2-weighted MRI. However, diffusion-weighted MRI is helpful in differentiating epidermoids from arachnoid cysts, because the former exhibit restricted diffusion (high signal, similar to brain parenchyma) and the latter exhibit normal diffusion (similar to CSF). Pineoblastomas, glioblastomas, and meningiomas are rarely confused with epidermoids (Osborn DN, pp. 633–635).

2. E. The most common brainstem tumor encountered in the pediatric population is an infiltrating astrocytoma. These are most commonly located in the pons (as in this case), and they are usually malignant. Pontine gliomas often present with cranial nerve palsies, extraocular muscle findings, and pyramidal signs. They rarely present with obstructive hydrocephalus, as this is usually a late finding that occurs after the tumors have grown considerably. Pontine gliomas are often hypointense on T1-weighted images and hyperintense on T2-weighted images, with variable enhancement. The prognosis for pontine tumors is much worse than for tumors located in the medulla or mesencephalon (Osborn DN, pp. 555–557).

3. C. Gradient echo sequences are the most sensitive in identifying any intracerebral lesions that exhibit chronic hemorrhage (such as cavernomas). Cavernomas often exhibit a "reticulated core" of mixed-signal intensity on T1-weighted images due to the presence of hemorrhage of varying ages. These lesions also often exhibit a hypointense rim on T1-weighted images, T2-weighted images, and gradient echo sequences that corresponds to hemosiderin deposits. Fast-spin echo sequences are T2-weighted sequences that are not very sensitive in the detection of chronic hemorrhage (Osborn DN, p. 313).

4. A. Optic nerve gliomas occur in 5 to 15% of all cases of NF-1. The majority of these tumors are low-grade (pilocytic) astrocytomas, and they can occur bilaterally. These lesions are usually hypo- to isointense on T1-weighted images and hyperintense on T2-weighted images with variable enhancement. Intracranial meningiomas are commonly observed in NF-2, and neurofibromas usually involve the spinal and peripheral nerves with NF-1 (Osborn DN, pp. 74–76).

5. C. This postcontrasted T1-weighted MRI study depicts an intracanalicular acoustic neuroma. Where there is an attempt to preserve the patient's hearing, either the suboccipital or middle fossa approach is used, because the translabyrinthine or transcochlear approaches sacrifice hearing. The suboccipital (retrosigmoid) approach is the most commonly used procedure by neurosurgeons for lesions mostly located within the CPA. It provides excellent control of the lower cranial nerves, brainstem, and vascular structures within the CPA. However, only the proximal two-thirds of the IAC can be safely exposed without traversing the inner ear. The middle fossa approach allows access to the labyrinthine segment of the facial nerve without sacrificing hearing and is the procedure most commonly used for small intracanalicular lesions. The dura is elevated from the floor of the middle fossa and the labyrinthine segment of the facial nerve identified medial to the geniculate ganglion. Access to the posterior fossa and CPA is somewhat limited and retraction of the temporal lobe is necessary for exposure. The transpetrosal infratemporal fossa corridor is not typically used for CPA tumors but instead for tumors of the jugular foramen such as paragangliomas and meningiomas (Bernstein, pp. 394–395, 430).

6. A. The primitive trigeminal artery (PTA) represents a persistence of the embryonic anastomosis between the cavernous segment of the internal carotid artery and the paired longitudinal neural arteries (vertebrobasilar system). The PTA is the most cephalad of the persistent fetal circulations; it is also the most common. The PTA is associated with an increased incidence of intracranial aneurysms. The persistent otic artery originates from the petrous ICA, the persistent hypoglossal artery originates from the cervical ICA, and the proatlantal intersegmental artery can originate from the internal or external carotid artery (Osborn DCA, pp. 65, 91–93).

7. D. *N*-acetyl aspartate (NAA) is a neuronal marker and is generally decreased in most CNS pathologic conditions. Total creatine is generally constant within the brain regardless of the presence of disease. Elevations of choline indicate increased plasma membrane turnover and synthesis, which is commonly observed with neoplasms. Thus, neoplasms are usually associated with decreases in NAA and elevations in choline and myoinositol (and lactate); total creatine is largely constant. The ratio of NAA to total creatine is thus decreased, whereas the ratios in A, B, C, and E are all increased with CNS neoplasms (Castillo et al., pp. 1–5).

8. E. Medulloblastomas are aggressive, primitive neuro-ectodermal tumors that occur primarily in the pediatric population. Medulloblastomas are found exclusively in the posterior fossa and usually reside in the midline (vermis). Occasionally these lesions are found in the lateral cerebellum, but this usually occurs in adults and older children. Medulloblastomas are aggressive tumors that frequently metastasize throughout the CNS via spinal fluid pathways. On MRI, medulloblastomas are generally isointense on T1-weighted images, with variable signal on T2-weighted images and intense enhancement with contrast. The lesions usually occupy most of the fourth ventricle and are often associated with communicating hydrocephalus. The history and MRI findings in this case are most consistent with a medulloblastoma. Choroid plexus papillomas are predominantly supratentorial lesions in the pediatric population, and pilocytic astrocytomas are usually cystic. Subependymomas do not typically enhance, and they are found almost exclusively in adults. Hemangioblastomas are also rare in children and occur most frequently in the brain parenchymas (Osborn DN, pp. 613–618).

9. E. Oligodendrogliomas generally exhibit mixed signal intensity on T1-weighted images and hyperintensity on T2-weighted images with mild heterogenous enhancement. These lesions exhibit calcification 70 to 90% of the time, are often associated with cysts, and frequently have evidence of chronic hemorrhage (Osborn DN, pp. 564–566).

10. A. Tuberous sclerosis (TS) is an autosomal dominant neurocutaneous disorder associated with the triad of seizures, mental retardation, and adenoma sebaceum. TS has variable expressivity and very high penetrance. Patients with TS often exhibit cortical tubers, subependymal nodules along the lateral ventricles, and benign foci of dysmyelination in the deep white matter on MRI. Subependymal giant cell astrocytoma develops in 15% of all patients with TS; it frequently occurs near the foramen of Monro and typically presents with obstructive hydrocephalus. TS is also associated with retinal phakomas, subungual fibromas, cardiac rhabdomyomas, and aneurysms (Osborn DN, pp. 93–98).

11. D. This angiogram illustrates a dural arteriovenous fistula (DAVF) with prominent retrograde cortical venous drainage. Most DAVFs originate from the transverse and sigmoid sinuses along the skull base, although the cavernous sinus is also frequently involved. The presence of retrograde cortical venous drainage places the patient at significant risk for subarachnoid hemorrhage, and mandates treatment. The treatment of DAVF usually consists of preoperative embolization followed by surgical obliteration of the nidus. Successful treatment entails disconnection of the cortical venous drainage from the nidus. Follow-up angiography may be appropriate with DAVF without retrograde cortical venous drainage but would be inappropriate in this case (Osborn DN, pp. 301–306).

12. C. Diffuse axonal injury most commonly involves the corticomedullary junction of the frontal and temporal lobes or the corpus callosum. DAI can also occur in the deep white matter (usually at gray-white junctions), dorsolateral brainstem, caudate nuclei, thalamus, and internal capsule. DAI rarely involves the cerebellum (Osborn DN, pp. 212–214).

13. A. Gangliogliomas are generally cystic supratentorial tumors that present in pediatric patients with seizures or elevated intracranial pressure. They are most commonly located in the temporal lobes and are hypointense on T1-weighted images and hyperintense on T2-weighted images, with variable enhancement patterns. Pleomorphic xanthoastrocytoma (PXA) can also present in children with epilepsy, although it is more typically found in a superficial location adjacent to the leptomeninges. PXA is usually cystic with an enhancing mural nodule. Germ cell tumors (including germinomas) are usually found in the pineal or paraphenol regions, and pilocytic astrocytomas are usually located in the posterior fossa or third ventricle in children (Osborn DN, pp. 580–581).

14-D; 15-A; 16-B; 17-B; 18-C; 19-A; 20-C. Refer to Table 5.14–5.20A. The appearance of hyperacute hematomas (up to 4 to 6 hours) on MRI is due to the presence of large amounts of oxyhemoglobin, which is diamagnetic and does not influence T1 and T2 relaxation times. Hyperacute clots have a high concentration of water, which renders them isointense on T1-weighted images and hyperintense on T2-weighted images. Acute hematomas (7 to 72 hours) consist primarily of deoxyhemoglobin, which is paramagnetic and has pronounced effects upon T2 relaxation times but no significant effects on T1 relaxation time. Acute hematomas are therefore isointense on T1-weighted images and hypointense on T2-weighted images. The precise reason for the dramatic T2 effect remains unclear but is believed to result from phase dispersion and subsequent preferential T2 proton relaxation enhancement. During this stage, the red blood

TABLE 5.14–20A   General MRI appearance and blood clot age

STAGE	T1-WEIGHTED IMAGE	T2-WEIGHTED IMAGE
Hyperacute (up to 4–6 hours)	Isointense	Hyperintense
Acute (7–72 hours)	Isointense	Hypointense
Early subacute (4–7 days)	Hyperintense	Hypointense
Late subacute (1–4 weeks)	Hyperintense	Hyperintense
Early chronic (weeks to months)	Hyperintense	Hyperintense
Late chronic (months to years)	Hypointense	Hypointense

cells shrink, lose their spherical shapes, become trapped in blood vessels, and acquire irregular spiculated projections and form "echinocytes." Early subacute hematomas (4 to 7 days) consist of intracellular methemoglobin, which is paramagnetic and renders subacute hematomas hyperintense on T1-weighted images and hypointense on T2-weighted images. With late subacute hematomas (1 to 4 weeks), methemoglobin becomes mostly extracellular (secondary to hemolysis), resulting in a progressively more hyperintense clot on T2-weighted images. Early chronic hematomas (months) generally consist of a pool of dilute-free methemoglobin surrounded by a ferritin- and hemosiderin-containing vascularized wall. At this stage, clots are generally similar in appearance to late subacute clots (hyperintense on both T1- and T2-weighted images), with a thin-rimmed wall of pronounced hypointensity on T2-weighted images (ferritin and hemosiderin deposits). With time (late chronic hematomas, months to years), ferritin- and hemosiderin-containing substances are further deposited throughout the clot, producing hypointense T1- and T2-weighted images (Osborn DN, pp. 154–172).

21. D. This CT scan illustrates perimesencephalic subarachnoid hemorrhage, which usually involves subarachnoid blood within the prepontine, interpeduncular, crural, or ambient cisterns. This is generally a benign entity, thought to result from rupture of a small vein. Angiography is required, however, because ruptured basilar apex aneurysms can exhibit a similar hemorrhage pattern. Patients with perimesencephalic hemorrhage can exhibit cardiac and electrolyte abnormalities. Although this disease is not associated with intraventricular hemorrhage, approximately 1% of cases can eventually develop hydrocephalus. Empiric calcium channel blockers, anticonvulsants, and hyperdynamic therapy is not indicated due to the rarity of vasospasm and seizures with this entity. Repeat angiography is controversial and is generally not indicated if the diagnosis is clear (Greenberg, pp. 793–795).

22. C. Cavernous malformations are circumscribed, multilobulated vascular lesions that often exhibit hemorrhage in various stages of evolution. The center of a cavernoma frequently contains a mixed-signal region known as a "reticulated (popcorn-like) core." The periphery of cavernomas is usually surrounded by a low-signal rim on T2-weighted images that corresponds to a peripheral rim of hemosiderin deposition from remote hemorrhages. Cavernomas can be located anywhere within the brain, although 80% are supratentorial parenchymal lesions, and they are often multiple. Gradient echo sequences are the most sensitive for detecting cavernomas. Capillary telangiectasias are usually small lesions that are hypointense on T2-weighted images and rarely exhibit hemorrhage. Venous angiomas are radial collecting veins that drain normal brain and rarely hemorrhage. Venous angiomas are occasionally associated with cavernous

malformations. Although oligodendrogliomas and choriocarcinoma can exhibit hemorrhage, the presence of a reticulated core and surrounding hemosiderin rim is more consistent with a cavernoma (Osborn DN, pp. 311–313).

23. C. This patient's symptoms consist largely of postural headaches that occurred shortly after a lumbar puncture. The patient's MRI shows evidence of diffuse pachymeningeal thickening with enhancement. These features are consistent with primary intracranial hypotension as a consequence of lumbar puncture. Meningeal carcinomatosis can exhibit similar features on MRI; however, this is unlikely in light of the negative cytologic examination of the CSF. Additionally, although melanoma frequently metastasizes to the CNS, this is unlikely in the absence of any other systemic metastases. Therefore an epidural blood patch will likely treat the source of the intracranial hypotension and result in cessation of headaches. The lack of focal neurologic signs and symptoms makes the diagnosis of CNS vasculitis unlikely; thus, cerebral angiography would not be indicated (Greenberg, pp. 63–64; Zaatreh et al., pp. 1342–1346).

24. B. The tentorial artery is a branch of the meningohypophyseal artery of the cavernous segment of the internal carotid artery; it is also known as the artery of Bernasconi and Cassinari, or the Italian artery. This artery was classically described in reference to a tentorial meningioma, but it is commonly observed with dural arteriovenous malformations of the tentorium as well (Wilkins, pp. 911, 918–919).

25. C. Juxtafacet (synovial) cysts commonly exhibit hyperintense signal on T2-weighted images with a hypointense capsule. These cysts originate from the facet joint and can present with lumbar radiculopathy secondary to nerve root compression. The signal intensity of the cyst contents is variable on MRI and depends largely upon the protein concentration within the cyst. Synovial cysts occasionally enhance with contrast administration (Osborn DN, pp. 843–845).

26. E. This MRI depicts ossification of the posterior longitudinal ligament (OPLL). OPLL occurs in 0.12% of all North Americans, and 2.4% of all Japanese and accounts for 27% of all cases of cervical myelopathy in Japan. OPLL involves the cervical spine in 70% of cases and the thoracic (15%) and lumbar (15%) regions less frequently. OPLL is more common in men and usually presents in the fifth to sixth decade with symptoms of progressive myelopathy. OPLL cannot be visualized with plain spinal x-rays; MRI or CT myelography is required to demonstrate the pathology and cord compression. Complications of anterior cervical decompression for OPLL include worsening myelopathy, durotomy, and radiculopathy. Postoperative C5 radiculopathy has been reported in up to 17% of all patients undergoing anterior decompressive procedures for OPLL. Posterior decompressions, with or without concomitant fusion, have also been utilized in the treatment of OPLL, with variable success rates (Osborn DN, p. 848; Wilkins, pp. 3783–3786).

27. D. Glioblastoma multiforme (GBM) is usually observed in the fifth to sixth decades of life and is most commonly located in the deep white matter of the frontal or temporal lobes. GBM often exhibits a central hypointense (necrotic) core on T1-weighted images with surrounding "ring enhancement" and prominent peritumoral edema. GBM can be multifocal, as depicted above, in approximately 1 to 5% of all cases. GBM is associated with exposure to hydrocarbons and radiation and often results in progressive neurologic symptoms and signs. Metastases are frequent in the adult population, and they can exhibit variable enhancement patterns on CT and MRI. Metastases, however, are most commonly located at the gray-white junction. Oligodendrogliomas usually exhibit heterogenous signal patterns on T1-weighted MRI, with patchy enhancement and calcification. CNS lymphoma is also often multiple and is usually found in the periventricular white matter or basal ganglia. CNS lymphoma is usually iso- to hypointense on T1-weighted images with variable enhancement patterns. The ring enhancement, prominent peritumoral edema, demographics, and the acute onset of a focal neurologic deficit are most consistent with a GBM (Osborn DN, pp. 541–544, 563–566, 620–622).

28. D. Colloid cysts are cystic, encapsulated lesions that occur at the foramen of Monro in the anterior aspect of the third ventricle. These lesions are usually hyperdense on CT scans (66%), hyperintense to cortex on T1-weighted images, and hypointense to cortex on T2-weighted images, although the MRI characteristics of these cysts are quite variable. Colloid cysts do not exhibit calcification or malignant degeneration; however, they occasionally show mild peripheral enhancement. Colloid cysts are derived from endoderm and usually present with intermittent or chronic headaches. Vertigo, memory loss, diplopia, and even sudden death can also occur with these lesions (Osborn DN, pp. 642–645).

29. D. Central neurocytoma is a lobulated, intraventricular tumor that usually occurs adjacent to the septum pellucidum or at the foramen of Monro within the lateral ventricle. Central neurocytoma usually presents in the second to third decades and is iso- to slightly hyperdense on CT scans. Central neurocytoma is generally isointense on T1-weighted images and iso- to hyperintense on T2-weighted images, with minimal to mild heterogenous enhancement patterns. Supratentorial ependymomas are generally extraventricular and exhibit prominent enhancement. Additionally, choroid plexus papillomas and intraventricular meningiomas also exhibit prominent enhancement on MRI. Intraventricular pilocytic astrocytomas are generally cystic lesions that exhibit heterogenous enhancement. The presence of an

intraventricular mass adjacent to the septum pellucidum that is isointense to surrounding brain on T1-weighted MRI without enhancement is most consistent with a central neurocytoma (Osborn DN, pp. 570, 582–584).

30. D. Aneurysmal bone cysts (ABCs) are benign lesions that can occur in all parts of the skeleton and often involve the posterior elements of the cervical and thoracic spine. ABCs usually occur in patients less than 20 years of age, and present with pain, edema, symptoms of neurologic compression, or pathologic fractures. ABCs are osteolytic lesions that often contain multiple lobulations and fluid-fluid levels secondary to hemorrhage at various stages of evolution. Eosinophilic granuloma, osteosarcoma, and osteoid osteoma rarely exhibit fluid-fluid levels and multiple lobulations. Giant cell tumors are also highly vascular, lytic lesions, however, they usually involve the vertebral body and present in patients in the third to fourth decades of life. The CT scan above exhibits prominent fluid-fluid levels within an osteolytic lesion, which is most consistent with an aneurysmal bone cyst (Osborn DN, pp. 881, 884–885).

31-F; 32-D; 33-A; 34-B. The central sulcus (A) is generally the most prominent sulcus that approaches the interhemispheric fissure, and it is usually located adjacent to or just anterior to the pars marginalis (E). The precentral gyrus (primary motor cortex) is generally thicker than the postcentral gyrus and exhibits a sigmoid-shaped "hook" laterally (F) that corresponds roughly to the motor hand region. The postcentral sulcus is generally bifid (D) and is intersected by the intraparietal sulcus laterally. The superior frontal sulcus (B) generally courses posteriorly to join the precentral sulcus (Naidich et al., pp. 313–338).

35. A. Sturge-Weber syndrome (encephalotrigeminal angiomatosis) is a sporadic neurocutaneous syndrome that is associated with development of a port-wine stain in the distribution of the trigeminal nerve and multiple thin-walled capillaries and venules along the convexity of the ipsilateral cerebral hemisphere. Sturge-Weber syndrome (SWS) has a predilection for involving the parietal and occipital regions, and is associated with prominent gyral calcification ("tramtrack" pattern), progressive cortical atrophy, ipsilateral calvarial thickening, enlargement of the paranasal sinuses, and prominent subependymal veins. On MRI, SWS often exhibits prominent enhancement of the pial angioma and subependymal veins of the involved hemisphere, as depicted here (Osborn DN, pp. 98–103).

36. D. Moyamoya (idiopathic progressive arteriopathy of childhood) is a progressive cerebrovascular disease that results in the progressive stenosis/occlusion of the distal internal carotid arteries and proximal segments of the anterior and middle cerebral arteries. Moyamoya usually presents with signs of progressive cerebral ischemia, although hemorrhagic variants can also occur. The angiographic hallmarks of moyamoya include stenoses and occlusions of the distal ICA and proximal ACA/MCA, along with the development of prominent leptomeningeal collaterals and enlarged lenticulostriate arteries, which resembles a "puff of smoke." (Osborn DN, pp. 371–372).

37. C. FDG PET imaging techniques usually exhibit focal hypometabolism in regions of radiation necrosis, low-grade neoplasms, and epileptic foci. In contrast, recurrent or high-grade neoplasms usually exhibit hypermetabolism (Juhasz et al., pp. 705–716).

38. D. Congenital cytomegalovirus (CMV) infection usually results in premature delivery and is associated with seizures, mental retardation, hydrocephalus, hearing loss, and optic atrophy. MRI characteristics of congenital CMV infection include encephalomalacia, ventriculomegaly, calcifications of the periventricular and basal ganglia, delayed myelination, and subependymal paraventricular cysts. CMV is considered one of the TORCH agents, along with toxoplasmosis, rubella, and herpes. The above T2-weighted image illustrates prominent bilateral basal ganglia calcifications (hypointense), ventriculomegaly, and encephalomalacia (Osborn DN, pp. 674–675).

39. C. See Table 5.14–5.20A. Subacute hematomas initially consist largely of intracellular methemoglobin, which results in hyperintensity on T1-weighted images. This hyperintense signal is largely peripheral with early subacute hematomas and gradually progresses toward the isointense central region of the hematoma. Early subacute hematomas are markedly hypointense on T2-weighted and gradient echo sequences. Late subacute hematomas are largely characterized by extracellular methemoglobin, which results in hyperintensity on both T1- and T2-weighted MRI sequences (Osborn DN, pp. 166–167).

40. C. Germinomas present in patients between the second and fourth decades and usually involve the pineal or suprasellar regions (midline locations). Suprasellar germinomas often present with headaches, diabetes insipidus, and panhypopituitarism in children. Germinomas are usually isointense on both T1- and T2-weighted sequences, and they exhibit intense, homogenous enhancement. Germinomas rarely occur off of the midline, and the presence of this lesion in nonmidline locations usually indicates metastasis, although the thalamus and basal ganglia are occasionally involved from local invasion. The MRI in this case exhibits synchronous suprasellar and pineal lesions, which can occur in 10% of all intracranial germinomas (Osborn DN, pp. 476, 607–610).

41. D. Embolic strokes often exhibit an abrupt vessel cutoff on angiography, with occasional wedge-shaped regions that

are devoid of blood flow and surrounding luxury perfusion (vascular blush) on late arterial phases. Occasionally an intravascular thrombus is also visualized, with slow distal antegrade flow. This lateral angiogram demonstrates a marked paucity of filling of the candelabra of the MCA, which is most consistent with embolic occlusion (Osborn DCA, pp. 383–388).

42. E. Toxoplasmosis is the most common opportunistic infection of the CNS in AIDS patients. Toxoplasmosis usually involves the basal ganglia or gray-white junction, and is iso- to hypointense on T1-weighted images. Toxoplasmosis exhibits prominent ring enhancement, as well as a central enhancing region that imparts a "target" appearance, as depicted here. This target appearance is not commonly observed with cryptococcomas, tuberculomas, or lymphoma (Osborn DN, pp. 698–700).

43. B. Vein of Galen malformations (VOGM) often present in neonates with macrocephaly, hydrocephalus, and high-output congestive heart failure. VOGMs appear as iso- to hyperdense midline masses located posterior to the third ventricle on CT scan, often with associated hydrocephalus. Neonatal teratomas can also involve the third ventricle, however, they usually exhibit heterogenous density and intensity on CT and MRI, respectively. Germinomas rarely occur in the neonatal population (Osborn DN, pp. 320–323, 612).

44. D. Chordomas arise from the clivus in approximately 35% of all cases and are typically slow-growing, lobulated extradural lesions. Calcification is often observed in chordomas; they are usually heterogenous lesions with hypointensity on T1-weighted images and hyperintensity on T2-weighted images, with variable enhancement patterns. The sella is not expanded in this example, which eliminates pituitary neoplasms from the differential, and en plaque meningiomas of the clivus are typically less lytic and invasive than chordomas. The surrounding hyperintensity (edema) of the clivus is consistent with a chordoma arising from within the clivus itself (Osborn DN, pp. 887–890).

45. A. Cephalhematomas generally result from hemorrhage between the skull and the overlying periosteum at delivery. Cephalhematomas are initially hard and typically exhibit progressive softening as the hematoma is absorbed. Approximately 3 to 5% of all cephalhematomas exhibit calcification, usually after 6 weeks, which can require surgical resection. Cephalhematomas do not cross suture lines. The AP skull radiograph in this case illustrates a calcifying cephalhematoma. Dermoid tumors often exhibit surrounding calcification and are located in the midline. Osteochondromas typically involve long bones or the spine, and eosinophilic granuloma often exhibits beveled nonsclerotic margins surrounding a lytic lesion involving the inner and outer tables (Osborn DN, p. 516; Wilkins, pp. 2739–2740).

46. A. Far lateral (extraforaminal) disc herniations typically compress the nerve root that is exiting at that level, as opposed to typical paracentral disc herniations, which often impinge upon the nerve root exiting at the level below. CT myelography does not typically identify far lateral disc herniations (Greenberg, p. 304).

47-D; 48-H; 49-B; 50-A; 51-F. Germinoma accounts for approximately 66% of all germ cell tumors of the pineal region and 40% of pineal region neoplasms overall. The most common posterior fossa tumor in children is the pilocytic astrocytoma; in adults, it is the hemangioblastoma (cerebellum). Approximately 75% of all cerebellopontine angle tumors are acoustic schwannomas. Tumors of the atrium are most commonly choroid plexus papillomas in children and meningiomas or lymphoma in adults (Osborn DN, pp. 412, 429–430, 434–436, 441, 607–608).

52. A. The appearance of acute epidural hematomas is generally hyperdense on noncontrasted CT scans. The observance of central regions of low density in an epidural hematoma is usually secondary to the rapid accumulation of unretracted semiliquid blood clots and is known as the "swirl sign." The lack of clear fluid-fluid levels and clot density helps eliminate subacute and chronic hematomas (Osborn DN, pp. 158–160).

53. D. Ankylosing spondylitis (Marie-Strümpell disease) is an inflammatory disorder that primarily affects the spine of young males and is associated with HLA B27. Autofusion of the apophyseal joints and anterior and posterior longitudinal ligaments is commonly observed in ankylosing spondylitis. This progressive ossification is often referred to as a "bamboo" spine, which is depicted in this case. Patients with ankylosing spondylitis are prone to develop spinal fractures and craniocervical instability over time (Osborn DN, p. 849; Merritt, p. 884).

54. D. Myxopapillary ependymomas are located in the conus medullaris or filum terminale and are usually isointense to spinal cord on T1-weighted images and iso- to hyperintense on T2-weighted images, with prominent enhancement. Myxopapillary ependymomas exhibit clusters of cuboidal cells with occasional hyalinized blood vessels among a prominent mucoid matrix (Osborn DN, pp. 906–909).

55. D. Rathke's cleft cysts (RCC) result from persistence of a cleft that is found between the pars distalis and pars nervosa during the development of the pituitary gland. RCC are usually asymptomatic, and they often contain both intrasellar and suprasellar components. The appearance of RCC on MRI is variable, but they are usually hyperintense to cortex on T1- and T2-weighted images without enhancement. RCC can be differentiated from craniopharyngiomas by the lack of calcification and from pituitary adenomas by the lack of enhancement (Osborn DN, pp. 645–646).

56. A. Arteriovenous malformations (AVMs) exhibit prominent flow voids on T2-weighted images with minimal observable intervening brain tissue and prominent enhancement. AVMs are not associated with surrounding edema unless they have recently hemorrhaged, although variable signal intensities can be observed in and around the nidus due to the presence of microhemorrhages of various ages and vascular thrombosis. The prominent flow voids, lack of surrounding edema, and lack of significant intranidal brain parenchyma helps distinguish AVMs from vascular tumors (Osborn DN, pp. 294–298).

57. C. Hemangioblastomas are well-circumscribed, often cystic lesions that are usually (80%) located within the cerebellum. Hemangioblastomas typically present in adults in the third to fifth decades of life, and they represent the most common primary neoplasm of the cerebellum in adults and often occur in conjunction with von Hippel-Lindau syndrome. Hemangioblastomas usually exhibit a cyst that is hypointense on T1-weighted images and hyperintense on T2-weighted images. The cystic component is usually associated with a mural nodule that is isointense to brain on T1-weighted images and hyperintense on T2-weighted images, with occasional flow voids. Solid hemangioblastomas often exhibit prominent enhancement, and the mural nodule of cystic lesions usually enhances as well. Choroid plexus papillomas can also occur in the fourth ventricle in adults, although they are usually solid, lobulated masses with homogenous, intense enhancement. Pilocytic astrocytomas can also exhibit prominent cyst formation with an enhancing mural nodule, although they usually occur in children and young adults (Osborn DN, pp. 555, 574, 605–607).

58. E. Osteochondromas are pedunculated lesions that can arise from the spinous or transverse processes of the cervical or thoracic spine. Osteochondromas are rarely symptomatic, usually present in the third to fourth decade of life, and a cartilaginous cap that exhibits calcification covers them. Osteoblastoma is an expansile lytic mass that usually involves the neural arch, is associated with night pain, and exhibits matrix mineralization. Osteoid osteoma is similar to osteoblastoma, although smaller (< 2 cm) and usually associated with more prominent surrounding sclerosis. Osteosarcoma is an aggressive lesion associated with prominent surrounding bony destruction/invasion and has a very poor prognosis. The lesion depicted in this x-ray is exophytic and originates from the neural arch, which is most consistent with osteochondroma (Osborn DN, pp. 879–883).

59. D. Nodular heterotopias are neuronal migration disorders that exhibit prominent subcortical collections of gray matter in various locations. Nodular heterotopias are often located in periventricular regions, as exhibited on the MRI above. Nodular heterotopias resemble normal gray matter on all sequences and do not enhance. These disorders can be differentiated from tuberous sclerosis (TS) because the cortical tubers of TS are often calcified, slightly hyperintense to cortex, and exhibit mild enhancement. The presence of a normal septum pellucidum eliminates holoprosencephaly and septo-optic dysplasia from the differential (Osborn DN, pp. 42–51).

60. D. Neurofibromatosis type 1 (NF-1) is associated with optic nerve gliomas, hamartomas of the basal ganglia and deep white matter, plexiform neurofibromas, spinal cord neurofibromas, kyphoscoliosis, meningoceles, intramedullary astrocytomas, and scalloping of the posterior aspects of the vertebral bodies. Spinal and cranial schwannomas are not observed in NF-1, however (Kaye and Laws, pp. 71–72; Osborn DN, pp. 73–84).

61. D. The patient's MRI exhibits enhancement of the mucous membranes of the frontal sinus with an adjacent subdural empyema that has spread laterally along the convexity and along the interhemispheric fissure. Subdural empyemas are associated with a high rate of cortical vein thrombosis and cerebritis, which results in their relatively high mortality (10 to 20%). Emergent surgical evacuation is indicated in almost all cases of subdural empyema, especially with the development of neurologic symptoms. Approximately two-thirds of all cases of subdural empyema result from adjacent spread of infections of the frontal sinus. Nonsurgical management has been reported in asymptomatic patients with the initiation of early IV antibiotics and close ICU observation, however, most authorities advocate early surgical drainage in all cases (Greenberg, pp. 223–225; Osborn DN, pp. 684–686).

62. A. Wyburn-Mason syndrome is a neurocutaneous syndrome that is characterized by the presence of multiple intracranial AVMs, cutaneous vascular nevi, and vascular malformations of the retina and optic nerves. The presence of multiple, discrete intracranial AVMs is extremely rare (2% of all cases), and usually occurs in the context of Wyburn-Mason syndrome or Rendu-Osler-Weber syndrome (hereditary hemorrhagic telangiectasia). Involvement of the optic pathways and mesencephalon, however, is more characteristic of Wyburn-Mason syndrome. Meningioangiomatosis is a rare neurocutaneous disorder that is characterized by prominent fibroblastic proliferation along the meninges and Virchow-Robin spaces. Blue rubber bleb nevus syndrome is also a rare neurocutaneous disorder that is characterized by vascular malformations of the skin, GI tract, and CNS. The CNS manifestations of blue rubber bleb nevus syndrome include the development of hemangiomas, sinus pericranii, and venous angiomas. True AVMs are not observed with this disorder (Osborn DN, pp. 106–109, 287).

63. C. Diastematomyelia (split-cord malformation) is characterized by the presence of two hemicords in a single or separate dural enclosure. When the hemicords occupy different dural enclosures, they are often separated by a septum consisting of bone, fibrous, or osteocartilaginous tissue. The hemicords usually reunite into a solitary spinal cord above and below the level of the diastematomyelia. Cutaneous stigmata often overlie the level of the split cord malformation, and it usually occurs between the levels of T9 and S1. Diastematomyelia is associated with Chiari II malformations, hemivertebrae, intersegmental laminar fusion, spina bifida, scoliosis, tethered cord, and narrowed disc spaces (Osborn DN, pp. 811–813).

64. B. This noncontrasted CT scan exhibits prominent intraluminal thrombus within the right MCA, which is known as the "hyperdense MCA sign." This CT scan was obtained approximately 4 hours after symptom onset, which consisted of a moderate left hemiparesis and hemisensory loss (Osborn DN, pp. 344–345).

65. C. This angiogram illustrates an aneurysm along one of the distal branches of the middle cerebral artery. Aneurysms of the distal MCA are infrequent, and are usually secondary to infections of the arterial wall (mycotic aneurysm). Traumatic aneurysms that result from blunt trauma usually occur at the skull base (ICA) or along the falx (A2 segment of the ACA) (Osborn DN, pp. 271–273).

66. D. Agenesis of the corpus callosum can be partial or complete and is associated with several disorders, including Chiari II malformations, Dandy-Walker malformation, Aicardi syndrome, holoprosencephaly, heterotopias, schizencephaly, intracranial lipomas, encephaloceles, and trisomy 13, 15, and 18. Agenesis of the corpus callosum is not typically associated with Klippel-Feil syndrome (Osborn DN, pp. 29–32).

67. E. Skull films in patients with Sturge-Weber syndrome often exhibit prominent gyral ("tram-track") calcifications, and secondary signs of cortical hemiatrophy (thick calvarium, elevated petrous temporal bone, enlarged frontal sinus) (Osborn DN, pp. 98–99).

68. A. Basilar impression (BI) is characterized by upward displacement of the foramen magnum margins and cervical spine (odontoid process) into the posterior fossa. Some may refer to BI as the upward displacement of the odontoid process only. It may be associated with Down's syndrome, Klippel-Feil syndrome, Chiari malformation, syringomyelia, rheumatoid arthritis, and trauma. It is the most common congenital (not acquired) anomaly of the craniocervical junction. McRae's line is described as a line drawn across the foramen magnum from the tip of the clivus to opisthion (should be > 19 mm, average 35 mm). No part of the odontoid should be above this line (most accurate for BI) (Greenberg, pp. 570–571).

69. A. Schwannomas, neurofibromas, ganglioneuromas, paragangliomas, meningiomas, and neurofibrosarcomas of the spine are typically intradural extramedullary lesions. Ependymomas, astrocytomas, and hemangioblastomas are typically intramedullary lesions (Osborn DN, pp. 895–899).

70-D; 71-A; 72-B; 73-D; 74-C. Pituitary macroadenomas are generally isointense to gray matter on all MRI sequences, with intense, heterogenous enhancement. Microadenomas generally exhibit less rapid enhancement than the surrounding normal pituitary gland, which renders them hypointense on contrasted T1-weighted MRI. Mixed-density pituitary adenomas often exhibit hemorrhage, cyst formation, or necrosis; however, calcification is rare. Rathke's cleft cysts are most commonly hyperintense on T1-weighted and T2-weighted MRI, with no enhancement, although their appearance is variable. Rathke's cleft cysts are usually intrasellar lesions with suprasellar extension, and they lack calcification (Osborn DN, pp. 645–646, 650–652).

75. B. Thoracolumbar burst fractures are secondary to axial compression injuries, and they usually occur between the levels of T12 and L2. Burst fractures can result in significant retropulsion of bony fragments (as depicted here), with concomitant neurologic deficits (Wilkins, pp. 2987–2989).

76. D. Hypoxic injury often involves the basal ganglia (caudate and lentiform nuclei), as depicted on this axial FLAIR MRI (Osborn DN, pp. 355–360).

77. C. Hemangioblastomas are highly vascular lesions that exhibit prominent, prolonged tumor blushes on angiography with large draining veins (Osborn DN, p. 915).

78. D. Meningiomas are generally vascular, dural-based tumors that receive their blood supply solely from meningeal vessels. Convexity and parasagittal meningiomas (as depicted here) are usually fed by an enlarged anterior falcine or middle meningeal artery in a radial ("sunburst") pattern. Occasionally large meningiomas also receive blood supply from pial vessels (dual vascular supply) (Osborn DN, pp. 589–590).

79. C. Saethre-Chotzen syndrome is one of the acrocephalosyndactyly syndromes and is an autosomal dominant disorder that is characterized by early fusion of the cranial sutures, often in an asymmetric fashion, low-set hairline, syndactyly, brachydactyly, ptosis, and septal deviations. This plain skull x-ray illustrates the typical "cotton beaten" skull that is characteristic of the syndrome. Patients with Saethre-Chotzen syndrome generally exhibit normal IQs (Wilkins, pp. 3432, 3694).

80. A. Multiple sclerosis plaques are generally iso- to hypointense on T1-weighted images and hyperintense on T2-weighted images. MS plaques can be located anywhere within the CNS, and they are commonly observed in periventricular regions and within the corpus callosum. Extension of calloseptal plaques along veins into the deep white matter is common and is known as "Dawson's fingers." More severe cases of MS exhibit hypointensity within the basal ganglia, which corresponds to the deposition of iron. MS plaques can also enhance during the active demyelinating stage as well (Osborn DN, pp. 756–761).

81. E. Parietal foramina are normally 1 to 2 mm in diameter and contain emissary veins. Occasionally, these foramina are larger and are covered by fibrous tissue that is continuous with the pericranium. The majority of parietal foramina are incidental findings that require no treatment. Cranioplasty is reserved for large foramina that persist beyond the ages of 3 to 4 years (Wilkins, p. 3570).

82. C. Arteriovenous malformations of the parenchyma usually appear as focal collections of arterial feeders with tortuous draining veins on angiography. The angiographic hallmark of AVMs is early filling of draining veins during the arterial phases of the study. Venous stenosis or occlusions are occasionally observed adjacent to the AVM nidus. Cavernous malformations are generally angiographically occult, and venous angiomas exhibit radial medullary veins located around an enlarged transcortical draining vein ("caput medusae"). Occasionally vascular, high-grade neoplasms can exhibit early draining veins as well, although the focal collection of multiple arterial feeders without intervening tissue on imaging studies is more consistent with an AVM (Osborn DN, pp. 287–291).

83. A. Pituitary macroadenomas are generally isointense to surrounding brain on all sequences and exhibit prominent, heterogenous enhancement with contrast. Craniopharyngiomas are most commonly hypointense on T1-weighted images and hyperintense on T2-weighted images, with heterogenous enhancement. Craniopharyngiomas are often cystic and calcified and usually present in children. A smaller proportion of craniopharyngiomas present in the fifth to sixth decades of life. The signal of craniopharyngiomas on T1-weighted images is often heterogenous; they are suprasellar lesions that often exhibit extension into the sella. This MRI exhibits a homogenous, predominantly intrasellar isointense mass with suprasellar extension, sellar expansion, and heterogenous enhancement. These MRI findings in a 72-year-old are most consistent with a pituitary adenoma (Osborn DN, pp. 649–657).

84. A. This MRI exhibits hypoplasia of the left sphenoid wing, with concomitant herniation of the temporal lobe into the orbit. This is characteristic of NF-1, which is inherited in an autosomal dominant fashion (Osborn DN, pp. 82–83).

85. D. Fibromuscular dysplasia (FMD) is a disorder that commonly involves medium-sized arteries, particularly the cervical carotid, vertebral, and renal arteries. FMD usually presents in women between the fourth to sixth decades with symptoms of ischemia, transient ischemic attacks, or even subarachnoid hemorrhage (increased incidence of intracranial aneurysms). The classic angiographic appearance of FMD is alternating regions of stenosis and dilatation ("string of beads"), as depicted in this angiogram. Catheter-induced vasospasm can occasionally mimic the angiographic appearance of FMD (Osborn DCA, pp. 341–346).

86. B. Arachnoid cysts resemble CSF on all MR sequences and are thus hypointense on T1-weighted images and hyperintense on T2-weighted images without enhancement. Arachnoid cysts are usually located in the middle cranial fossa (50 to 65%), suprasellar cistern (5 to 10%), quadrigeminal cistern (5 to 10%), or cerebellopontine angle (5 to 10%) (Osborn DN, pp. 640–642).

87. E. The most common neoplasms to occur at the trigone in adults are intraventricular meningiomas, lymphoma, and metastases. The most common trigonal mass in children is the choroid plexus papilloma, although ependymomas and astrocytomas are also observed at this location in this population. This MRI exhibits a homogenously enhancing intraventricular meningioma. Approximately 2% of all meningiomas arise within the ventricles, and these lesions are thought to originate from the tela choroidea or choroid plexus stromal cells (Osborn DN, pp. 429–430, 588).

88. C. This MRI exhibits a focal region of encephalomalacia in the distribution of the left middle cerebral artery. Ipsilateral ventricular dilatation accompanies the temporal lobe atrophy. It is this prominent lack of mass effect that helps distinguish a chronic infarct from a neoplasm or an acute infarction (Osborn DN, pp. 353–354).

89. C. Fibrous dysplasia is characterized by the presence of prominent sclerotic bone on CT scan ("ground glass" appearance) with occasional cystic components early in the disease course. Bony lesions of fibrous dysplasia are generally hypointense on both T1- and T2-weighted images, with variable enhancement patterns. Fibrous dysplasia is usually monostotic; however, polyostotic forms are also fairly common (Osborn DN, pp. 509–510).

90. A. Primary CNS lymphoma is generally hyperdense on CT scans and is often located in the corpus callosum, basal ganglia, and periventricular regions. Primary CNS lymphoma is often multifocal. It is generally isointense to gray matter on T1-weighted images and slightly hyperintense on T2-weighted images (Osborn DN, pp. 620–622).

91. A. This axial CT scan depicts bilateral jumped (locked) facets, with a concomitant fracture of the lamina. Bilateral jumped facets result from severe hyperflexion injuries and are usually associated with concomitant spinal cord injury. With jumped facets, the facet capsule, apophyseal joints, ligamentum flavum, and interspinous ligaments are disrupted. Unilateral jumped facets result from flexion/rotation injury mechanisms (Greenberg, pp. 712–713).

92. E. Gangliogliomas are often located within the temporal lobe and result in poorly controlled epilepsy in children and young adults. The imaging characteristics of ganglioglioma are variable and include solid enhancing masses or cystic masses with enhancing mural nodules, usually with prominent calcification. Most gangliogliomas are hypointense to surrounding brain parenchyma on T1-weighted images and hyperintense on T2-weighted images. Gangliogliomas are rarely associated with significant surrounding edema or hemorrhage. Dysembryoplastic neuroepithelial tumors can also involve the temporal lobe; they are usually hypointense on T1-weighted images and hyperintense on T2-weighted images with variable enhancement. Pleomorphic xanthoastrocytoma is also a cystic tumor that can occur in the temporal lobe, and it is predominantly hypointense on T1-weighted images and hyperintense on T2-weighted images, with prominent enhancement of solid portions of the tumor. Pilocytic astrocytomas are usually found in the cerebellum or hypothalamic region in children, and they are generally hypointense (or isointense) on T1-weighted images and hyperintense on T2-weighted images with variable enhancement (Osborn DN, pp. 556, 561, 580–582).

93. B. Acoustic neuromas are generally slightly hypointense to brain on T1-weighted images and hyperintense on T2-weighted images. Acoustic neuromas usually exhibit uniform, prominent enhancement, although heterogenous enhancement is occasionally observed. Acoustic neuromas can exhibit cystic degeneration, and rarely hemorrhage within the neoplasm. Smaller acoustic neuromas can be confined within the internal auditory canal (Osborn DN, pp. 629–630).

94. C. The patient's MRI demonstrates obliteration of the T12-L1 disc space secondary to a prior history of discitis. The patient has subsequently developed a kyphotic deformity at this level. This patient's history of diabetes mellitus makes the diagnosis of discitis more likely (Osborn DN, pp. 820–821).

95. B. The patient experienced a transient ischemic attack after blunt injury to the neck and was found to have a pseudoaneurysm of the internal carotid artery on angiography secondary to blunt dissection. The most appropriate initial treatment of this lesion is systemic anticoagulation, initially with heparin and subsequently with warfarin (Coumadin). Endovascular treatment is reasonable if the lesion does not resolve with systemic anticoagulation; however, this should not be the initial treatment modality of choice. Acute pseudoaneurysms are unstable lesions and the wall of these structures often contains subintima. This makes stent deployment more dangerous in the acute setting. Repeat angiography should be performed; however, the initial treatment entails systemic anticoagulation. Antiplatelet agents should be reserved for patients who have undergone endovascular stent placement or those in whom systemic anticoagulation is contraindicated (Osborn DCA, pp. 410–411).

96. C. It can be very difficult to visualize impingement on cranial nerve V with imaging studies, although on this axial MRI there is a clear discrepancy in the appearance of the trigeminal nerves bilaterally. The fifth cranial nerve is well illustrated on the left (large arrow), whereas on the right, it is being pushed medially by what appears to be a blood vessel, as suggested by the flow voids (smaller arrow). Most patients being evaluated for trigeminal neuralgia do not require imaging studies to confirm a diagnosis, as most patients typically present with paroxysmal lancinating pain, often triggered by sensory stimuli, confined to the distribution of one or more branches of the trigeminal nerve, with no neurologic deficit. (Greenberg, pp. 373–380).

97-D; 98-B; 99-A; 100-C. Refer to Table 5.97–5.100A. (Osborn DN, pp. 688–693; Greenberg, pp. 217–223).

101-B; 102-A; 103-C; 104-E; 105-G. This coronal CT of the face depicts the anatomy of the right globe as well as the adjacent paranasal sinuses. Of note, the levator palpebrae superioris muscle (A), innervated by the oculomotor nerve (CN III), originates superiorly to the annulus tendineus, inserts into the tarsal plate of the superior eyelid, and acts to draw the eyelid upward when the eyeball is elevated. Additionally, the muscles most frequently involved in thyroid ophthalmopathy are the inferior (E) and medial (D) recti. Other muscles of the globe include the superior rectus (G), lateral rectus (F), superior oblique (C), and inferior oblique (not shown) (Grant, p. 491; Adams, p. 1134; April, pp. 460–462).

106-C; 107-C. Note the homogeneously enhancing lesions involving the periventricular region in this patient with primary CNS lymphoma (PCNSL, CD20, and CD79a positive). PCNSL represents approximately 1% of intracranial neoplasms in immunocompetent patients and has been described in up to 50% of AIDS patients. The precise role of Epstein-Barr virus (EBV) in the pathogenesis of PCNSL remains unclear, although many authors have reported that between 5 and 38% of PCNSL tumors contained EBV in immunocompetent patients, while up to 100% of tumors in AIDS-related patients contained the EBV virus (Greenberg, pp. 231–234, 238, 441–444; Kaye and Laws, pp. 915–927).

108-C; 109-B; 110-E; 111-B. Note the multiple spinal neurofibromas with concomitant enlarged neural foramina on this contrasted, sagittal MRI depicting a patient with NF-1 (autosomal dominant inheritance). Plexiform neurofibromas are diagnostic of NF-1, and they occur in approximately 33% of cases. Bilateral acoustic neuromas are the hallmark of NF-2 (Greenberg, pp. 476–478; Ramsey, pp. 225–229).

112-B; 113-E; 114-A. This gradient echo MR sequence demonstrates a multilobulated lesion with a "popcornlike" pattern of high signal intensity, which is most consistent with a cavernoma. The etiology/pathogenesis of this lesion is

TABLE 5.97–100A   Histologic/radiographic staging of cerebral abscess

STAGE	HISTOLOGIC/IMAGING CHARACTERISTICS
1	Early cerebritis (days 1–3). Early infection and inflammation, poorly demarcated mass of congested vessels with PMNs and edema, toxic neurons, perivascular infiltrates, scattered necrotic foci. Ill-defined subcortical hyperintense zone on T2WI. Postcontrast T1WI discloses poorly delineated enhancing areas within the isointense to mildly hypointense edematous regions.
2	Late cerebritis (days 4–9): Reticular matrix (collagen precursor) and developing necrotic center, ring enhancement usually appears by this stage on postcontrast T1WI, may be difficult to differentiate from early capsular stage on imaging. The central necrotic zone is typically hyperintense on T2WI.
3	Early capsule (days 10–13): Collagen and reticulin continue to form a well-delineated capsule around a liquefied and necrotic core, capsule thin and incomplete, especially adjacent to ventricle. Capsule evident even on unenhanced scans as a thin-walled, well-delineated isointense to slightly hyperintense ring that is hypointense on T2WI.
4	Late capsule (day > 14): Well-formed collagen capsule, necrotic center, gliotic reaction surrounding abscess, abscess consists of three layers: an inner inflammatory layer of granulation tissue and macrophages, a middle collagenous layer, and an outer gliotic layer.

uncertain, although in some cases it has been shown to arise de novo adjacent to a venous malformation. Multiple lesions are more common in patients of Hispanic origin and have been linked to a mutation in a gene on chromosome 7q. Isolated cavernomas are associated with venous malformations in 30 to 50% of cases. Angiography is usually negative, although a subtle vascular blush may occur in a small number of cases (Ramsey, pp. 272–276).

115. A. This lateral angiogram demonstrates a PICA aneurysm between the posterior medullary and supratonsillar (telovelotonsillar) segments of the PICA. The first segment of PICA (anterior medullary) courses posterolaterally within the medullary cistern at the level of the olivary nucleus. The second segment (lateral medullary) continues posteriorly in the cerebellomedullary fissure and loops caudally for a variable distance along the lateral surface of the medulla. The third segment (posterior medullary or tonsillomedullary segment) is formed when the PICA passes through the fibers of cranial nerves IX, X, and XI to reach the posterior margin of the medulla and ascend behind the posterior medullary velum. The fourth segment (supratonsillar or telovelotonsillar) represents the cranial loop of the PICA as it courses above the cerebellar tonsil. The apex of this loop is known as the choroidal point, and represents the origin of the aneurysm depicted here. The PICA then turns downward in the retrotonsillar fissure and terminates by dividing into the hemispheric and vermian branches. Unlike the proximal three segments, the distal segments do not give rise to brainstem perforators, a fact that may allow clinicians to sacrifice the PICA distal to the choroidal point in some specific instances (Osborn DCA, pp. 176–184; Ramsey, pp. 598–599; Kaye and Black, pp. 1043–1049).

116. C. Note the increased signal and atrophy of the left hippocampus compared to the normal appearing right hippocampus on this FLAIR MRI sequence depicting mesial temporal lobe sclerosis. Although reports indicate a higher incidence of complicated febrile seizures in patients with temporal lobe epilepsy and mesial temporal sclerosis, the precise etiology remains unclear. There is usually hypometabolism of the affected temporal lobe with interictal fluorodeoxyglucose PET scanning (Greenberg, p. 255).

117. B. A number of disorders are thought to develop due to faulty secondary neurulation, including myelocystocele, meningocele, and split-cord malformations. Generally, there are two types of split-cord malformations, as proposed by Pang et al.: type I and type II. Type I split-cord malformation (often referred to as diastematomyelia) consists of two hemicords, each housed within a separate dural tube and separated by a median bony septum. Treatment consists of removing the bony septum, untethering the spinal cord, and reconstructing a single dural tube. Type II split cord

malformations (diplomyelia) consist of two hemicords within a single dural tube separated by a nonrigid fibrous septum. Treatment consists of untethering the spinal cord at the level of the spina bifida occulta and in some cases at the level of the split (Osborn DN, p. 12; Greenberg, pp. 160–161; American Society of Pediatric Neurosurgeons, pp. 54–61).

118. D. Note the prominent involvement of the basal ganglia and adjacent white matter bilaterally on this noncontrasted CT scan depicting carbon monoxide poisoning (Ramsey, pp. 351–353).

119-D; 120-B. Epidermoids are usually hypointense on T1-weighted imaging, hyperintense on T2-weighted imaging, and exhibit restricted diffusion (increased signal) on DWI sequences (as depicted here). Arachnoid cysts are hypointense on DWI sequences. The fatty areas of dermoid tumors and lipomas will saturate out with fat-suppression sequences and produce a chemical shift artifact, whereas fat saturation sequences do not appreciably affect epidermoids (Ramsey, pp. 118–120).

121. D. This contrasted, axial T1-weighted MRI depicts an ovoid lesion centered over the left CPA, which enhances intensely and homogenously and is most consistent with a meningioma. Dural metastases are often multiple and may incite an adjacent inflammatory reaction. Vestibular schwannomas typically extend into the IAC, have areas of cyst formation, and often enhance heterogenously. Hemangiopericytomas cannot be differentiated from meningiomas on neuroimaging alone, but are more scarce then meningiomas (Ramsey, pp. 115–117).

122-B; 123-E; 124-C. Note the presence of multiple meningiomas on this contrasted T1-weighted MRI, which is most consistent with NF-2, an autosomal dominant condition that results from mutations on chromosome 22. Multiple intradural spinal cord tumors are also common in this condition including ependymomas (most common), schwannomas, and meningiomas. The incidence of NF-2 is 1 per 20,000 to 50,000, while the incidence for NF-1 is approximately 1 per 3000 (Greenberg, p. 47).

125-C; 126-E. Note the cyst contiguous with the fourth ventricle, the elevation of the torcula, and absence of all cerebellar tissue in this patient with a Dandy-Walker malformation. Dandy-Walker malformation is differentiated from other posterior fossa anomalies such as arachnoid cysts and mega cisterna magna by the presence of the vermis in these other anomalies. Cardiac defects are common extra-CNS anomalies seen associated this disorder (Albright, pp. 134–139).

127-D; 128-D. Note the presence of multiple flow voids on this sagittal T2-weighted MRI, which is most consistent with a spinal arteriovenous malformation. The next diagnostic test performed should be an angiogram for better evaluation of the region of interest, arterial supply, and venous drainage of this malformation (Albright, pp. 1071–1087).

129. E. Note the porencephalic cleft lined predominately by gliotic white matter (Osborn DN, pp. 54–56).

130. A. This sagittal MRI shows descent of the tonsils through the foramen magnum without other accompanying brain malformations, which is most consistent with Chiari I malformation. Osseous abnormalities may be seen in up to 25% of all patients with Chiari I malformation and include atlanto-occipital assimilation, platybasia, basilar invagination, and fused cervical vertebrae (Osborn DN, pp. 16–18).

131. A. Herpes simplex encephalitis (HSE) typically results from infection with herpes simplex virus (HSV) 2 in neonates and HSV 1 in children and adults. Neonatal HSE is a diffuse encephalitis that is often hemorrhagic and causes significant morbidity and mortality. HSE that is caused by HSV 1 is usually a focal infection that involves the limbic system (temporal lobes, cingulate gyri, and insular cortex). HSE type 1 often shows subtle low density in the temporal lobes early in the disease course on CT scans and often exhibits hemorrhage later in the disease course. On MRI, early HSE type 1 exhibits hyperintensity within the temporal lobe on T2-weighted images and gyral enhancement on T1-weighted images, as depicted here. Later in the disease course, contrast enhancement, subacute hemorrhage, and progressive limbic system involvement can be observed on MRI (Ramsey, pp. 157–160).

132. B. Note the multiple periventricular white matter lesions without mass effect in this patient with multiple sclerosis (Ramsey, pp. 335–338).

133. B. Note the longitudinal occipitoatlantal dissociation with a significant amount of surrounding soft tissue swelling (Harris, pp. 88–89).

134. B. The ADI does not usually exceed 3 mm in an adult (Harris, pp. 20–22).

135-B; 136-A. This lumbar meningocele contains prominent meninges and CSF, but lacks any neural tissue. It is most often the result of faulty secondary neurulation (4 to 5 weeks) where the notochord and mesodermal elements induce the formation of dura, pia, vertebrae, and skull (Osborn DN, pp. 12–13).

137-B; 138-A; 139-A. Note the presence of multiple regions of increased signal intensity (cortical tubers) and the presence of subependymal nodules within the ventricular walls in this patient with tuberous sclerosis. It is inherited in an auto-

somal dominant fashion and is frequently associated with subependymal giant cell astrocytoma (15% of cases) near the region of the foramen of Monro (Osborn DN, pp. 93–98).

140-B; 141-E. Note the anastomosis between the proximal cervical ICA and the vertebral artery on this lateral angiogram, depicting a proatlantal intersegmental artery (Osborn DN, pp. 65–71).

142-B; 143-E. Note the classic "polka dot" appearance of this hemangioma, which is most often an incidental finding that requires no treatment (Osborn DN, pp. 877–879).

144. D. Acute intracerebral hematomas are markedly hypointense to surrounding brain on T2-weighted MRI (Osborn DN, p. 166).

145. C. The fourth ventricle is the most common location for choroid plexus papillomas in adults, whereas the lateral ventricle is more common in children (Ramsey, pp. 75–77).

146. E. Shunted hydrocephalus, as well as chronic phenytoin therapy, can result in generalized skull thickening as opposed to regional or focal thickening (Osborn DN, p. 515).

147. D. Note the prominent dorsal epidural fat (high signal intensity) in a patient with epidural lipomatosis and chronic steroid use for asthma (Osborn DN, pp. 885–887)

148-C; 149-A. Eosinophilic granuloma of the spine is most often seen as a lytic lesion without surrounding sclerosis and is the classic cause of a single collapsed vertebral body in patients between the ages of 5 and 10 years, as depicted here. Giant cell tumors are highly destructive, lytic masses in patients between the ages of 20 and 40 years, while hemangiomas have the characteristic "polka dot" vertebral body pattern (Osborn DN, pp. 877–886).

150. B. Note the absence of the sacrum below S2 on this lateral plain radiograph depicting caudal regression syndrome, which results from faulty secondary neurulation (Osborn DN, p. 809).

151-A; 152-B. Note the marked narrowing of the proximal internal carotid artery (distal to the bulb) with a prominent, elongated, contrast-filled outpouching of the more distal part of the vessel. This patient has a carotid dissection with pseudoaneurysm formation. Typically, spontaneous dissection of the cervical carotid artery manifests with symptoms of headache (most common) and transient ischemic attacks or strokes. The mainstay of treatment includes anticoagulation, although carotid artery angioplasty and stenting is a viable initial treatment option in select patients. Direct surgical repair is seldom warranted, although surgical options may include superficial temporal artery to middle cerebral artery bypass versus high-flow saphenous vein graft bypass, depending on the intracranial blood flow deficit (Youmans, pp. 1684–1686).

153. D. The incidence of cerebral metastasis from prostate and gastric cancer is exceedingly low compared to lung, breast, renal, and skin (melanoma) cancer (Greenberg, p. 464).

154-C; 155-E; 156-E. Note the upward displacement of the odontoid process through the foramen magnum in this patient with Chiari II malformation (basilar invagination). Another pertinent finding on this MRI is the spinal cord syrinx, which is partly seen behind the C7 and T1 vertebral bodies. There are several lines used to evaluate the craniovertebral junction including McRae's line (line drawn across the foramen magnum), Chamberlain's line (line from posterior hard palate to posterior foramen magnum or opisthion), McGregor's line (line from posterior hard palate to most caudal point of occiput), Wackenheim's clivus-canal line (line along posterior surface of clivus), Fischgold's digastric line (line joining digastric notches), and Fischgold's bimastoid line (line joining tips of mastoid process). No part of the odontoid should be above McRae's or Wackenheim's line, while if more than 6 mm and 4.5 mm of odontoid lie above Chamberlain's and McGregor's lines, respectively, a cervicomedullary abnormality is likely to be present (Wilkins, pp. 3587–3591).

157. C. The use of contrast material can often help differentiate a recurrent disc fragment from scar formation following a microdiscectomy. In general, only the peripheral margin of a recurrent herniated disc exhibits enhancement following surgery (as in this case), whereas, scar tissue often exhibits homogenous enhancement secondary to the abundance of granulation tissue present. The enhancement around the periphery of a herniated disc is thought to result from granulation tissue surrounding the disc, which develops because of the reaction to the disc. If arachnoiditis is present, the study often reveals clumping of the nerve roots around the peripheral margins of the thecal sac in a very characteristic pattern (see question 8.201). In a chronically herniated disc, the capillary ingrowth may extend through the herniated fragment and result in homogeneous enhancement, which is similar to the appearance of a scar, while with chronic retracted scars, there may only be peripheral enhancement. Therefore clinical history and physical examination are extremely important for accurate diagnosis (Ramsey, pp. 637–639).

158. A. Systemic hypertension often weakens blood vessels, which can rupture in the setting of acute elevations of blood pressure. Some implicate microaneurysms of deep perforating vessels (Charcot-Bouchard) in the genesis of these hemorrhages, although this remains controversial. This CT

scan shows a characteristic putaminal hemorrhage secondary to hypertension (Ramsey, pp. 264–267).

159. C. Note the cystic structure in the middle cranial fossa on the left that parallels CSF in signal intensity and is most consistent with an arachnoid cyst. Unlike tumors, it has no internal structure and does not enhance, although occasionally hemorrhage or a high protein count may complicate its appearance and make diagnosis difficult. It can be differentiated from epidermoid tumors by the fact that epidermoids engulf adjacent arteries and nerves, whereas arachnoid cysts displace them. Schizencephalic clefts are lined by heterotopic gray matter, whereas enterogenous cysts are rare intraspinal masses that occur even less often intracranially (Osborn DN, pp. 639–649).

160. D. This skull radiograph demonstrates an enlarged parietal foramen, which is most often an incidental finding. In many instances, parietal foramina are no larger than a burr hole and rarely require treatment. Occasionally, they may be large enough to put the brain at risk of mechanical injury, and cranioplasty may be indicated (Albright, p. 214).

161-C; 162-E. Note the abrupt ACA angulation as it returns to the midline under the falx in this patient with subfalcine herniation. This angiographic appearance is usually caused by a holotemporal lobe mass and is described as a "square" ACA shift, as opposed to the "round" ACA shift often seen with deep frontal, insular, or basal ganglionic masses (less abrupt return of the ACA toward the midline) (Osborn DCA, pp. 314–325).

163-E; 164-C; 165-C; 166-A; 167-B; 168-F; 169-D. Refer to Table 5.163–5.169A (Ramsey, pp. 176–193; Greenberg, pp. 232–233).

170-B; 171-A. Note the presence of a left optic nerve glioma with diffuse enlargement of the optic nerve in this patient with NF-1 (unenhanced T1-weighted MRI) (Osborn DN, pp. 553–559).

172. B. This axial noncontrasted CT scan through the lateral ventricles and basal ganglia reveals a small, agyric brain with a relatively thin cortical mantle, bilateral calcifications, atrophy, and ventriculomegaly. These findings are most consistent with an intrauterine TORCH infection affecting sulcation and cellular migration (Osborn DN, pp. 44–46).

173-C; 174-B. Alobar holoprosencephaly (AH) is the most severe form of this disorder and consists of a monoventricle, fused thalami and a peripheral rim of undifferentiated cerebral tissue. AH is associated with severe craniofacial abnormalities, renal dysplasia, polydactyly, and trisomy 13. Lobar

TABLE 5.163–169A   Imaging characteristics of HIV and associated opportunistic infections and neoplasms

DISEASE	CT FINDINGS	MRI FINDINGS
HIV encephalitis	Cerebral atrophy; low density regions in deep white matter/periventricular regions	Symmetric patchy or confluent areas of high signal intensity on T2-weighted images involving the centrum semiovale and periventricular/deep white matter regions; frontal predominance; no evidence of mass effect or enhancement
Progressive multifocal encephalopathy (PML)	Asymmetric areas of hypodensity in periventricular/deep white matter regions	Asymmetric, multifocal areas of T1 and T2 prolongation in the periventricular and/or peripheral white matter without sparing of subcortical U fibers; parieto-occipital regions mostly affected; mass effect, enhancement, and/or hemorrhage absent or mild
Toxoplasmosis	"Eccentric target" sign; multifocal lesions with surrounding edema; basal ganglia commonly involved	Similar to CT findings
Cryptococcal disease	Frequently normal or mild communicating hydrocephalus; multiple round hypodensities resulting from expansion of perivascular spaces due to accumulation of mucinous material, inflammatory cells, and organisms, "gelatinous pseudocysts"	"Gelatinous pseudocysts" appear as punctate hyperintensities on T2-weighted images and hypo- to isointense on T1-weighted images, most common in midbrain and basal ganglia; cryptococcomas may be seen
Cytomegalovirus	Relatively insensitive; may demonstrate white matter hypodense regions or ependymal enhancement	Generalized ependymal/subependymal hyperintensity; thin linear enhancement along ventricular wall in 20–30% of cases
Lymphoma	Greater tendency for multiplicity in AIDS patients; may appear similar to toxoplasmosis	Ependymal enhancement is more nodular and irregular; often enhances; typically hypo- to isointense on T2-weighted images

holoprosencephaly is the mildest form of this disorder and consists of a nearly complete falx with separation of the basal ganglia and absence of the septum pellucidum (Osborn DN, pp. 38–43).

175. A. The most common location for cellular spinal ependymomas is the cervical spine, while myxopapillary ependymomas are often in the region of the cauda equina (Osborn DN, pp. 906–910).

Neurosurgery Questions

QUESTIONS 1–5

Scenario: A 54-year-old female was taken to an emergency room after collapsing at work. She was alert and communicative, with a severe headache, photophobia, nuchal rigidity, and blurry vision. Computed tomography (CT) of the brain revealed diffuse subarachnoid blood in the basal cisterns, mild hydrocephalus, and no intraparenchymal hematoma. Her angiogram is depicted below (Figure 6.1–6.5Q).

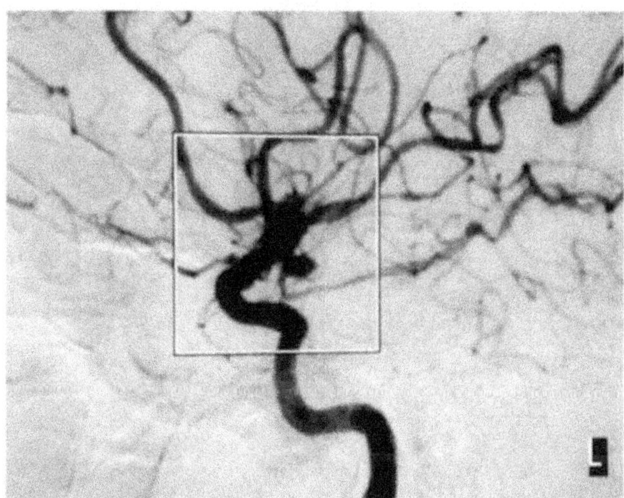

FIGURE 6.1–5Q

1. What is the clinical Hunt and Hess grade of this patient?

- **A.** Grade I
- **B.** Grade II
- **C.** Grade III
- **D.** Grade IV
- **E.** Grade V

2. Some posterior communicating artery (PComA) aneurysms do not produce any third nerve deficit. Why should special attention be given to the angiogram in these cases?

- **A.** If the aneurysm is projecting posterolaterally rather than in a more common medial position, there is an increased risk of injuring the perforating vessels from the PComA during microdissection
- **B.** An aneurysm projecting laterally onto the medial edge of the temporal lobe argues against premature retraction of the temporal lobe
- **C.** The angiogram may reveal a ventral carotid wall aneurysm instead of a PComA lesion, which is often better managed with coiling
- **D.** To look for any other associated aneurysms and/or vasospasm
- **E.** It may help with surgical planning, as medially projecting lesions are better approached through the carotid-oculomotor triangle

3. The patient is taken to the operating room for aneurysm clipping. Proximal and distal control of the internal carotid artery is obtained with temporary clip placement prior to aneurysmal neck dissection. Despite this maneuver, the aneurysm ruptures during microdissection and significant bleeding is encountered, which significantly hinders visualization. What preventative maneuver could have been employed prior to aneurysmal rupture to decrease the amount of intraoperative bleeding?

- **A.** Blunt surgical microdissection
- **B.** Obtaining proximal control of the internal carotid artery in the neck
- **C.** Releasing the dome of the aneurysm from the temporal lobe prior to temporary clip placement to prevent traction on the fundus
- **D.** Identifying the distal posterior communicating artery medial to the internal carotid artery for temporary clip placement if possible
- **E.** Temporary clip placement on the ophthalmic artery to prevent retrograde bleeding from the orbit

4. Postoperatively, the patient wakes up with contralateral weakness, numbness, and homonymous hemianopia. A CT scan of the brain shows an infarct in the posterior limb of the internal capsule and in the adjacent white matter (above the temporal horn of the lateral ventricle). This complication might possibly have been avoided by

- **A.** Identifying the anterior choroidal artery prior to aneurysm clipping in order to prevent damage or incorporation of this vessel into the clip construct
- **B.** Increasing temporary occlusion time to prevent hasty microdissection
- **C.** Limiting the sylvian fissure dissection to the sphenoidal portion in order to prevent unnecessary dissection adjacent to PComA artery perforators, which supply the posterior limb of the internal capsule
- **D.** Obtaining an intraoperative angiogram to confirm proper clip placement
- **E.** Identifying and preserving the recurrent artery of Heubner

5. Postoperatively, the patient sustained damage to the frontal branch of the facial nerve. What is the most likely reason for the frontal branch facial nerve injury?

- **A.** The supraorbital nerve was not identified in detaching the scalp from the supraorbital rim
- **B.** The incision was started less than 1 cm anterior to the tragus
- **C.** There was nerve neuropraxia from postoperative swelling
- **D.** The nerve in the subgaleal fat pad was injured during surgical dissection
- **E.** The nerve between the superficial and deep layers of the temporalis fascia was injured with monopolar cautery

End of set

QUESTIONS 6–9

Scenario: A 28-year-old male was involved in a motorcycle accident. About 1 week after being discharged from the hospital he began experiencing fevers, severe retroorbital headaches, diplopia, and left eye proptosis, which prompted a visit to the emergency department. A computed tomography (CT) scan of the brain showed a resolving 2- by 3-cm left frontal contusion underlying a minimally displaced frontal bone fracture, which was sustained at the time of initial injury. His erythrocyte sedimentation rate (ESR) and C-reactive protein (CRP) were mildly elevated. The angiogram is depicted below (Figures 6.6–6.9Q A, B).

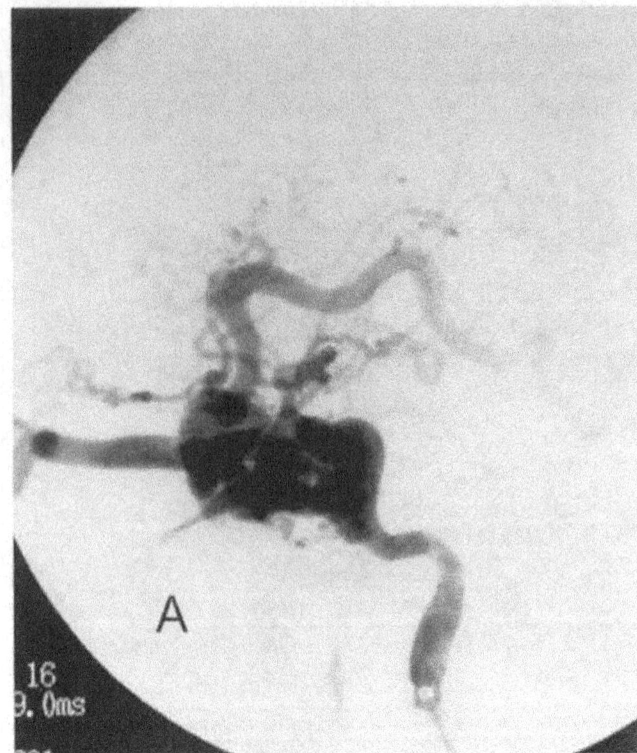

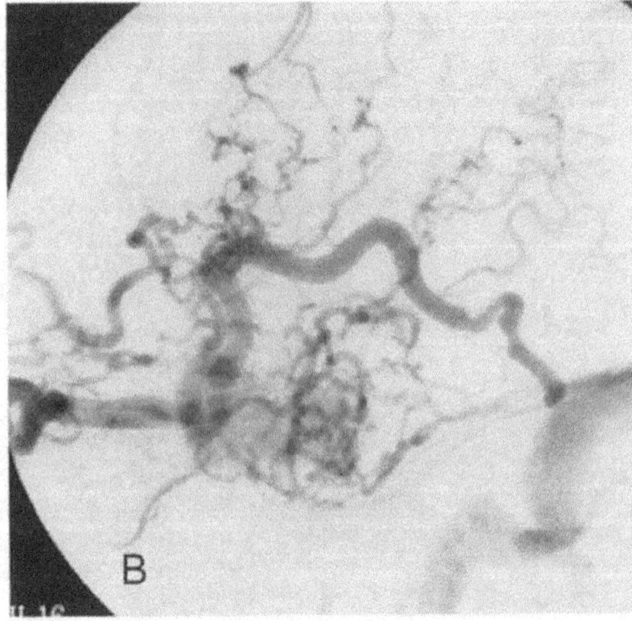

FIGURE 6.6–9Q

6. What is the most likely diagnosis?

A. Superior orbital fissure syndrome

B. Incidental meningioma originating from the medial aspect of the sphenoid ridge

C. Arterial-venous fistula

D. Occlusion of the internal carotid artery proximal to the ophthalmic artery origin

E. Cavernous sinus thrombosis

7. The signs/symptoms of this disease process depend mostly upon

A. The size and location of the tumor relative to the optic nerve

B. The direction of venous drainage and rate of blood flow through the shunt

C. The extent of the inflammatory reaction adjacent to the cavernous sinus

D. The extent of the inflammatory reaction adjacent to the superior orbital fissure

E. The extent of collateral flow from the opposite internal carotid artery and external meningeal feeders

8. What should be the initial treatment of choice for this patient?

A. Six weeks of antibiotics followed by repeat angiography

B. Glue embolization of major arterial feeders followed by tumor resection

C. Carotid artery sacrifice

D. Transarterial detachable balloon embolization

E. Heparin infusion

9. If the desired treatment strategy fails, what would be another potential treatment option?

1. Surgical debridement of the infection

2. Direct surgical packing of the cavernous sinus with either Gelfoam, Surgicel, platinum coils, or strands of cotton

3. Preoperative glue embolization of arterial feeders followed by tumor resection

4. Endovascular procedure for internal carotid artery sacrifice

A. 1, 2, and 3 are correct

B. 1 and 3 are correct

C. 2 and 4 are correct

D. Only 4 is correct

E. All of the above

End of set

10. What finding in the pathologic process depicted by the angiogram below (Figure 6.10Q) would mandate urgent treatment?

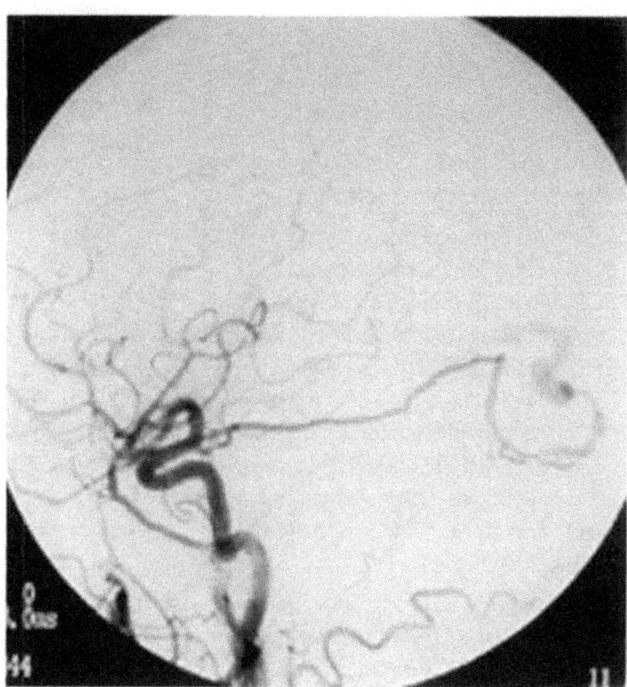

FIGURE 6.10Q

A. Retrograde cortical venous drainage

B. Multiple meningeal artery feeders

C. Dual internal and external carotid artery supply

D. Embolic stroke

E. Venous sinus occlusion

QUESTIONS 11–16

Scenario: A 67-year-old male with a history of diabetes mellitus and hypertension presents to the emergency department with right arm weakness and numbness. He is found to have > 90% stenosis of the left internal carotid artery and restricted MR diffusion in portions of the brain supplied by the left middle cerebral artery. He elects to proceed with surgery for his carotid stenosis but is found to have a high-riding carotid artery bifurcation.

11. Surgical maneuvers that may increase surgical exposure of a high-riding carotid artery bifurcation during carotid endarterectomy include all of the following EXCEPT?

A. Medial mobilization of the ansa cervicalis

B. Dividing the posterior belly of the digastric muscle

C. Mandibular osteotomy or disarticulation of the mandible at the temporomandibular joint

D. Judicious cautery and ligation of select vessels (occipital artery, common facial vein) hindering exposure

E. Transverse sectioning of the clavicular head of the sternocleidomastoid muscle at the level of the hyoid bone for better visualization of the carotid artery lateral to the jugular vein

12. What cranial nerve is at most risk of injury when exposing a high-riding carotid artery bifurcation?

   A. VII

   B. IX

   C. X

   D. XI

   E. XII

13. What is the order of clamp placement on the arteries during carotid endarterectomy?

   A. External, internal, common

   B. Internal, common, external

   C. External, common, internal

   D. Common, external, internal

   E. Common, internal, external

14. After clamp placement and arteriotomy, the surgeon notices continued bleeding from the back wall of the carotid artery, which severely hinders visualization during the surgical procedure. What is the most likely reason for the continued bleeding?

   A. Incomplete clamping of the common carotid artery

   B. Backbleeding from the superficial temporal artery

   C. Backbleeding from the ascending pharyngeal artery

   D. Venous bleeding from the adventitia of the internal carotid artery

   E. Clotting abnormality from heparin infusion

15. During surgical dissection adjacent to the carotid artery, the anesthesiologist notices that the patient becomes hypotensive and bradycardic. The next course of management should include

   A. Obtain an immediate arterial blood gas (ABG) to determine if the patient is suffering from a pulmonary embolus

   B. Check cardiac enzymes, as the patient is likely suffering from an anterior myocardial wall infarction

   C. The nerve to the carotid sinus (nerve of Hering) should be anesthetized with 0.5 mL of 2% lidocaine

   D. Begin dobutamine, check central venous pressures, and obtain a lactate level, as the patient is likely to be volume-depleted

   E. 100 IU/kg of heparin should be infused intravenously to prevent further emboli

16. Postoperatively, the patient awoke with right-sided hemiplegia and lethargy. The next logical course of management should include

   A. Immediate CT angiography to assess the patency of the right carotid artery

   B. Immediate selective angiography of the right carotid artery

   C. Antiplatelet therapy for 1 week, followed by repeat angiography

   D. Stent placement across the arteriotomy site to reinforce the closure

   E. Immediate surgical reexploration for thrombectomy

End of set

QUESTIONS 17–18

A 15-year-old female undergoes uncomplicated resection of the lesion depicted below (Figure 6.17–6.18Q). Four days later she develops lethargy, fever, meningismus, and photophobia. A cerebrospinal fluid (CSF) sample reveals a protein level of 86 mg/dL (reference range, 12 to 60 mg/dL), a glucose level of 61 mg/dL (reference range, 40 to 70 mg/dL), 16 red blood cells/mL, and 126 white blood cells/mL with a differential of 11% neutrophils, 82% lymphocytes, and 7% histiocytes. Gram stain and culture of CSF were sterile and remained so for the presence of organisms.

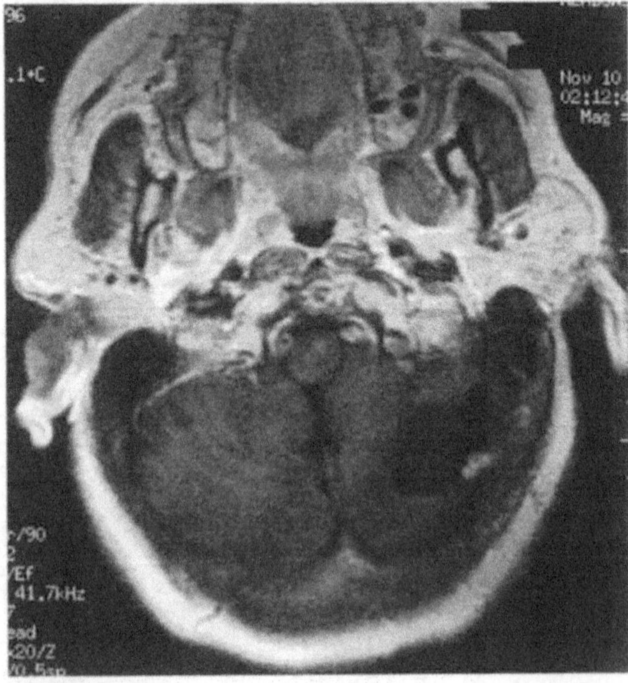

FIGURE 6.17–18Q

17. What is the most likely diagnosis?

   A. Bacterial meningitis
   B. Aseptic meningitis
   C. Hydrocephalus
   D. Postmeningitis syndrome
   E. Viral encephalitis

18. What is the natural history of this problem?

   A. Requires a 10-day course of antibiotics despite negative cultures to cover for slow-growing bacterial species
   B. Patients frequently require steroid therapy followed by repeat lumbar punctures
   C. Usually self-limited and requires no treatment
   D. Patients show drastic improvement with shunting
   E. Usually favorable once any synthetic material placed during surgery (e.g., dural graft) is removed

End of set

19. A 62-year-old female undergoes microvascular decompression for hemifacial spasm. Postoperatively, she has complete ipsilateral deafness but no other neurologic deficits. The most likely cause of this deficit was injury to one of the blood vessels that originated from which artery?

   A. Posterior cerebral artery (PCA)
   B. Superior cerebellar artery (SCA)
   C. Anterior inferior cerebellar artery (AICA)
   D. Posterior inferior cerebellar artery (PICA)
   E. Vertebral artery

20. A 14-year-old girl with progressive loss of vision in her right eye was recently diagnosed with a 2.0- by 3.5-cm right optic nerve glioma extending to the optic chiasm. During surgery, the portion of the tumor on the optic nerve was successfully resected, but the tumor adjacent to the optic chiasm was left behind. What is the maximal dose of single-fraction radiosurgery that can safely be employed to the optic chiasm?

   A. 4 to 7 Gy
   B. 9 to 10 Gy
   C. 11 to 13 Gy
   D. 14 to 16 Gy
   E. 21 Gy

21. A surgeon decides to utilize an infratentorial-supracerebellar corridor to approach a pineal region mass. What blood vessel is frequently cauterized and divided for better exposure of the posterior surface of the tumor during this approach?

   A. Vein of Galen
   B. Ipsilateral basal vein of Rosenthal
   C. Posterior cerebral artery (PCA)
   D. Precentral cerebellar vein
   E. Superior petrosal sinus

22. During translabyrinthine exposure for acoustic neuroma resection, surgeons find themselves exposing Trautmann's triangle. All of the following structures delineate this area EXCEPT?

   A. A triangular patch of dura on the posterior aspect of the temporal bone facing the cerebellopontine angle
   B. The sigmoid sinus laterally
   C. The superior petrosal sinus above
   D. The jugular bulb below
   E. The foramen magnum medially

23. One of the earliest procedures performed for Parkinson's disease was ligation of what blood vessel?

   A. Anterior choroidal artery
   B. Medial posterior choroidal artery
   C. Recurrent artery of Heubner
   D. Tentorial artery of Bernasconi and Cassarini
   E. Medial lenticulostriate artery

24. Vagal nerve stimulation is reserved for select patients with epilepsy. Why is it performed on the left side?

   A. To avoid injuring the recurrent laryngeal nerve, which follows a more torturous route on the right
   B. To avoid damage to the dominant superior laryngeal nerve on the right
   C. To avoid damage to cranial nerve X, which supplies the heart mainly from the right
   D. To avoid injuring the thoracic duct
   E. Less chance of vocal cord paralysis and hoarseness from the left

25. What is the treatment of choice for chronic, intractable brachial plexus avulsion injury?

   A. Cordotomy
   B. Dorsal root entry zone (DREZ) lesioning
   C. Morphine pump placement
   D. Midline myelotomy
   E. Ventroposterior lateral (VPL) thalamic deep brain stimulation

26. What basal cistern(s) contain portions of the vein of Rosenthal?

   1. Crural   **A.** 1, 2, and 3 are correct
   2. Quadrigeminal   **B.** 1 and 3 are correct
   3. Ambient   **C.** 2 and 4 are correct
   4. Quadrigeminal   **D.** Only 4 is correct
                           E. All of the above

27. A 3-month-old boy is brought to your office for an abnormally shaped head. The child is noted to have a flat occiput on the left, a left ear that is anterior to the right, and a prominent forehead and malar eminence on the left. What is the most likely etiology of this deformity?

   A. Left lambdoid synostosis
   B. Right lambdoid synostosis
   C. Sagittal suture synostosis
   D. Skull molding
   E. Right coronal suture synostosis

28. All of the following are suboptimal conditions for placement of an odontoid screw EXCEPT?

   A. Old fractures (> 6 weeks)
   B. Diagonal fractures through the odontoid process
   C. Barrel-chested patient
   D. Odontoid fracture that is displaced anteriorly
   E. An intact transverse ligament

29. A 56-year-old female underwent clipping of the aneurysm depicted on the angiogram below (Figure 6.29Q). Upon awakening from surgery, she was noted to have greater weakness in her left arm than in her left leg. What is the most likely reason for this new deficit?

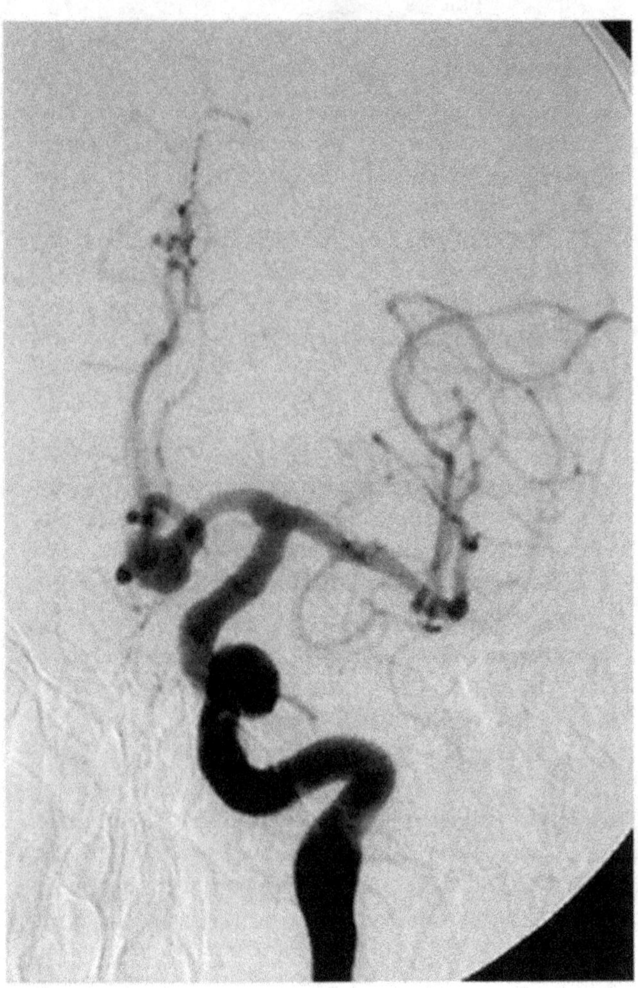

FIGURE 6.29Q

   A. Injury of a blood vessel originating from the A2 segment of the anterior cerebral artery
   B. Venous infarct from excessive frontal lobe retraction
   C. Injury to the small perforating blood vessels originating from the anterior communicating artery
   D. Posterior internal capsule infarction from microemboli originating from the internal carotid artery
   E. Mesial temporal lobe retraction

30. Basilar skull fractures can be associated with cranial nerve palsies, bilateral periorbital ecchymosis, mastoid ecchymosis, hemotympanum, and rhinorrhea. Nasal drainage that is not clearly CSF can be assayed for __________, which is unique to CSF and __________.

   A. α-Fetoprotein, saliva
   B. β_2-Transferrin, vitreous fluid of the eye
   C. β_2-Transferrin, tears
   D. Hypoglycorrhachia, nasal secretions
   E. Sodium, peritoneal fluid

31. A 4-month-old male fell from his crib and suffered a growing skull fracture. All of the following are true of this disease entity EXCEPT?

- **A.** May be associated with late neurologic deficits
- **B.** A dural laceration is always present
- **C.** There may be ongoing damage to underlying brain from continued herniation of brain through the defect
- **D.** CSF diversion is often the only treatment required for this fracture pattern
- **E.** May be associated with leptomeningeal cyst development

32. A 54-year-old female completed radiation therapy for breast cancer. She has been complaining of weakness in her left arm over the past 3 months and is concerned there may be recurrence of her cancer. How can her physician distinguish between radiation-induced plexopathy and cancerous invasion of the brachial plexus?

- **A.** Radiation-induced plexopathy is frequently accompanied by pain and lack of edema
- **B.** Cancerous invasion of the brachial plexus is accompanied by lymphedema, painless weakness, and sensory loss
- **C.** Radiation-induced plexopathy is frequently reversible
- **D.** Myokymia on EMG favors radiation-induced plexopathy
- **E.** Prolonged H latency is typically seen only with brachial plexopathy secondary to radiation damage

QUESTIONS 33–36

Scenario: A 42-year-old male falls 25 feet while at work and arrives at the emergency department with a Glasgow Coma Scale (GCS) score of 5, a dilated and nonreactive right pupil, and a mean arterial blood pressure of 80. After airway management and fluid resuscitation, his GCS improves to 7, but his right hemiparesis and nonreactive pupil remain unchanged. The patient also sustained a pelvic fracture, a left humeral fracture, splenic and liver lacerations, and multiple fractures of the cervical spine.

33. Initial management of this patient should include

1. Begin hyperventilation to decrease the pCO_2
2. Administer mannitol on arrival to the emergency department because of clinical evidence of an asymmetric exam
3. Complete the primary survey, obtain cervical spine films and chest x-ray, and then move directly to CT scan
4. The patient should be started on pentobarbital for elevated intracranial pressure immediately after completion of the primary survey if no mass lesion is found on CT

- **A.** 1, 2, and 3 are correct
- **B.** 1 and 3 are correct
- **C.** 2 and 4 are correct
- **D.** Only 4 is correct
- **E.** All of the above

34. The CT scan of the brain is depicted below (Figure 6.34Q). Why did this patient develop hemiparesis on the same side as the hematoma?

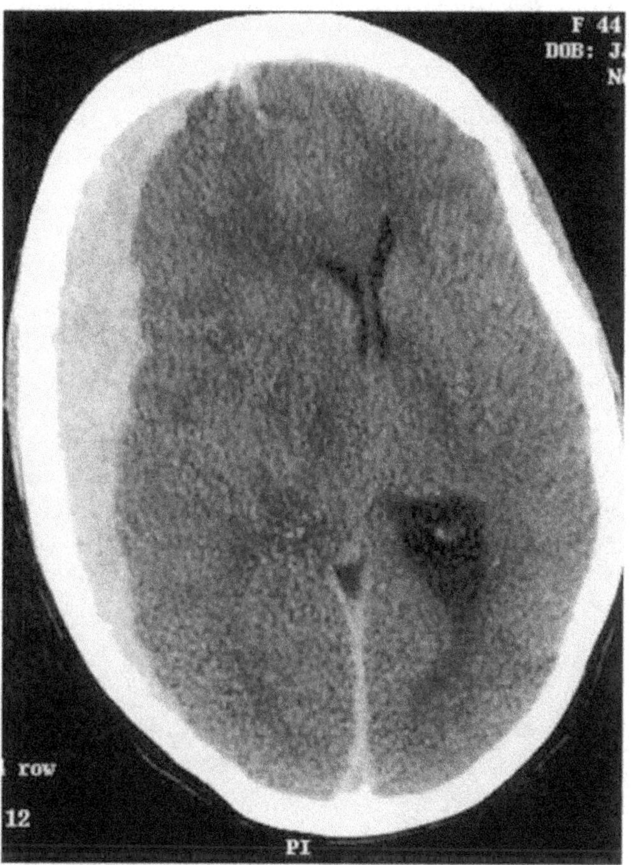

FIGURE 6.34Q

- **A.** Shift of the brainstem away from the mass producing compression of the contralateral cerebral peduncle against the tentorium
- **B.** The patient likely suffered a Duret hemorrhage
- **C.** There was likely a contusion in the underlying motor cortex on the contralateral side that was not detected on the initial CT scan
- **D.** The patient likely had a left internal carotid artery dissection that subsequently showered emboli to the distal vasculature
- **E.** There was an associated fracture of the transverse foramen on the left, which produced a vertebral artery dissection and small infarct in the ventral pons

35. Which of the following are possible complications of mannitol administration?

1. Aggravation of vasogenic edema
2. Development of a hyperosmolar nonketotic state
3. Acute tubular necrosis
4. Hypotension

   A. 1, 2, and 3 are correct
   B. 1 and 3 are correct
   C. 2 and 4 are correct
   D. Only 4 is correct
   E. All of the above

36. After surgery for evacuation of the right subdural hematoma, CT angiogram was obtained to rule out a vertebral artery injury because of the multiple fractures of the cervical spine extending through the transverse foramina. The study was inconclusive, and a follow-up angiogram (Figure 6.36Q) was obtained later that evening after hematoma evacuation. What would be the most reasonable treatment strategy at this point for this multisystem trauma patient? Consider that the patient adequately fills the posterior circulation from the right vertebral artery.

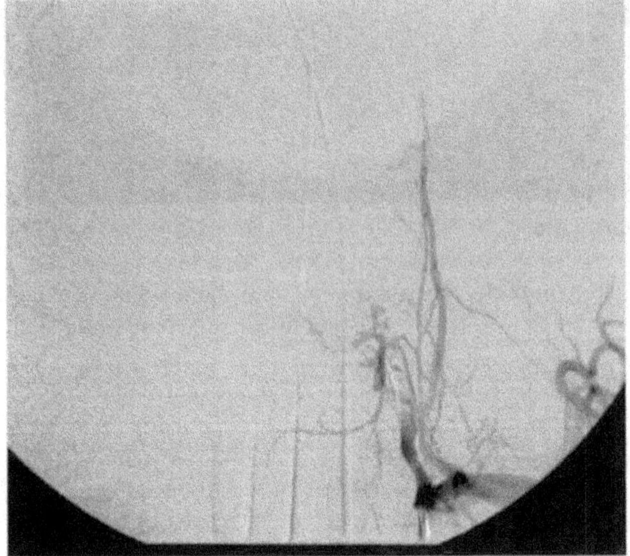

FIGURE 6.36Q

1. Commencement of a heparin infusion with a goal of keeping the PTT approximately two times the normal level
2. Antiplatelet therapy
3. Intravenous t-PA
4. Endovascular sacrifice of the occluded vertebral artery

   A. 1, 2, and 3 are correct
   B. 1 and 3 are correct
   C. 2 and 4 are correct
   D. Only 4 is correct
   E. All of the above

End of set

QUESTIONS 37–39

Scenario: A 45-year-old male presents to an emergency room with fever, nausea, vomiting, and severe headache. CT of the brain is normal. Lumbar puncture reveals slightly elevated red blood cells, but normal protein, glucose, white blood cell count, and no xanthochromia. His angiogram is depicted below.

37. What is the most likely etiology of the abnormality depicted in the angiogram below (Figure 6.37–6.39Q)?

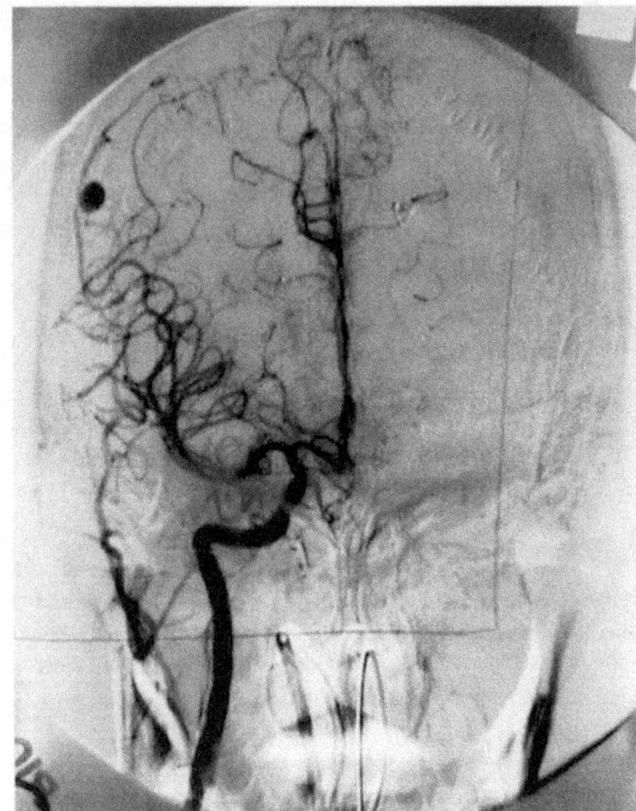

FIGURE 6.37–39Q

   A. Head trauma
   B. Infection
   C. Genetic predisposition
   D. Collagen vascular disease
   E. Hypertension

38. This finding occurs most frequently in what condition?

   A. Alcoholism
   B. Ehlers-Danlos disease
   C. Subacute bacterial endocarditis
   D. Marfan's syndrome
   E. Polycystic kidney disease

39. How should this problem be treated?

A. Observation followed by repeat angiography in 6 months
B. Antibiotics followed by repeat angiography
C. Emergent surgery
D. Stent/coiling followed by blood pressure control
E. Steroids

End of set

QUESTIONS 40–43

Scenario: A 15-month-old girl was brought to the emergency department for lethargy, nausea, and vomiting and was found to have aqueductal stenosis on brain MRI.

40. What is the best treatment strategy for this patient?

A. Observation
B. Placement of a subgaleal shunt
C. Placement of a ventriculoperitoneal shunt followed by endoscopic third ventriculostomy if shunting fails
D. Endoscopic third ventriculostomy
E. Endoscopic third ventriculostomy followed by septostomy

41. All of the following are advantages of endoscopic third ventriculostomy (ETV) over shunting EXCEPT?

A. Lower rate of subdural hematoma formation with ETV
B. Higher rate of craniosynostosis with ETV
C. Lower infection rate with ETV
D. Physiologic CSF diversion with ETV
E. Higher chance of overdrainage with shunt placement

42. All of the following are true about preoperative planning for ETV EXCEPT?

A. It is relatively straightforward to accurately determine the future function of the subarachnoid pathways and patency of the ETV as long as a high resolution MR cisternogram is obtained preoperatively that identifies the level of the block
B. MRI can accurately delineate the anatomy of the foramen of Monro, third ventricle, and massa intermedia
C. The position of the basilar artery and the thickness of the third ventricular floor can be verified on most preoperative MRIs
D. A prior history of CSF infection may decrease the success rate of ETV
E. A prior history of a shunt is not an absolute contraindication for ETV

43. What is the optimal site for fenestrating the floor of the third ventricle during ETV?

A. Posterior to the mammillary bodies
B. Anterior to the infundibular recess, posterior to the prechiasmatic space
C. In the most translucent area of the floor of the third ventricle
D. Anterior to the mammillary bodies, posterior to the infundibular recess
E. Anterior to the pulsations of the basilar artery

End of set

QUESTIONS 44–47

44. The borders of the lateral recess include all of the following EXCEPT?

A. Pedicle
B. Superior articular facet
C. Inferior articular facet
D. Vertebral body
E. Spinal canal/thecal sac

45. The underlying cause of lateral recess stenosis is osteophyte formation originating from what structure?

A. Inferior articular process
B. Pedicle
C. Superior articular process
D. Ligamentum flavum hypertrophy
E. Vertebral body

46. Although quite similar to the symptoms of radiculopathy secondary to discogenic disease, lateral recess stenosis can be differentiated from discogenic disease by which of the following?

A. Pain in the lateral recess syndrome is exacerbated by walking or standing
B. Failure of coughing or sneezing to aggravate pain in discogenic disease
C. Positive straight leg raising in lateral recess syndrome
D. Pain in lateral recess syndrome is relieved by postures accentuating lumbar lordosis
E. There is a slightly higher incidence of bladder incontinence with lateral recess stenosis

47. What is the best surgical strategy for patients with lateral recess stenosis?

A. Laminectomy
B. Laminectomy with resection of the medial third of the hypertrophied facet (medial facetectomy)
C. Microdiscectomy
D. Laminectomy and fusion
E. None of the above

End of set

QUESTIONS 48–54

Directions: Match each of the following procedures with the potential complication using each answer once, more than once, or not at all.

- **A.** Cordotomy
- **B.** Periaqueductal gray stimulation
- **C.** Percutaneous trigeminal electrocautery
- **D.** Sympathectomy
- **E.** Bilateral thalamotomy
- **F.** Pallidotomy
- **G.** Commisural myelotomy

48. Dysarthria and cognitive decline

49. Hemiparesis, homonymous hemianopia

50. "Ondine's curse"

51. Eye movement disorder, pupillary dilation, feeling of fear

52. Horner's syndrome

53. Anesthesia dolorosa

54. Leg weakness, dysesthesias, bladder dysfunction

End of set

55. All of the following are established procedures for the treatment of trigeminal neuralgia EXCEPT?

- **A.** Glycerol rhizolysis
- **B.** Balloon decompression
- **C.** Radiofrequency thermocoagulation
- **D.** Microvascular decompression
- **E.** Peripheral alcohol injection

QUESTIONS 56–58

Scenario: A 58-year-old male with rheumatoid arthritis presents to the emergency department with intolerable neck pain and cervical myelopathy. On MRI, he is found to have superior migration of the odontoid (SMO) process through the foramen magnum (cranial settling) and compression of the brainstem by the odontoid process itself.

56. All of the following information is important to gather preoperatively in patients with craniocervical junction (CCJ) abnormalities EXCEPT?

- **A.** The evaluation of craniocervical stability
- **B.** EMG and nerve conduction studies (NCS) to identify the extent of peripheral nerve damage
- **C.** Whether there is an associated syrinx
- **D.** The extent of ventral compression
- **E.** Presence of abnormal ossification centers and epiphyseal growth plates in children, as this may alter treatment strategies

57. Dynamic imaging studies of the craniocervical junction reveal instability. The neurosurgeon elects to employ gentle cervical traction for 3 days with good success in reducing the abnormality. After 3 days of traction, the patient's neck pain significantly improves, and MRI reveals minimal brainstem compression in the reduced position. What should be the next course of management?

  A. Posterior cervical laminectomy
  B. Posterior cervical laminectomy, suboccipital craniectomy, and fusion
  C. Cervical traction for another week to attempt to further reduce the abnormality before embarking on any surgical procedure
  D. Immobilization alone with posterior cervical fusion without a decompression
  E. Transoral odontectomy followed by posterior cervical decompression, suboccipital craniectomy, and fusion

58. One year later the patient experiences progressive weakness in his legs, ataxia, and bladder incontinence. His strength in the upper extremities is preserved, and he has no evidence of cranial nerve abnormalities. Plain films and CT scan of the craniocervical junction are unremarkable. What should be the next diagnostic test employed?

  A. CT of the brain to look for hydrocephalus
  B. EMG and NCS to identify the extent of peripheral nerve damage
  C. Screening MRI of the spine
  D. Bladder urodynamic testing
  E. Dynamic films of the cervical spine to evaluate for pseudoarthrosis and instability

End of set

QUESTIONS 59–61

59. A surgeon utilizes an infratemporal fossa approach to remove a large infiltrating tumor of the cranial base. He comes across the shaded structure depicted by the arrow below (Figure 6.59–6.61Q). How many muscles attach to this structure?

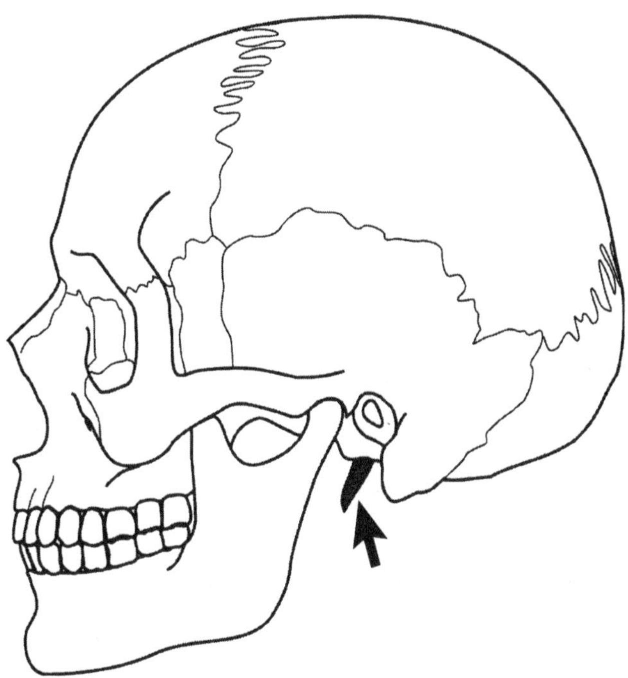

FIGURE 6.59–61Q

  A. 2
  B. 3
  C. 4
  D. 5
  E. 6

60. Which cranial nerves innervate these muscles?
  A. VII, IX
  B. VII, IX, XII
  C. IX, X, XII
  D. V, VII, IX
  E. X, XII

61. How many ligaments attach to this structure?

- **A.** 1
- **B.** 2
- **C.** 3
- **D.** 4
- **E.** 5

End of set

QUESTIONS 62–69

Directions: Match each of the following questions with the most likely fracture pattern (letterhead) depicted in Figure 6.62–6.69Q, using each answer once, more than once, or not at all.

62. Most likely to cause weakness of the extensor muscles of the wrist and hand; extension of forearm typically not affected; sensation of dorsal hand affected

63. May result in teres minor weakness

64. Weakness of flexion and adduction of wrist, paralysis of hypothenar muscles and most deep muscles of the hand, some weakness in thenar muscles

65. Shoulder abduction weakness

66. High likelihood of ulnar nerve injury only

67. Median nerve damage, paralysis of hypothenar muscles, some thenar muscles, and most of the deep muscles of the hand; flexion and adduction of wrist spared

68. Can be associated with brachial plexus injuries

69. Most likely to cause combined radial, medial, and ulnar nerve injuries

End of set

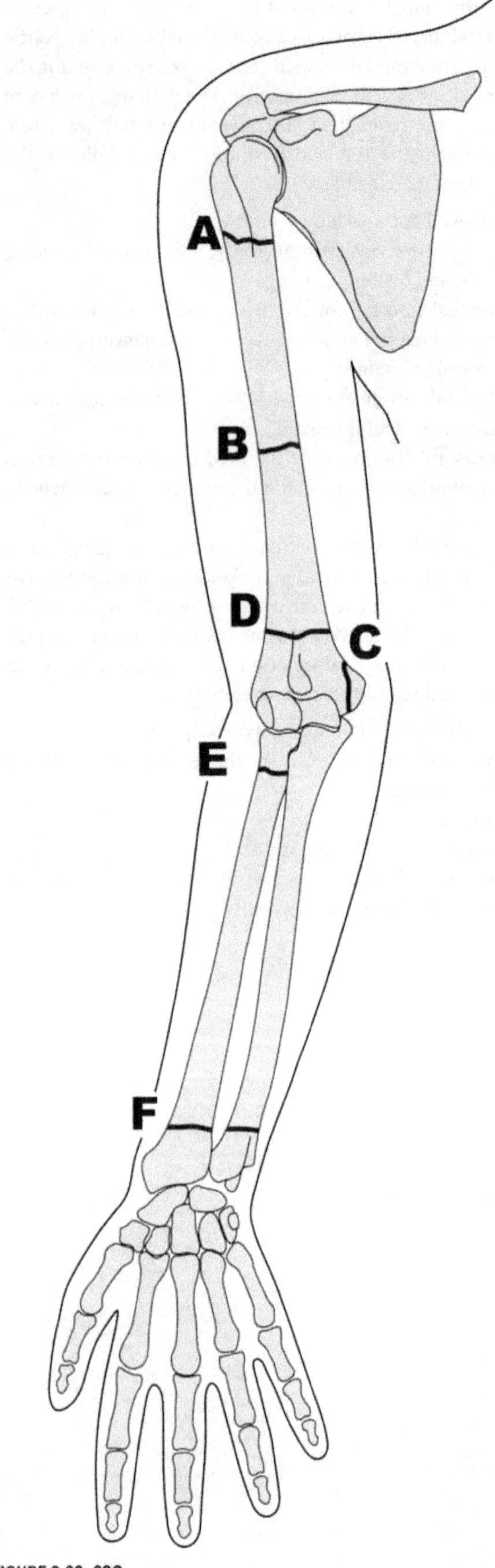

FIGURE 6.62–69Q

70. A 9-year-old girl presented to her pediatrician with headaches and a bitemporal field cut. Her MRI is depicted below (Figure 6.70Q). Which of the following would be true regarding the endocrine outcome after surgical resection of this tumor?

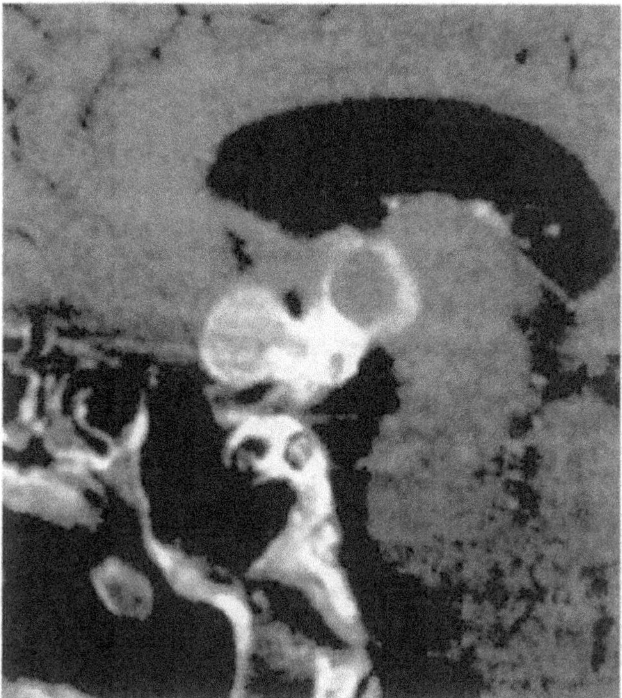

FIGURE 6.70Q

- **A.** There is a 30% chance that she will develop diabetes insipidus
- **B.** The most serious and disabling problem is the development of obesity, which occurs in about 50% of these patients after surgery
- **C.** Approximately 90% of patients will not require maintenance corticosteroid and thyroid replacement therapy
- **D.** Approximately 10% of patients will require growth hormone replacement therapy
- **E.** The endocrine outcome after surgery is very unpredictable

71. A 42-year-old female was recently diagnosed with spontaneous intracranial hypotension. All of the following are frequently associated with this problem EXCEPT?

- **A.** The headaches often resemble a post–lumbar puncture headache
- **B.** MRI scans with contrast may reveal enhancement of the dura over the cerebral and cerebellar convexities
- **C.** Spontaneous improvement is rarely seen, since CSF leaks are often identified adjacent to nerve roots
- **D.** Spinal fluid may reveal elevated protein and pleocytosis
- **E.** Analgesics containing caffeine may be helpful

72. All of the following lesions are appropriate for stereotactic radiosurgery EXCEPT?

- **A.** A 3-cm³ arteriovenous malformation in the brainstem
- **B.** A 1-cm right frontal and 2-cm left parietal metastatic carcinoma from the lung
- **C.** Recurrent glioblastoma of the left temporal lobe (2 cm³)
- **D.** A 1-cm cavernoma of the right caudate nucleus that previously hemorrhaged
- **E.** Bilateral thalamic arteriovenous malformations (3 cm³)

73. All of the following would reduce pain conduction or a patient's reaction to pain EXCEPT?

- **A.** Stimulation of the periaqueductal gray
- **B.** Prefrontal lobotomy
- **C.** Cingulotomy
- **D.** Hippocampectomy
- **E.** Ventrolateral cordotomy

74. A 34-year-old female is involved in a motor vehicle collision, suffers a severe closed head injury (Figure 6.74Q), and develops a significant posttraumatic tremor in the right arm. Although posttraumatic tremors are generally difficult to manage, which surgical procedure may help control tremors, which are otherwise refractory to medical therapy?

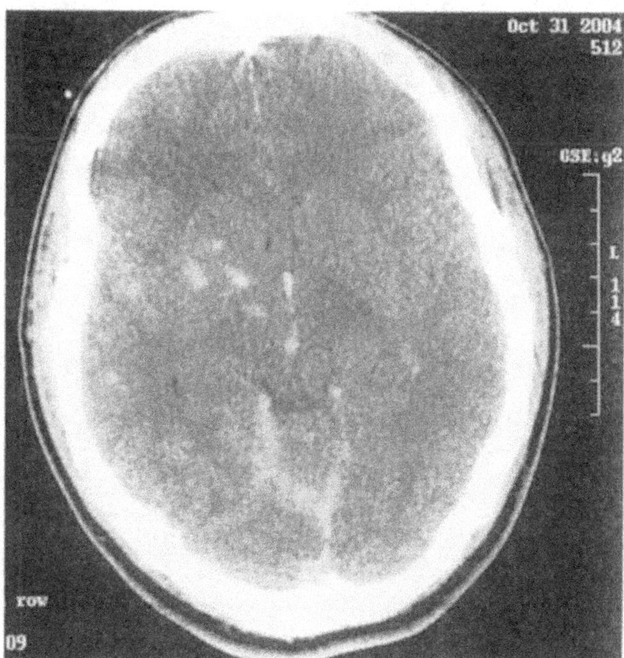

FIGURE 6.74Q

- **A.** Thalamic stimulation
- **B.** Subthalamic nucleus stimulation
- **C.** Motor cortex stimulation
- **D.** Capsulotomy
- **E.** Multiple subpial transections

75. A 36-year-old female has a complex aneurysm that requires the use of cardiac arrest and profound hypothermia during surgery. All of the following are potential physiologic effects of profound hypothermia EXCEPT?

A. Increased blood viscosity
B. Hyperglycemia
C. Decreased corticosteroid release
D. Complement-mediated pneumonitis
E. Hypercoagulable state

76. What is the most common physical manifestation of the abnormality depicted by the angiogram below (Figure 6.76Q)?

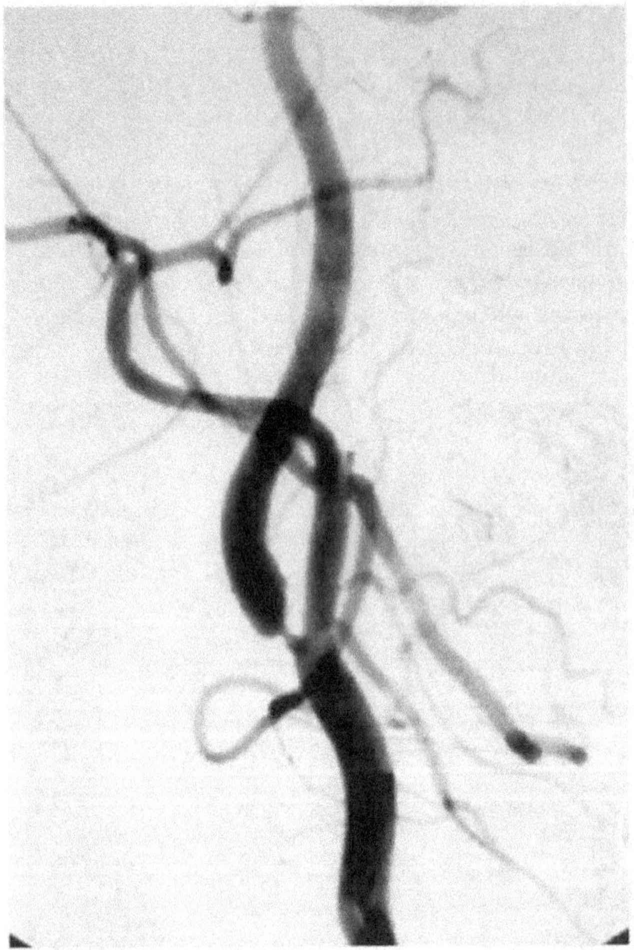

FIGURE 6.76Q

A. Neck pain
B. Cervical bruit
C. Contralateral arm weakness or numbness
D. Dysesthesia
E. Transient vision loss

QUESTIONS 77–79

77. Refer to Figure 6.77–6.79Q. What is the most likely diagnosis?

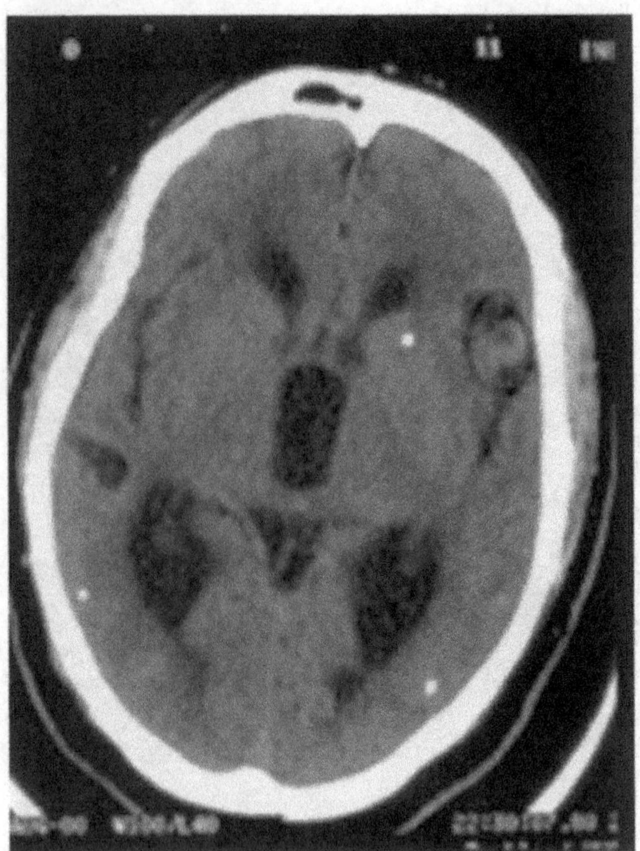

FIGURE 6.77–79Q

A. *Echinococcus* infection
B. Neurocysticercosis
C. *Cryptococcus* infection
D. Cytomegalovirus infection
E. Trichinosis

78. This patient is most likely to present with?

A. Headaches
B. Obtundation
C. Cranial nerve palsies
D. Fevers
E. Seizure

79. This disorder is caused by

A. *Borrelia burgdorferi*
B. *Echinococcus granulosa*
C. *Toxoplasma gondii*
D. *Treponema pallidum*
E. *Taenia solium*

End of set

80. What is the most likely diagnosis depicted by the angiogram below (Figure 6.80Q)?

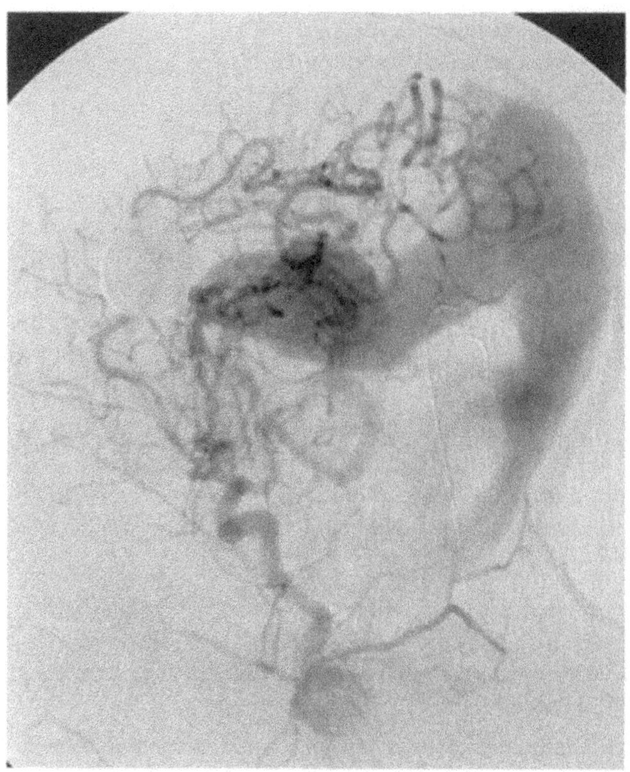

FIGURE 6.80Q

- **A.** Blue rubber bleb nevus syndrome
- **B.** Vein of Galen aneurysm
- **C.** Carotid-cavernous fistula
- **D.** Intracranial hemangioblastoma of infancy
- **E.** Sinus pericranii

81. The posterior interosseous nerve supplies all of the following muscles EXCEPT?

- **A.** Supinator
- **B.** Extensor carpi ulnaris
- **C.** Abductor pollicis longus
- **D.** Extensor digitorum
- **E.** Pronator quadratus

82. The ability to create irregularly shaped radiosurgical volumes is important to achieve conformal irradiation of target tissue. Which of the following techniques can be employed to create such plans?

- **A.** Combine multiple isocenters of irradiation in different planes
- **B.** Individual isocenters can be weighted variably to change their relative shape
- **C.** Individual radiation beams can be blocked to restrict dose away from critical structures, such as the optic chiasm
- **D.** A and B only
- **E.** All of the above

QUESTIONS 83–84

83. A 45-year-old female undergoes a C5-6 and C6-7 anterior cervical discectomy and fusion. Postoperatively, she awakens with a Horner's syndrome. The most likely etiology of this finding was related to damage of what structure(s)?

- **A.** Sympathetic nerves running along the carotid artery during neck dissection
- **B.** Injury of the T1 nerve root during the discectomy
- **C.** Interruption of the sympathetic chain located on the anterior surface of the longus colli muscles
- **D.** Spinal cord injury during surgery
- **E.** A small hypothalamic infarct during surgery

84. A left-sided approach decreases the risk of recurrent laryngeal nerve palsy during anterior cervical procedures, but at lower levels in the neck a left-sided approach runs the risk of injuring what structure?

- **A.** Inferior laryngeal nerve
- **B.** Thyrocervical artery
- **C.** Thoracic duct
- **D.** C5 nerve root
- **E.** Dominant cardiac accelerator nerves

End of set

85. Degenerative spondylolisthesis is most common at what level in the lumbar spine?

- **A.** L1-2
- **B.** L2-3
- **C.** L3-4
- **D.** L4-5
- **E.** L5-S1

86. A 72-year-old female with rheumatoid arthritis is found to have a reducible atlantoaxial dislocation after 36 hours of cervical traction. There is minimal ventral compression from pannus formation, no cranial settling, and no foramen magnum stenosis noted on MR scan. What is the best treatment strategy for this patient?

- **A.** Transarticular screw fixation and fusion if the lateral atlantal masses are intact with good-quality bone
- **B.** Transoral odontectomy followed by posterior occipital-cervical decompression and fusion
- **C.** Laminectomy
- **D.** Transoral odontectomy followed by observation
- **E.** Halo placement

87. The ideal bone graft provides all of the following elements for successful healing EXCEPT?

- **A.** Osteoconductive matrix
- **B.** Osteoinductive factors
- **C.** To support viable osteogenic cells
- **D.** Structural support
- **E.** Osteoblasts for bone healing

88. Interfering with uptake of which ion into cells during severe closed head injury has resulted in a significant clinical benefit?

    A. Ca^{2+}
    B. Na^+
    C. Cl^-
    D. K^+
    E. None of the above

89. Surgical therapies used for dystonia have traditionally included all of the following EXCEPT?

    A. Peripheral denervation
    B. Pallidotomy
    C. Thalamotomy
    D. Dorsal column stimulation
    E. Motor cortex stimulation

90. All of the following surgical procedures have been employed to treat neuropsychiatric illness and behavioral disorders EXCEPT?

    A. Arcuate fasciculotomy
    B. Subcaudate tractotomy
    C. Limbic leukotomy
    D. Anterior capsulotomy
    E. Anterior cingulotomy

91. The superior semicircular canal projects into the floor of the middle cranial fossa as what structure often seen during a subtemporal approach for acoustic neuroma resection?

    A. Arcuate eminence
    B. Tegmen tympani
    C. Vestibule
    D. Vertical crest
    E. Vestibular prominence

QUESTIONS 92–94

Scenario: A 45-year old male undergoes a subtemporal approach for tumor resection with elevation of the dura from the middle fossa floor and petrous bone.

92. Structures visible on the floor of the middle cranial fossa during this exposure may include all of the following EXCEPT?

    A. Middle meningeal artery
    B. Trigeminal nerve (V3)
    C. Lesser superficial petrosal nerve
    D. Hypoglossal nerve
    E. Greater superficial petrosal nerve

93. Postoperatively, the patient has decreased lacrimation on the ipsilateral side. What is the most likely etiology of this problem?

    A. Lesser petrosal nerve injury
    B. Greater petrosal nerve injury
    C. Geniculate ganglion injury
    D. Chorda tympani injury
    E. Injury of Jacobson's nerve

94. During surgery, additional exposure is needed to access the upper petroclival region for tumor resection. Which maneuver may assist the surgeon in accomplishing this task?

    A. Further drilling of Glasscock's triangle
    B. Additional exposure through Kawase's quadrilateral
    C. Further drilling of the arcuate eminence
    D. Identifying Trautmann's triangle and exposing medially to this landmark
    E. Modifying the approach by utilizing a presigmoid corridor

End of set

95. What is the most likely mechanism accounting for the Cushing response?

    A. Herniation of the cerebellar tonsils through the foramen magnum
    B. Brainstem distortion
    C. Large hemispheric insult
    D. Hypoxia of the brainstem
    E. Posterior fossa mass

QUESTIONS 96–97

96. What is the most common clinical manifestation of the abnormality depicted on the angiogram below (Figure 6.96–6.97Q)?

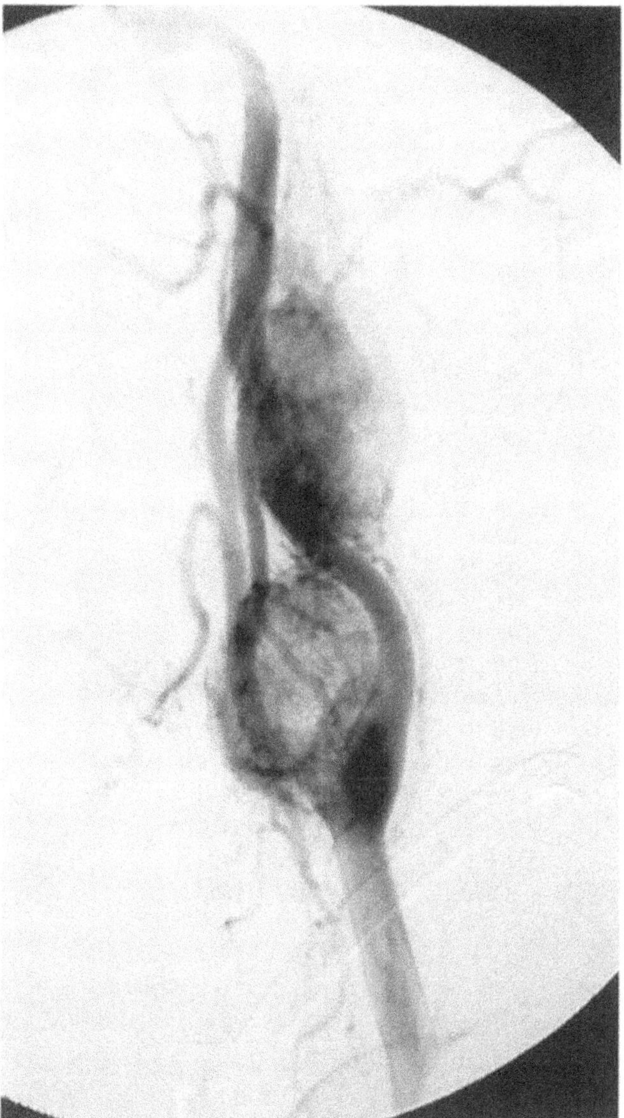

- **A.** Hoarseness
- **B.** Dysphagia
- **C.** Unilateral tongue atrophy
- **D.** Palpable neck mass
- **E.** Hypertension

97. Clinicians must be aware of what endocrine comorbidity in evaluating patients with this tumor?

- **A.** Diabetes insipidus
- **B.** Pheochromocytoma
- **C.** Hyperprolactinemia
- **D.** Phenylketonuria
- **E.** None of the above

End of set

98. A 45-year-old male has a long history of epilepsy from seizure foci originating in the right premotor cortex and extending into the adjacent motor cortex. His seizures have remained refractory to a variety of antiepileptic drugs, and he was referred to a neurosurgeon to discuss surgical options. EEG recordings reveal a seizure focus in the left premotor region that extends to the adjacent motor cortex. Which of the following surgical procedures may be performed concomitantly during lesionectomy to avoid major injury to the motor cortex and help control his seizures?

- **A.** Topectomy
- **B.** Limited lesionectomy
- **C.** Motor cortex stimulation
- **D.** Multiple subpial transections
- **E.** Vagal nerve stimulation

99. What is the most common neurologically related complication after vagal nerve stimulator placement?

- **A.** Facial numbness
- **B.** Bradycardia
- **C.** Dysphonia
- **D.** Hypotension
- **E.** Short-lived arrhythmia

100. Which of the following statements concerning stabilization of the lumbar spine with segmental pedicle screw fixation is correct?

- **A.** The lateral stability is significantly enhanced if the pedicle screw angle is 30 degrees or greater
- **B.** The use of transfixation increases the rotational but not the lateral load stability of the construct
- **C.** Without a transfixator, the vertebral column is stable in lateral load
- **D.** None of the above
- **E.** All of the above

Neurosurgery Answer Key

1. B	21. D	41. B	61. B	81. E
2. B	22. E	42. A	62. B	82. E
3. D	23. A	43. D	63. A	83. C
4. A	24. C	44. C	64. C	84. C
5. D	25. B	45. C	65. A	85. D
6. C	26. B	46. A	66. C	86. A
7. B	27. D	47. B	67. F	87. E
8. D	28. E	48. E	68. A	88. E
9. C	29. A	49. F	69. D	89. E
10. A	30. B	50. A	70. B	90. A
11. E	31. D	51. B	71. C	91. A
12. E	32. D	52. D	72. D	92. D
13. B	33. B	53. C	73. D	93. B
14. C	34. A	54. G	74. A	94. B
15. C	35. E	55. B	75. E	95. D
16. E	36. C	56. B	76. B	96. D
17. B	37. B	57. D	77. B	97. B
18. C	38. C	58. C	78. E	98. D
19. C	39. B	59. B	79. E	99. C
20. B	40. D	60. B	80. B	100. A

Neurosurgery Answers

1-B; 2-B; 3-D; 4-A; 5-D. Refer to Table 6.1–6.5A. Patients with posterior communicating artery (PComA) aneurysms typically present with subarachnoid hemorrhage (SAH) and partial or complete third nerve palsies (ptosis, dilated pupil, extraocular muscle abnormalities) due to compression of the third nerve by the aneurysm. Another common presentation of PComA aneurysms is the development of a third nerve deficit in the absence of SAH. The appearance of an enlarged pupil with or without involvement of other third nerve functions should be taken as diagnostic of a PComA aneurysm until proven otherwise. After the aneurysm is clipped, it should be punctured not only to ensure complete obliteration but also to achieve maximal decompression of the third nerve. Most patients with third nerve palsies improve within 6 months and frequently sooner. Some PComA aneurysms will not produce any oculomotor nerve deficit. Special care must be taken in interpreting the angiograms of these patients, since the aneurysms often project laterally onto the medial edge of the temporal lobe rather than in more common posterolateral or downward directions. This is relevant during operative planning, since early retraction of the temporal lobe may result in premature aneurysmal rupture.

TABLE 6.1–5A
Hunt and Hess clinical grading scale after subarachnoid hemorrhage

GRADE	CLINICAL FINDINGS
Grade I	Awake, mild headache and/or nuchal rigidity
Grade II	Awake, moderate to severe headaches and nuchal rigidity
Grade III	Drowsy or confused, with or without focal deficits
Grade IV	Stuporous, mild to moderate hemiparesis and signs of increased intracranial pressure
Grade V	Comatose, severe disability, severe increased intracranial pressure

It is important during surgery to identify the distal PComA for temporary clip placement, if possible, because obtaining proximal and distal control of the internal carotid may not be enough to halt back bleeding from the PComA if intraoperative rupture occurs. Frequently this can significantly impair vision and make further microdissection and aneurysm clipping difficult. Moreover, if the PComA is not identified prior to clip placement, the surgeon runs the risk of incorporating this vessel into the clip construct, especially when vision is impaired by intraoperative rupture. If the territory supplied by the PComA is small, sacrificing it or incorporating this vessel into the clip construct may not result in any adverse sequelae; however, if the PComA is fetal or there is a hypoplastic P1, it may result in a significant PCA infarct. Along the same lines, it is also important to identify the anterior choroidal artery prior to aneurysm clipping to prevent incorporating this vessel into the clip construct as well, especially with PComA aneurysms arising further distally on the internal carotid artery. Patients with anterior choroidal artery infarcts sustained during surgery may wake up with contralateral hemiplegia, numbness, and homonymous hemianopia. Although the majority develop varying degrees of these deficits, patients with infarcts of the PCA or PComA perforators generally do not present with this constellation.

The frontotemporal branch of the facial nerve exits the parotid gland and divides into three rami: the anterior, middle, and occipital branch. The anterior ramus innervates the corrugator supercilii and orbicularis oculi muscles, the middle ramus innervates the frontalis muscle, and the occipital ramus has minimal significance in humans. The approximate point where the frontotemporal branch of the facial nerve gives off the anterior and middle rami is located about 1.1 cm below the zygomatic arch and about 2.4 cm anterior to the tragus. Therefore, as a general rule, keeping the incision approximately 1 cm anterior to the tragus and at the level of the zygoma should avoid damage to this nerve. The middle ramus courses in the subcutaneous tissues over the zygomatic arch approximately 1 cm anterior to the superficial temporal artery. Above the zygomatic arch, it travels in the subgaleal space in the same plane as the subgaleal fat pad, although occasionally it may enter the interfascial space between the superficial and deep layers of the superficial temporal fascia. Dissection between the superficial and deep temporalis fascia deep to the interfascial fat pad significantly reduces the chance of nerve injury (Kaye and Black, pp. 126, 967–972, 969–970; Youmans, pp. 1916–1918; Wilkins, pp. 2204–2205, 2306–2307; Samson, pp. 58–67).

6-C; 7-B; 8-D; 9-C. Carotid-cavernous fistulas (CCFs) can be divided into posttraumatic and spontaneous types. They are direct shunts between the ICA or ECA and cavernous sinus and usually occur after trauma or spontaneous aneurysmal rupture. Traumatic CCFs often present in a delayed fashion; like spontaneous fistulas, they often present with retro-orbital pain, chemosis, pulsatile proptosis, ocular or cranial bruit, decreased visual acuity, diplopia, and rarely epistaxis and subarachnoid hemorrhage. The symptoms depend on the direction of venous flow and quantity of blood flow through the fistula. There are four types of CCFs: type A is a direct, high-flow shunt between the ICA and cavernous sinus (as in this case), and types B to D are low-flow shunts between the cavernous sinus and meningeal branches of the internal carotid artery, external carotid artery, or both, respectively. Approximately 50% of low-flow fistulas spontaneously thrombose without treatment. The main treatment option has traditionally included transarterial balloon embolization through the ICA for type A fistulas, although accessing the fistula transvenously (i.e., inferior petrosal sinus) is also commonly performed, especially for indirect types B to D. A direct surgical approach is indicated if transarterial or transvenous approaches fail. Radiosurgery has been proposed as an option for some of the low-flow fistulas, although it would not be the best strategy for the high-flow symptomatic fistula seen in this patient. Figure A depicts nearly complete capture of the blood from the internal carotid artery, and fistulous drainage primarily from the superior ophthalmic and superior petrosal veins. Figure B depicts a later venous run with superior petrosal vein drainage into the transverse-sigmoid sinus junction as well as some venous drainage into the superior sagittal sinus (Kaye and Black, pp. 1132; Greenberg, pp. 811–812; Youmans, pp. 2341–2352; Wilkins, pp. 2529–2535).

10. A. The natural history of DAVF is variable and includes spontaneous resolution, recruitment of meningeal arterial feeders, and the development of intracranial hypertension. DAVF can present with pulsatile tinnitus, visual symptoms, papilledema, hydrocephalus, and intracranial hemorrhage. The presence of retrograde cortical venous drainage indicates the potential for intracranial hemorrhage and mandates urgent treatment of the DAVF. Intracranial hemorrhage from a DAVF in the absence of retrograde cortical venous drainage has not been reported. Hemorrhage from a DAVF is associated with a high morbidity and mortality (approximately 30%). Ectatic dilation or venous occlusion of the involved sinus, multiple or dual ICA/ECA arterial feeders, or embolic stroke, in the absence of retrograde cortical venous drainage has not been reported to increase hemorrhage rates of DAVFs (Kaye and Black, pp. 1125–1135; Greenberg, p. 811; Youmans, pp. 2171–2173; Wilkins, pp. 2523–2527).

11-E; 12-E; 13-B; 14-C; 15-C; 16-E. Attempts to gain additional exposure for a high-riding carotid artery bifurcation include mobilization of the ansa cervicalis, sectioning the posterior belly of the digastric muscle, cautery and ligation of the occipital artery, and mandibular osteotomy or disarticulation of the jaw at the temporomandibular joint. This type of exposure places the hypoglossal nerve at particular risk, although segments of cranial nerves VII, IX, X, and XI can

also be injured during carotid endarterectomy (CEA). Patients who become hypotensive and bradycardic during surgery often do so as a result of manipulation of the nerve of Hering near the carotid bulb. This is not uncommon with CEA and can often be addressed with lidocaine infusion adjacent to the carotid bulb. Placing the clamps on the internal carotid artery first, followed by the common and then the external carotid artery often ensures that the clot will pass through the external carotid artery instead of the internal carotid artery. The order for clamp removal should be just the opposite, as this should again ensure that any accumulated blood clot will be more likely to pass through the external rather than internal carotid circulation. It is not uncommon during CEA to have some backbleeding into the surgical field by the ascending pharyngeal artery after clamp placement on the major vessels. If the extent of bleeding is severe and hinders the operation, identification, clamping (aneurysm clip), or ligation of this vessel may drastically improve visibility. A patient who awakens with a major neurologic deficit is likely to have suffered thrombosis at the arteriotomy site, which usually warrants immediate attention (surgical exploration) rather than time-consuming diagnostic studies, as some case reports describe a significant neurologic improvement if flow is re-established within 45 minutes. For later-onset deficits, workup (i.e., CT, angiogram) may be indicated. CT may help to identify hemorrhage and an angiogram may reveal whether the ICA is occluded or if the deficit is from another cause (emboli) that would not necessarily require surgical re-exploration (Kaye and Black, pp. 1179–1187; Greenberg, pp. 837–841; Youmans, pp. 1631–1645; Wilkins, pp. 2113–2114).

17-B; 18-C. Aseptic meningitis (AM) is a well-recognized complication after posterior fossa surgery but is typically self-limited and requires no treatment. It has generally been attributed to one or more irritants released into the subarachnoid space during surgery, including blood breakdown products, tumor, muscle, and brain. Lowering of intracranial pressure with lumbar puncture and dexamethasone is the mainstay of treatment in certain patients with continued, problems. Bacterial meningitis and postmeningitic syndrome are unlikely, considering that an organism was not isolated from the CSF, although this is not always the case. Moreover, the CSF profile was more consistent with aseptic meningitis than bacterial meningitis. Hydrocephalus is unlikely, since fever, meningismus, and photophobia rarely accompany this diagnosis, and encephalitis would be very uncommon in this situation (Carmel et al., pp. 276–280; Youmans, pp. 3645, 3659; Kaye and Black, p. 868; Wilkins, p. 3965).

19. C. Complications of microvascular decompression for hemifacial spasm include CSF leak, facial weakness, facial anesthesia, corneal anesthesia, intracranial hemorrhage, and infarction. Complete ipsilateral deafness is associated with disruption or coagulation of the labyrinthine artery, which is most commonly a branch of either the AICA (45%), SCA (25%), or basilar artery (16%) (Kaye and Black, pp. 1652–1653; Osborne DN, p. 186; Greenberg, pp. 358–360; Youmans, pp. 3013–3014; Wilkins, pp. 3227–3233).

20. B. The maximal safe dose of single-shot radiosurgery that the optic chiasm can tolerate is approximately 9 to 10 Gy (Alexander, p. 171).

21. D. Cauterizing and dividing the precentral cerebellar vein will often expose the posterior surface of pineal region tumors. The veins of Galen and Rosenthal should be preserved during this operation, as well as the vermian vein, which often can be spared in this approach. The choroidal arteries may supply feeders to the tumor but rarely need to be cauterized and ligated for adequate tumor resection (Kaye and Black, pp. 815–824; Youmans; pp. 1017–1021, Wilkins, p. 1029).

22. E. There are two goals of the translabyrinthine approach for acoustic neuroma resection that may help achieve maximal tumor resection. The first is to remove enough bone to identify the nerves lateral to the tumor as they course through the IAC, and the second is to expose the dura of the posterior aspect of the temporal bone that faces the cerebellopontine angle (CPA). This triangular patch of dura facing the CPA is called Trautmann's triangle and extends from the sigmoid sinus laterally, the superior petrosal sinus above, and the jugular bulb below. The foramen magnum is not included in Trautmann's triangle (Kaye and Black, pp. 851–860; Youmans, pp. 1155–1156; Wilkins, pp. 1067–1071).

23. A. Neurosurgical therapies for Parkinson's disease (PD) have been utilized in patients with progressive disease despite maximal medical therapy. An early procedure performed for PD was ligation of the anterior choroidal artery, with subsequent infarction of the pallidum. Due to the variable distribution of this vessel outside the confines of the pallidum, results were too unpredictable and this procedure lost favor. In the 1950s, anterodorsal pallidotomy became an accepted procedure, but the long-term benefits were mostly for rigidity, while tremor and dyskinesia did not improve. Subsequently, the ventrolateral thalamus became the preferred target for lesioning, but this procedure also lost favor, as patients were often still left with bradykinesia and/or rigidity. Moreover, this procedure reduced tremor only in the contralateral half of the body, and bilateral thalamotomies were not recommended due to an unacceptably high risk of postoperative dysarthria and gait disturbances. Thalamotomy procedures fell off dramatically in the late 1960s with the introduction of L-DOPA.

More recently, dramatic and beneficial effects of both subthalamic nucleus (STN) and globus pallidus interna (Gpi) deep brain stimulation (DBS) have been consistently observed. Both interventions appear to result in significant improvements in both motor fluctuations and dyskinesias. The DBS study group, in a large multicenter study, reported that on time without dyskinesia during the waking hours increased from 25 to 30% at baseline to 65 to 75% 6 months postoperatively. In a complementary fashion, these procedures also markedly decreased off time and on time without dyskinesia. Although some preliminary studies suggest STN DBS may be a superior intervention, no large randomized controlled trial comparing STN and Gpi DBS has been conducted to compare the efficacy of these treatments. The most consistent finding has been the reduction in antiparkinson medication following STN DBS compared to Gpi DBS. (Greenberg, p. 751; Tarsy, p. 191).

24. C. Vagal nerve stimulation must be performed on the left side so that the cardiac innervation of CN X is unaffected (Youmans, pp. 2644–2645).

25. B. Dorsal root entry zone (DREZ) lesioning involves radiofrequency ablation along the dorsolateral sulcus of the spinal cord. The DREZ procedure is most effective in the treatment of brachial and lumbar plexus avulsion pain. Direct sectioning of the spinothalamic tract (cordotomy) is very effective for unilateral pain below the upper chest region; however, it is associated with many complications and is usually performed only in terminally ill patients. Complications of cordotomy include hemiparesis, respiratory depression ("Ondine's curse" with bilateral procedures), and dysesthesias. Midline myelotomies can also be performed to interrupt the decussating fibers of the spinothalamic tract, and this can be quite effective in the treatment of chronic pelvic pain secondary to cancer. Intrathecal narcotic administration is typically used for the treatment of chronic pain associated with malignancy or failed low back syndrome. Deep brain stimulation of the VPL and VPM nuclei of the thalamus as well as the periaqueductal gray have been performed in the treatment of thalamic pain states, postherpetic neuralgia, and causalgia. Chronic low-threshold stimulation of the motor cortex is also utilized in the treatment of thalamic pain syndromes; it is thought to work by retrograde thalamic stimulation pathways (Kaye and Black, pp. 1521–1537; Greenberg, pp. 365–370; Youmans, pp. 3025–3030, 3045–3048, 3068–3070, 3101, 3125, 3128–3129; Wilkins, pp. 4036–4038, 4055–4059).

26. B. The ambient and crural cisterns contain portions of the basal vein of Rosenthal (Youmans, pp. 36–39).

27. D. Lambdoid synostosis is among the rarest forms of suture synostosis, while sagittal synostosis is the most common. After the American Academy of Pediatrics published its recommendations that all children sleep on their back, the incidence of skull molding increased. Most infants sleep on their backs and spend the rest of the day sitting in a car seat or infant seat. Children with this condition are often noted to have a flat occiput, one ear that is anterior to the other in an axial plane, and a prominent forehead and malar eminence. Many infants may also have a mild torticollis due to a shortened sternocleidomastoid muscle on one side, as well as decreased range of motion in the neck. The skull deformity usually responds very well to behavioral modification, which includes having the parents turn the infant or child from side to side during sleep and reducing the amount of time spent in a car seat. If this is unsuccessful, a molding helmet or band is often helpful. For nonresponders, a variety of occipital remolding surgical procedures are available (Committee on Education in Neurological Surgery, pp. 43, 137; Pattisapu, pp. 178–179).

28. E. An intact transverse ligament must be confirmed preoperatively prior to placement of an odontoid screw. Old fractures in which a nonunion has already formed, diagonal fractures through the odontoid process, and comminuted odontoid fractures do not allow for proper odontoid screw placement due to suboptimal arthrodesis rates and inadequate screw purchase and compression effects (Kaye and Black, pp. 2048–2050; Youmans, pp. 4943–4945; Benzel, pp. 225–228).

29. A. The recurrent artery of Heubner usually originates from the A2 segment of the anterior cerebral artery (ACA). Injury of this vessel during surgery is generally witnessed on the first postoperative day, as evidenced by a hypodensity on CT scan. Although injury to this vessel during surgery often presents with arm weakness greater than leg weakness on the nondominant side and cognitive deficits from injury on the dominant side, a percentage of patients do not have any adverse neurologic sequelae after injury of this vessel. Identifying this vessel early in the dissection may prevent later injury (Greenberg, pp. 103–104).

30. B. β_2-transferrin is present in the CSF but absent in the tears, saliva, peritoneal fluid, nasal exudates, and serum (except for newborns or those with liver disease). The only other source is the vitreous humor of the eye. Other commonly employed tests include measuring the glucose level of the fluid (CSF glucose > 30 mg %, whereas lacrimal and mucous secretions are < 5 mg%) or placing the fluid on a piece of linen (bed sheet, pillowcase) and seeing whether a ring of blood surrounded by a larger concentric ring of clear fluid develops ("ring" or "halo" sign) (Greenberg, pp. 168–169).

31. D. Growing skull fractures occur in children, are always associated with underlying dural lacerations, and almost always require surgical treatment. Early surgical correction of growing fractures is often necessary because these types of fractures almost never heal spontaneously and late neuro-

logic deterioration can occur. The pathophysiology requires a fracture with enough force to cause a tear in the dura (which is always present) and an underlying constant force such as a growing brain, leptomeningeal cyst, hydrocephalus, or porencephaly. The precise etiology of late neurologic deficits remains unclear but is believed to occur by one of two mechanisms. There may be ongoing brain damage from brain herniation and pulsations of the brain against the bone edges. Alternatively, some have proposed that there may be vascular compromise of blood vessels at the bone edges. Although some authors have recommended a CSF diversion procedure for growing skull fractures, direct repair of the fracture is the definitive treatment (Youmans, pp. 3468–3469; Wilkins, pp. 2757–2761).

32. D. Myokymia (quivering of muscles) on EMG strongly favors radiation-induced changes of the brachial plexus. Lymphedema, painless paresis, and numbness suggest radiation-induced injury (irreversible), whereas pain and lack of edema suggest recurrent tumor. When ancillary studies are inconclusive, surgical exploration of the plexus may have to be considered (Merritt, p. 459)

33-B; 34-A; 35-E; 36-C. Current head injury research guidelines suggest that mannitol and hyperventilation may exacerbate cerebral ischemia after head injury. However, mannitol and hyperventilation are recommended for those patients with acute head injury as a temporary measure to control elevated intracranial pressure. Hyperventilation may be commenced immediately, but mannitol should be withheld until the primary survey is complete and adequate intravascular volume and urine output are realized. The mechanism of action of mannitol is still debated, but it is believed to have the following beneficial effects. First, it acts to immediately expand the plasma by reducing hematocrit and blood viscosity (improved rheology), which improves CBF and O_2 delivery. This reduces ICP very quickly, which is most marked in patients with CPP < 70 mm Hg. Second, it draws edema from the adjacent cerebral parenchyma into the intravascular compartment (osmotic effect), an effect that may last up to 6 hours. And last, it is a possible free-radical scavenger. Despite these short-lived but beneficial effects, the administration of mannitol is not without risks. It opens the blood-brain barrier and can potentially draw fluid into the CNS and aggravate vasogenic cerebral edema. It should also be used cautiously with concomitant administration of steroids and phenytoin (Dilantin), as it may cause a nonketotic hyperosmolar state, with high mortality. With overuse, it can also result in hypertension and increased CBF if cerebral autoregulation is defective. And last, high doses carry a significant risk for the development of acute renal failure, especially with coexisting sepsis, concomitant nephrotoxic drug use, serum osmolarity > 320, or pre-existing kidney disease. Some patients with mass lesions on one side may not uniformly develop contralateral hemiparesis, as expected. In some cases, brainstem shift away from the mass lesion (e.g., EDH, SDH) may produce compression of the opposite cerebral peduncle against the tentorium, which results in hemiparesis on the same side as the lesion (Kernohan's notch phenomenon), a false localizing sign.

Injury to the vertebral artery (VA) after trauma can result in various abnormalities. The most severe is total occlusion of the vessel, which can result in infarction if there is not adequate collateral blood flow. One major risk (besides acute infarction) of traumatic vertebral artery occlusion is the potential for recanalization and embolization to downstream vessels. Although the precise incidence of recanalization and downstream embolization remains unknown, many favor sacrificing the artery via an endovascular approach to prevent this occurrence if collateral circulation is adequate. Moreover, this may potentially decrease the need for anticoagulation or antiplatelet therapy during the acute period in high-risk, multisystem-trauma patients. Others opt for less drastic strategies for dealing with this problem, such as observation or starting antiplatelet therapy, as compared to anticoagulation and t-PA, which may carry a higher hemorrhage risk in traumatized patients.

Patients with spontaneous or traumatic partial occlusion, dissection, or pseudoaneurysm formation of the vertebral or carotid arteries may also pose a difficult treatment dilemma, especially if there is bleeding in other locations from trauma. Each institution usually has its own guidelines, based on the literature, for managing such patients. Nevertheless, optimal treatment has not yet been determined. For patients without serious bleeding in other locations, many authors advocate anticoagulation with IV heparin for 1 to 2 weeks followed by warfarin (Coumadin) for an additional 4 to 12 weeks, as most arterial injuries have been noted to heal with recanalization within 6 weeks. For patients at high risk for bleeding with anticoagulation, some advocate aspirin and/or clopidogrel bisulfate (Plavix) therapy as an alternative to anticoagulation, which may (potentially) be associated with less risk of bleeding. Further studies are warranted to determine the best strategy for these types of injuries (Youmans, pp. 1692–1693, 5057–5059, 5095–5098, 5125–5137, 5157, 5158; Greenberg, pp. 648–655, 845–850).

37-B; 38-C; 39-B. Mycotic or infective aneurysms account for about 4% of intracranial aneurysms and are most commonly found along the distribution of the distal middle cerebral artery (MCA). Patients with head trauma also are at risk of developing aneurysms, although these are most frequently located along the distal anterior cerebral artery distribution. Mycotic aneurysms occur in about 3 to 15% of patients with subacute bacterial endocarditis (SBE), and the most common organism isolated from the blood is *Streptococcus viridans* species. Patients that are IV drug abusers or immunodeficient (HIV) are at increased risk of developing

this disease entity. Most cases are treated with 4 to 6 weeks of antibiotics followed by repeat angiography to document effectiveness of therapy. Delayed clipping may be feasible for patients with subarachnoid hemorrhage, an increase in the size of the aneurysm on antibiotics, or failure to reduce in size after completion of antibiotics (Kaye and Black, pp. 1050–1060; Youmans, pp. 2101–2106; Greenberg, pp. 790–791).

40-D; 41-B; 42-A; 43-D. ETV is a commonly performed procedure for patients with aqueductal stenosis (AS). Although there is some controversy about the age at which this procedure should first be employed, results indicate high success rates for properly selected patients. Complications of shunting may include slit ventricle syndrome, intracranial hypotension, subdural hematomas, craniosynostosis, microcephaly, and overdrainage, which are typically not noted after endoscopy. The precise location to fenestrate the floor of the third ventricle may vary on a case-by-case basis, but perforating the floor anterior to the mamillary bodies and posterior to the infundibulum seems to a popular approach. Performing a septostomy in conjunction to a third ventriculostomy does not improve results in patients with AS, as the obstruction is downstream to the foramen of Monro. A patient with scarring or a cyst obstructing one foramen of Monro would likely benefit from this ancillary procedure. Predicting the success rate of ETV by preoperative imaging studies has proven to be very difficult, although identifying relevant anatomy (thickness of the floor of the third ventricle, location of basilar artery) to help guide the operation has proven to be effective (Kaye and Black, pp. 789–797; Youmans, pp. 3429–3430; Wilkins, pp. 541–542).

44-C; 45-C; 46-A; 47-B. Compression of nerve roots in the lateral recess (lateral recess syndrome) can occur between a hypertrophied superior articular facet (dorsally), the pedicle (laterally), and the inferior vertebral body (ventrally). Medially, the lateral recess opens toward the spinal canal/thecal sac. The characteristic feature of lateral recess syndrome is that of radicular symptoms that occur mainly when the patient is walking or standing and are relieved by sitting, squatting forward, lying on either side, and/or postures that accentuate lumbar kyphosis. This is opposite to what is seen with patients harboring discogenic disease, who are uncomfortable while sitting. With the lateral recess syndrome, adequate decompression involves laminectomy with resection of the medial third of the hypertrophied facet (medial facetectomy), which is usually the superior articular process (Wilkins, pp. 3841–3845).

48-E; 49-F; 50-A; 51-B; 52-D; 53-C; 54-G. Direct sectioning of the spinothalamic tract (cordotomy) is very effective for unilateral pain below the upper chest region, however, it is associated with many complications and is usually performed only in terminal patients. Complications of cordotomy include hemiparesis, respiratory depression (Ondine's curse with bilateral procedures), and dysesthesias. Midline myelotomies can also be performed to interrupt the decussating fibers of the spinothalamic tract. This can be quite effective in the treatment of chronic pelvic pain secondary to cancer but is associated with leg weakness, dysesthesias, and bladder dysfunction. Chronic deep brain stimulation of the VPL and VPM nuclei of the thalamus as well as the periaqueductal gray (PAG) has been performed in the treatment of thalamic pain states, postherpetic neuralgia, and causalgia. Stimulation of the PAG has been associated with eye movement disorders, pupillary dilation, and the feeling of fear. Complications of pallidotomy include injury to the adjacent internal capsule (hemiparesis) and optic tract (homonymous hemianopsia), while complications of bilateral thalamotomy include speech problems and congnitive decline. Horner's syndrome, pneumothorax, intercostal neuralgias, and spinal cord injury can occur after sympathectomy, while anesthesia dolorosa has been reported to occur after percutaneous trigeminal electrocautery (Kaye and Black, pp. 1431–1445, 1481; Greenberg, pp. 352–354, 361, 365–370, 373–380; Youmans, pp. 3025–3030, 3045–3048, 3067–3070, 3101–3102; Wilkins, pp. 4055–4059).

55. B. Peripheral alcohol injection, glycerol rhizolysis, radiofrequency thermocoagulation, and microvascular decompression are all established procedures for the treatment of trigeminal neuralgia. Peripheral balloon compression instead of decompression is a modification of the observation that open surgical decompression of the ganglion could lead to significant pain relief in trigeminal neuralgia (Kaye and Black, pp. 1616–1633; Greenberg, pp. 373–380).

56-B; 57-D; 58-C. Refer to Figure 6.56–6.58A. Craniocervical junction (CCJ) abnormalities can often be very difficult to manage, with the primary goal being to relieve the compression at the cervicomedullary junction. They are commonly seen in patients with Chiari malformation or rheumatoid arthritis. With reducible lesions, stabilization is essential to maintain neural decompression, while for irreducible lesions, decompression at the site of encroachment (ventral or posterior) as well as stabilization are often required.

Patients with rheumatoid arthritis are at risk for developing atlantoaxial instability (AAI); superior migration of the odontoid process (SMO), also known as cranial settling; and subaxial subluxations (SAS). For rheumatoid patients with reducible lesions, immobilization alone with posterior spinal or craniospinal fusion without decompressive procedures is the mainstay of treatment.

Late-onset deterioration in patients with rheumatoid arthritis or Chiari malformations in the pattern seen in this patient is concerning for syrinx or syringomyelia formation (Kaye and Black, pp. 1755–1770; Wilkins, pp. 3789–3790; Youmans, pp. 4569–4580).

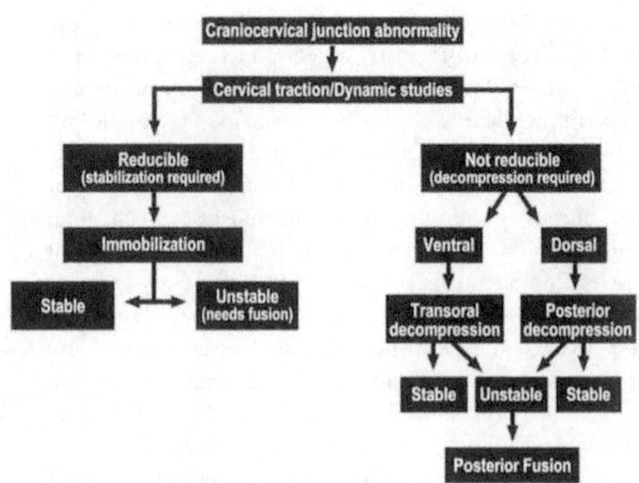

FIGURE 6.56–58A Algorithm for managing craniocervical junction abnormalities.

59-B; 60-B; 61-B. The styloid process gives rise to the stylohyoid (VII), styloglossus (XII), and stylopharyngeal muscles (IX) of the visceral neck as well as the stylomandibular and stylohyoid ligaments. It is a remnant of the second brachial arch (Youmans, p. 36).

62-B; 63-A; 64-C; 65-A; 66-C; 67-F; 68-A; 69-D. Fracture of the proximal humerus (A) can result in injury to the axillary nerve (C5-6), which innervates the teres minor and deltoid muscles. This can result in sensory loss at the shoulder as well as shoulder abduction weakness. There is also a chance of concomitant brachial plexus injury with such a fracture due to the proximity of the proximal humerus to the brachial plexus. The radial nerve runs down the posterior aspect of the arm and is at risk for injury during fractures of the midhumeral shaft as it winds around the spiral groove (B). This could cause paralysis of the wrist and hand extensor muscles. Since the fibers that innervate the triceps muscle often arise proximal to the spiral groove, extension of the forearm may not be affected by midhumeral fractures, and some supination is possible due to an intact biceps brachii muscle. Fracture in the vicinity of the medial epicondyle may result in ulnar nerve damage only (C), which can produce weakness of flexion and adduction of wrist, paralysis of hypothenar muscles and most deep muscles of the hand, as well as some weakness in select thenar muscles. Injury of the ulnar nerve by fracture of the distal ulna can result in weakness or paralysis of hypothenar, some thenar, and intrinsic hand muscles but often spares innervation of the wrist (flexion, adduction), since these nerves often arise more proximally. If there is also a concomitant distal radial fracture, injury to the median nerve may accompany the ulnar nerve injury (F) and produce loss of sensation of the lateral side of the palm without sensory loss on the palmar sides of the first, second, and third digits (superficial branch of the median nerve) as well as marked weakness of thumb flexion and abduction, inability to oppose the thumb, inability to fully extend the second and third digits, and sensory loss along the palmar side of the first, second, and third digits (deep branch in carpal tunnel). A fracture of the distal humerus (D) is most likely to result in combined radial, median, and ulnar nerve injuries (Fitzgerald, pp. 258, 276, 286, 293, 302–313; Greenberg, pp. 535–543; Youmans, pp. 3671–3675).

70. B. A significant number of children with craniopharyngiomas will have a significant endocrine abnormality after surgery, which is quite predictable. The most serious complication appears to be obesity, which develops in about 50% of patients. These patients are unable to control their appetite secondary to damage to the hypothalamic satiety center. Growth hormone may benefit these patients, as it appears to reduce body fat and increase lean body mass. Nearly 50% of patients will require GH-replacement therapy. Diabetes insipidus occurs in about 90% of patients and is often permanent. Moreover, about 90% of patients will require hydrocortisone and thyroid replacement therapy after surgery (Kaye and Black, pp. 741–748; Committee on Education in Neurological Surgery, pp. 26, 116; Curtis et al., pp. 24–27).

71. C. The headaches of spontaneous intracranial hypotension often resemble post–lumbar puncture headaches. Headaches are usually worse in the upright position and are generally relieved when the patient is lying down. The diagnosis is established by lumbar puncture, which reveals low opening pressure or dry tap. It is not uncommon to have elevated protein and pleocytosis. It is postulated that this syndrome results from leakage of CSF to the outside neuraxis, often around nerve roots. MR cisternography is often capable of demonstrating the leak. Jugular compression will elevate intracranial pressure but usually makes the headache worse, suggesting that low pressure may not be the only factor responsible for the headaches. MRI scans often reveal dural enhancement over the cerebral and cerebellar convexities, tentorium, and falx, which usually resolves with resolution of the symptoms. Treatment should be conservative, since there is often spontaneous improvement. Analgesics containing caffeine and adequate hydration seem to help. In some cases an epidural patch may be required; surgical closure of the fistula is rarely required (Committee on Education in Neurological Surgery, pp. 17, 105; Kosmosky, pp. 79–83).

72. D. A long history of radiosurgical treatment for arteriovenous malformations exists. The best responses are often obtained for lesions with volumes less than 4 cm³. Multiple metastatic lesions are also amenable to this treatment modality, as are recurrent gliomas located in a variety of locations including the brainstem, thalamus, or other eloquent areas. There is, however, controversy about the radiosurgical treatment of cavernomas. While disease control has been documented, some authors are concerned with the potential of treatment-related complications such as recurrent hemorrhage after radiosurgery (Committee on Education in Neurological Surgery, pp. 108–109; Friedman, pp. 832–841; Lunsford, pp. 404–444; Black, pp. 367S–369S).

73. D. Prefrontal lobectomy, cingulotomy, ventrolateral cordotomy, and periaqueductal gray stimulation may interrupt pain pathways or the response to painful stimuli. Hippocampectomy does not interrupt these pathways but may decrease the severity of complex partial seizures (Youmans, pp. 3025–3030; Greenberg, pp. 364–370).

74. A. Traumatic injury to the brainstem including the superior cerebellar peduncles and their connections can result in severe tremor that may be delayed by weeks to months following the brain injury. In some cases, improvement or resolution occurs spontaneously, so some authors have recommended a period of observation before considering surgery. The largest published series for secondary tremors is among patients with multiple sclerosis, although a growing body of information is now available for patients with posttraumatic tremors. With posttraumatic tremors, thalamic stimulation (Vim) may be considered for those who are refractory to medical management, although results have been mixed. Thalamotomy is another treatment option for this group of patients, although postoperative dysarthria or worsening pre-existing dysarthria is an especially troubling complication in some of these studies (Tarsy, pp. 244–254; Youmans, pp. 2748–2750).

75. E. Profound hypothermia during circulatory arrest can result in various physiologic effects including increasing blood viscosity, metabolic acidosis (underperfused tissue), hyperglycemia (secondary to hypoinsulinemia), decreased corticosteroid secretion, complement-mediated pneumonitis, renal failure (due to transient decrease in glomerular filtration rate, hemolysis, and blood product reactions), hepatic failure, and hypothermia-induced coagulopathy (due to platelet dysfunction and slowing of the enzymatic clotting cascade) (Youmans, p. 1532).

76. B. The most common physical manifestation of extracranial carotid artery disease is a cervical bruit. The degree of stenosis necessary to produce a bruit has been reported to be as low as 25%, but in various studies its presence has been found to indicate a significant level (> 50%) of stenosis on angiography in at least 70% of patients. False-positive rates of 10 to 40% and false-negative rates of 30 to 70% have been reported for cervical bruits. The Framingham Study found that the risk of stroke and TIAs in patients with bruits was two to three times the risk for patients without bruits. Such patients were also about 2.5 times more likely to have a heart attack and 1.9 times more likely to die during the study period (Youmans, p. 1622).

77-B; 78-E; 79-E. Neurocysticercosis (NCC) is the most common parasitic infection of the central nervous system (CNS) worldwide. Humans are the definitive host for the adult tapeworm *Taenia solium*, which thrives in the small intestine without consequence. Fecal shedding of eggs usually leads to ingestion of eggs in contaminated water or food by an intermediate host, typically humans or pig. Once inside the intestine, the eggs are released and produce primary larvae that enter the circulatory system. Hematogenous spread to muscular, ocular, and neural tissue then occurs. Once inside the brain, the primary larvae develop into secondary larvae, the cysticerci. Clinical manifestations of the neural form of the disease are varied and nonspecific. This pleomorphism is related to the number, size, and topography of the lesions. Parenchymal disease (as in this case) is most common and presents with seizures in 50 to 80% of patients. Treatment typically includes antiepileptics, albendazole, or praziquantel, as well as a short course of steroids to reduce the inflammatory reaction during antihelminthic treatment. Niclosamide may be given orally to treat adult tapeworms in the GI tract. Fluconazole is an antifungal and not used to treat this disease process. The colonization of the ventricular system often presents with rapid clinical deterioration due to increased intracranial pressure from obstructive hydrocephalus. There is still controversy about the best treatment for this form of the disease, but most authors advocate either a trial of antihelminthic medication, endoscopic cyst resection, or microsurgery. Subarachnoid disease is usually more difficult to manage because the cysts are usually multiple, attain larger sizes, and produce severe basal meningitis, but antihelminthic medications are typically first-line therapy for this form of the disease. From the many tests performed, current data indicate that enzyme-linked immunosorbent assay (ELISA) and electroimmunotransfer blot (EITB) tests are the most effective laboratory tests for diagnosis. Peripheral white blood cells, ova and parasites in stool, and eosinophilia are inconsistent and unreliable markers of disease. This patient also harbored a fourth ventricular cyst and obstructive hychocephalus, which accounts for the rounded third ventricle (Greenberg, pp. 236–239).

80. B. A neonate suffering high-output cardiac failure, hyperdynamic precordium, dilated cervical and cranial veins, and arteries with a "machine-like" bruit heard over the head and neck is most likely harboring a vein of Galen aneurysm. Vascular tumors, CC fistula, blue rubber bleb nevus syndrome, and sinus pericranii do not typically present with this constellation of problems. Although transcranial ultrasonography is an excellent way to diagnose these lesions, the "gold standard" is cerebral angiography. In infants, a transarterial and transvenous route to eliminate the high-flow shunt is often employed. This technique may not lead to complete obliteration but often converts high-output cardiac failure to a persistent fistula. In an older child or adult, the treatment is frequently gradual and entails graded elimination of the shunt with endovascular surgery, usually via a transarterial route (Kaye and Black, pp. 174–176; Youmans, pp. 3433–3445).

81. E. The deep branch of the radial nerve passes through a slit in the supinator muscle (arcade of Frohse) to the posterior forearm. After passing this slit, the nerve is called the posterior interosseous nerve and supplies the supinator, extensor carpi radialis brevis, extensor digitorum, extensor digiti minimi, extensor carpi ulnaris, abductor pollicis longus, extensors pollicis longus and brevis, and extensor indicis muscles. The anterior interosseous nerve, a branch of the median nerve, supplies the pronator quadratus (Greenberg, pp. 523, 542–543).

82. E. The ability to create irregularly shaped radiosurgical volumes is important to achieve conformal irradiation of target tissue, as all tumors or lesions are rarely perfect spheres. The following techniques can be used to create an irregularly shaped plan during radiosurgery. First, combine multiple isocenters of irradiation in different planes. For example, a series of 4-mm isocentors of irradiation is often used to tailor radiation to the porus acusticus for schwannomas. Second, individual isocenters can be weighted variably to change their relative shape. Finally, individual radiation beams can be blocked to restrict dose away from critical structures, such as the optic chiasm (Youmans, pp. 4118–4119).

83-C; 84-C. A rare complication after anterior cervical procedures is the development of a Horner's syndrome (anhidrosis, miosis, ptosis) from interruption of the sympathetic chain located on the anterior surface of the longus colli muscle. The thoracic duct enters the subclavian vein on the left and is particularly vulnerable to injury during left-sided anterior cervical procedures (Youmans, pp. 4442–4443, 4451).

85. D. Degenerative spondylolisthesis is most common in women at the L4-5 level, but may also be seen at the L3-4 level. Because this often occurs with sacralization of L5 in many patients, the facet degeneration may be explained as a hypermobility syndrome (Youmans, pp. 4545–4546).

86. A. Irreducible pathologic conditions affecting the cervicomedullary junction in patients with rheumatoid arthritis frequently require an anterior cervical procedure to remove the offending pathology (frequently pannus formation), followed by dorsal fixation and fusion. Reducible atlantoaxial dislocation is best managed by a posterior fusion and fixation procedure. Usually transarticular screw fixation is desirable if the bone quality is good and the lateral masses of the atlas are intact; but if this is not the case, placement of a rectangle of bone between the posterior arch of C2 and C1 followed by wiring may be an option. This, however, has been associated with higher failure rates in some studies.

These patients often required further reinforcement with cervical immobilization techniques such as halo placement. Dorsal occipitocervical fusion is almost always required for patients with rheumatoid cranial settling and in those following rheumatoid pannus resection. Transoral odontectomy with or without posterior fusion is not required for this patient since there was a reducible lesion. Laminectomy alone would likely further destabilize this patient, while halo placement without fusion would run a very high risk of failure (Youmans, pp. 4578–4550; Wilkins, pp. 3789–3790).

87. E. The ideal bone graft provides the following elements for successful healing: osteoconductive matrix, osteoinductive factors, viable osteogenic cells, and structural support. Only fresh autografts contribute viable osteogenic cells to the developing fusion. Processed allografts frequently have no living cellular elements and are mainly derived from the tissues of the recipient bed (Youmans, pp. 4615–4616).

88. E. Although traumatic brain injury (TBI) has been shown to result in increases of calcium flux into cells with subsequent cell injury, no clinical benefit has been observed in clinical trials attempting to attenuate this response in patients with TBI. A subset of patients with subarachnoid hemorrhage, however, did show a benefit. Calcium may enter cells via ion channels influenced by excitatory amino acids (glutamate, aspartate). Unfortunately clinical trials to antagonize these receptors have been discouraging in TBI (Youmans, pp. 5025–5027).

89. E. Surgical therapies including cerebellar stimulation, dorsal column stimulation, peripheral denervation, thalamotomy, and pallidotomy have been used in the past to treat various forms of dystonia. Although the thalamus has been the primary target for years, more recently many surgeons are targeting the globus pallidus with good results. Medications such as anticholinergics, muscle relaxants, and benzodiazepines are of limited use to patients. Botulism toxin is a safe and effective therapy for many focal dystonias but has not proven effective for patients with segmental dystonia, hemidystonia, or generalized dystonia (Youmans, pp. 2795–2801).

90. A. The surgical management of psychiatric disease can be helpful for select patients with treatment-refractory major affective disorders, obsessive-compulsive disorder, and chronic anxiety states. Surgical interventions have included anterior capsulotomy, limbic leukotomy, subcaudate tractotomy, and anterior cingulotomy but not arcuate fasciculotomy (Youmans, pp. 2853–2862).

91. A. The superior semicircular canal projects into the floor of the middle cranial fossa as the arcuate eminence (Tew, pp. 48–49; Wilkins, pp. 1071–1073).

92-D; 93-B; 94-B. Structures often visible on the middle fossa floor during subtemporal approach include the middle meningeal artery (often sacrificed by cautery and packing of the foramen spinosum), trigeminal nerve (V3), lesser superficial petrosal nerve, greater superficial petrosal nerve, ICA (if there is a small dehiscence in the bone), as well as the arcuate eminence, which overlies the superior semicircular canal. Decreased tearing after surgery most likely resulted from injury of the greater superficial petrosal nerve, which provides parasympathetic supply to the lacrimal and nasal gland. Additional exposure to the posterior fossa during a subtemporal approach may be gained by removing the bone of Kawase's quadrilateral located in the medial petrous apex, medial to Glasscock's triangle. Kawase's quadrilateral is bounded laterally by the greater superficial petrosal nerve, medially by the petrous ridge and V3 of the trigeminal nerve, and at its base by the arcuate eminence. Glasscock's triangle is bounded laterally by a line from the foramen spinosum to the facial hiatus, medially by the GSPN, and at its base by the mandibular division of the trigeminal nerve (Tew, pp. 48–49, 385–395).

95. D. The Cushing response consists of the triad of hypertension, bradycardia, and an irregular breathing pattern. According to many authors, the most likely mechanism accounting for this response is reduction in oxygenation in an area just rostral to the medulla. For this reason it is also called the ischemic response (Greenberg, p. 642; Committee on Education in Neurological Surgery, pp. 58, 155).

96-D; 97-B. The most common clinical presentation of carotid body tumors is a palpable neck mass in the high cervical region. Less commonly patients present with hoarseness, dysphagia, and unilateral tongue atrophy and weakness due to the tumors' proximity to the vagus and hypoglossal nerves. These tumors are generally benign, although they do tend to locally invade adjacent tissue, which can make their resection difficult. An evaluation of the endocrine system may be warranted, especially in patients with hypertension and tachycardia. Some patients may harbor a pheochromocytoma-like lesion that secretes excess catecholamines. In such patients, α-adrenergic blockade must be started about 2 weeks preoperatively to control hypertension, tachycardia, and the potential for arrhythmia. Preoperative planning is critical in these patients to reduce comorbidity. Some may require preoperative embolization to reduce the amount of bleeding during surgery (Youmans, pp. 1677–1681).

98. D. Multiple subpial transection (MST) was developed as a procedure to address seizure activity that extends beyond the area of resection and into eloquent cortex. The cerebral cortex has functional vertical columns, with its vertical orientation of incoming and outgoing fibers. Seizures, however, are believed to spread horizontally through the cortex. MST involves disconnecting the vertical columns of the cerebral cortex, which inhibits synchronization and spread of the seizure focus with minimal injury to the cortex. The most common problem faced by patients after this procedure includes subtle, transient deficits corresponding to the area of resection that typically improve. Permanent complication rates after this procedure are in the order of 5% (Youmans, pp. 2635–2642).

99. C. The most common surgical complication after vagal nerve stimulator (VNS) placement is infection. Transient vocal cord paralysis with hoarseness and swallowing problems is the second most common surgical complication of VNS. Temporary lower face numbness and weakness occur in about 0.7% of patients, likely related to high cervical incisions and superficial nerve injury (Youmans, pp. 2649–2650).

100. A. The internal stabilization of two adjacent segments of the lumbar spine with a pedicle screw construct having a pedicle-to-pedicle screw angle of zero and no transfixitor is not stable in lateral or rotational load, as each of the screws are free to turn in their screw holes in the body. Stability can be enhanced by the application of a transfixitor or angling the screws inward to form a pedicle-to-pedicle screw angle of 30 degrees (Carson, pp. 893–901; Committee on Education in Neurological Surgery, pp. 36, 128).

CHAPTER 7

Critical Care and Clinical Skills Questions

1. What is the half-life of phenobarbital?

  A. 6 hours
  B. 12 hours
  C. 24 hours
  D. 100 hours
  E. 140 hours

2. What is the initial treatment of choice in a patient with symptomatic hyperkalemia associated with ECG changes?

  A. Furosemide
  B. Insulin/glucose
  C. Bicarbonate
  D. Kayexalate
  E. Calcium gluconate

3. What is the treatment of choice for paroxysmal supraventricular tachycardia (SVT)?

  A. Electric cardioversion
  B. Adenosine
  C. Calcium antagonists
  D. β blockers
  E. Digoxin

4. Which of the following disorders is most commonly associated with prominent leukocyte casts on microscopic urinalysis?

  A. Acute interstitial nephritis
  B. Acute tubular necrosis
  C. Minimal change disease
  D. Cryoglobulinemia
  E. None of the above

QUESTIONS 5–9

Directions: Match the following clinical characteristics with the corresponding electrolyte abnormality, using each answer once, more than once, or not at all.

  A. Hyponatremia
  B. Hypocalcemia
  C. Hypomagnesemia
  D. Hypokalemia
  E. Hypophosphatemia
  F. Hypochloremia

5. Muscle weakness, altered mental status, U waves on ECG

6. Associated with other electrolyte abnormalities and torsades de pointes

7. Muscle weakness, decreased cardiac output, hemolytic anemia

8. Decreased cardiac output, hyperreflexia, tetany

9. Encephalopathy, cerebral edema, and seizures

End of set

QUESTIONS 10–15

Directions: Match the most effective anticonvulsant with the corresponding seizure disorder. Answers may be used once, more than once, or not at all.

  A. Absence
  B. Infantile spasms
  C. Complex partial
  D. Neonatal seizures
  E. Generalized tonic-clonic
  F. Lennox-Gastaut syndrome
  G. None of the above

10. Ethosuximide

11. Valproic acid

12. ACTH

13. Phenytoin

14. Phenobarbital

15. Carbamazepine

End of set

16. Which of the following characteristics is NOT applicable to synchronized intermittent mandatory ventilation (SIMV)?

  A. Delivers volume-cycled breaths
  B. Often combined with pressure support to overcome the resistance of the ventilator circuit tubing
  C. Allows spontaneous breaths between ventilator-delivered breaths
  D. Associated with a decreased work of breathing
  E. Associated with impaired ventricular filling

17. Which of the following characteristics is NOT associated with extrinsic positive end-expiratory pressure (PEEP)?

A. Facilitates alveolar recruitment
B. Reduces pulmonary edema
C. Increases mean intrathoracic pressure
D. Decreases intrapulmonary shunt
E. Reduces cardiac output

18. All of the following are associated with acute respiratory distress syndrome (ARDS) EXCEPT?

A. Hypoxia
B. Diffuse pulmonary infiltrates
C. Hypercapnia
D. The addition of positive end-expiratory pressure (PEEP) prevents alveolar collapse and allows for reduction of the FiO_2 to nontoxic levels
E. Often exhibits a PAO_2/FiO_2 ratio > 200 mmHg

19. Which of the following characteristics is NOT associated with auto-PEEP (intrinsic PEEP or hyperinflation)?

A. Large inflation volumes
B. Lower respiratory rates
C. Inverse ratio ventilation
D. Asthma
E. Pneumothorax

20. Which of the following ECG changes can be observed in patients with pulmonary emboli?

1. Tachycardia
2. Nonspecific ST changes
3. Large Q wave in lead III
4. Inverted T wave in lead III

A. 1, 2, and 3 are correct
B. 1 and 3 are correct
C. 2 and 4 are correct
D. Only 4 is correct
E. All of the above are correct

21. Which of the following is the first-line agent of choice in the treatment of multifocal atrial tachycardia?

A. IV magnesium
B. Verapamil
C. Metoprolol
D. Lidocaine
E. Electric cardioversion

22. Which of the following characteristics is associated with cardiac tamponade?

1. Jugular venous distention
2. Hypotension
3. Muffled heart sounds
4. A rise in the systolic blood pressure (> 10 mmHg) with inspiration onset

A. 1, 2, and 3 are correct
B. 1 and 3 are correct
C. 2 and 4 are correct
D. Only 4 is correct
E. All of the above are correct

23. A 48-year-old female with three children experiences the acute onset of a fever three hours after receiving a blood transfusion. What precautions should be taken prior to the administration of a second transfusion?

A. Administer washed red cells
B. Administer leukocyte-poor red cells
C. Pretreatment with Tylenol
D. Investigate for the presence of IgA deficiency
E. None of the above

24. Which of the following laboratory tests is abnormally prolonged with von Willebrand's disease?

1. Prothrombin time
2. Partial thromboplastin time
3. Prothrombin 1:1 dilution
4. Bleeding time

A. 1, 2, and 3 are correct
B. 1 and 3 are correct
C. 2 and 4 are correct
D. Only 4 is correct
E. All of the above are correct

QUESTIONS 25–27

Directions: Match the following shock syndromes with the appropriate Swan-Ganz catheter measurements/vital signs, using each answer once, more than once, or not at all. Note- CVP- central venous pressure (mm Hg), PCWP- pulmonary capillary wedge pressure (mm Hg), CI- cardiac index ($L/min/m^2$), SVR- systemic vascular resistance ($dynes/cm^2$).

A. Hypovolemic shock
B. Cardiogenic shock
C. Septic shock

25. CVP 16, PCWP 20, CI 1.2, SVR 1250

26. CVP 4, PCWP 6, CI 4.5, SVR 350

27. CVP 2, PCWP 5, CI 2.0, SVR 1400

End of set

28. Which of the following characteristics is NOT associated with multiple endocrine neoplasia type 2 (Sipple syndrome)?

  A. Autosomal dominant inheritance
  B. Pheochromocytomas
  C. Pituitary adenomas
  D. Medullary thyroid carcinoma
  E. Parathyroid hyperplasia

29. Which of the following characteristics are associated with intraoperative venous air embolism?

  1. High incidence in the sitting position
  2. Most sensitive diagnostic modality is transesophageal echocardiography
  3. Associated with decreases in end tidal CO_2
  4. The patient should be placed rapidly in the right lateral decubitus position

  A. 1, 2, and 3 are correct
  B. 1 and 3 are correct
  C. 2 and 4 are correct
  D. Only 4 is correct
  E. All of the above are correct

QUESTIONS 30–34

Directions: Select which of the following characteristics is most commonly observed with cerebral salt wasting/syndrome of inappropriate ADH secretion (SIADH).

  A. Cerebral salt wasting
  B. SIADH
  C. Both of the above
  D. None of the above

30. Hypovolemia

31. Hypervolemia

32. Elevated serum osmolality

33. Hypouricemia

34. Treatment entails free water restriction

End of set

35. Which of the following agents is associated with the development of tension pneumocephalus?

  A. Propofol
  B. Isoflurane
  C. Etomidate
  D. Nitrous oxide
  E. Lorazepam

36. All of the following characteristics are associated with barbiturates EXCEPT?

  A. Dose-dependent EEG burst suppression
  B. Associated with decreases in cerebral blood flow
  C. Effects are terminated primarily by redistribution
  D. Can result in prominent peripheral vasoconstriction
  E. Dose-dependent myocardial suppression

37. Which of the following agents exhibits the highest selectivity for β_1 receptors?

  A. Dobutamine
  B. Dopamine
  C. Epinephrine
  D. Phenylephrine
  E. Isoproterenol

QUESTIONS 38–44

Directions: Match the following metal intoxications with their appropriate characteristics/therapies. Some answers may be used once, more than once, or not at all.

  A. Arsenic poisoning
  B. Lead poisoning
  C. Mercury poisoning
  D. Iron poisoning
  E. Succimer (DMSA)
  F. Penicillamine
  G. Thallium
  H. Deferoxamine
  I. Manganese poisoning
  J. None of the above

38. Encephalopathy, peripheral neuropathy, hypochromic anemia

39. Gingivostomatitis, peripheral neuropathy, psychiatric disturbances

40. Treatment of choice for iron poisoning

41. Treatment of choice for lead poisoning in children

42. Cardiomyopathy, pancytopenia, hypotensive shock

43. Treatment of choice for Wilson's disease

44. Sometimes treated with L-DOPA

End of set

45. What is the maximum expected correction of a patient with symptomatic hyponatremia over a 24-hour period (mEq/L)?

  A. 4
  B. 8
  C. 12
  D. 16
  E. 20

46. At what point in time after injury does a healing wound contain the maximum collagen content?

- **A.** Two days
- **B.** Two weeks
- **C.** Two months
- **D.** Two years
- **E.** None of the above

47. Which of the following anesthetics lower seizure threshold?

1. Enflurane
2. Propofol
3. Methohexital
4. Diazepam

- **A.** 1, 2, and 3 are correct
- **B.** 1 and 3 are correct
- **C.** 2 and 4 are correct
- **D.** Only 4 is correct
- **E.** All of the above are correct

48. A 34-year-old female presents with secondary amenorrhea, normal visual fields, and a prolactin level of 560 ng/mL. The patient's MRI showed evidence of an enhancing pituitary macroadenoma, and she was initiated on oral bromocriptine therapy. Over the subsequent several months the patient's prolactin level normalized, her macroadenoma decreased significantly in size, and she eventually underwent a successful pregnancy. The patient was lost to follow up and then presented acutely five years later with complaints of visual loss. Repeat MRI showed a recurrent macroadenoma, and the patient reported amenorrhea and galactorrhea. Routine serum prolactin level was 39 ng/mL. What is the most likely explanation for the patient's current prolactin level?

- **A.** Stalk effect
- **B.** The macroadenoma no longer synthesizes prolactin
- **C.** Hook effect
- **D.** Prior bromocriptine therapy favored the growth of non-hormone-producing neoplastic pituitary cells (null-cell adenoma)
- **E.** None of the above

49. All of the following characteristics are consistent with the high-dose dexamethasone suppression test (2 mg q 6 h × 8 doses) EXCEPT?

- **A.** Distinguishes Cushing's disease from cortisol-producing adrenal adenomas
- **B.** Urine free cortisol levels will exhibit 90% suppression of baseline with Cushing's disease
- **C.** 17-Hydroxysteroids are suppressed to < 50% of baseline with Cushing's disease
- **D.** Adrenal adenomas exhibit 25 to 50% suppression of urine free cortisol baseline levels
- **E.** None of the above

50. Which of the following characteristics is consistent with induced barbiturate coma in patients with closed head injuries?

1. Adequate burst suppression on EEG is associated with maximal reductions in cerebral metabolism ($CMRO_2$)
2. Barbiturates improve global cerebral perfusion
3. Barbiturates can result in myocardial depression
4. Barbiturates are associated with immunosuppression

- **A.** 1, 2, and 3 are correct
- **B.** 1 and 3 are correct
- **C.** 2 and 4 are correct
- **D.** Only 4 is correct
- **E.** All of the above are correct

51. Which of the following should be utilized in the treatment of coagulopathy resulting from von Willebrand's disease?

1. Fresh frozen plasma
2. Desmopressin
3. Platelets
4. Cryoprecipitate

- **A.** 1, 2, and 3 are correct
- **B.** 1 and 3 are correct
- **C.** 2 and 4 are correct
- **D.** Only 4 is correct
- **E.** All of the above are correct

52. Which of the following characteristics is NOT associated with perioperative gastrointestinal bleeding?

- **A.** Patients with severe closed head injuries
- **B.** Patients with > 30% body surface area burns
- **C.** Hypotensive shock
- **D.** Early postoperative enteral feeds
- **E.** Incidence is decreased with utilization of H_2 blockers and sucralfate

53. Which of the following acute phase reactants are typically increased during periods of acute systemic inflammation?

1. C-reactive protein
2. Fibrinogen
3. Haptoglobin
4. Albumin

- **A.** 1, 2, and 3 are correct
- **B.** 1 and 3 are correct
- **C.** 2 and 4 are correct
- **D.** Only 4 is correct
- **E.** All of the above

54. Which of the following agents act as pyrogens at the hypothalamus?

1. Interleukin-6
2. Tumor necrosis factor
3. Interleukin-1
4. Prostaglandin E2

- **A.** 1, 2, and 3 are correct
- **B.** 1 and 3 are correct
- **C.** 2 and 4 are correct
- **D.** Only 4 is correct
- **E.** All of the above

55. Which of the following parameters is the best indicator of adequate tissue perfusion?

- **A.** Systolic blood pressure
- **B.** Urine output
- **C.** Heart rate
- **D.** Gastrointestinal pH
- **E.** Oxygen saturation

56. Which of the following features is NOT typically associated with septic shock?

- **A.** Mental status changes
- **B.** Respiratory acidosis
- **C.** Hyperglycemia
- **D.** Increased pulse pressure
- **E.** Elevated white blood cell count

57. Which of the following metabolic complications is NOT typically associated with the administration of total parenteral nutrition?

- **A.** Hyperglycemia
- **B.** Essential fatty acid deficiency
- **C.** Metabolic alkalosis
- **D.** Hypophosphatemia
- **E.** Hepatic cholestasis

58. Which of the following characteristics are consistent with pseudomembranous colitis?

- **1.** Prior antibiotic administration
- **2.** Development of toxic megacolon
- **3.** Watery diarrhea
- **4.** Enzyme-linked immunosorbent assays (ELISA) for *C. difficile* toxins represent the gold standard in laboratory diagnosis

- **A.** 1, 2, and 3 are correct
- **B.** 1 and 3 are correct
- **C.** 2 and 4 are correct
- **D.** Only 4 is correct
- **E.** All of the above

59. Which of the following studies has the highest positive predictive value in the diagnosis of acute pulmonary embolism?

- **A.** Pulmonary angiogram
- **B.** High resolution helical computed tomographic angiography
- **C.** Nuclear scintigraphic ventilation-perfusion lung scan
- **D.** Venous duplex ultrasound
- **E.** None of the above

60. Warfarin (Coumadin) administration inhibits synthesis of which of the following clotting factors/anticoagulant proteins?

- **1.** Factor VII
- **2.** Factor II
- **3.** Factor IX
- **4.** Protein C

- **A.** 1, 2, and 3 are correct
- **B.** 1 and 3 are correct
- **C.** 2 and 4 are correct
- **D.** Only 4 is correct
- **E.** All of the above

61. Which of the following medications can result in a decrease in the bioavailability of warfarin during coadministration?

- **1.** Barbiturates
- **2.** Cimetidine
- **3.** Rifampin
- **4.** Metronidazole

- **A.** 1, 2, and 3 are correct
- **B.** 1 and 3 are correct
- **C.** 2 and 4 are correct
- **D.** Only 4 is correct
- **E.** All of the above

62. Which of the following characteristics is NOT observed with primary aldosteronism (Conn's syndrome)?

- **A.** Hypertension
- **B.** Hyperkalemia
- **C.** Low plasma renin activity
- **D.** Metabolic alkalosis
- **E.** Hypomagnesemia

63. A 22-year-old male is brought to the emergency department after sustaining injuries in a motor vehicle collision. The patient has a heart rate of 122, respiratory rate of 28, systolic blood pressure of 86, oxygen saturation of 88%, and mild tracheal deviation to the left. What is the immediate next step in management of this condition?

- **A.** Emergent needle thoracocentesis
- **B.** Placement of a thoracostomy tube
- **C.** Portable chest x-ray
- **D.** Obtain an arterial blood gas
- **E.** CT scan of the chest

QUESTIONS 64–66

Scenario: A 46-year-old male with no prior surgical history is intubated and placed under general anesthesia for an elective anterior cervical discectomy and fusion. Shortly after intubation, the patient exhibits a prominent increase in end tidal CO_2, tachycardia, and an elevated temperature.

64. What is the immediate next step in management?

- **A.** STAT portable chest x-ray
- **B.** Immediate cessation of inhalational anesthetics
- **C.** Heparin anticoagulation
- **D.** Increase in ventilatory rate
- **E.** None of the above

65. Which of the following features are likely to develop with delays in diagnosis and treatment of the above malady?

- **1.** Hypoxia
- **2.** Metabolic acidosis
- **3.** Rhabdomyolysis
- **4.** Disseminated intravascular coagulation

- **A.** 1, 2, and 3 are correct
- **B.** 1 and 3 are correct
- **C.** 2 and 4 are correct
- **D.** Only 4 is correct
- **E.** All of the above are correct

66. Administration of what medication is effective in halting the progression of the above disorder in the majority of cases?

A. Propofol
B. Etomidate
C. Lorazepam
D. Dantrolene
E. Heparin

End of set

67. Which of the following is effective in the treatment of hypercalcemia?

1. Furosemide
2. Isotonic saline
3. Calcitonin
4. Pamidronate

A. 1, 2, and 3 are correct
B. 1 and 3 are correct
C. 2 and 4 are correct
D. Only 4 is correct
E. All of the above are correct

68. Which of the following characteristics are consistent with fat embolism?

1. Global cerebral dysfunction
2. Renal dysfunction
3. Conjunctival petechiae
4. Treatment involves avoidance of positive pressure ventilation

A. 1, 2, and 3 are correct
B. 1 and 3 are correct
C. 2 and 4 are correct
D. Only 4 is correct
E. All of the above

69. Which of the following pathogens are most likely to cause early (less than 2 weeks) and late (greater than 6 months) shunt infections, respectively?

A. *Staph. aureus, Staph. epidermidis*
B. *Staph. epidermidis, Strep. pneumonia*
C. *Staph. epidermidis, Staph. epidermidis*
D. *Staph. epidermidis, P. acnes*
E. *Staph. epidermidis, Staph. aureus*

QUESTIONS 70–74

Directions: Match the following anesthetic agents with their most appropriate characteristic. Some letters may be used once, more than once, or not at all.

A. Etomidate
B. Propofol
C. Lorazepam
D. Halothane
E. Isoflurane
F. Nitrous oxide
G. Fentanyl
H. Pentobarbital
I. None of the above

70. Increases both cerebral metabolism and cerebral blood flow

71. Markedly increases CBF and can disrupt autoregulation

72. Reduces cerebral metabolism and increases CSF absorption

73. Reduces CBF and ICP, suppresses cortisol production with prolonged infusions

74. Uncouples CBF and cerebral metabolism, minimal effects on evoked potentials

End of set

75. An 18-year-old male suffers a moderate closed head injury with a concomitant fracture of the skull base. The patient exhibits prominent meningeal signs with a fever and leukocytosis one week after the injury. Which of the following organisms is the most likely to be identified on CSF culture?

A. *Haemophilus influenzae*
B. *Moraxella catarrhalis*
C. *Strep. pneumoniae*
D. *Klebsiella pneumonia*
E. *Staph. epidermidis*

76. Which of the following side effects is NOT typically associated with administration of BCNU (carmustine)?

A. Interstitial pneumonitis
B. Hepatitis
C. Bone marrow suppression
D. Nausea
E. Hemorrhagic cystitis

77. Which of the following agents is most appropriate for the treatment of urinary retention?

A. Oxybutynin
B. Bethanecol
C. Imipramine
D. Atropine
E. Methacholine

78. Which of the following is most likely to account for cases of nosocomial pneumonia in patients on mechanical ventilation?

A. Gram-positive cocci
B. Gram-positive rods
C. Gram-negative cocci
D. Gram-negative rods
E. None of the above

79. Which of the following characteristics are consistent with disseminated intravascular coagulation (DIC)?

1. Associated with diffuse microvascular thrombosis
2. Associated with widespread release of tissue factor
3. Often results in fulminant ARDS
4. Heparin is contraindicated with onset of DIC

A. 1, 2, and 3 are correct
B. 1 and 3 are correct
C. 2 and 4 are correct
D. Only 4 is correct
E. All of the above

80. Which of the following agents has been associated with precipitating thyrotoxicosis (Jodbasedow effect)?

A. Iodinated radiographic contrast dye
B. Propylthiouracil
C. Hydrocortisone
D. Propranolol
E. None of the above

81. Which of the following paralytics is associated with the development of hyperkalemia?

A. Rocuronium
B. Vecuronium
C. Pancuronium
D. Succinylcholine
E. None of the above

82. Which of the following vitamins is often coadministered with isoniazid to prevent a relative deficiency?

A. Thiamine
B. Vitamin K
C. Pyridoxine
D. Vitamin B_{12}
E. Vitamin D

83. Which of the following is NOT characteristic of atropine toxicity?

A. Mydriasis
B. Xerostomia
C. Delirium
D. Bradycardia
E. Cutaneous flushing

84. A 56-year-old male complains of severe chest pain on postoperative day 1 after undergoing elective lumbar microdiscectomy. The patient's blood pressure is 163/82 with a pulse of 48, respiratory rate of 18, and oxygen saturation of 98% on 2 L of oxygen via nasal cannula. The patient's ECG shows evidence of ST elevations of 0.5 to 2.0 mm in three successive leads. Which of the following medications should be administered (i.e., are NOT contraindicated) at this time?

1. Aspirin
2. β blockers
3. Nitroglycerin
4. Tissue plasminogen activator (t-PA)

A. 1, 2, and 3 are correct
B. 1 and 3 are correct
C. 2 and 4 are correct
D. Only 4 is correct
E. All of the above

QUESTIONS 85–89

Directions: Match the appropriate vasopressor with the appropriate characteristics. Answers may be used once, more than once, or not at all.

A. Isoproterenol
B. Dopamine
C. Dobutamine
D. Epinephrine
E. Norepinephrine
F. None of the above

85. Inotropic agent of choice for treatment of acute severe heart failure

86. Primarily α receptor agonist for shock states

87. Augments cerebral blood flow at low doses

88. Mainly α1 activity

89. Primarily β receptor agonist that increases cardiac output and decreases diastolic blood pressure

End of set

90. A 62-year-old male is admitted to the ICU for the acute management of severe hypertension after subendocardial myocardial infarction. The patient's hypertension is refractory to intravenous labetalol, hydralazine, and nitroglycerin, however, it responds well to continuous nitroprusside infusion. The patient is then initiated on oral antihypertensive therapies. The following day the patient experiences the acute onset of confusion, tinnitus, nausea, tachycardia, abdominal pain, and blurred vision. What is the most appropriate next course of action?

    A. Obtain an arterial blood gas
    B. Obtain a serum sodium level
    C. Administration of IV lorazepam
    D. Administration of IV methylene blue
    E. Administration of IV hematin

91. Which of the following are useful in the treatment of SIADH?

    1. Fluid restriction   **A.** 1, 2, and 3 are correct
    2. 3% saline infusion   **B.** 1 and 3 are correct
    3. Demeclocycline   **C.** 2 and 4 are correct
    4. Hemodialysis   **D.** Only 4 is correct
        E. All of the above

92. What is the free water deficit of an 80 kg male (lean body mass) with a serum sodium level of 148 mEq/L?

    A. 1.4 L
    B. 2.7 L
    C. 3.5 L
    D. 4.8 L
    E. 6.0 L

93. Which of the following is a necessary cofactor in the synthesis of collagen?

    A. Vitamin D
    B. Thiamine
    C. Vitamin B_{12}
    D. Vitamin C
    E. Pyridoxine

94. Acute toxicity of which of the following vitamins can result in headache, blurry vision, nausea, emesis, and papilledema (elevated intracranial pressure)?

    A. Vitamin A
    B. Vitamin D
    C. Vitamin E
    D. Thiamine
    E. Folate

95. Which of the following characteristics is NOT typically observed with Cushing's syndrome?

    A. Muscle weakness
    B. Plethora
    C. Loss of diurnal rhythm of cortisol secretion
    D. High serum ACTH level
    E. Solitary adrenal adenoma

QUESTIONS 96–100

Directions: Match the following arterial blood gas values with the appropriate acid/base disorder. Letters may be used once, more than once, or not at all.

    A. Respiratory acidosis
    B. Respiratory alkalosis
    C. Metabolic acidosis
    D. Metabolic alkalosis
    E. Combined respiratory acidosis and metabolic acidosis
    F. Combined respiratory alkalosis and metabolic alkalosis

96. pH 7.27, $PaCO_2$ 52 mmHg, HCO_3^- 23 mEq/L

97. pH 7.48, $PaCO_2$ 45 mmHg, HCO_3^- 32 mEq/L

98. pH 7.35, $PaCO_2$ 48 mmHg, HCO_3^- 28 mEq/L

99. pH 7.31, $PaCO_2$ 34 mmHg, HCO_3^- 19 mEq/L

100. pH 7.28, $PaCO_2$ 40 mmHg, HCO_3^- 19 mEq/L

End of set

Critical Care and Clinical Skills Answer Key

1. D	21. A	41. E	61. B	81. D
2. E	22. A	42. A	62. B	82. C
3. B	23. C	43. F	63. A	83. D
4. A	24. C	44. I	64. B	84. B
5. D	25. B	45. C	65. E	85. C
6. C	26. C	46. C	66. D	86. E
7. E	27. A	47. B	67. E	87. B
8. B	28. C	48. C	68. A	88. F
9. A	29. A	49. D	69. C	89. A
10. A	30. A	50. E	70. F	90. D
11. F	31. B	51. C	71. D	91. E
12. B	32. D	52. D	72. G	92. B
13. E	33. B	53. A	73. A	93. D
14. D	34. B	54. E	74. H	94. A
15. C	35. D	55. D	75. C	95. D
16. D	36. D	56. B	76. E	96. A
17. B	37. A	57. C	77. B	97. D
18. E	38. B	58. A	78. D	98. A
19. B	39. C	59. A	79. A	99. C
20. E	40. H	60. E	80. A	100. E

Critical Care and Clinical Skills Answers

1. D. The half-life of phenobarbital is generally between 98 and 120 hours in the average adult. Phenobarbital is largely metabolized by the liver, although 20 to 30% of the drug can be excreted unchanged in the urine. Barbiturates bind the $GABA_A$ receptor in the CNS, which facilitates Cl-mediated inhibitory postsynaptic potentials. Phenobarbital is often used in the treatment of partial and generalized tonic-clonic seizures in neonates (Katzung, pp. 37, 358–359, 393–394).

2. E. Calcium gluconate is the initial treatment of choice for symptomatic hyperkalemia because it rapidly antagonizes the effects of hyperkalemia directly at the plasma membrane level. The effects of calcium gluconate are short-lived, however, and other therapies should be instituted simultaneously. Loop diuretics (furosemide) can increase renal potassium excretion, Kayexalate enhances gastrointestinal potassium excretion, and bicarbonate and insulin/glucose induce intracellular shifts of potassium primarily into muscle cells. Sodium bicarbonate is less effective in patients with renal failure, however, and can actually bind calcium; therefore its utility is limited. The definitive treatment for patients with chronic hyperkalemia is hemodialysis (Marino, pp. 655–658).

3. B. Paroxysmal supraventricular tachycardia (AV-nodal re-entrant tachycardia) results from re-entry of impulses from an ectopic source. Adenosine blocks the positive inotropic effects of catecholamines, slows conduction at the AV node, and dilates coronary arteries. Additionally, the effects of adenosine are short-lived, so it does not elicit significant myocardial depression. It is these characteristics of adenosine that make it the drug of choice in the treatment of paroxysmal SVT over calcium antagonists (Marino, pp. 329–330).

4. A. Acute interstitial nephritis (AIN) is a common cause of acute renal failure and is usually associated with infections or hypersensitivity drug reactions. AIN is characterized by a decrease in the glomerular filtration rate, often with oliguria. Urinalysis often exhibits hematuria, mild proteinuria, an elevated fractional excretion of sodium, eosinophilia, and leukocyte casts with AIN. Acute tubular necrosis (ATN) most commonly results from renal hypoperfusion and is characterized by acute renal failure, an elevated fractional excretion of sodium, and granular casts on urinalysis. Cryoglobulinemia can result in acute renal insufficiency secondary to the deposition of immunoglobulins in the renal parenchyma and is usually associated with the nephrotic syndrome. Minimal change disease is associated with proteinuria and the nephrotic syndrome as well (Cecil, pp. 579, 581–583; Marino, pp. 621–622, 626).

5-D; 6-C; 7-E; 8-B; 9-A. Symptomatic hyponatremia (usually 120 mEq/L or less) can result in generalized seizures, metabolic encephalopathy, depressed level of consciousness, acute respiratory distress syndrome, muscle weakness, and even cerebral edema and elevated intracranial pressure. Hypokalemia can result in muscle weakness, altered mental status, and ECG changes (prominent U waves, T-wave inversion, prolonged QT interval); however, isolated hypokalemia does not result in significant cardiac arrhythmias. Hypomagnesemia is very common in the ICU setting and is often associated with depletion of other electrolytes (phosphate, calcium, potassium). Symptomatic hypomagnesemia has been associated with digitalis cardiotoxicity, torsades de pointes, tremors, hyperreflexia, and generalized seizures. Hypocalcemia can result in decreased cardiac output, hypotension, ventricular ectopy, hyperreflexia, generalized seizures, and tetany. Mild to moderate hypophosphatemia is often asymptomatic, while severe phosphate depletion can be associated with decreased cardiac output, hemolytic anemia, impaired tissue oxygen availability, and muscle weakness (Marino, pp. 643–644, 650–651, 662–665, 677, 683–685).

10-A; 11-F; 12-B; 13-E; 14-D; 15-C. Isolated absence seizures (petit mal epilepsy) are generally treated with ethosuximide; however, valproic acid is the agent of choice if the patient also experiences generalized tonic-clonic seizures. Lennox-Gastaut syndrome is a heterogenous disorder characterized by mental retardation, seizures, and generalized spike-and-wave complexes at 1 to 2 Hz on EEG. Valproic acid is the initial treatment of choice for this disorder; however, less than 10% of all patients with Lennox-Gastaut syndrome achieve effective seizure control with single-agent anticonvulsant therapy. Infantile spasms (West syndrome) occur in children less than 6 months of age and are associated with tuberous sclerosis, cerebral malformations, and metabolic disorders. The treatment of choice for infantile spasms is ACTH. Several anticonvulsants are utilized in the treatment of generalized tonic-clonic seizures; however, phenytoin is the traditional first-line agent. Phenobarbital is the drug of choice in the treatment of neonatal seizures, but phenytoin and lorazepam are often added with inadequate seizure control. Carbamazepine is the agent of choice in the treatment of complex partial seizures and is particularly effective in preventing secondary generalization (Merritt, pp. 813–826).

16. D. SIMV was developed secondary to complications (e.g., hyperinflation and overventilation) that can arise in patients on assist-control ventilation (ACV) with rapid respiratory rates. SIMV delivers volume-cycled breaths at a preselected rate that are synchronized to the patient's spontaneous breaths. Additionally, SIMV allows spontaneous breaths to occur between ventilator-delivered breaths. Spontaneous breaths during SIMV occur through a high-resistance circuit with a unidirectional valve, which results in an increased work of breathing and potential for respiratory muscle fatigue. The addition of pressure support facilitates spontaneous breaths and can limit increases in work of breathing (and respiratory muscle fatigue) with SIMV. Any form of positive-pressure mechanical ventilation can be associated with impaired ventricular filling and concomitant reductions in cardiac output (Marino, pp. 434–438).

17. B. Normally, the alveolar pressure at the end of expiration is equal to atmospheric pressure. The addition of PEEP (extrinsic PEEP) results in an elevated alveolar pressure at the end of expiration by stopping exhalation when the preselected pressure is reached. PEEP results in increases in end-expiratory and mean intrathoracic pressures. PEEP tends to prevent alveolar collapse and facilitate alveolar reopening (recruitment), which results in improved gas exchange (decreased intrapulmonary shunt) and increased lung compliance. The addition of PEEP can result in decreased cardiac filling and cardiac output, especially in hypovolemic patients; this effect is independent of the absolute value of the extrinsic PEEP. The increases in mean intrathoracic pressure that are secondary to extrinsic PEEP are directly related to the observed decreases in cardiac output. The application of PEEP does not reduce pulmonary edema and can, in fact, exacerbate pulmonary edema secondary to alveolar overdistention and impaired pulmonary lymphatic drainage (Marino, pp. 382–383, 441–445).

18. E. ARDS is characterized by the acute onset of diffuse pulmonary infiltrates and hypoxemia that is refractory to elevations in FiO_2. Lung-protective ventilatory strategies with ARDS include the utilization of lower tidal volumes (7 to 10 cc/kg) than with other traditional forms of ventilation to keep peak inspiratory pressures less than 35 cm H_2O. The addition of PEEP with ARDS prevents alveolar collapse (with the lower tidal volumes) and allows the reduction of the FiO_2 to nontoxic levels (< 60%). Patients with ARDS who exhibit refractory hypoxemia or hypercapnia are often placed on inverse-ratio ventilation (IRV), which results in prolonged lung inflation times and concomitant alveolar recruitment (Marino, pp. 381–383, 440).

19. B. Intrinsic PEEP (occult PEEP) results from incomplete alveolar emptying during expiration. The development of intrinsic PEEP is associated with large inflation volumes, rapid respiratory rates, decreases in exhalation time (inverse ratio ventilation), and airway obstruction (e.g., asthma and COPD). High levels of intrinsic PEEP are associated with decreased cardiac output, alveolar rupture (volutrauma) with possible pneumothorax, increased work of breathing, and elevations in plateau pressures (Marino, pp. 462–464).

20. E. ECG changes in acute pulmonary emboli include sinus tachycardia (most common), inverted T waves in leads V_1 to V_3, right axis deviation, right bundle branch block, and atrial arrhythmias. The classic findings of "S_1, Q_3, T_3" refers to the presence of a wide S complex in lead I, a large Q wave in lead III, and an inverted T wave in lead III, although these findings are not very sensitive in the diagnosis of acute pulmonary embolism. All of these ECG changes are usually transient findings that resolve once the pulmonary arterial pressure has normalized after the acute ictus (Cecil, p. 424).

21. A. Multifocal atrial tachycardia (MAT) exhibits multiple P-wave morphologies and variable PR intervals on ECG, with an irregular ventricular rate. MAT is associated with chronic lung disease and theophylline, and has been associated with hypokalemia, acute myocardial infarction, pulmonary embolism, and congestive heart failure. MAT should initially be treated with IV magnesium; theophylline should be discontinued and any underlying hypokalemia corrected. If these therapies are ineffective, verapamil or metoprolol should be administered (Marino, pp. 328–329).

22. A. Cardiac tamponade is associated with Beck's triad (jugular venous distention, muffled heart sounds, hypotension) and pulsus paradoxus (drop in systolic blood pressure of at least 10 mm Hg with the onset of inspiration). Diastolic pressures (CVP, PCWP, pulmonary artery diastolic pressure) are often equalized with cardiac tamponade, and the diagnosis is often confirmed with transesophageal echocardiography. The treatment of cardiac tamponade entails emergent pericardiocentesis (Marino, pp. 255–256).

23. C. Febrile nonhemolytic reactions are extremely common and accompany approximately 1% of all transfusions. These reactions are secondary to antibodies in the recipient blood that react to donor leukocytes and are more common in multiparous women and a history of prior transfusions. The fever usually occurs between 1 and 6 hours after the transfusion and is not associated with other symptoms. The majority of patients who experience a febrile nonhemolytic reaction will not experience a second fever with repeat transfusion; however, leukocyte-poor red cells can be utilized in patients with repetitive febrile nonhemolytic reactions. Patients with IgA deficiency can exhibit more severe hypersensitivity reactions to transfusions, including rash and anaphylaxis (Marino, pp. 702–703).

24. C. Von Willebrand's disease results in prolongations of the partial thromboplastin time (PTT) and bleeding time because von Willebrand factor stabilizes factor VIII and mediates platelet adhesion (Cecil, pp. 993).

25-B; 26-C; 27-A. Hypovolemic shock is characterized by decreased central venous and intracardiac pressures, decreased cardiac output, elevated SVR (> 1200 dynes/cm^2), and concomitant hypotension and tachycardia, with a dampened Swan-Ganz catheter waveform. Cardiogenic shock is characterized by a decreased cardiac index (less than 1.8 L/min/m^2), elevated PCWP (> 18 mm Hg) and CVP, elevated SVR, and decreased systolic blood pressure (< 100 mm Hg). Septic shock is characterized by low filling pressures, decreased SVR (although early septic shock can exhibit an elevated SVR), and normal or increased cardiac output. Normal Swan-Ganz catheter parameters are as follows: CVP 1 to 6 mm Hg, PCWP 6 to 12 mm Hg, CI 2.4 to 4.0 L/min/m^2, SVR 900 to 1200 dynes/cm^2 (Marino, pp. 164, 505–509).

28. C. Multiple endocrine neoplasia (MEN) type 2 (Sipple syndrome) is an autosomal dominant disorder that localizes to chromosome 10 and is characterized by the development pheochromocytomas and medullary thyroid carcinoma. MEN-2 can be further subdivided into a type A (associated with parathyroid hyperplasia or adenomas) and type B (associated with multiple mucosal neuromas). Pituitary adenomas are associated with MEN type 1 (Cecil, p. 1254).

29. A. Intraoperative venous air embolism (VAE) has a high incidence during procedures performed in the sitting position (up to 25 to 45% of all cases). VAE is characterized by the development of bronchoconstriction, hypoxia, hypercarbia, hypotension, shock, cardiac arrhythmias, increased airway pressures, and decreased end-tidal CO$_2$ (secondary to increased dead space). Transesophageal echocardiography is the most sensitive diagnostic modality for VAE, detecting volumes as small as 0.02 mL/kg of air entering the venous system. The immediate treatment of suspected VAE entails rapid hemostasis with concomitant irrigation of the surgical field, lowering of the patient's head with left lateral decubitus positioning, increasing the FiO$_2$ to 100%, stopping any concomitant nitrous oxide administration, manual occlusion of the jugular veins, and aspiration of air from a multiorifice CVP catheter (Greenberg, p. 602; Youmans, pp. 614–615; Wilkins, pp. 409–410).

30-A; 31-B; 32-D; 33-B; 34-B. Cerebral salt wasting (CSW) is characterized by hyponatremia (< 135) and hypovolemia secondary to renal sodium loss. CSW is associated with either normal or decreased serum osmolality (< 280), elevated urine sodium levels (> 20 mEq/L), elevated urine osmolality, decreased PCWP and CVP (hypovolemia), and normal or elevated serum potassium levels. SIADH is characterized by the presence of hyponatremia and hypervolemia secondary to plasma volume expansion. SIADH is associated with a decreased serum osmolality (< 280), increases in urine sodium and osmolality levels (greater than plasma osmolality), elevated PCWP and CVP (hypervolemia), and normal or decreased serum potassium levels. It is the presence of hypervolemia with SIADH that primarily distinguishes it from CSW, although hypouricemia tends to be observed in a delayed fashion with SIADH. The treatment of SIADH is free water restriction, whereas the treatment of CSW is volume and salt replacement. CSW can accompany aneurysmal subarachnoid hemorrhage and must be recognized and treated appropriately in this patient population, especially in the presence of vasospasm, to prevent the delayed development of ischemic deficits (Youmans, pp. 1829–1830; Greenberg, pp. 17–19).

35. D. Nitrous oxide increases cerebral blood flow and thus intracranial pressure when intracranial compliance is altered. Nitrous oxide can also diffuse into intracranial air faster than nitrogen can escape, which can contribute to the development of tension pneumocephalus (Greenberg, p. 2; Youmans, p. 1508; Wilkins, p. 405).

36. D. Barbiturates are anticonvulsants that result in prominent decreases in CBF and CMRO$_2$, dose-dependent EEG burst suppression, dose-dependent myocardial suppression, and peripheral vasodilation. Barbiturates are lipid-soluble and their CNS effects are primarily terminated by redistribution. At higher dosages, barbiturates can actually result in decreases in cerebral perfusion pressure if decreases in mean arterial pressure exceed the decrease in intracranial pressure (Katzung, p. 410; Youmans, pp. 1508, 1521; Greenberg, pp. 2, 776–777; Wilkins, p. 404).

37. A. See Table 7.37A. Dobutamine is relatively selective for β_1 receptors, which makes it the agent of choice in the treatment of severe systolic heart failure. Isoproterenol is also a β-selective agent but has clinically insignificant actions on α_1 and α_2 receptors as well (Katzung, p. 128; Marino, pp. 278–298; Greenberg, pp. 7–9).

38-B; 39-C; 40-H; 41-E; 42-A; 43-F; 44-I. Refer to Table 7.38–7.44A. Arsenic neuropathy is the most common of all the heavy metal–induced neuropathies. Gastrointestinal (GI) symptoms such as nausea, vomiting, and diarrhea occur when large quantities are ingested, but these symptoms are often absent if arsenic is taken parenterally or taken in small amounts over a protracted period of time. In acute poisoning, the onset of symptoms usually takes 4 to 8 weeks to develop, but the evolution of polyneuropathy is slower in chronic

TABLE 7.37A   Adrenergic agonists and actions

DRUG	RECEPTOR SPECIFICITY	THERAPEUTIC USES
Epinephrine	$\alpha 1, \alpha 2$ $\beta 1, \beta 2$	Management of cardiac arrest associated with pulseless ventricular tachycardia, ventricular fibrillation, asystole, and pulseless electrical activity Acute asthma Open-angle glaucoma Anaphylactic shock Use with local anesthetics
Norepinephrine	$\alpha 1, \alpha 2$ $\beta 1$	Shock states
Isoproterenol	$\beta 1, \beta 2$	Bronchodilator in asthma Cardiac stimulant
Dopamine	Low doses : Affects dopaminergic receptors in renal (increased sodium and water excretion), mesenteric, and cerebral circulations Intermediate doses: β receptors in the heart and peripheral circulation (increase cardiac output) High doses: dose-dependent activation of α receptors in the systemic and pulmonary circulations	Cardiogenic shock states and circulatory shock syndromes associated with systemic vasodilation (sepsis) In lower dose rates, can preserve renal blood flow and promote urine output in patients with oliguric acute renal failure
Dobutamine	$\beta 1$	Low-output heart states due to systolic dysfunction
Phenylephrine	$\alpha 1$	Nasal decongestant Supraventricular tachycardia

poisoning. Numbness in a stocking-and-glove distribution with impaired position and vibration sensation is the early finding, followed by weakness that progresses to flaccid paralysis. Pigmentation and hyperkeratosis of the skin and nails (Mees' lines) are frequently present, and arsenic can often be detected in the urine, hair, and nails. Large ingestions of inorganic arsenic compounds are usually rapidly fatal due to hypotensive shock. The treatment of arsenic poisoning entails the use of dimercaprol or DMPS.

Lead neuropathy occurs almost exclusively in adults, while children often experience encephalopathy. It can cause abdominal distress, retention of urate crystals and gout, hypochromic anemia, and weakness in the distribution of the radial nerve (often sparing the brachioradialis muscle), which can produce wrist drop. Sensory symptoms are often absent, and laboratory findings include anemia with basophilic stippling of red blood cells, increased serum uric acid, a slight elevation of CSF protein, and increased urinary lead and porphobilinogen excretion. Treatment of lead poisoning entails the use of dimercaptosuccinic acid or DMSA (succimer) in children and EDTA or succimer in adults.

Inorganic mercury can be absorbed through the GI tract, while elemental mercury may be directly absorbed through the skin or lungs. Mercury poisoning can produce weakness and wasting more than sensory symptoms. It is characterized by neuropsychiatric symptoms, gingivostomatitis, peripheral neuropathy, acute tubular necrosis, and acrodynia. Treat-

ment of mercury intoxication involves the use of succimer or penicillamine. Manganese poisoning can result in a parkinsonian type of syndrome that is often responsive to L-DOPA. Deferoxamine is a chelator that is used primarily to treat iron poisoning, and penicillamine is the treatment of choice for Wilson's disease (copper accumulation) (Katzung, pp. 957–966; Merritt, pp. 622–625; Levin, pp. 663–664).

45. C. Symptomatic hyponatremia (generally < 125 mEq/L) should be corrected at a maximal rate of 0.5 mEq/L/h (thus 12 mEq/L/24 h) to avoid central pontine myelinolysis (Marino, p. 644; Greenberg, pp. 15–16).

46. C. Wound healing occurs in primarily three phases: the inflammatory, the proliferative, and the remodeling phases. The inflammatory phase occurs during the first week and is characterized by hemostasis as well as neutrophil and macrophage infiltration. The proliferative phase occurs from approximately 5 days to 3 weeks and consists of neovascularization, wound contraction (myofibroblasts), extracellular matrix synthesis (fibroblasts), and cellular migration (epithelialization). The third phase (remodeling) occurs from approximately 4 weeks to 2 years and consists of the aggregation and alignment of collagen fibers, with a progressive increase in wound tensile strength for the first 6 to 8 months until it plateaus. The wound contains the maximum collagen content approximately 2 to 3 months after injury, during the

TABLE 7.38–44A   Heavy metal toxicity

METAL	ACUTE SYMPTOMS	CHRONIC SYMPTOMS	THERAPY
Aluminum	GI: constipation	CNS: dementia, seizures, myoclonus Pulmonary: fibrosis	Deferoxamine
Arsenic	GI: bloody diarrhea CV: arrhythmia Renal: hematuria, anuria General: fever, anorexia	CV: Arteritis, cardiomyopathy GI: cirrhosis Skin: melanosis, hyperkeratosis, alopecia, carcinoma CNS: peripheral neuropathy Heme: pancytopenia	Dimercaprol DMPS
Lead	GU: reversible renal dysfunction	GU: nephropathy CNS: peripheral neuropathy, encephalopathy Heme: hypochromic anemia	CNS: Dimercaprol, calcium disodium edentate Non-CNS: calcium disodium edentate followed by penicillamine
Manganese	Pulmonary: fibrosis	CNS: Parkinson-like syndrome, psychiatric disorder GI: cirrhosis	L-DOPA
Thallium	GI: irritation CNS: ascending paralysis, psychiatric disturbances, dementia	Skin: alopecia CNS: neuropathy GI: liver necrosis GU: nephritis Pulmonary: edema	
Inorganic mercury	Pulmonary: pneumonitis GI: gingivostomatitis, bloody diarrhea GU: kidney damage	CNS: spasms, tremors, psychiatric ("mad hatter syndrome") GI: excess salivation GU: glomerular disease	Dimercaprol, DMPS, Penicillamine, calcium disodium edentate, dialysis
Organic mercury		CNS: paresthesias, ataxia, dysarthria, deafness	Chelation not helpful

early portion of the proliferative phase (Robbins, pp. 74–76; Wilkins, pp. 519–520; Youmans, pp. 564–565).

47. B. Enflurane is an inhaled general anesthetic that actually lowers seizure threshold; methohexital is a barbiturate that also lowers seizure threshold. This property renders these two agents unsuitable for most neurosurgical procedures (Greenberg, pp. 2, 47; Katzung, p. 417; Youmans, pp. 1508–1512).

48. C. The Hook effect results in false-negative lab assays for prolactin in the presence of extremely high prolactin levels. This is secondary to inhibition of formation of the normal prolactin-antibody complexes due to the presence of extremely high prolactin levels. In these cases, a 1:100 prolactin dilution should be obtained to effectively rule out a prolactinoma. Stalk effect results from compression of the adjacent hypothalamus or pituitary stalk by non-prolactin-secreting macroadenomas and commonly results in prolactin levels of 25 to 150 ng/mL. Pituitary adenomas are typically monoclonal neoplasms; thus it is unlikely that a null cell adenoma has arisen in a patient with a prior known prolactinoma. The diagnosis of a prolactinoma generally requires a serum prolactin level of > 200 ng/mL (Greenberg, pp. 420–426; Kaye and Laws, pp. 206–210).

49. D. The high-dose dexamethasone suppression test helps distinguish Cushing's disease (ACTH-secreting pituitary adenoma) from ectopic sources of ACTH and cortisol-producing adrenal adenomas. Pituitary adenomas will exhibit suppression with this test, with concomitant decreases in 17-hydroxysteroids to < 50% of baseline and urine free cortisol levels to < 90% of baseline. Adrenal adenomas are ACTH-independent and thus do not respond to the high-dose dexamethasone suppression test (Cecil, p. 1217; Youmans, pp. 1196–1197).

50. E. High-dose barbiturates uncouple cerebral blood flow and cerebral metabolism, thus resulting in decreases in $CMRO_2$ and increases in CBF. Burst suppression on EEG results in maximal reductions in $CMRO_2$ with continuous barbiturate infusions. High-dose barbiturate therapy is associated with myocardial depression and hypotension, and patients often require concomitant vasopressor therapy to maintain an adequate mean arterial pressure during barbiturate infusions. Other effects of high-dose barbiturate infusion include immunosuppression, impaired gastric motility, increased lysosomal stability, and improved free-radical scavenging. Global cerebral perfusion is improved with barbiturate infusions, and it is thought that blood is "shunted" from normal brain regions to damaged (ischemic) regions. Although barbiturate infusions can lower ICP, improvements in overall outcomes in patients with closed head injuries undergoing high-dose barbiturate therapy is controversial (Greenberg, pp. 653–654; Wilkins, p. 353).

51. C. Von Willebrand's disease (VWD) results in prolongation of the partial thromboplastin time (PTT) and bleeding time. Coagulopathy resulting from VWD is typically treated with cryoprecipitate, which is rich in both factor VIII and von Willebrand factor as well as desmopressin (DDAVP), which facilitates the release of von Willebrand factor from epithelial cells (Cecil, p. 994).

52. D. Superficial stress ulcers in the gastric/duodenal mucosa are a result of regional decreases in blood flow and are exacerbated by the presence of H⁺. Patients in the highest risk category for GI hemorrhages are those with severe closed head injuries (Cushing's ulcer) and those with burns over > 30% body surface area (Curling's ulcer). Superficial stress ulcers can lead to nosocomial sepsis and occult GI bleeding, although overt hemorrhage occurs in only 5% of all cases of stress ulcers. The risk of perioperative GI bleeding can be decreased with the administration of H₂ blockers and sucralfate, maintenance of adequate systemic blood pressure and oxygen transport, and initiation of early enteral feedings (Marino, pp. 94–101).

53. A. Acute-phase reactants are a group of proteins that are largely synthesized by the liver. Synthesis of the acute-phase reactants is altered during periods of systemic inflammation, which results in prominent increases in several plasma proteins including C-reactive protein, serum amyloid A, fibrinogen, von Willebrand factor, α_1-antitrypsin, haptoglobin, ceruloplasmin, and several complement proteins. Serum plasma levels of albumin and transferrin are typically decreased during periods of acute inflammation (Cecil, pp. 1535–1537).

54. E. There are several different proteins that act at the anterior hypothalamus to induce a systemic fever (pyrogens), including interleukin-1, interleukin-6, tumor necrosis factor, interferon-α, and some bacterial toxins. All of these substances induce local increases in prostaglandin E2 levels in the anterior hypothalamus to increase the temperature set point (Cecil, pp. 1533–1535).

55. D. In shock states, blood is selectively shunted away from the GI tract, which results in decreases in the local gastric pH. GI pH normalizes after adequate resuscitation and is thus an excellent indicator of regional perfusion.

Normal systolic blood pressure, heart rate, and even urine output can all be observed in inadequately resuscitated patients who are in states of compensated shock (Marino, pp. 198–200; Brown et al., pp. 569–585).

56. B. Septic shock is usually a result of bacteremia with gram-positive or gram-negative organisms, although it can also occur with fungal and anaerobic infections. Septic shock often exhibits fever, mental status changes, tachypnea, tachycardia, an increased pulse pressure, hyperglycemia, and an elevated white blood cell count. Septic shock results in tachypnea and a concomitant respiratory alkalosis early in the disease course, although late in the disease course a concomitant metabolic acidosis can occur from lactate accumulation (hypoperfusion). Septic shock is also accompanied by tachycardia and an increased cardiac output initially, although cardiac output and stroke volume are often decreased in the later stages of septic shock. Most patients with sepsis exhibit an elevated white blood cell count and hyperglycemia (glucocorticoid release), although marked decreases in the white blood cell count and hypoglycemia (with prominent bacteremia) are also occasionally observed (Marino, pp. 505–510).

57. C. Metabolic complications of total parenteral nutrition (TPN) include volume overload, hyperglycemia, hypophosphatemia, hyperchloremic metabolic acidosis, hypomagnesemia, hypokalemia, trace element deficiency, and essential fatty acid deficiency. Patients on long-term TPN are also at risk to develop hepatic cholestasis and vitamin deficiencies. Other complications of TPN include complications related to central line placement (e.g., pneumothorax, hemothorax) and the presence of an indwelling central catheter (e.g., venous thrombosis and sepsis) (Marino, pp. 759–763).

58. A. Pseudomembranous colitis (PMC) is a relatively common cause of severe diarrhea and colitis in the ICU population and results from toxins produced by *Clostridium difficile*. PMC is usually associated with prior exposure to third-generation cephalosporins, clindamycin, or one of the penicillins, although many different antibiotics have been implicated in the development of this disorder. *C. difficile* produces two different toxins (toxin A and toxin B) that ultimately result in disruption of colonic mucosal integrity, with subsequent fluid secretion, inflammation, and edema. Findings of PMC include fever, leukocytosis, watery diarrhea, abdominal pain/cramping, dehydration, hypoalbuminemia, and even the development of sepsis and toxic megacolon (with colonic perforations). The "gold standard" laboratory study for the diagnosis of PMC is direct cytotoxic assay of stool filtrate for *C. difficile* toxin. ELISA tests for *C. difficile* toxin are also available; however, they exhibit low sensitivity. Direct culture of the bacterium is the most sensitive laboratory assay, but it is rarely performed due to time and cost constraints and the inability to differentiate between normal and toxic strains of *C. difficile*. The treatment of PMC includes discontinuation of causative antibiotics, fluid and electrolyte repletion, and the administration of oral metronidazole (Flagyl) (Marino, pp. 534–537).

59. A. Pulmonary angiography continues to be the gold standard in the diagnosis of acute pulmonary embolism (PE), with close to a 100% positive predictive value and 90% negative predictive value. High-resolution helical CT angiography is evolving as a more accurate diagnostic modality for acute pulmonary embolism, although its sensitivity and specificity are not as well defined. Nuclear scintigraphic ventilation-perfusion (V/Q) lung scan is often the initial diagnostic study of choice in patients with small pulmonary emboli, although approximately 40% of all patients with an acute PE will exhibit a nondiagnostic (indeterminate) V/Q scan. Lower extremity duplex ultrasound can often confirm the source of a PE, although a negative result does not significantly reduce the likelihood of a PE (Marino, pp. 112–115).

60. E. Warfarin (Coumadin) inhibits the synthesis of the vitamin K–dependent clotting factors (factors II, VII, IX, X) and the anticoagulant proteins C and S (Katzung, p. 552).

61. B. Barbiturates, rifampin, and cholestyramine administration can all result in decreased levels of warfarin (and thus decreases in INR). Cimetidine, metronidazole, trimethoprim-sulfamethoxazole, fluconazole, amiodarone, and disulfiram all result in increased levels of coumadin (and thus increases in INR) (Katzung, p. 554).

62. B. Primary aldosteronism (Conn's syndrome) is characterized by hypertension, hypernatremia, hypokalemia, metabolic alkalosis, and low plasma renin activity. Excessive aldosterone levels promote retention of sodium, water, and bicarbonate in the distal renal tubules, with concomitant losses of potassium and magnesium. The majority of cases of Conn's syndrome result from excessive production of aldosterone by an adrenal adenoma (Cecil, p. 1249).

63. A. Tension pneumothorax is a life-threatening condition that often exhibits tracheal deviation to the side opposite the pneumothorax. The marked increases in intrathoracic pressure that accompany tension pneumothorax can result in prominent decreases in venous blood return to the heart, with concomitant hypotension and shock, as in this case. ATLS guidelines recommend immediate empiric treatment of suspected tension pneumothorax with needle thoracocentesis, followed by placement of a definitive thoracostomy tube (American College of Surgeons Committee on Trauma, pp. 128–129).

64-B; 65-E; 66-D. Malignant hyperthermia is a heritable disorder that is characterized by skeletal muscle hyperme-

tabolism secondary to decreased calcium sequestration in the sarcoplasmic reticulum. Malignant hyperthermia is associated with the administration of succinylcholine and some inhalational anesthetics (e.g., halothane, cyclopropane). This disorder is characterized by the acute onset of an increase in end-tidal CO_2, tachycardia, muscle rigidity, and an elevated temperature. With disease progression, arrhythmias, hypoxia, metabolic acidosis, pulmonary edema, disseminated intravascular coagulation, rhabdomyolysis, hypotension, and even cardiac arrest can occur. The mortality of malignant hyperthermia is as high as 30%. Suspected cases should be treated initially by the immediate cessation of the suspected offending agent, followed by the administration of IV dantrolene until symptoms cease (Greenberg, pp. 4–5).

67. E. Hypercalcemia is quite rare in the ICU setting and is usually secondary to the presence of hyperparathyroidism, thyrotoxicosis, or malignancy. Medications that are effective in the treatment of hypercalcemia include furosemide (promotes urinary excretion), isotonic saline (corrects hypovolemia and promotes calcium excretion), calcitonin (inhibits bone resorption), hydrocortisone, bisphosphonates (e.g., pamidronate), and plicamycin (mithramycin). Hemodialysis is also an effective treatment for hypercalcemia (Marino, pp. 679–681).

68. A. Fat embolism is characterized by pulmonary, cerebral, hepatic, and renal involvement. Cerebral symptoms are usually global, and pulmonary symptoms usually dominate the clinical presentation. Occasionally petechiae of the chest and conjunctivae are observed. Treatment entails aggressive oxygenation with positive-pressure ventilation, volume resuscitation, and the administration of corticosteroids (Robbins, pp. 110–111; Wilkins, pp. 2704–2705).

69. C. *Staphylococcus epidermidis* is the most common pathogen to result in shunt infections in both an early and late fashion (Greenberg, p. 214).

70-F; 71-D; 72-G; 73-A; 74-H. Etomidate is often used for induction or cerebral protection during aneurysm surgery; it is a potent cerebral vasoconstrictor that reduces CBF and ICP. Etomidate can also suppress cortisol synthesis with prolonged infusions. Halothane is an inhalational anesthetic that increases CBF (often as high as 100%), decreases CSF absorption, and disrupts autoregulation, all of which can contribute to elevated ICP. Nitrous oxide increases both CBF and cerebral metabolism and increases the risk of developing tension pneumocephalus in patients with underlying pneumocephalus. Narcotics (e.g., fentanyl) in general increase CSF absorption and decrease cerebral metabolism. Barbiturates (e.g., pentobarbital) uncouple cerebral metabolism from CBF, as they decrease cerebral metabolism and increase CBF. Barbiturates also exhibit minimal effects upon evoked potentials (Greenberg, pp. 1–3; Katzung, pp. 417, 420–422).

75. C. *Streptococcus pneumoniae* is associated with approximately 50 to 70% of all cases of meningitis occurring after traumatic skull fractures. After the appropriate antibiotics are administered and the patient recovers from meningitis, a thorough evaluation for the presence of a CSF fistula, with possible surgical repair, should be entertained (Wilkins, p. 3305; Greenberg, p. 213).

76. E. BCNU is associated with alopecia, bone marrow suppression, dysphagia, encephalopathy, nausea, diarrhea, hepatitis, and renal failure. Some of the most important side effects of BCNU are dose-dependent pulmonary complications, including interstitial pneumonitis and pulmonary fibrosis (Katzung, pp. 888–889).

77. B. Bethanechol is a muscarinic agonist that facilitates detrusor contraction and inhibits contraction of the bladder sphincter and trigone, thus effectively treating urinary retention. Methacholine is also a muscarinic agonist, however, it is typically used to facilitate the diagnosis of hyperactive airway disease (e.g., asthma) due to its potent bronchoconstrictive effects (Greenberg, p. 116; Katzung, pp. 94, 96, 100).

78. D. While gram-positive cocci (e.g., *Streptococcus pneumoniae*) account for the majority of cases of community-acquired pneumonias, gram-negative rods account for the majority of cases of nosocomial pneumonia. Gram-negative rods account for 46% of all cases of nosocomial pneumonia in ward patients and 83% of all patients on mechanical ventilation. *Pseudomonas* species are the most common bacteria to account for ventilator-associated nosocomial pneumonia (30% of all cases) (Marino, pp. 516–517).

79. A. DIC is often a result of sepsis and severe systemic trauma, which results in endothelial cell damage and release of tissue factor. The presence of large amounts of tissue factor can result in the diffuse activation of both the fibrinolytic and coagulation pathways. Clinically, DIC is characterized by diffuse microvascular thrombosis, thrombocytopenia, and hemorrhage (especially GI bleeding). As DIC progresses, oliguric renal failure, ARDS, and even death from multiple organ failure can ensue. DIC often exhibits elevations of fibrin split products (D-dimer), decreases in fibrinogen, prolongations of the PT and PTT, and thrombocytopenia. Although not contraindicated, heparin is often ineffective in controlling the diffuse microvascular thrombosis that is inherent to DIC because antithrombin III levels are concomitantly decreased (Marino, pp. 712–713).

80. A. The Jodbasedow effect refers to the precipitation of thyrotoxicosis in patients with toxic nodular goiter (or occasionally Graves' disease) who are exposed to large levels of iodine acutely. Common precipitating agents include iodinated radiographic contrast dye and amiodarone (Cecil, pp. 1235–1236).

81. D. Succinylcholine usually results in mild elevations in serum potassium levels and is rarely associated with severe hyperkalemia (Greenberg, p. 49; Katzung, p. 444).

82. C. Isoniazid is associated with the development of peripheral neuropathy that occurs secondary to a relative pyridoxine deficiency (excessive excretion). Administration of pyridoxine during isoniazid therapy is effective in preventing the development of peripheral neuropathy (Katzung, p. 773).

83. D. Atropine is an antimuscarinic agent that blocks almost all parasympathetic effects at high concentrations. Symptoms of atropine toxicity include delirium, mydriasis, cycloplegia, xerostomia, tachycardia, cutaneous flushing, and fever. Treatment of atropine toxicity involves the judicious use of physostigmine (Katzung, pp. 113–114).

84. B. Morphine, nitroglycerin, aspirin, oxygen, and β blockers are often administered in the setting of an acute myocardial infarction (MI). The administration of thrombolytics have been shown to improve outcome in patients with acute MI who exhibit chest pain (for > 30 minutes and < 12 hours), ST elevation of at least 0.1 mm in two contiguous leads, or new left bundle branch block and no evidence of heart failure or hypotension. Although the patient meets the criteria for the administration of t-PA, the recent surgical procedure makes this option less appealing due to the associated bleeding risk. Additionally, aspirin is universally recommended for the treatment of acute MI and would not be contraindicated approximately 48 hours after a simple microdiscectomy. The use of β blockers in this patient is contraindicated because the patient's pulse is less than 50 (Marino, pp. 304–305, 309–310).

85-C; 86-E; 87-B; 88-F; 89-A. Refer to Table 7.37A. Isoproterenol is a potent β agonist that results in prominent increases in cardiac output and decreases in diastolic blood pressure (peripheral vasodilation, β_2). Isoproterenol promotes both positive inotropic and chronotropic actions. Dopamine primarily activates dopaminergic receptors in the renal, mesenteric, and cerebral vasculature at low dosages, augmenting flow to these regions. At high dosages, dopamine acts primarily as a vasoconstrictor, activating peripheral α receptors. Dobutamine is primarily a β_1 agonist that is the inotropic agent of choice in acute, severe systolic heart failure. Epinephrine stimulates both α and β receptors. At low dosages, epinephrine stimulates primarily β receptors; at high dosages, α receptors are primarily stimulated. As opposed to dopamine, however, epinephrine is a potent renal vasoconstrictor, even at low dosages. Norepinephrine is an α-receptor agonist that results in prominent vasoconstriction (Katzung, pp. 127–128; Marino, pp. 281–286, 295–296).

90. D. Prolonged nitroprusside infusions are associated with the accumulation of cyanide, which gradually exhausts thiosulfate and methemoglobin reserves and can result in cyanide toxicity. Cyanide accumulation can result in delirium, ataxia, tinnitus, abdominal pain, blurry vision, muscle spasms, nausea, emesis, and dyspnea. Without treatment, cyanide toxicity can progress to metabolic acidosis, hypotension, coma, and death. Treatment of nitroprusside-induced cyanide toxicity includes cessation of the medication and IV methylene blue. Sodium nitrite, sodium thiosulfate, and hemodialysis are also effective therapies (Marino, pp. 838–841).

91. E. First-line therapy for asymptomatic patients with hyponatremia secondary to SIADH entails fluid restriction. The treatment of severe, symptomatic hyponatremia (typically Na < 120 mEq/L) secondary to SIADH involves more aggressive correction with 3% saline infusions, which are generally discontinued when the patient's symptoms resolve or the serum sodium reaches 128 to 130 mEq/L. The treatment of chronic SIADH often involves demeclocycline; the treatment of SIADH in association with congestive heart failure or renal failure often involves hemodialysis (Greenberg, pp. 17–19; Marino, p. 643).

92. B. To calculate free water deficit, total body water (TBW) must be calculated initially. TBW is 0.5 times lean body mass (in kilograms) for a female and 0.6 times lean body mass for a male. Free water deficit is then calculated by multiplying TBW by $(S_{Na}-140)/140$. Thus, the free water deficit in this patient is 2.7 L (Greenberg, p. 19).

93. D. Vitamin C is a necessary cofactor in the synthesis of collagen. Vitamin C is important in the intracellular hydroxylation of proline and lysine residues in the procollagen molecule (Robbins, pp. 456–459; Wilkins, pp. 519–520).

94. A. Acute vitamin A toxicity can result in symptoms of elevated intracranial pressure (headache, nausea, emesis, blurry vision, papilledema), hepatomegaly, and ascites. These symptoms are usually transient and typically resolve after discontinuing the excessive intake of vitamin A; however, severely symptomatic patients occasionally require serial lumbar punctures (to treat the elevated intracranial pressure) and restoration of any underlying electrolyte abnormalities (e.g., hypercalcemia) (Robbins, p. 441).

95. D. Cushing's syndrome usually results from iatrogenic steroid administration or adrenal adenomas. Under these circumstances, the diurnal rhythm of cortisol secretion is lost and serum ACTH levels are markedly depressed. Rarely, ectopic ACTH production by a malignant tumor occurs (e.g., oat cell carcinoma of the lung); this can result in Cushing's syndrome with concomitant high serum ACTH levels. Cushing's disease results from an ACTH-producing pituitary adenoma. The clinical symptomatology of Cushing's syndrome and Cushing's disease is similar and consist of truncal obesity, abdominal striae, acne, muscle weakness, hirsuitism, depression, lethargy, "moon facies," and plethora (Greenberg, pp. 420–421).

96-A; 97-D; 98-A; 99-C; 100-E. The normal range for pH is 7.36 to 7.44; for PCO_2 36 to 44 mm Hg; and for HCO_3 22 to 26 mEq/L. The initial step in the interpretation of acid-base disorders involves determining whether the disorder is primarily respiratory or metabolic. With primary metabolic acid-base disorders, the changes in pH and PCO_2 occur in the same direction. With primary respiratory disorders, the changes in pH and PCO_2 occur in opposite directions. The absolute value of the PCO_2 and the change in the pH are then used to determine whether there is a superimposed respiratory or metabolic acid-base disorder as well. The expected compensatory change in PCO_2 for metabolic acidosis is 1.5 $HCO_3 + (8 \pm 2)$. The expected compensatory change in PCO_2 for metabolic alkalosis is 0.7 $HCO_3 + (21 \pm 2)$. If the PCO_2 is normal, higher (respiratory acidosis) or lower (respiratory alkalosis) than the expected value, a superimposed respiratory acid-base disorder is also present. With primary respiratory acid-base disorders, the expected change in pH can be calculated to determine whether a metabolic acid-base disorder is also present. With acute respiratory acidosis, the expected change in pH is $0.008 \times (PCO_2 - 40)$. With acute respiratory alkalosis, the expected change in pH is $0.008 \times (40 - PCO_2)$. If the change in pH exceeds 0.008 times the change in PCO_2, a superimposed metabolic acid-base disorder exists. In addition, with chronic (fully compensated) respiratory disorders, the change in pH is 0.003 times the change in PCO_2. In question 96, the values are consistent with an acute respiratory acidosis without renal compensation. Question 97 represents metabolic alkalosis with partial respiratory compensation. Question 98 is fully compensated respiratory acidosis. Question 99 is metabolic acidosis with partial respiratory compensation. Question 100 is combined respiratory and metabolic acidosis (Marino, pp. 581–586).

Multidisciplinary Self-Assessment Examination

1. Clinical features of the Brown-Séquard syndrome include all of the following EXCEPT?

- **A.** Contralateral loss of pain and temperature sensation beginning one to two spinal segments below the lesion
- **B.** Ipsilateral loss of proprioception and vibratory sense below the level of the lesion
- **C.** Ipsilateral Horner's syndrome if the lesion is cervical
- **D.** Ipsilateral loss of crude touch below the level of the lesion
- **E.** Ipsilateral loss of sweating below the level of the lesion

2. What is depicted in the photomicrograph below (Figure 8.2Q)?

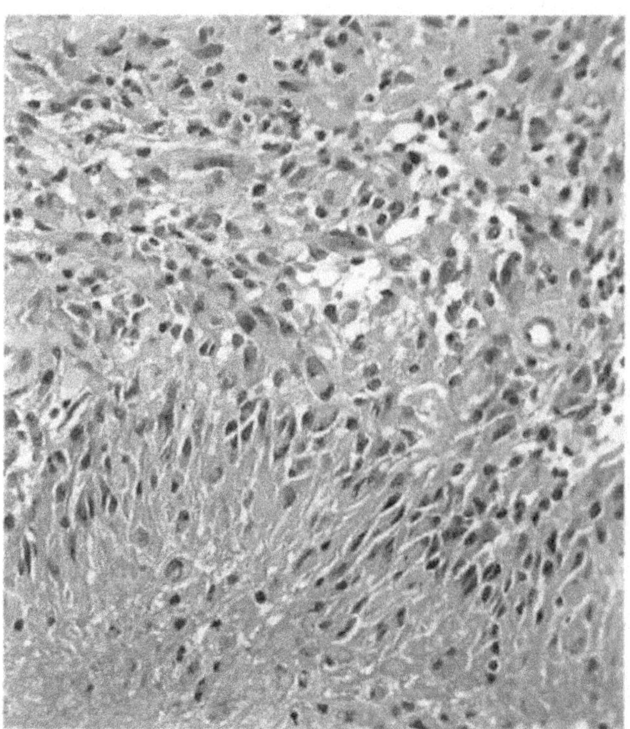

FIGURE 8.2Q

- **A.** Palisading cells around a necrotic region in a patient with glioblastoma
- **B.** Spongiform change in a patient with prion disease
- **C.** Homer-Wright rosette in a 3-year-old male with medulloblastoma
- **D.** Acute infarct in a patient with myoclonic epilepsy with ragged red fibers (MERRF)
- **E.** Fibrinoid necrosis in a patient with acute hemorrhagic leukoencephalopathy

3. What is the most sensitive laboratory test for the detection of neurocysticercosis (NCC)?

- **A.** Peripheral eosinophil count
- **B.** Complete serum white blood cell count
- **C.** Stool for ova and parasites
- **D.** Enzyme-linked immunosorbent assay (ELISA)
- **E.** Electroimmunotransfer blot (EITB)

QUESTIONS 4–9

Directions: Match each of the following spinal cord lesions with the appropriate clinical syndrome (Figure 8.4–8.9Q), using each answer once, more than once, or not at all.

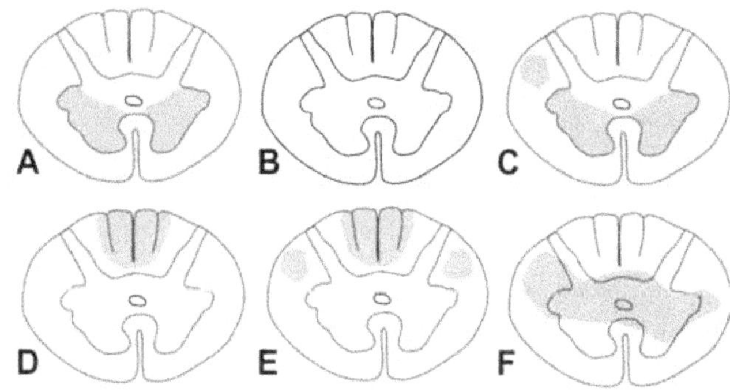

FIGURE 8.4–9Q

4. Early subacute combined degeneration

5. Syringomyelia

6. Tabes dorsalis

7. Poliomyelitis

8. Amyotrophic lateral sclerosis

9. Familial spastic paraplegia

End of set

10. Which of the following tumors may share certain histopathologic features with the lesion depicted below (Figure 8.10Q)?

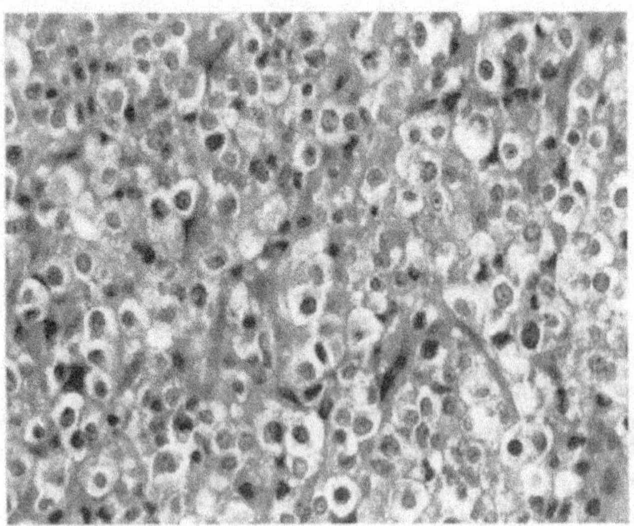

FIGURE 8.10Q

1. Clear cell ependymoma
2. Central neurocytoma
3. Dysembryoplastic neuroepithelial tumor
4. Fibrous meningioma

A. 1, 2, and 3
B. 1 and 3
C. 2 and 4
D. Only 4 is correct
E. All of the above

11. Which of the following abdominal wall layers will best hold suture (highest tensile strength) during placement of a ventriculoperitoneal shunt?

A. Colles fascia
B. Cruveilhier's fascia
C. Buck's fascia
D. Scarpa's fascia
E. Camper's fascia

12. Refer to Figure 8.12Q. What is the diagnosis?

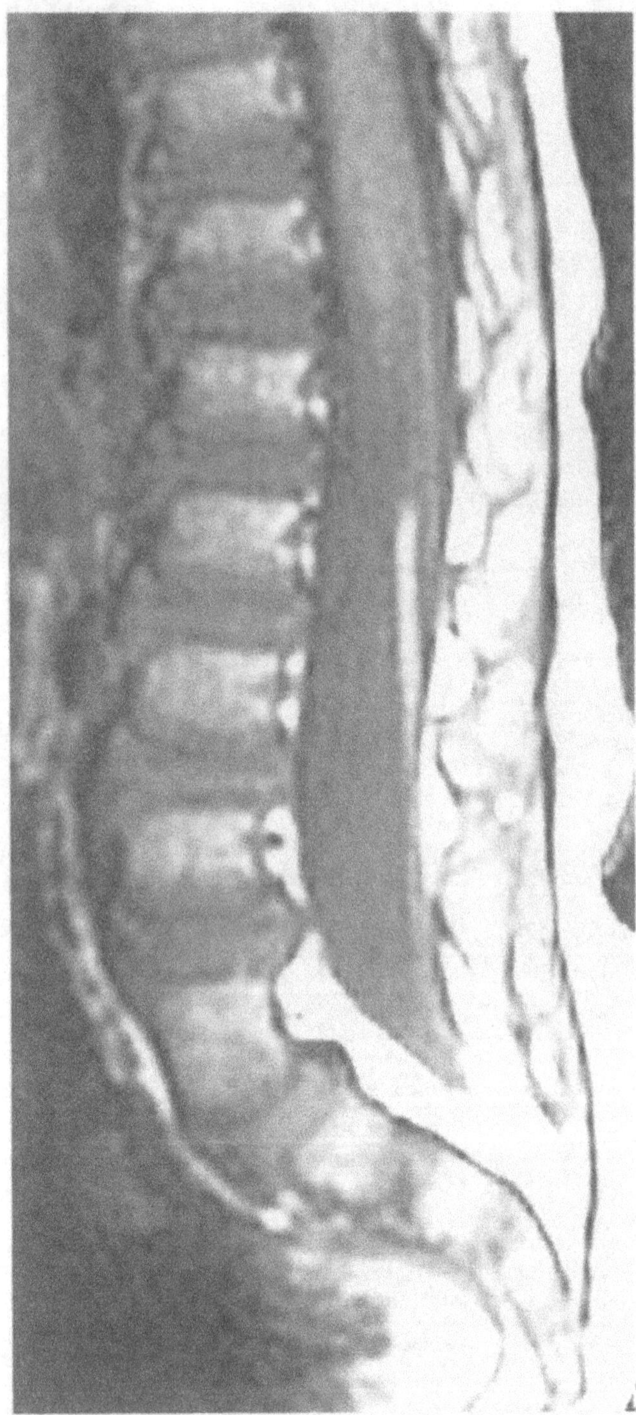

FIGURE 8.12Q

A. Fatty filum with tethered cord
B. Myxopapillary ependymoma
C. Dermal sinus tract
D. Epidural hematoma
E. Dermoid tumor

13. Which of the following is correct about the lesion depicted on the angiogram below (Figure 8.13Q)?

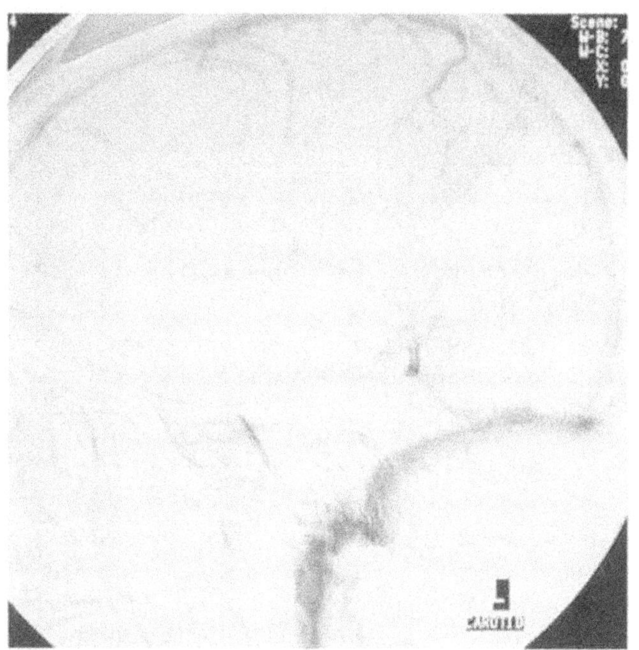

FIGURE 8.13Q

A. Annual risk of bleeding is approximately 3% per year
B. Associated with cranial bruit and congestive heart failure during the neonatal period
C. The loss of a tumor suppressor gene on chromosome 22
D. This lesion is usually found within normal brain parenchyma
E. Represents an extreme anatomic variant of cortical arterial blood supply

14. Which of the following structures are connected by the stria medullaris thalami?

A. Nucleus basalis (of Meynert) and septal nuclei
B. Septal nuclei and habenular nuclei
C. Habenular nuclei and occipital cortex
D. Septal nuclei and anterior thalamic nuclei
E. Pineal gland and anterior commissure

15. Which retinal cell provides a mechanism for mediating opposite responses in adjacent groups of photoreceptor cells that is used to enhance contrast between objects?

A. Plexiform cells
B. Amacrine
C. Horizontal cells
D. Ganglion
E. Bipolar cells

16. What deficit may result from damage to Exner's area?

A. Alexia
B. Aphasia
C. Agraphia
D. Anosmia
E. Apathy

QUESTIONS 17–24

Directions: Match the following structures with the appropriate letterhead on the following axial CT scans (Figures 8.17–8.24Q a, b, c) of the right petrous temporal bone, using each answer only once.

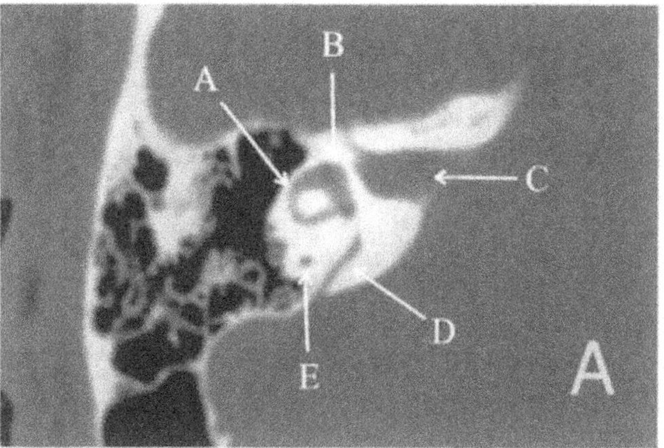

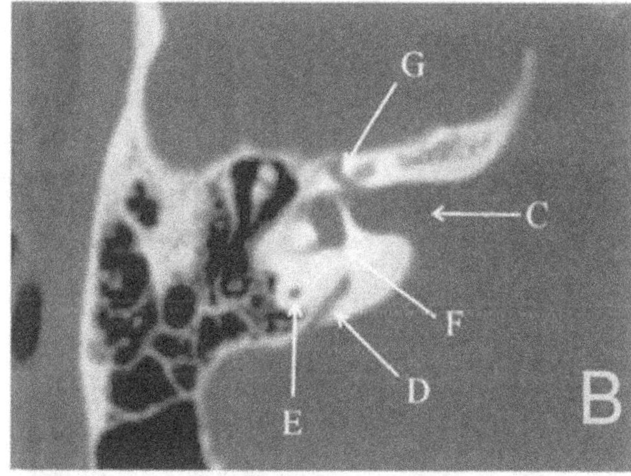

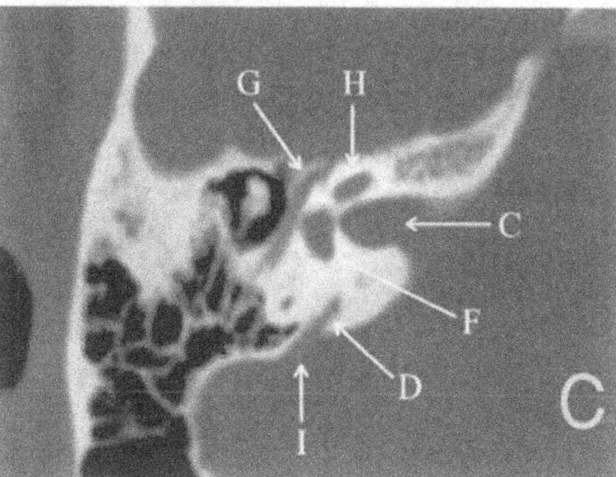

FIGURE 8.17–24Q

17. Vestibule

18. Cochlea

19. Posterior semicircular canal

20. Lateral semicircular canal

21. Vestibular aqueduct

22. Facial nerve

23. Superior semicircular canal

24. Endolymphatic duct

End of set

25. Which of the following is a flow-regulated valve?

    A. Orbis-Sigma valve
    B. PS Medical Delta valve
    C. Cordis horizontal-vertical valve
    D. Codman Hakim programmable valve
    E. Holter-Hausner valve

QUESTIONS 26–27

26. Refer to Figure 8.26–8.27Q. What is the diagnosis?

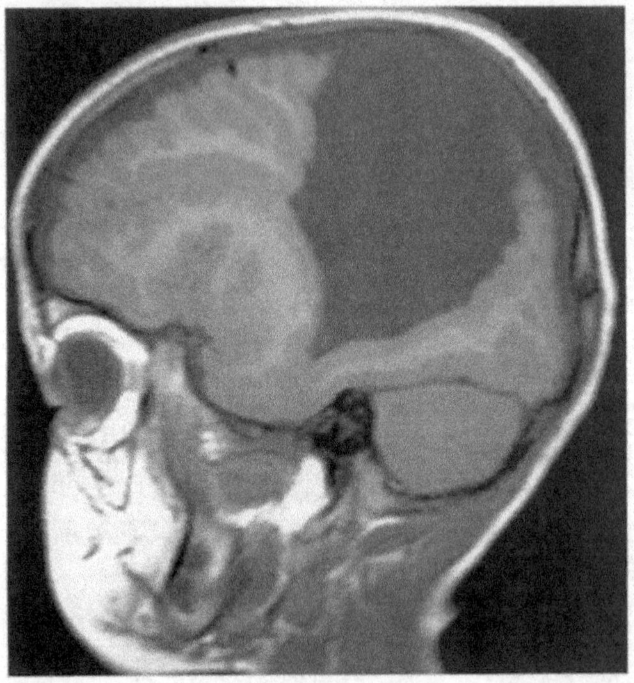

FIGURE 8.26–27Q

    A. Porencephaly
    B. Cortical dysplasia
    C. Open-lip schizencephaly
    D. Arachnoid cyst
    E. Closed-lip schizencephaly

27. This abnormality is believed to result from failure of what embryologic stage of development?

    A. Primary neurulation
    B. Secondary neurulation
    C. Disjunction
    D. Cellular migration
    E. Myelination

End of set

28. All of the following are derived from a common precursor EXCEPT?

    A. ACTH
    B. Melanocyte-stimulating hormone
    C. Beta lipotropin
    D. Beta endorphin
    E. Leucine-enkephalin

29. A 62-year-old female undergoes uncomplicated transsphenoidal resection of a pituitary macroadenoma and is recovering in the intensive care unit. Postoperatively, she develops increased thirst, nausea, elevated urine output (> 300 mL for 3 consecutive hours), hypernatremia (149 mEq/L), and a serum osmolarity of 323 mEq/L. At this point, optimal treatment for this patient should include what?

    A. Fludrocortisone acetate
    B. Urea
    C. Oral desmopressin acetate (DDAVP)
    D. Arginine vasopressin (aqueous Pitressin) intravenously
    E. Pitressin in tannic oil suspension intramuscularly

30. What is depicted on the EEG below (Figure 8.30Q)?

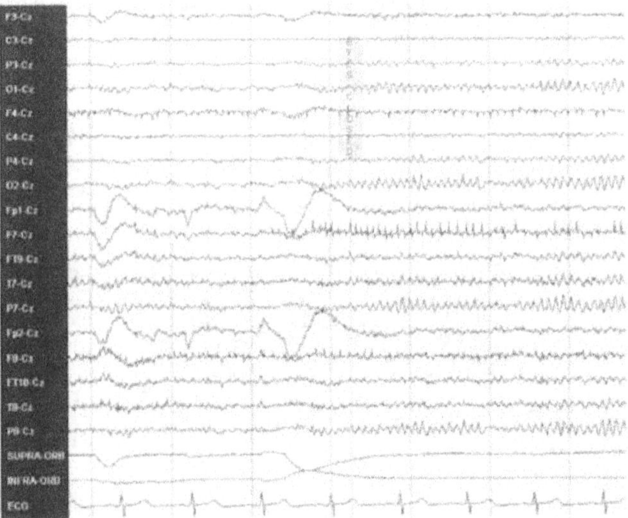

FIGURE 8.30Q

    A. Absence seizure
    B. Left temporal lobe spike-and-wave discharges
    C. Alpha rhythm
    D. Theta rhythm
    E. K complexes

31. A 54-year-old female awakens from surgery for an elective right ophthalmic artery aneurysm clipping with complete right eye blindness and no other neurologic deficit. A cerebral angiogram reveals incorporation of the ophthalmic artery origin into the clip construct. What other finding(s) may be present on the angiogram?

- **A.** Occlusion of the right internal carotid artery with inadequate posterior or anterior communicating artery collaterals
- **B.** Vasospasm of the right internal carotid artery
- **C.** Poor collateral filling of the right globe from the maxillary and facial arteries
- **D.** Inadequate ascending pharyngeal artery collateral flow to the right globe
- **E.** All of the above

QUESTIONS 32–33

32. A 28-year-old obese male presents with a 2-month history of headaches and diplopia. He is found to harbor the lesion depicted in the photomicrograph below (Figure 8.32–8.33Q). What should be the next course of treatment after surgical resection of this lesion?

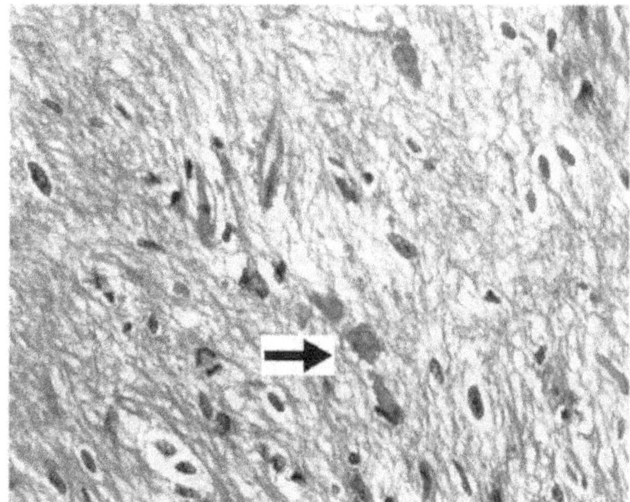

FIGURE 8.32–33Q

- **A.** Whole-brain radiation therapy
- **B.** Radiosurgery
- **C.** Chemotherapy
- **D.** Observation and serial MRI
- **E.** Proton-beam radiotherapy

33. What does the arrow in this photomicrograph depict?

- **A.** Capillary telangiectasia
- **B.** Gemistocytes
- **C.** Rosenthal fibers
- **D.** Normal blood vessels
- **E.** Melanin granules

End of set

34. An infant is able to transfer objects from hand to hand, bear some of his weight, lift his head off the table prior to being pulled up, and turn his head to voice. What is the approximate age of this child?

- **A.** 2 months
- **B.** 4 months
- **C.** 6 months
- **D.** 8 months
- **E.** 10 months

35. All of the following reflexes generally disappear by 4 to 6 months of age EXCEPT?

- **A.** Suck
- **B.** Palmar grasp
- **C.** Tonic neck
- **D.** Ventral suspension (Landau)
- **E.** Placing/stepping

QUESTIONS 36–37

36. What is the earliest visual field cut experienced by patients with ophthalmic artery aneurysms?

- **A.** Monocular inferior temporal quadrantanopsia
- **B.** Monocular superior temporal quadrantanopsia
- **C.** Monocular superior nasal quadrantanopsia
- **D.** Binocular inferior nasal quadrantanopsia
- **E.** Binocular temporal hemianopsia

37. Which of the following structures are usually either drilled or sectioned during surgical exposure of large ophthalmic artery aneurysms?

- **1.** Falciform ligament
- **2.** Distal dural ring
- **3.** Anterior clinoid process
- **4.** Optic strut

- **A.** 1, 2, and 3 are correct
- **B.** 1 and 3 are correct
- **C.** 2 and 4 are correct
- **D.** Only 4 is correct
- **E.** All of the above

End of set

38. A 42-year-old right-handed male presents to an emergency department with seizures. His CT and MRI studies show a fairly well circumscribed, heterogenously enhancing right frontal lesion with patchy calcification and surrounding edema suggestive of an oligodendroglioma. All of the following are true about this tumor EXCEPT?

- **A.** The polypeptide glial fibrillary acidic protein (GFAP) is not expressed by oligodendrocytes
- **B.** They account for approximately 5% of all primary intracranial neoplasms
- **C.** Identifying the oligodendroglial component on frozen section is usually facilitated by the classic "fried egg" appearance of the perinuclear halo
- **D.** The greater the degree of anaplasia, the shorter the survival
- **E.** There is a strong association between response to PCV (procarbazine, CCNU, and vincristine) chemotherapy and allelic loss on 1p/19q in anaplastic oligodendrogliomas

39. Which of the following structures contains second-order neurons of the spinocerebellar tracts?

    A. Clarke's nucleus
    B. Nucleus gracilis/cuneatus
    C. Accessory cuneate nucleus
    D. Inferior olives
    E. Both A and C

40. Where is the cortical representation of macular vision?

    A. Occipital poles
    B. Lower bank of the calcarine sulcus
    C. Temporoparieto-occipital junction
    D. Precuneus
    E. Superior bank of calcarine sulcus

41. What is the first site of binaural convergence within the auditory pathway?

    A. Dorsal cochlear nuclei
    B. Lateral lemniscus
    C. Superior olive
    D. Medial geniculate bodies
    E. Inferior colliculi

42. A 42-year-old male underwent a therapeutic interventional neuroradiologic procedure. What is depicted on his angiogram below (Figure 8.42Q)?

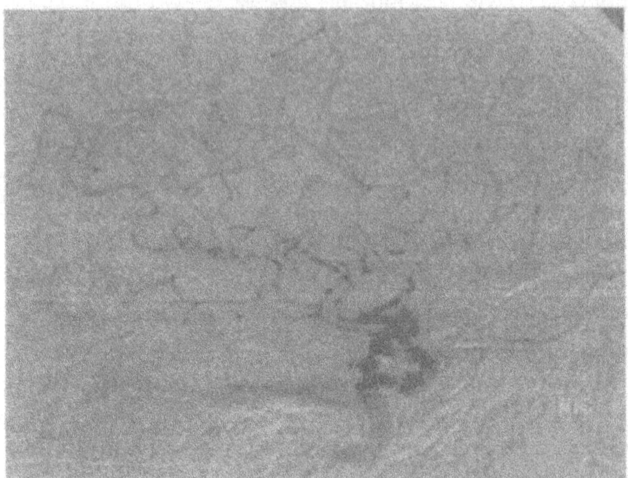

FIGURE 8.42Q

    A. Intraprocedural aneurysmal rupture
    B. Poor distal middle cerebral artery perfusion
    C. An enlarged tentorial artery supplying a lateral pontine arterial-venous malformation
    D. A dural arterial-venous fistula
    E. Type II carotid-cavernous fistula

43. What is depicted on the ECG below (Figure 8.43Q)?

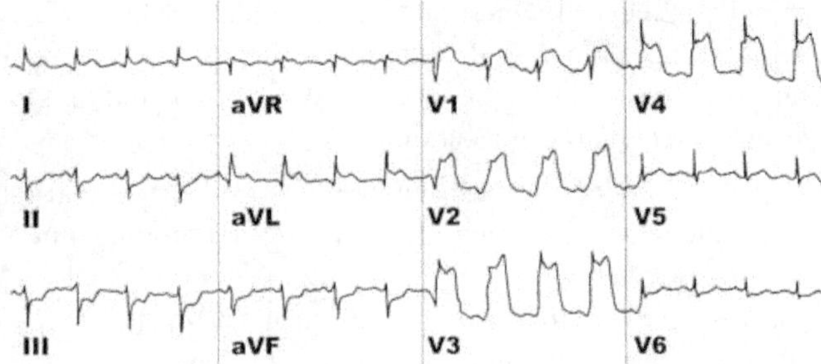

FIGURE 8.43Q

    A. Myocardial infarction
    B. Hyperkalemia
    C. Torsades de pointes
    D. Digoxin toxicity
    E. Atrial flutter

QUESTIONS 44–45

Scenario: A 16-year-old male with the MRI depicted below (Figure 8.44–8.45Q) is referred to your office for surgical evaluation. His laboratory studies reveal that he has hypothyroidism, cortisol deficiency, and a prolactin level of 69. His family states that they have noted behavior changes and a recent increase in his weight. He has no vision with the left eye and a dense temporal field cut of the right eye.

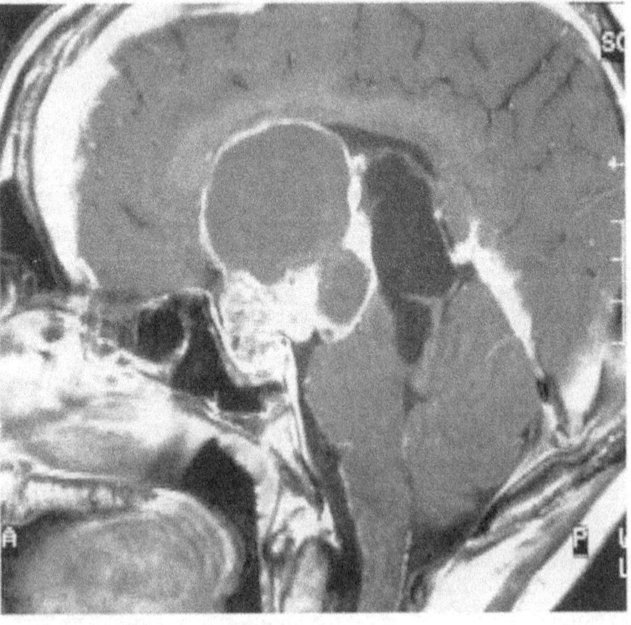

FIGURE 8.44–45Q

44. What is the most likely diagnosis?

    A. Pituitary macroadenoma
    B. Metastatic tumor invading the posterior pituitary gland
    C. Craniopharyngioma
    D. Sphenoid sinusitis
    E. Invasive mucocele of the sphenoid sinus

45. The prolactin level is elevated most likely secondary to what process?

   A. Hook effect
   B. Stalk effect
   C. Avengaard effect
   D. Tumor secretion
   E. Prolactin-secreting lung nodule

End of set

46. All of the following are typically associated with Behçet's syndrome EXCEPT?

   A. Uveitis
   B. Genital ulcers
   C. Aphthous stomatitis
   D. Arthritis
   E. Elevation of serum angiotensin-converting enzyme

QUESTIONS 47–51

Directions: Match the following questions with the associated EMG finding, using each answer only ONCE.

   A. Myasthenia gravis
   B. Lambert-Eaton syndrome
   C. Polymyositis
   D. Carpal tunnel syndrome
   E. Myotonia
   F. None of the above

47. Postexercise facilitation

48. Decremental motor response

49. "Dive bomber" frequency

50. Myopathic motor units, fibrillation, pseudomyotonia

51. Sensory > motor latencies

End of set

QUESTIONS 52–54

52. A 13-year-old boy with a lytic skull lesion presents with diabetes insipidus and the coronal MRI depicted below (Figure 8.52–8.54Q). What is the most likely diagnosis?

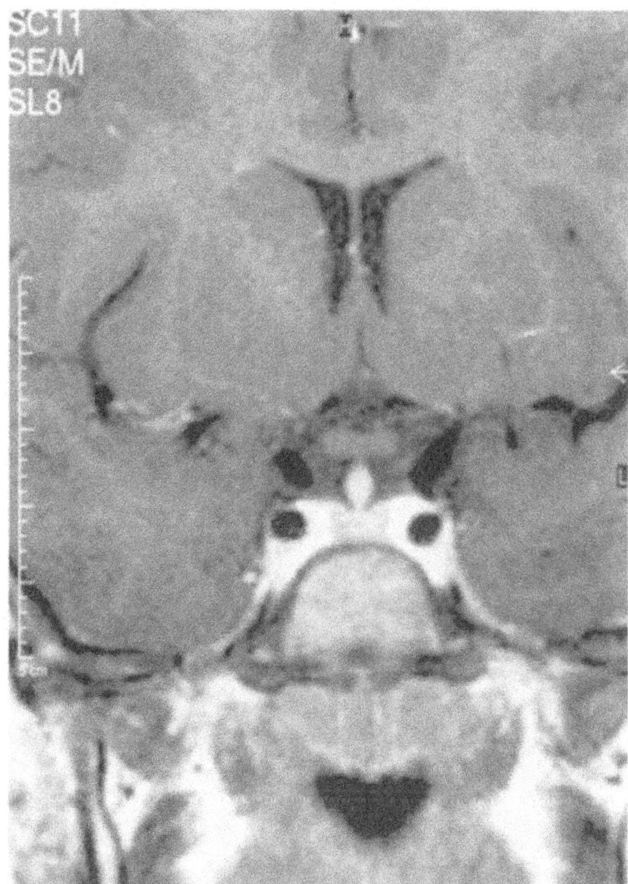

FIGURE 8.52–54Q

   A. Granular cell tumor
   B. Sarcoidosis
   C. Pituitary adenoma
   D. Langerhans' cell histiocytosis
   E. Germinoma

53. This disorder is marked by proliferation of what cell type?

   A. Fibroblasts
   B. T-cell lymphocytes
   C. Antigen-presenting dendritic cells
   D. Eosinophils
   E. Cells derived from Rathke's pouch

54. A pathognomonic finding of this condition on microscopy includes the presence of

- **A.** Birbeck granules
- **B.** Junctional complexes
- **C.** Cholesterol crystals
- **D.** Keratohyaline granules
- **E.** Stippled chromatin

End of set

QUESTIONS 55–56

55. What is depicted in the photomicrograph below (Figure 8.55–8.56Q)?

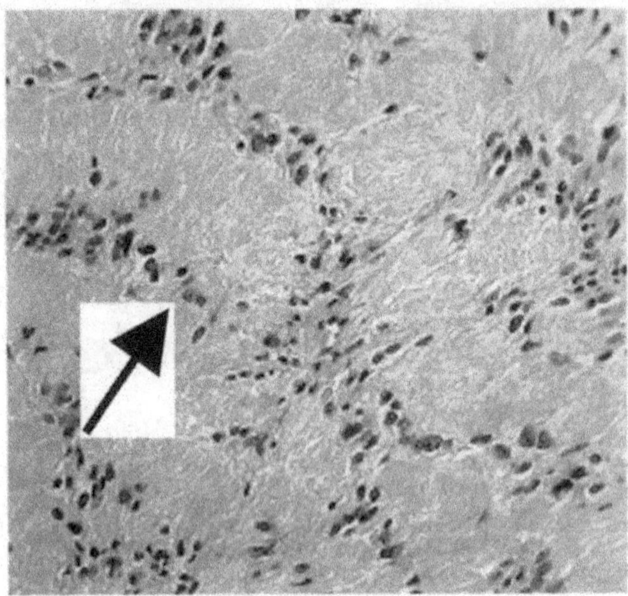

FIGURE 8.55–56Q

- **A.** Neurofibroma
- **B.** Transitional meningioma
- **C.** Acoustic neuroma
- **D.** Pilocytic astrocytoma
- **E.** Pleomorphic xanthoastrocytoma

56. What does the arrow depict?

- **A.** Verocay body
- **B.** Whorls
- **C.** Psammoma body
- **D.** Pseudopalisading
- **E.** Antoni B area

End of set

57. When a patient cannot adduct the right eye in attempting to look to the left but the eye adducts on convergence, the lesion is most likely in what location?

- **A.** Right medial longitudinal fasciculus
- **B.** Left medial longitudinal fasciculus
- **C.** Left abducens nucleus
- **D.** Right abducens nucleus
- **E.** Nucleus of cranial nerve III

QUESTIONS 58–63

Directions: Match the following peripheral nerve injuries with the appropriate hand abnormality (Figure 8.58–8.63Q), using each answer once, more than once, or not at all.

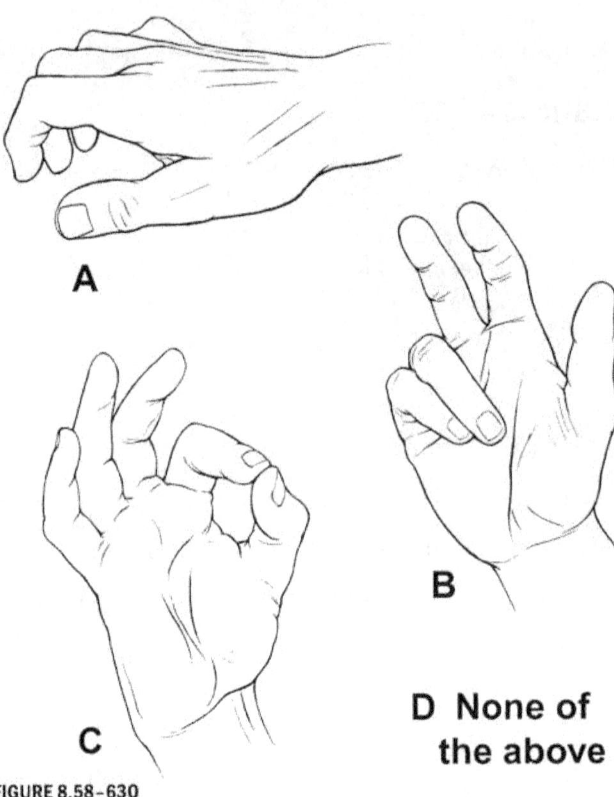

FIGURE 8.58–63Q

58. Injury of the median nerve at the level of the elbow

59. Injury of the ulnar nerve at the elbow

60. Injury of the ulnar nerve at the wrist

61. Anterior interosseous nerve injury

62. Klumpke's paralysis

63. C8 root lesion

End of set

QUESTIONS 64–69

Directions: Match each of the following lesion sites with the associated clinical deficit.

- **A.** Dressing apraxia
- **B.** Writing apraxia
- **C.** Speech apraxia
- **D.** Gait apraxia
- **E.** Prosopagnosia
- **F.** Astereognosis
- **G.** None of the above

64. Posterior end of the inferior frontal gyrus

65. Left angular gyrus

66. Posterior part of right parietal lobe

67. Diffuse cerebral disease

68. Medial inferior temporo-occipital region

69. Either parietal lobe

End of set

70. Where do afferent axons serving the muscle stretch reflex synapse?

- **A.** Dorsal root ganglia
- **B.** Dorsal horn neurons
- **C.** Ventral motoneuron
- **D.** Clarke's nucleus
- **E.** Rexed lamina III

71. A 35-year-old construction worker fell from a three-story building while at work and suffered a complete spinal cord injury at the C2 level. Which of the following functions may be preserved after a complete spinal cord injury at this level?

1. Micturition	**A.** 1, 2, and 3 are correct
2. Ejaculation	**B.** 1 and 3 are correct
3. Peristalsis	**C.** 2 and 4 are correct
4. Breathing	**D.** Only 4 is correct
	E. All of the above

72. A 15-year-old-girl sees her physician for a physical examination prior to the start of soccer season. The physician notices that the palate fails to elevate on the left side when the patient says "Ah." What other associated deficits may be seen in this patient?

1. Swallowing	**A.** 1, 2, and 3
2. Phonation	**B.** 1 and 3
3. Taste	**C.** 2 and 4
4. Salivation	**D.** Only 4 is correct
	E. All of the above

QUESTIONS 73–80

Directions: Match each of the spinal cord tracts with the appropriate clinical correlate (Figure 8.73–8.80), using each answer once, more than once, or not at all. Major ascending tracts are depicted on the left, while descending tracts are shown on the right.

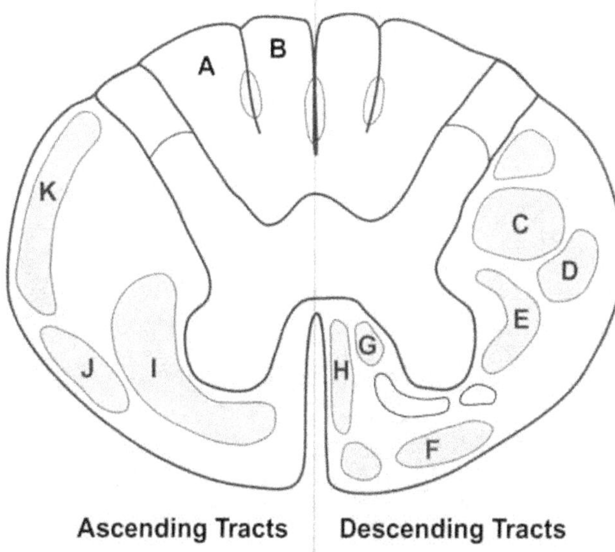

FIGURE 8.73–80Q

73. Small peripheral myelinated fibers of this pathway synapse in the substantia gelatinosa of the dorsal horn

74. These fibers pass through the superior cerebellar peduncle

75. This tract arises from Dieter's nucleus

76. Conscious proprioception from the legs is mainly transmitted in this tract

77. Carries fibers from medial and inferior vestibular nuclei, tectospinal tract, and interstitial nucleus of Cajal

78. Fibers from this tract originate from layer V of the cerebral cortex

79. Carries fibers that ascend to either the thalamus, periaqueductal gray, reticular formation, or superior colliculus

80. Uncrossed pyramidal fibers mainly supplying the axial musculature

End of set

81. Facial nerve displacement by an acoustic neuroma is most commonly (in decreasing order of frequency) in what direction?

- **A.** Inferior, followed by anterior, superior, and posterior
- **B.** Anterior, followed by superior, inferior, and posterior
- **C.** Anterior, followed by inferior, superior, and posterior
- **D.** Posterior, followed by anterior, inferior, and rarely superior
- **E.** Superior, followed by inferior, anterior, and posterior

82. Paralysis of pelvic floor muscles, symmetric saddle anesthesia, impaired erection and ejaculation, constipation, and an autonomous neurogenic bladder best describe what spinal cord lesion?

    A. Lesion of the first and second sacral segments
    B. Cauda equina syndrome
    C. Conus medullaris syndrome
    D. Tethered cord syndrome
    E. Syringomyelia

83. The finding depicted on the CT scan below (Figure 8.83Q) is most likely to occur after

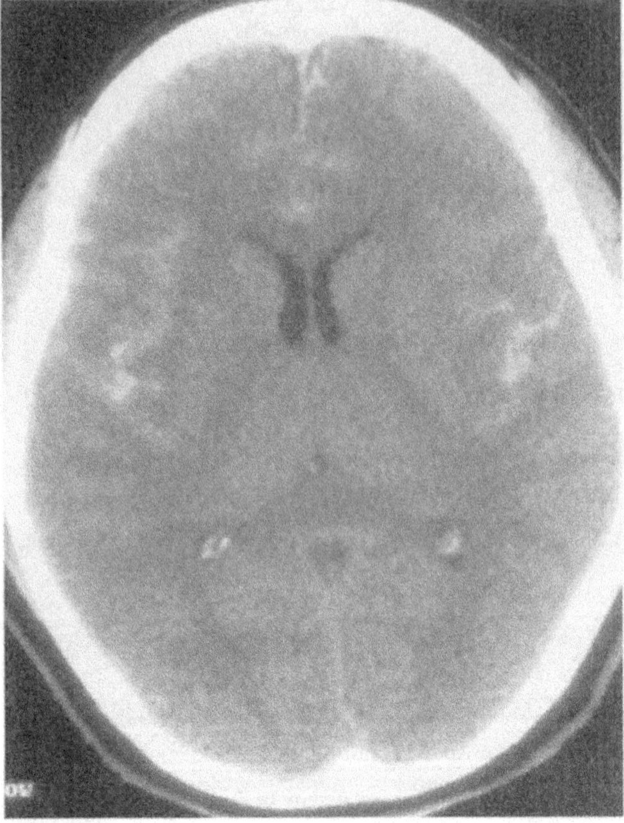

FIGURE 8.83Q

    A. Berry aneurysm rupture
    B. Infection
    C. Extradural carotid artery dissection
    D. Trauma
    E. Contrast administration

84. What is the region of cerebral cortex most closely associated with the conscious perception of smell?

    A. Temporal association cortex
    B. Cingulate gyrus
    C. Limbic system
    D. Orbitofrontal cortex
    E. Amygdala

QUESTIONS 85–86

85. Refer to Figure 8.85–8.86Q. What is the most likely diagnosis?

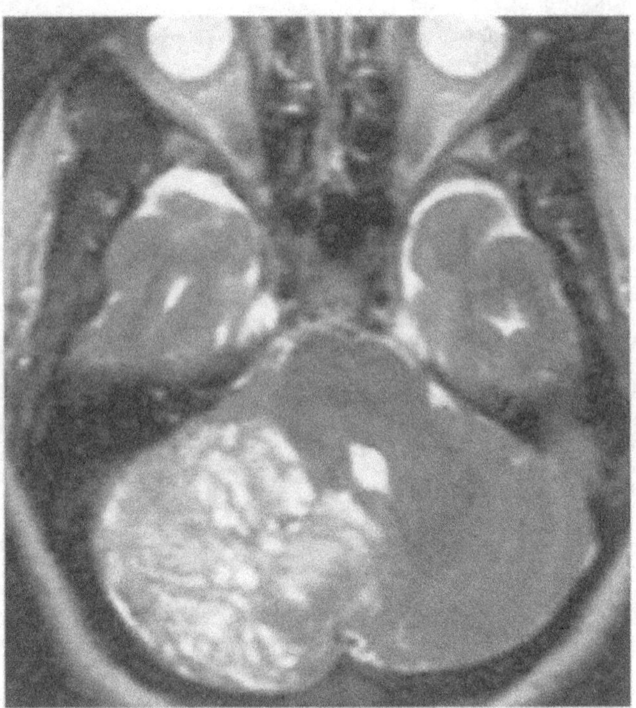

FIGURE 8.85–86Q

    A. Pilocytic astrocytoma
    B. Medulloblastoma
    C. Subacute infarct
    D. Lhermitte-Duclos disease
    E. Ependymoma

86. Which of the following best characterizes this abnormality?

    A. These lesions typically have an abundance of Rosenthal fibers
    B. Most often secondary to vertebral artery occlusion
    C. Hypertrophy of granular-cell neurons and axonal hypermyelination in the molecular layer
    D. Evidence of Homer-Wright rosettes on histopathologic sectioning
    E. Pseudorosettes on histopathologic sectioning

End of set

87. A 42-year-old female presents to the emergency department with staring spells and the T2-weighted MR image depicted below (Figure 8.87Q). What is the most likely diagnosis?

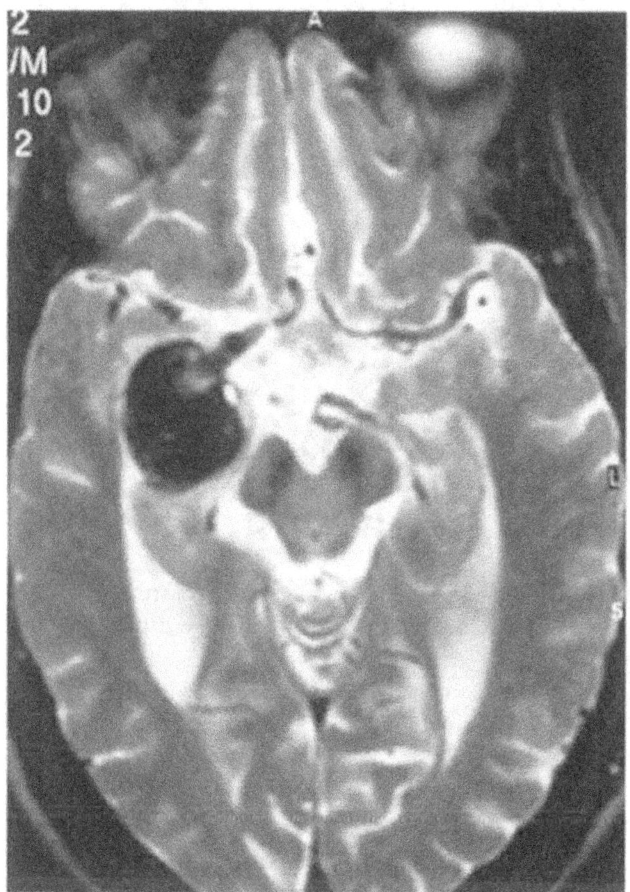

FIGURE 8.87Q

- **A.** Temporal lobe ganglioglioma
- **B.** Dysembryoplastic neuroepithelial tumor
- **C.** Epidermoid cyst
- **D.** Aneurysm
- **E.** Neurocysticercosis

QUESTIONS 88–95

Directions: Match each of the following types of nystagmus with the specific lesion areas, using each answer once, more than once, or not at all.

- **A.** Downbeat nystagmus
- **B.** Upbeat nystagmus
- **C.** Seesaw nystagmus
- **D.** Spasmus nutans
- **E.** Ocular bobbing
- **F.** Ocular flutter
- **G.** Convergence-retraction nystagmus
- **H.** Ocular myoclonus
- **I.** Abducting nystagmus
- **J.** Bruns nystagmus

88. Posterior diencephalon/pretectum (interstitial nucleus of Cajal); suprasellar region

89. Dorsal midbrain

90. Pons (medial longitudinal fasciculus)

91. Central pons

92. Ipsilateral inferior olive, red nucleus, contralateral dentate nucleus (Mollaret triangle)

93. Medulla, ventral tegmentum of pons, cerebellar pathway

94. Cervicomedullary junction

95. Pontomedullary junction, vestibular pathways

End of set

96. A patient suffers a closed head injury after a motor vehicle collision and is noted to have ecchymosis over the right eye, with diplopia when looking down and to the left. The diplopia most likely represents weakness of what muscle?

- **A.** Right superior oblique
- **B.** Left superior rectus
- **C.** Right inferior rectus
- **D.** Left inferior oblique
- **E.** Right inferior oblique

97. The lesion depicted on the photomicrograph below (Figure 8.97Q) may be associated with all of the following EXCEPT?

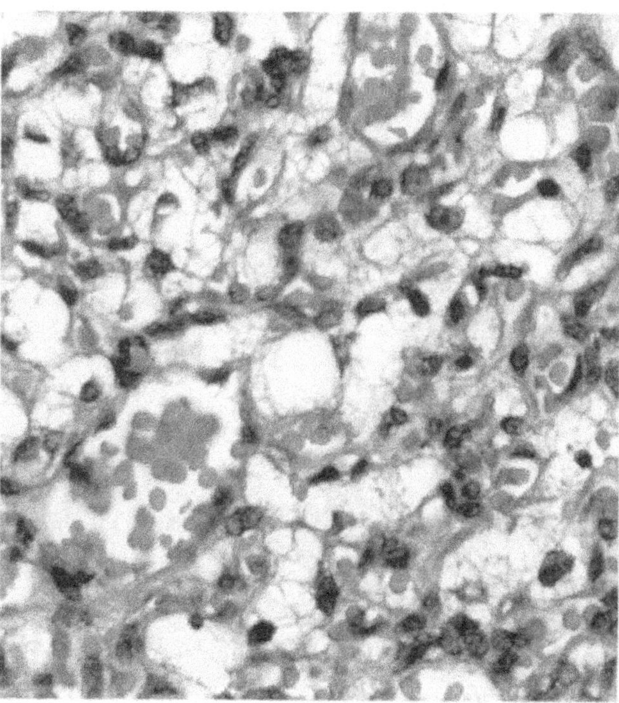

FIGURE 8.97Q

- **A.** Autosomal dominant inheritance
- **B.** Renal cell carcinoma
- **C.** Pancreatic cysts
- **D.** Overproduction of erythropoietin
- **E.** Tumor suppressor gene that maps to chromosome 9p25

QUESTIONS 98–99

Scenario: A 47-year-old female underwent clipping of a ruptured middle cerebral artery bifurcation aneurysm and required a blood transfusion while recovering in the ICU. The patient developed hypotension, fever, confusion, and back pain shortly after receiving the first unit of packed red blood cells (PRBCs).

98. What is the most likely etiology of these findings?

   A. A prior sensitization in a patient who had a non-detectable level of antibody at the time of blood typing
   B. ABO incompatibility
   C. Antileukocyte antibodies in a patient with a prior blood transfusion
   D. Viral contamination of the PRBCs
   E. None of the above

99. What should be the next course of management in this patient's care?

   A. The transfusion should be continued, but hemoglobin and bilirubin levels should be checked
   B. Administer diphenhydramine (25 mg) IV immediately and continue the transfusion
   C. Administer epinephrine (1:1000) 0.5 mg every 10 to 15 minutes until the adverse reaction subsides
   D. The transfusion should be stopped and the patient's blood sent for free hemoglobin, haptoglobin levels, and Coombs' test
   E. Stop the transfusion; administer acetaminophen and diphenhydramine 30 minutes prior to any subsequent blood transfusion

End of set

100. What is the most common intradural spinal cord tumor in patients with neurofibromatosis type II (NF-2)?

   A. Schwannoma
   B. Meningioma
   C. Paraganglioma
   D. Astrocytoma
   E. Ependymoma

101. Destruction of the pyramidal cells of Ammon's horn would most likely produce severe axonal projection loss to what structure?

   A. Subiculum and entorhinal cortex
   B. Premotor cortex
   C. Amygdala
   D. Ventrolateral thalamus
   E. Superior colliculus

102. What is depicted in the photomicrograph below (Figure 8.102Q)?

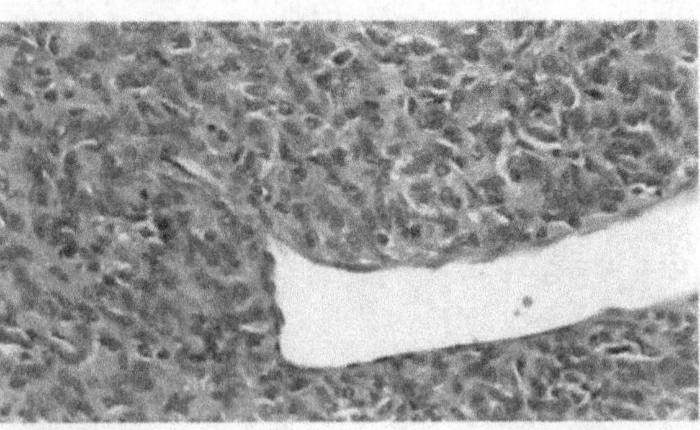

FIGURE 8.102Q

   A. Hemangiopericytoma
   B. Medulloblastoma
   C. Melanoma
   D. Rhabdoid tumor
   E. Germinoma

103. A patient presents to a neurologist with a 2-week history of weakness in the muscles of the lower right face. If this patient was also aphasic, what type of aphasia is most likely to accompany the facial weakness?

   A. Agraphia
   B. Alexia without agraphia
   C. Expressive aphasia
   D. Fluent aphasia
   E. Auditory word agnosia

104. A coronal section through the plane of the genu of the internal capsule would bisect what structure?

   A. Putamen
   B. Globus pallidus
   C. Caudate nucleus
   D. Hypothalamus
   E. Thalamus

105. The lesion depicted below (Figure 8.105Q) most likely originates from what blood vessel?

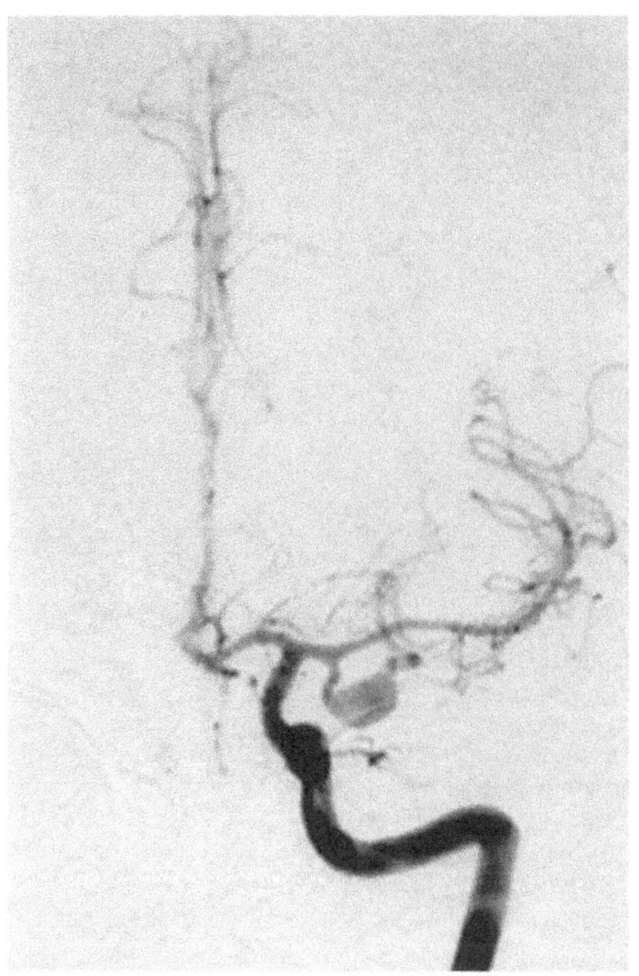

FIGURE 8.105Q

A. Accessory middle cerebral artery
B. Frontopolar artery
C. Anterior temporal artery
D. Posterior temporal artery
E. Lenticulostriate

106. What percentage of patients with subarachnoid hemorrhage secondary to aneurysmal rupture develops angiographic vasospasm at some time during their hospital course?

A. 20%
B. 30%
C. 70%
D. 80%
E. 90%

107. A 43-year-old female presents to your clinic with acromegaly and an MRI revealing a 3-cm pituitary macroadenoma with extension into the right cavernous sinus. The patient has normal vision and a serum growth hormone level after induced hyperglycemia of 220 mg/dL. The most appropriate next step in the management of this patient may include

A. Transsphenoidal surgery
B. Radiosurgery
C. Octreotide
D. Conventional radiation therapy
E. A and C

QUESTIONS 108–116

Directions: Figure 8.108–8.116Q depicts an endoscopic approach to the third ventricle. Match the following anatomic structures to the corresponding letterhead, using each answer either once, more than once, or not at all.

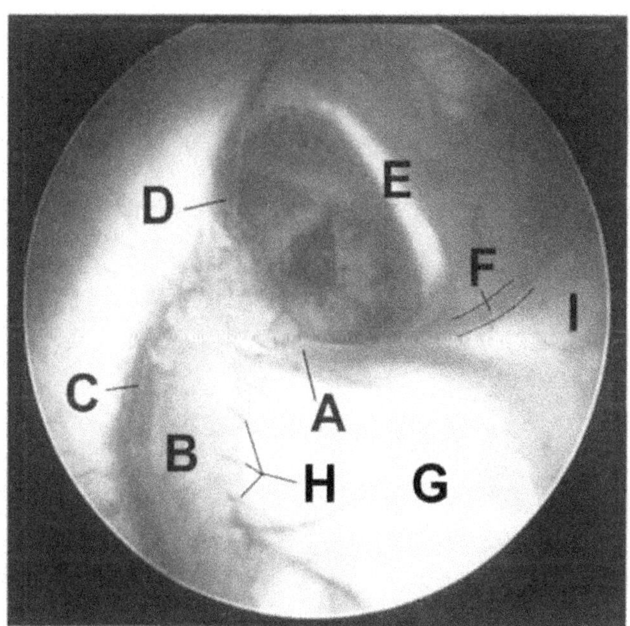

FIGURE 8.108–116Q

108. Thalamostriate vein

109. Septal vein

110. Thalamus

111. Choroid plexus

112. Anterior caudate vein

113. Superior choroidal vein

114. Fornix

115. Superior superficial thalamic veins

116. Caudate nucleus

End of set

117. Injury to the thalamostriate vein during surgery may produce which of the following complications?

1. Drowsiness
2. Hemorrhagic infarct in the basal ganglia
3. Hemiparesis
4. Mutism

A. 1, 2, and 3
B. 1 and 3
C. 2 and 4
D. Only 4 is correct
E. All of the above

118. Characteristic microscopic features of diffuse axonal injury (DAI) 12 to 24 hours after the insult may include

1. Astrogliosis
2. Axonal retraction balls
3. Hemosiderin-laden macrophages
4. Perivascular hemorrhages

A. 1, 2, and 3 are correct
B. 1 and 3 are correct
C. 2 and 4 are correct
D. Only 4 is correct
E. All of the above

119. How far below the iliac crest does the sciatic notch lie?

A. 3 to 4 cm
B. 4 to 5 cm
C. 7 to 8 cm
D. 10 to 12 cm
E. 14 cm

QUESTIONS 120–122

120. The etiology of the abnormality depicted on the MRI scan below (Figure 8.120–8.122Q) is most likely

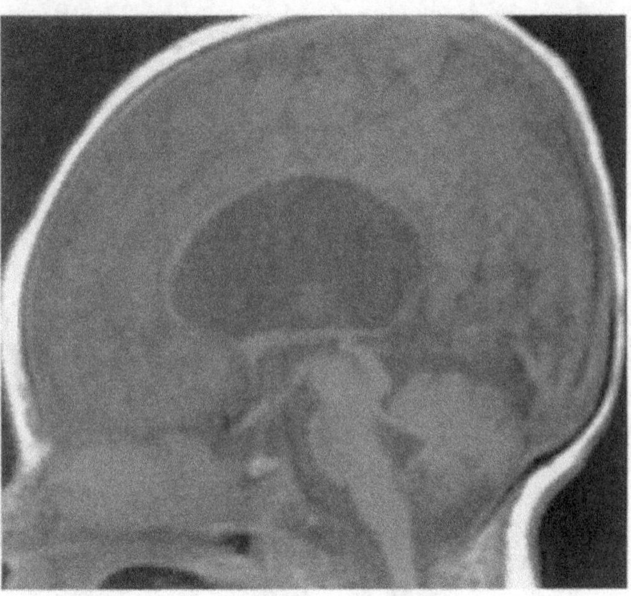

FIGURE 8.120–122Q

A. Iatrogenic
B. Infectious
C. Traumatic
D. Developmental
E. Neoplastic

121. What is the diagnosis?

A. Diffuse axonal injury
B. Obstruction of the aqueduct of Sylvius
C. Meningitis
D. Agenesis of the corpus callosum
E. Obstruction of the foramen of Monro

122. Associated conditions may include all of the following EXCEPT?

A. Schizencephaly
B. Chiari I malformation
C. Dandy-Walker malformation
D. Cephaloceles
E. Azygos anterior cerebral artery

End of set

123. What are the most important ligaments for maintaining atlantoaxial stability?

1. Transverse atlantal ligament (horizontal portion of cruciate ligament)
2. Apical ligament
3. Alar ligaments
4. Inferior band of cruciate ligament

A. 1, 2, and 3 are correct
B. 1 and 3 are correct
C. 2 and 4 are correct
D. Only 4 is correct
E. All of the above

QUESTIONS 124–125

Scenario: A 45-year-old telemarketing agent has noticed a gradual decline in his hearing over the course of a few months and, only recently, some right arm weakness. Physical exam discloses full extraocular motion, symmetric facial movements, a Weber test that lateralizes to the right, a Rinne test revealing bone conduction better than air conduction on the left side, a uvula that deviates slightly to the right, and a tongue that deviates to the left. His MRI is depicted below (Figure 8.124–8.125Q).

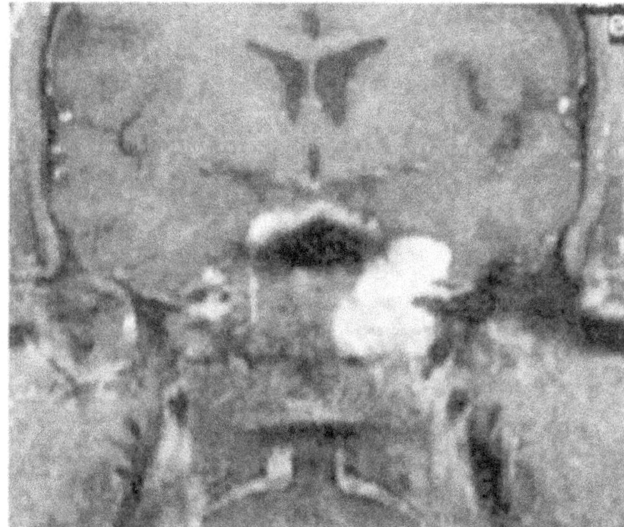

FIGURE 8.124–125Q

124. What is the most likely diagnosis?

A. Foramen magnum meningioma
B. Acoustic neuroma
C. Glomus jugulare tumor
D. Hemangiopericytoma
E. Chordoma

125. The best treatment strategy for this patient wound entail

A. Radiosurgery
B. Proton-beam radiation
C. Observation with serial MRI scans
D. Attempted gross total resection
E. Conventional external-beam radiation

End of set

QUESTIONS 126–127

126. What is the most likely mechanism accounting for the fracture pattern depicted in Figure 8.126–8.127Q)?

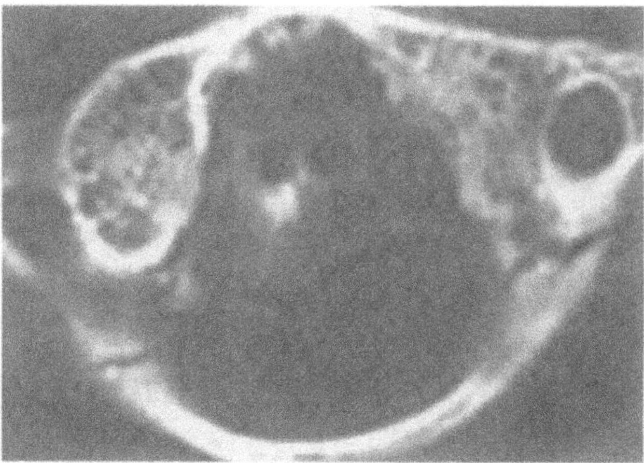

FIGURE 8.126–127Q

A. Direct axial load on a neutral neck
B. Direct axial load on a flexed neck
C. Distraction
D. Direct axial load on a laterally bent neck
E. Hyperextension

127. What amount of C1 lateral mass excursion beyond the axis indicates transverse ligament disruption?

A. 4 mm
B. 5 mm
C. 6 mm
D. 7 mm
E. 9 mm

End of set

QUESTIONS 128–129

128. A lesion of the facial nerve distal to the geniculate ganglion but proximal to the stylomastoid foramen will produce all of the following deficits EXCEPT?

A. Inability to wrinkle the forehead
B. Diminished corneal reflex
C. Impairment of sublingual and submandibular gland secretions
D. Hyperacusis
E. Impaired lacrimation

129. "Crocodile tears" results from aberrant regeneration of what fibers?

A. Parasympathetic fibers that previously projected to the submandibular ganglion may regrow and enter the greater petrosal nerve

B. Parasympathetic fibers that previously projected to the submandibular ganglion may regrow and enter the lesser petrosal nerve

C. Parasympathetic fibers from the Edinger-Westphal nucleus aberrantly project to the greater petrosal nerve

D. Trigeminal nerve fibers that aberrantly project to the superior salivatory nucleus

E. Parasympathetic fibers that previously projected to the lacrimal gland may regrow and enter the lesser petrosal nerve

End of set

130. The mammillothalamic tract contains fibers that project from the medial mammillary nucleus to what structure?

A. Pulvinar
B. Anterior thalamic nucleus
C. Dorsal and ventral tegmental nuclei
D. Centromedian (CM) nucleus of the thalamus
E. Ventral posterior thalamic nucleus

131. Crossed fibers from the fastigial nucleus emerge from the cerebellum through what structure?

A. Fastigial-tectal tract
B. Uncinate fasciculus (of Russell)
C. Juxtarestiform body
D. Middle cerebellar peduncle
E. Fastigial-rubral tract

132. Some excitatory effects of the sympathetic nervous system that lack parasympathetic opposition include

1. Splenic capsule contraction
2. Sweating and piloerection
3. Elevation of the upper eyelid
4. Constriction of the bladder wall

A. 1, 2, and 3 are correct
B. 1 and 3 are correct
C. 2 and 4 are correct
D. Only 4 is correct
E. All of the above

QUESTIONS 133–134

133. What is the most likely mechanism of injury of the abnormality depicted below (Figure 8.133–8.134Q)?

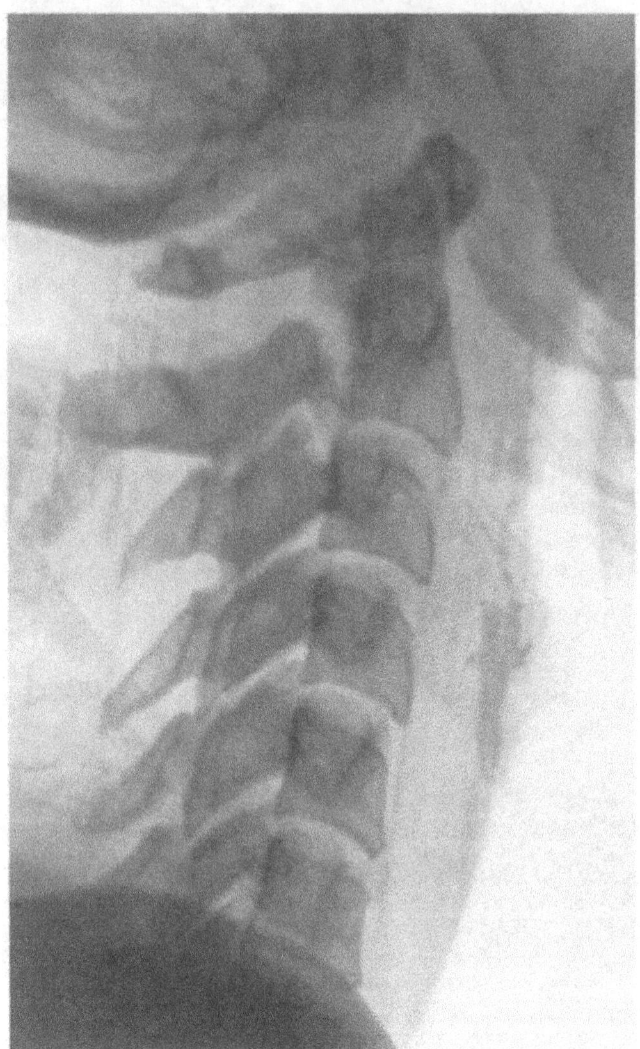

FIGURE 8.133–134Q

A. Hyperextension and axial loading
B. Axial load on a neutral neck
C. Axial loading on a laterally bent neck
D. Severe hyperflexion and axial loading
E. Hyperextension and distraction

134. Therapeutic options may include all of the following EXCEPT?

A. Cervical collar
B. Halo vest immobilization
C. Open reduction with internal fixation (C2 to C3)
D. Odontoid screw
E. SOMI brace

End of set

135. All of the following are associated with Klippel-Feil syndrome EXCEPT?

A. Sprengel's deformity
B. Unilateral absence of a kidney
C. Deafness
D. Scoliosis
E. Naevus flammeus

QUESTIONS 136–139

Directions: Match the fontanelle with the approximate age of closure, using each answer once, more than once, or not at all.

A. 2 to 3 months
B. 1 year
C. 2.5 years
D. None of the above

136. Anterior fontanelle

137. Posterior fontanelle

138. Sphenoid fontanelle

139. Mastoid fontanelle

End of set

140. Blood supply to the dura originates from what arteries?

1. Ophthalmic artery
2. Occipital artery
3. Vertebral artery
4. Maxillary artery

A. 1, 2, and 3 are correct
B. 1 and 2 are correct
C. 2 and 4 are correct
D. Only 4 is correct
E. All of the above

141. How many great vessels originate from the aortic arch?

A. 2
B. 3
C. 4
D. 5
E. 6

142. A 38-year-old female has been complaining of ptosis and intermittent diplopia for approximately 4 months. She has no extremity or respiratory muscle weakness, but antibodies to myofibrillar proteins were found during her workup. All of the following statements about this condition are true EXCEPT?

A. Diagnosis can be confirmed with the administration of edrophonium chloride, which reverses the muscle weakness
B. Single-fiber electromyography (EMG) may show "jitter" and "blocking"
C. Signs of denervation are often seen on standard EMG during the later stages of the disease
D. Antibodies to myofibrillar proteins may precede clinical symptomatology
E. Prednisone, plasmapheresis, and/or IVIG therapy may be used for patients with generalized disease or respiratory crisis

QUESTIONS 143–148

Directions: Match the disorder (mucopolysaccharidosis) with the enzyme abnormality, using each answer once, more than once, or not at all.

A. Hurler
B. Hunter
C. Sanfilippo A
D. Sanfilippo B
E. Morquio A
F. Morquio B
G. Maroteaux-Lamy
H. Sly
I. None of the above

143. Sulfatase B

144. β-Galactosidase

145. Sulfamidase

146. Galactose-6-sulfate sulfatase

147. Iduronate-2-sulfate sulfatase

148. α-L-Iduronidase

End of set

149. Which of the following structures sends the largest number of projections to the striatum?

A. Subthalamic nucleus
B. Cerebral cortex
C. Substantia nigra
D. Cerebellum
E. Spinal cord

QUESTIONS 150–154

Directions: Match each of the following lesion sites with the appropriate clinical picture, using each answer either once, more than once, or not at all.

A. Amygdala
B. Substantia nigra
C. Vicinity of red nucleus
D. Status marmoratus of the corpus striatum and thalamus
E. Subthalamic nucleus

150. Athetosis

151. Rigidity and resting tremor

152. CN III palsy and terminal tremor

153. Klüver-Bucy syndrome

154. Hemiballism

End of set

155. Arteries that supply the thalamus include?

1. Anterior choroidal artery
2. Posterior communicating artery
3. Medial posterior choroidal artery
4. Basilar artery

A. 1, 2, and 3 are correct
B. 1 and 3 are correct
C. 2 and 4 are correct
D. Only 4 is correct
E. All of the above

156. Refer to Figure 8.156Q. What is the most likely diagnosis?

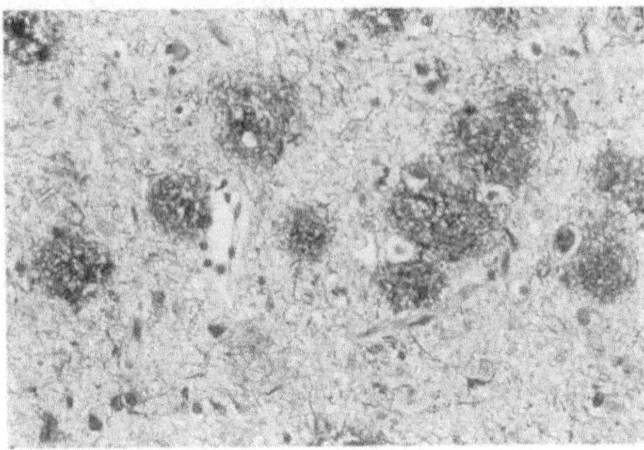

FIGURE 8.156Q

A. Toxoplasmosis
B. Alzheimer's disease
C. Neurocysticercosis
D. *Echinococcus*
E. Spinal cord injury

QUESTIONS 157–164

Directions: Match the cervical spine fracture with the most likely mechanism, using each response once, more than once, or not at all.

A. Axial loading/compression on neutral neck
B. Hyperextension and axial loading
C. Hyperextension and distraction
D. Hyperflexion and axial rotation
E. Hyperflexion and compression
F. Hyperflexion and distraction
G. Hyperflexion
H. Lateral bending and compression
I. None of the above

157. Teardrop fracture

158. Unilateral jumped facet

159. Burst fracture

160. Bilateral facet dislocation

161. Unilateral facet fracture

162. Compression wedge fracture

163. Occipital condylar fracture

164. Odontoid fracture

End of set

165. What is depicted in the photomicrograph below (Figure 8.165Q)?

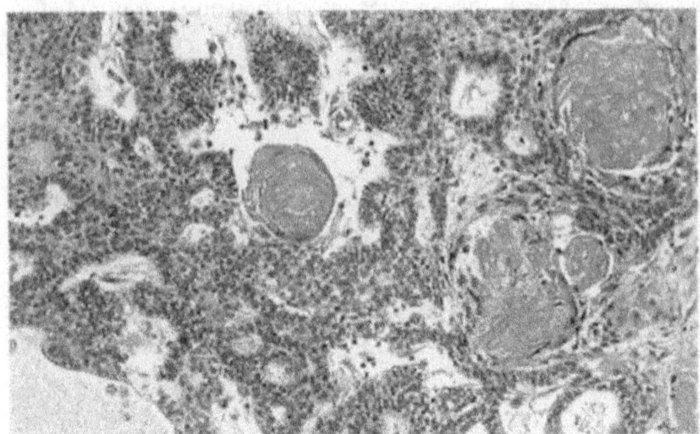

FIGURE 8.165Q

A. Choroid plexus papilloma
B. Ependymoma
C. Adamantinomatous craniopharyngioma
D. Chordoma
E. Angiomatous meningioma

166. All of the following entities may be considered in the differential diagnosis of vertigo of peripheral origin EXCEPT?

A. Ménière's disease
B. Benign paroxysmal positional vertigo
C. Secondary endolymphatic hydrops
D. Vestibular neuronitis
E. Craniovertebral junction abnormality

167. Primarily branches of what nerve(s) innervate the supratentorial dura?

1. Upper cervical spinal nerves
2. Glossopharyngeal nerve
3. Vagus nerve
4. Trigeminal nerve

A. 1, 2, and 3 are correct
B. 1 and 3 are correct
C. 2 and 4 are correct
D. Only 4 is correct
E. All of the above

QUESTIONS 168–169

168. A wedding singer from your town presents to your office with a 1-week history of neck pain and slight left arm and hand numbness. His MRI is depicted below (Figure 8.168–8.169Q). What is the most likely diagnosis?

(a)

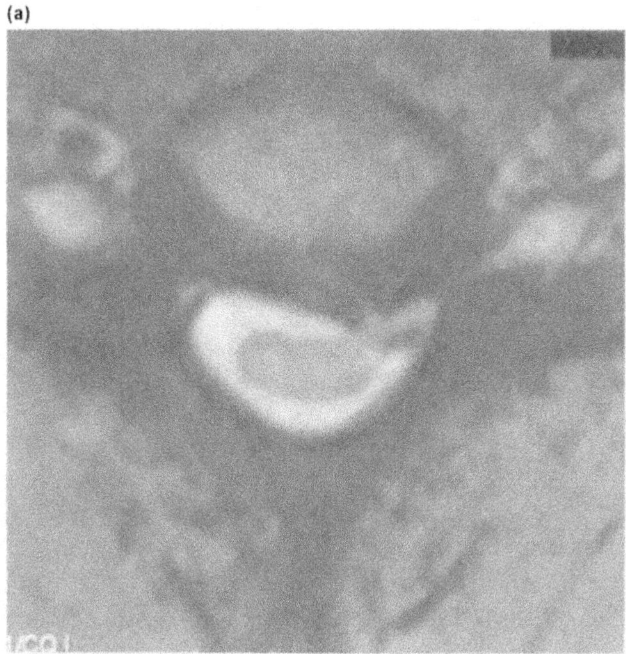

FIGURE 8.168–169Q

- **A.** Synovial cyst
- **B.** Juxtafacet cyst
- **C.** Hypertrophy of the ligamentum flavum
- **D.** Disc herniation
- **E.** Ossification of the posterior longitudinal ligament (OPLL)

(b)

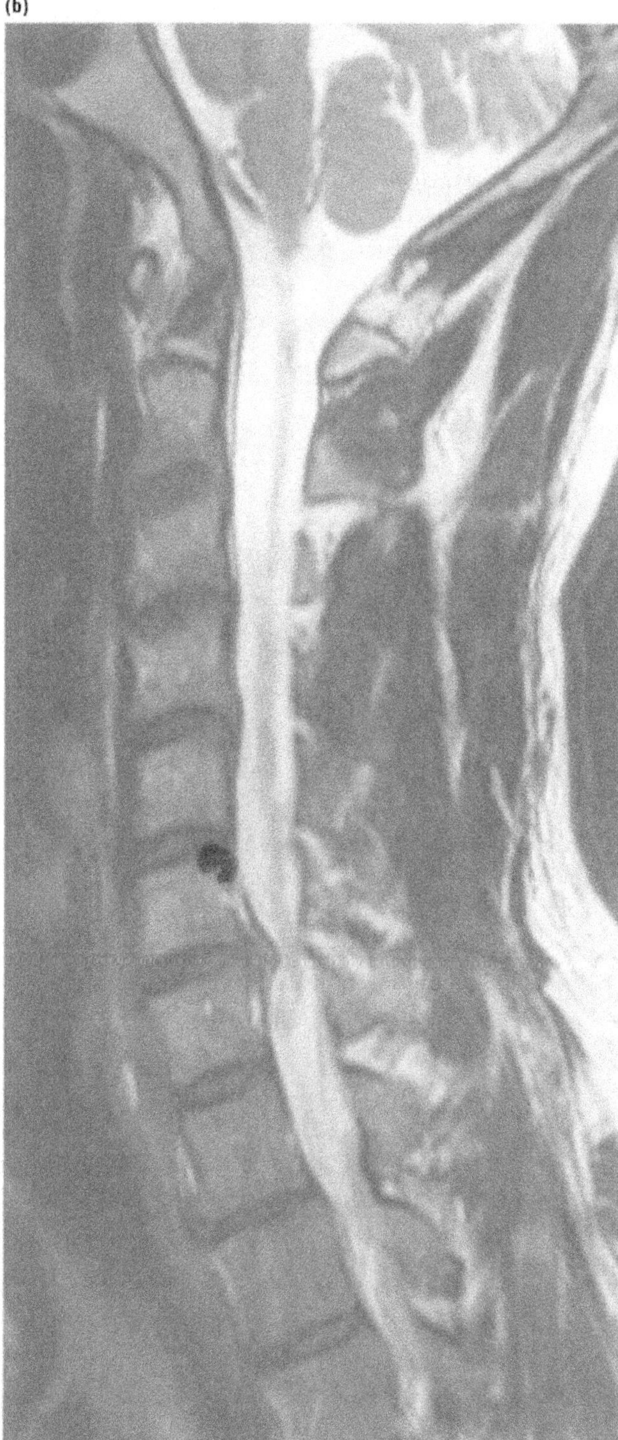

FIGURE 8.168–169Q Continued

169. The patient's symptomatology does not improve after 8 weeks of nonsurgical therapy. He returns to your office to explore surgical options. You inform him that the best surgical option for him should include what procedure, if possible?

    A. Anterior cervical discectomy and fusion
    B. Posterior cervical laminectomy
    C. Posterior keyhole laminotomy
    D. Anterior cervical corpectomy and fusion
    E. Costotransversectomy

End of set

170. Which of the following are associated with yolk sac tumors?

    1. AFP positivity
    2. β-HCG positivity
    3. Schiller-Duval bodies
    4. Placental alkaline phosphatase positivity

    A. 1, 2, and 3 are correct
    B. 1 and 3 are correct
    C. 2 and 4 are correct
    D. Only 4 is correct
    E. All of the above

171. Patients with acromegaly require a meticulous preoperative anesthetic workup because they may often have which of the following clinical findings?

    1. Macroglossia
    2. Elevated angiotensin-converting enzyme
    3. Cardiomyopathy
    4. Nasal telangiectasias

    A. 1, 2, and 3 are correct
    B. 1 and 3 are correct
    C. 2 and 4 are correct
    D. Only 4 is correct
    E. All of the above

172. Huntington's disease primarily affects which projections from the striatum to the external segment of the globus pallidus?

    A. Cholinergic
    B. Adrenergic
    C. GABA/enkephalin
    D. Glutamate
    E. Serotonin

173. What is depicted in Figure 8.173Q?

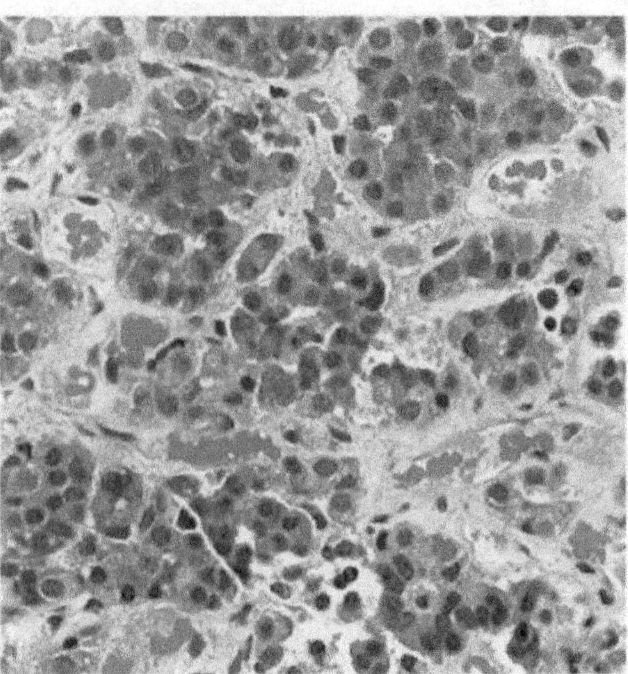

FIGURE 8.173Q

    A. Pleomorphic xanthoastrocytoma
    B. Ependymoma
    C. Choriocarcinoma
    D. Medulloblastoma
    E. Adenohypophysis

174. A newborn infant is diagnosed with Meckel-Gruber syndrome. What is the most likely etiology of this abnormality?

    A. Maternal diabetes
    B. Excessive alcohol consumption by the mother during the third gestational week
    C. Maternal hyperthermia on gestational days 20 to 26
    D. Folate deficiency
    E. None of the above

175. The release of a single quantum of acetylcholine produces what type of postsynaptic response?

    A. Endplate potential
    B. Temporal summation
    C. Spatial summation
    D. Miniature endplate potential
    E. Temporal dispersion

176. Nitric oxide (NO) results in the generation of what second messenger?

- **A.** cAMP
- **B.** cGMP
- **C.** Diacylglycerol (DAG)
- **D.** Inositol 1, 4, 5-triphosphate (IP_3)
- **E.** Protein kinase C

177. Functions of the Golgi complex include all of the following EXCEPT which?

- **A.** N- and O-linked glycosylation
- **B.** Proteoglycan formation
- **C.** Sulfation of arginine residues
- **D.** Attachment of fatty acids to proteins
- **E.** Polysaccharide phosphorylation

178. What is mainly responsible for the high selectivity of the blood-brain barrier (BBB)?

- **A.** Astrocytic foot processes covering fenestrated endothelial cells
- **B.** Tight junctions between nonfenestrated endothelial cells
- **C.** The extensive basal lamina that surrounds endothelial cells
- **D.** The basement membrane, capillary endothelium, and astrocytic foot processes
- **E.** The exclusion of foreign antigens by a superselective neuronal membrane

179. What structure of the brain has the highest concentration of substance P?

- **A.** Thalamus
- **B.** Pineal gland
- **C.** Hypothalamus
- **D.** Substantia nigra
- **E.** Amygdala

QUESTIONS 180–181

180. A 54-year-old male presents to the emergency department with a generalized tonic-clonic seizure and a 6-month history of behavioral changes. His lateral angiogram is depicted below (Figure 8.180–8.181Q). What is the most likely diagnosis?

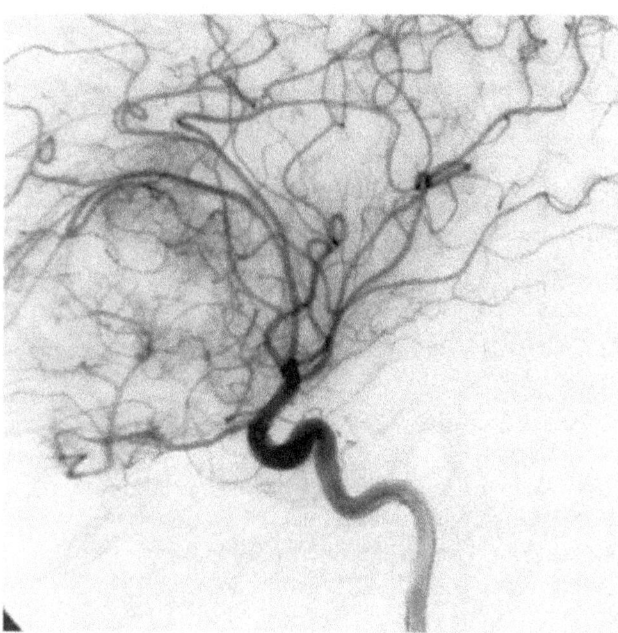

FIGURE 8.180–181Q

- **A.** Hydrocephalus from a third ventricular tumor obstructing the foramen of Monro
- **B.** Glioblastoma
- **C.** Olfactory groove meningioma
- **D.** Craniopharyngioma
- **E.** Arterial-venous malformation

181. The most common blood supply to this lesion originates from what blood vessel(s)?

- **A.** Superior hypophyseal artery
- **B.** Anterior meningeal branches from the maxillary artery
- **C.** Superficial temporal artery
- **D.** Anterior meningeal branches from the cavernous internal carotid artery
- **E.** The anterior and posterior ethmoidal arteries

End of set

QUESTIONS 182–186

Directions: Match the disorder with the most common inheritance pattern, using each answer once, more than once, or not at all.

  A. X-linked recessive
  B. Autosomal dominant
  C. Autosomal recessive

182. Duchenne muscular dystrophy (DMD)

183. Fascioscapulohumeral muscular dystrophy (FSHMD)

184. Myotonic muscular dystrophy (MD)

185. Charcot-Marie-Tooth disease

186. Dejerine-Sottas disease

End of set

187. Which of the following is/are correct about the common peroneal nerve?

  1. Arises from the dorsal divisions of the sacral plexus (L4, L5, S1, and S2)
  2. Begins at the rostral margin of the popliteal fossa
  3. Follows the medial border of the biceps femoris muscle
  4. Leaves the popliteal fossa by passing superficial to the lateral head of the gastrocnemius muscle

  A. 1, 2, and 3 are correct
  B. 1 and 3 are correct
  C. 1 and 4 are correct
  D. Only 4 is correct
  E. All of the above

188. The most common pathology in mesial temporal lobe epilepsy is hippocampal sclerosis. The least amount of damage is usually seen in what sector(s) of the hippocampus?

  A. CA1
  B. CA2
  C. CA3
  D. CA4
  E. A and D are correct

189. All of the following are correct about proximal (type II) renal tubular acidosis EXCEPT?

  A. The proximal renal tubule cannot reabsorb HCO_3^- properly
  B. There is usually low to normal serum K^+
  C. Nephrocalcinosis can accompany this disorder
  D. Urine pH < 6 during periods of acidosis
  E. Often caused by toxic injury to the renal tubules (heavy metals, Bence Jones proteins)

QUESTIONS 190–192

190. What is the diagnosis of the lesion depicted in this photomicrograph (Figure 8.190–8.192Q)?

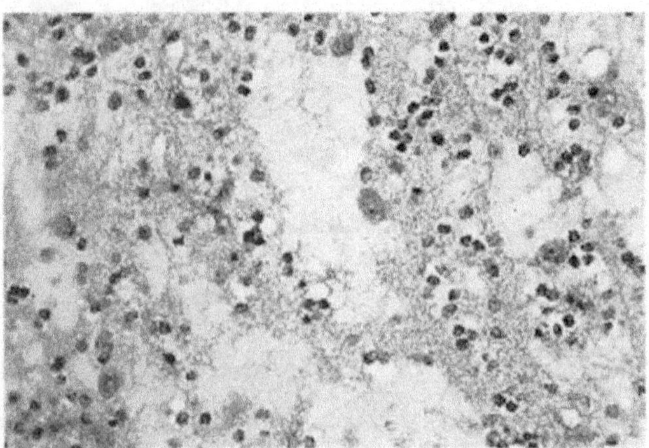

FIGURE 8.190–192Q

  A. Dysembryoplastic neuroepithelial tumor (DNT)
  B. Central neurocytoma
  C. Pleomorphic xanthoastrocytoma (PXA)
  D. Giant cell astrocytoma (GCA)
  E. Chordoid glioma of the third ventricle

191. What is the histologic hallmark of this lesion?

  A. Rosenthal fibers
  B. Alzheimer II astrocytes
  C. Glioneuronal element
  D. Synaptophysin reactivity
  E. Bizarre-appearing nucleated cells

192. Patients harboring this lesion typically present with

  A. Meningitis
  B. Seizures
  C. Hemorrhage
  D. Leptomeningeal dissemination
  E. Hydrocephalus

End of set

193. All of the following may be seen with hypochromic microcytic anemia EXCEPT?

  A. Low mean corpuscular volume (MCV)
  B. Poikilocytosis
  C. Elevated total iron-binding capacity (TIBC)
  D. Early decrease in mean corpuscular hemoglobin concentration (MCHC)
  E. Low serum ferritin

194. The serum level of valproate may increase following the administration of which of the following medications?

1. Phenytoin
2. Clozapine
3. Phenobarbital
4. Ethosuximide

A. 1, 2, and 3 are correct
B. 1 and 3 are correct
C. 2 and 4 are correct
D. Only 4 is correct
E. All of the above

195. All of the following are true about polymyositis and inclusion body myositis (IBM) EXCEPT?

A. IBM is more likely to affect the distal muscles of the legs thin polymyositis
B. IBM is less often seen in association with collagen vascular or autoimmune diseases
C. Polymyositis rarely responds to steroids, whereas IBM may respond in some cases
D. IBM affects older patients
E. Muscle biopsy in patients with IBM demonstrates inflammation and inclusion bodies with "rimmed vacuoles" that contain amyloid

196. All of the following may cause carpal tunnel syndrome EXCEPT?

A. Rheumatoid arthritis
B. Pregnancy
C. Acromegaly
D. Amyloidosis
E. Graves' disease

197. A high school gymnast develops a sudden headache, dizziness, left-sided arm and leg clumsiness, and left facial and right body numbness following a practice session. What is the most likely diagnosis?

A. Labyrinthitis
B. Benign paroxysmal positional vertigo
C. Vertebral artery dissection
D. Complex migraine headache
E. Multiple sclerosis

198. What is the primary ligand that binds to epidermal growth factor receptor (EGFR) in gliomas?

A. Fibronectin
B. Epidermal growth factor (EGF)
C. Tumor growth factor (TGF-α)
D. Vascular endothelial growth factor (VEGF)
E. Fibroblast growth factor (FGF)

199. All of the following neurochemical and cellular mediators may be elevated after severe closed head injury EXCEPT?

A. TNF-α
B. IL-1β
C. IL-6
D. Potassium
E. Magnesium

200. After denervation, the first evidence of fibrillation potentials in human muscle usually occurs how many days after the insult?

A. 5 to 10 days
B. 14 to 21 days
C. 24 to 32 days
D. 42 days
E. 6 months

201. This axial CT scan (Figure 8.201Q) demonstrates

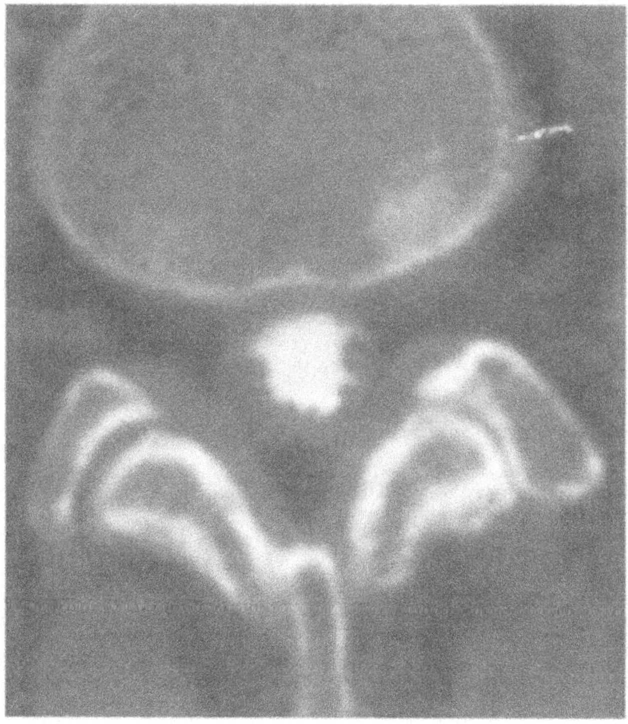

FIGURE 8.201Q

A. Arachnoiditis
B. Hypertrophy of the ligamentum flavum
C. Synovial cyst
D. Laminar fracture
E. Hemangioma

202. Which of the following is/are true about diagnostic studies for neurosarcoidosis?

1. Elevation in IgG and IgG index
2. Elevated angiotensin-converting enzyme levels
3. CNS granulomas on MRI
4. Oligoclonal bands found in CSF

A. 1, 2, and 3 are correct
B. 1 and 3 are correct
C. 2 and 4 are correct
D. Only 4 is correct
E. All of the above

203. The EEG below (Figure 8.203Q) is most consistent with?

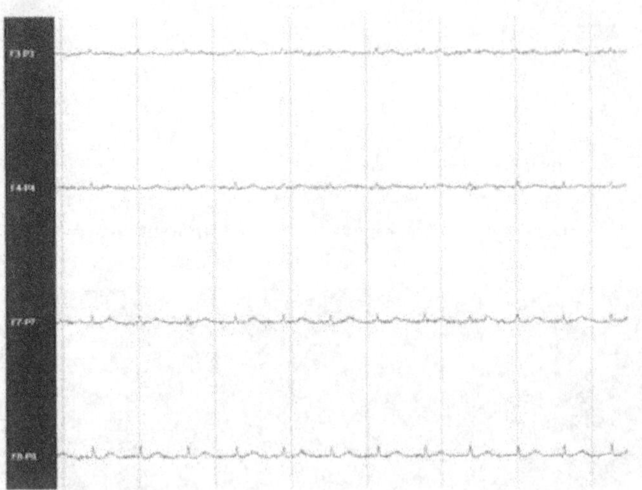

FIGURE 8.203Q

   A. Alcohol intoxication
   B. Left frontal lobe mass
   C. A lethal closed head injury
   D. Hepatic encephalopathy
   E. Delta rhythm

204. What abnormality is depicted on the ECG below (Figure 8.204Q)?

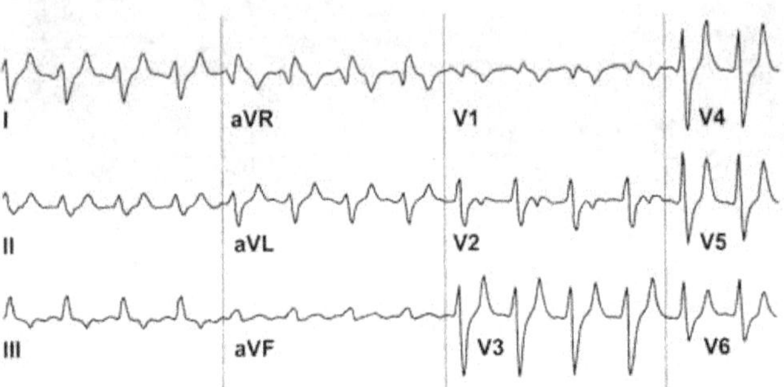

FIGURE 8.204Q

   A. Torsades de pointes
   B. Hyperkalemia
   C. Digoxin toxicity
   D. First-degree heart block
   E. Multifocal atrial tachycardia

QUESTIONS 205–209

Directions: Match the visual field cut (Figure 8.205–8.209Q) with the most likely lesion site.

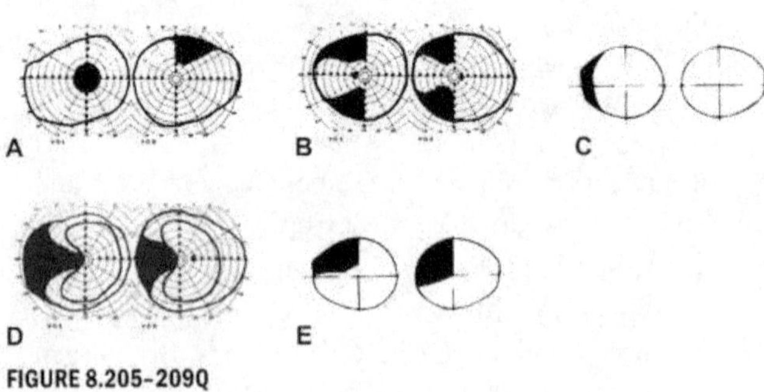

FIGURE 8.205–209Q

205. Temporal lobe

206. Lateral posterior choroidal artery

207. Anterior chiasm

208. Anterior calcarine cortex

209. Anterior choroidal artery

End of set

210. The musculocutaneous nerve controls what muscle actions?

   1. Elbow flexion
   2. Forearm pronation
   3. Forearm supination
   4. Wrist flexion

   A. 1, 2, and 3 are correct
   B. 1 and 3 are correct
   C. 2 and 4 are correct
   D. Only 4 is correct
   E. All of the above

211. Where is the lesion that may cause ipsilateral upper extremity weakness and contralateral leg weakness (cruciate paralysis) most likely located?

   A. Ventrolateral pons
   B. Basis pontis
   C. Posterior internal capsule
   D. Cervicomedullary junction
   E. Ventral lateral pons

QUESTIONS 212–213

212. Refer to Figure 8.212–8.213Q. What is the diagnosis?

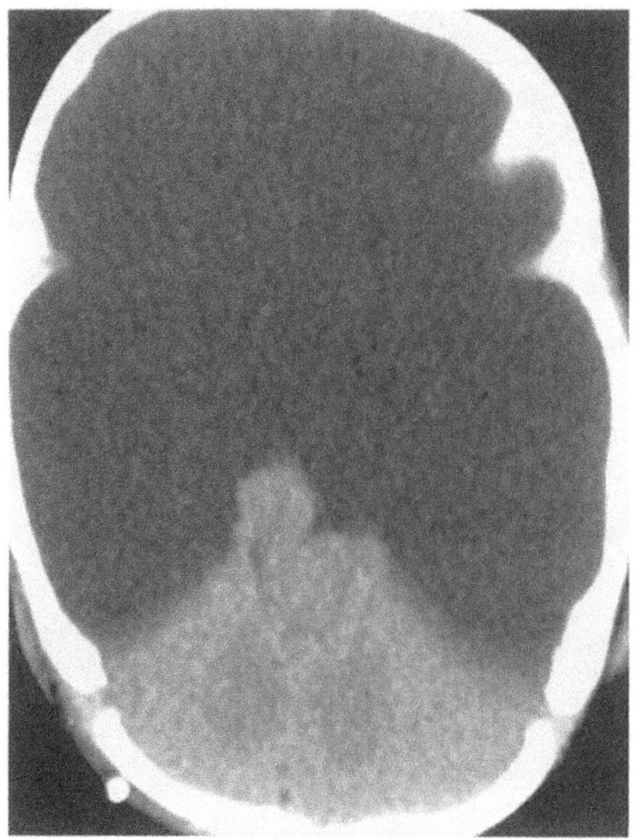

FIGURE 8.212–213Q

A. Alobar holoprosencephaly
B. Lobar holoprosencephaly
C. Hydranencephaly
D. Severe hydrocephalus
E. Anencephaly

213. What is the most likely etiology of this finding?

A. Obstructive hydrocephalus
B. Failure of disjunction
C. Disorder of cellular migration
D. Bilateral in utero disruption of the anterior circulation
E. Failure of neural tube closure

End of set

214. Diagnostic peritoneal lavage (DPL) is relatively fast, safe, and reliable for patients with blunt injury and stab wounds to the anterior abdominal wall. This diagnostic procedure is considered positive with all of the following EXCEPT?

A. Greater than 10 mL of gross blood is aspirated from the abdomen
B. Microscopic evaluation of fluid aspirate reveals > 100,000/mm^3 of red blood cells
C. Greater than 500/mm^3 white blood cells
D. Presence of bile or particulate matter in aspirate
E. An amylase level that is less than the normal serum level

215. What is depicted by the photomicrograph below (Figure 8.215Q)?

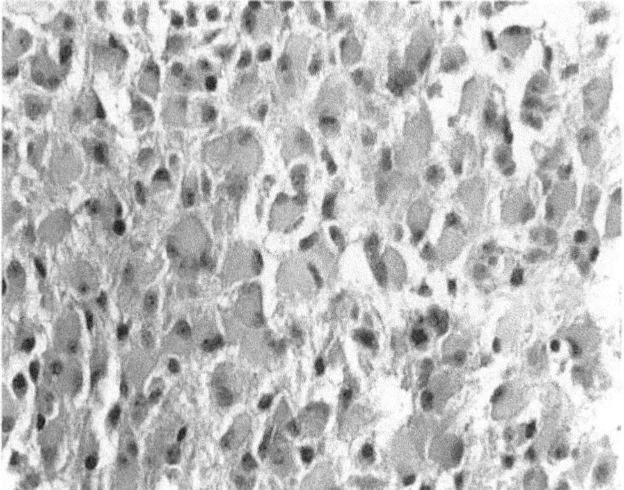

FIGURE 8.215Q

A. Gemistocytic astrocytoma
B. Hemangioblastoma
C. Chordoma
D. Clear cell meningioma
E. Desmoplastic medulloblastoma

216. In a patient with conductive hearing loss on the right, which of the following apply?

A. Weber lateralizes to the left, Rinne is negative (b > a), Schwabach test is normal
B. Weber lateralizes to the right, Rinne is positive (a > b), Schwabach test is normal
C. Weber lateralizes to the right, Rinne is negative, Schwabach test is normal or slightly prolonged
D. Weber lateralizes to the right, Rinne is positive, Schwabach test is abnormal
E. Weber lateralizes to the left, Rinne is positive, Schwabach test is abnormal

217. In performing the Nylén-Bárány maneuver, all of the following suggest peripheral disease EXCEPT?

   A. Latency of appearance of nystagmus of 2 to 12 seconds

   B. The vertigo and nystagmus usually disappear 10 to 15 seconds after their appearance

   C. Change in direction of nystagmus with the head down and persistence of nystagmus

   D. Habituation of the response with repeated maneuvers

   E. The reproducibility of abnormalities noted with this maneuver becomes inconsistent

218. A 35-year-old male with the photomicrograph depicted below (Figure 8.218Q) presents with fever, chills, and a seizure. What is the diagnosis?

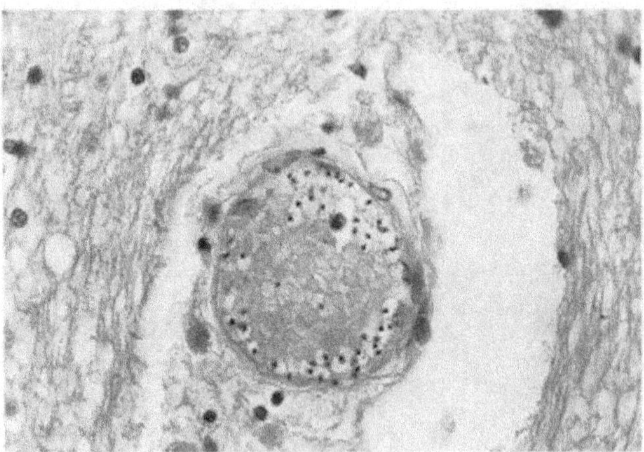

FIGURE 8.218Q

   A. Creutzfeldt-Jakob disease

   B. Herpes encephalitis

   C. Malaria

   D. Ganglioglioma

   E. Lymphoma

219. The lesion depicted below (Figure 8.219Q) is most often associated with what other abnormality?

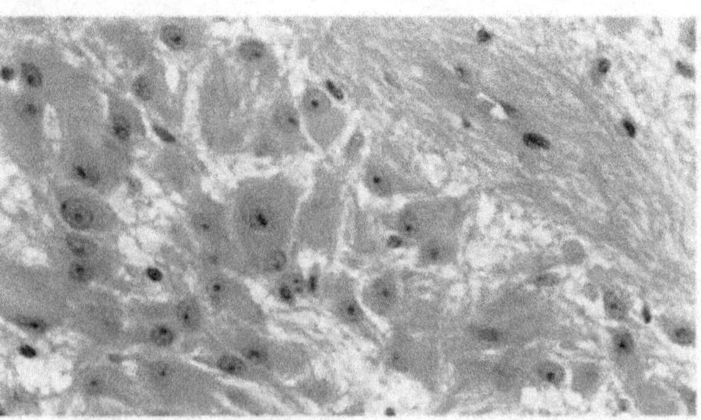

FIGURE 8.219Q

   A. Castleman's syndrome

   B. Tuberous sclerosis

   C. Temporal lobe epilepsy

   D. Café au lait spots

   E. Cobblestone skin pattern

220. Paralysis of upward gaze, light-near dissociation of pupil response, convergence retraction nystagmus, and pathologic lid retraction are most consistent with what abnormality?

   A. Hydrocephalus

   B. A 3-cm meningioma of the falx

   C. Pituitary adenoma

   D. Temporal lobe porencephalic cyst

   E. Occipital lobe arterial-venous malformation

221. All of the following are true of the secondary somatosensory cortex (SII) EXCEPT?

   A. Lies along the superior bank of the lateral sulcus and extends posteriorly into the parietal lobe

   B. Representation of body parts is in the reverse sequence to that found in the primary somesthetic area with the two face areas adjacent

   C. Representation of the body is bilateral in SII, although contralateral predominates

   D. The efferent cortical projections are mainly to SI and the primary motor cortex

   E. Lesions typically cause contralateral weakness

222. In the callosal syndrome (interhemispheric disconnection syndrome) due to surgery, all of the following may be seen in a left hemisphere–dominant patient EXCEPT?

   A. Inability to name objects (kept from view) palpated by the right hand

   B. Inability to name objects presented to the left hemifield

   C. No interference with most activities of daily living

   D. Inability to copy a complex design with the right hand

   E. Unable to execute a command with the left hand

223. Which one of the following correctly identifies the most to least common locations for hypertensive intracranial hemorrhage?

- **A.** Pons, thalamus, putamen, cerebellum, lobar
- **B.** Putamen, thalamus, pons, cerebellum, lobar
- **C.** Putamen, thalamus, cerebellum, pons, lobar
- **D.** Thalamus, putamen, cerebellum, lobar, pons
- **E.** Thalamus, putamen, cerebellum, pons, lobar

224. All of the following are characteristics of normal pressure hydrocephalus EXCEPT?

- **A.** Wide-based "magnetic" gait
- **B.** Bradyphrenia
- **C.** Incontinence
- **D.** Headaches
- **E.** Transient increases in intracranial pressure with continuous monitoring

225. The EEG below (Figure 8.225Q) is most consistent with what diagnosis?

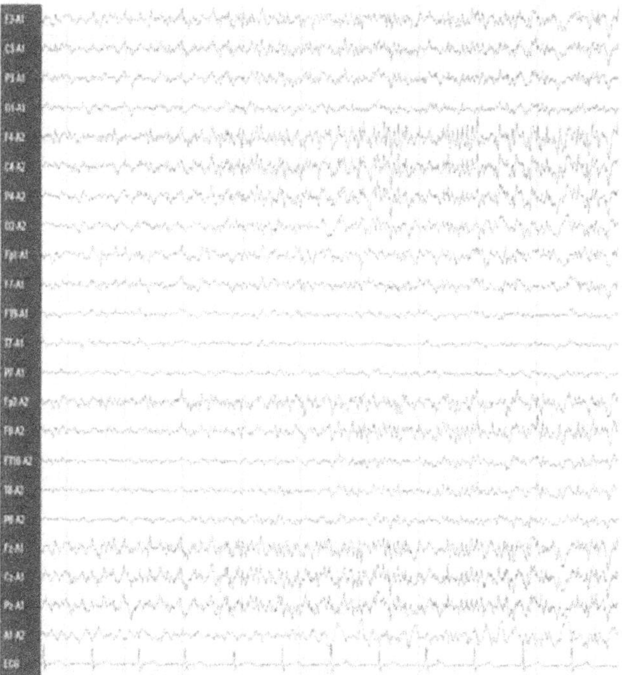

FIGURE 8.225Q

- **A.** Right frontal tumor
- **B.** Left occipital tumor
- **C.** Uremia
- **D.** Sleep
- **E.** Large hemispheric insult

QUESTIONS 226–231

Directions: The following is a schematic diagram through the pallidofugal fiber system in a coronal plane. Match the fibers (numbered items) with the appropriate letterhead (Figure 8.226–8.231Q), using each answer either once, more than once, or not at all.

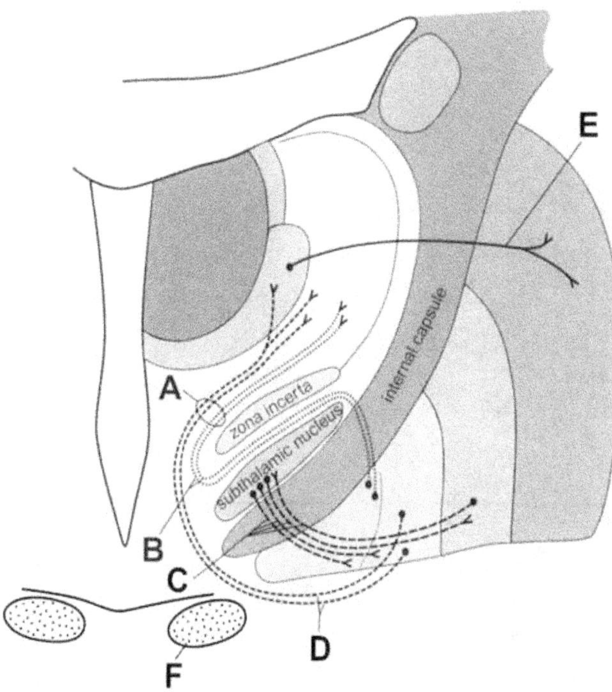

FIGURE 8.226–231Q

226. Ansa lenticularis

227. Thalamostriate fibers

228. Optic tract

229. Subthalamic fasciculus

230. Thalamic fasciculus (H1)

231. Lenticular fasciculus (H2)

End of set

232. A 31-year-old immunocompromised male with a history of intravenous drug abuse presents with back pain. His sagittal postcontrasted T1-weighted MRI is depicted below (Figure 8.232Q). What is the most likely diagnosis?

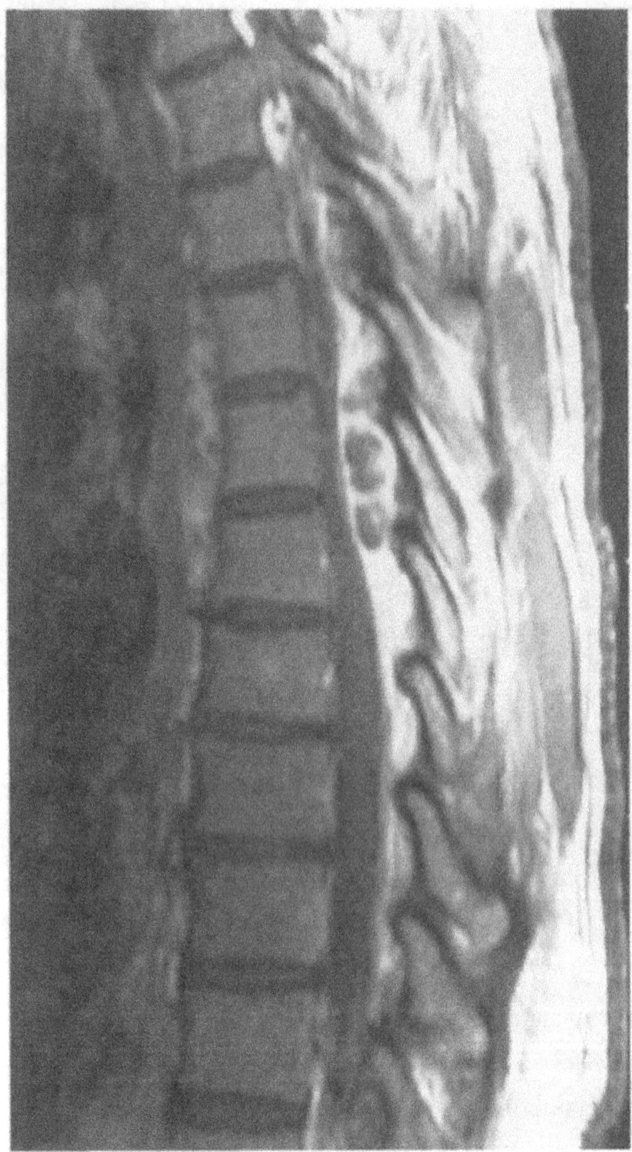

FIGURE 8.232Q

  A. Leukemia
  B. Lymphoma
  C. Epidural abscess
  D. Epidural lipomatosis
  E. Hemangioblastoma

233. Necrotizing wound infections are most commonly produced by what organism(s)?

  1. *Clostridium*
  2. *Staphylococcus*
  3. β-hemolytic streptococci
  4. *Corynebacterium*

  A. 1, 2, and 3 are correct
  B. 1 and 3 are correct
  C. 2 and 4 are correct
  D. Only 4 is correct
  E. All of the above

234. All of the following blood vessels originate from the intracavernous internal carotid artery (ICA) EXCEPT?

  A. Tentorial artery (of Bernasconi and Cassinari)
  B. Dorsal meningeal artery
  C. Inferior hypophyseal artery
  D. Vidian artery
  E. McConnell's capsular artery

235. One day after a high school football game, the starting quarterback presents to the emergency department complaining of diffuse right shoulder pain. The pain is centered over the lateral scapula and posterior shoulder and is aggravated by right upper arm abduction (first 15 degrees) and external rotation (particularly when the elbow is held in 90 degrees of flexion). What nerve is most likely injured?

  A. Suprascapular
  B. Axillary
  C. Spinal accessory
  D. Posterior interosseous
  E. Dorsal scapular

236. A 33-year-old male has a 5-month history of dull low back pain that is exacerbated at night. An axial CT scan of the lumbar spine reveals a 1.4-cm lytic lesion in the vertebral body and pedicle of L4 that is most consistent with an osteoid osteoma. Why does the pain associated with these lesions typically respond to aspirin?

  A. Aspirin decreases the amount of PDGF secreted by tumor cells
  B. Aspirin decreases prostaglandin synthesis in fibroblasts adjacent to the tumor
  C. Aspirin halts the production of prostaglandin by the tumor cells
  D. Aspirin decreases the amount of substance P in the dorsal horn of spinal cord cells
  E. Aspirin significantly reduces prostaglandin synthesis in the vasculature supplying the lesion

237. A 4-year-old male continues to have medically refractory generalized seizures ("drop attacks") despite being placed on numerous anticonvulsant medication regimens. What would be the best surgical option for this patient at this point?

  A. Anatomic hemispherectomy
  B. Functional hemispherectomy
  C. Sectioning of the corpus callosum
  D. Multiple subpial transection
  E. Depth electrode placement for monitoring

QUESTIONS 238–239

Scenario: A 67-year-old female is referred to your office for a left shoulder droop that she has experienced since undergoing a recent lymph node biopsy. She has difficulty raising her arm above the horizontal and has some numbness in the occiput behind the ear on the right.

238. What is the most likely diagnosis?

A. Axillary nerve injury
B. Suprascapular nerve injury
C. Dorsal scapular nerve injury
D. Spinal accessory nerve injury
E. Brachial plexopathy

239. What is the most likely reason for the numbness behind the right ear?

1. Greater auricular nerve injury
2. Lesser auricular nerve injury
3. Lesser occipital nerve injury
4. Lesser auricular nerve injury

A. 1, 2, and 3 are correct
B. 1 and 3 are correct
C. 2 and 4 are correct
D. Only 4 is correct
E. All of the above

End of set

240. All of the following are advantages of magnetoencephalography (MEG) over electroencephalography (EEG) EXCEPT?

A. MEG provides better spatial and temporal resolution for localization of cortical neuronal activity
B. Mass lesions or other pathologic changes do not significantly distort the signal detected by MEG
C. MEG signals are not as readily attenuated as compared to EEG signals
D. MEG includes data points from below the surface, whereas EEG reflects only the cortical surface
E. MEG includes both a tangential and radial component of neuronal current, whereas EEG includes only a tangential component, which significantly reduces the complexity of the signal

QUESTIONS 241–242

241. Refer to Figure 8.241–8.242Q. What is the most likely diagnosis of this patient?

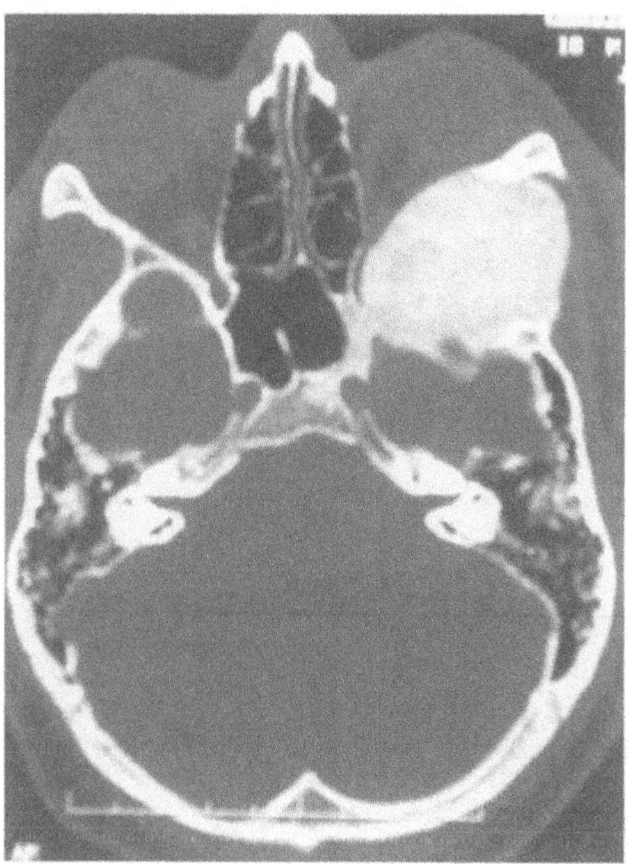

FIGURE 8.241–242Q

A. Sphenoid wing meningioma
B. Chondrosarcoma
C. Fibrous dysplasia
D. Esthenioblastoma
E. Osteochondroma

242. Malignant degeneration of this lesion is most likely to produce what type of neoplasm?

A. Osteochondroma
B. Osteoblastoma
C. Chloroma
D. Osteosarcoma
E. Neuroblastoma

End of set

243. The stylopharyngeus muscle is derived from which brachial arch?

- **A.** First
- **B.** Second
- **C.** Third
- **D.** Fourth
- **E.** Sixth

244. An 18-year-old male presents to the emergency department with morning headaches associated with nausea and right arm numbness; his CT scan showed a low-density area in the left parietal region. The angiogram is depicted below (Figure 8.244Q). What is the most likely diagnosis?

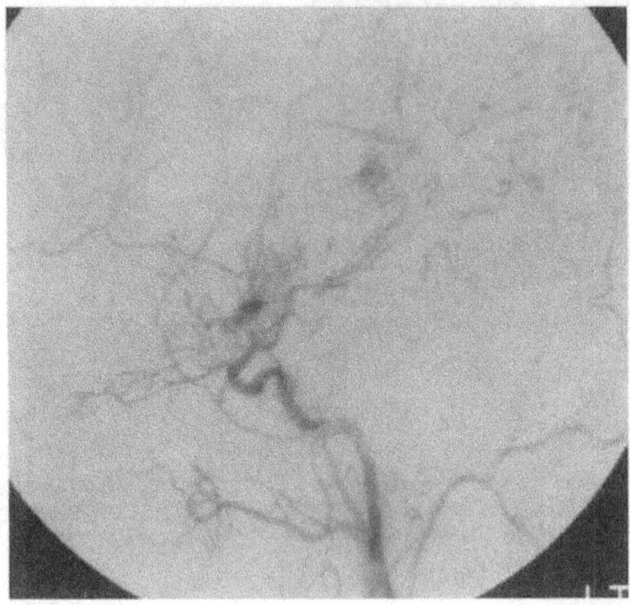

FIGURE 8.244Q

- **A.** Atherosclerosis
- **B.** Malignant brain tumor
- **C.** Fibromuscular dysplasia
- **D.** Moyamoya disease
- **E.** Embolic infarct

245. Which of the following cells give rise to axons that compose the optic nerve?

- **A.** Rods and cones of the retina
- **B.** Bipolar cells
- **C.** Ganglion cells
- **D.** Horizontal cells
- **E.** Amacrine cells

QUESTIONS 246–249

Directions: Match the questions with the most likely type of nerve injury, using each letterhead either once, more than once, or not at all.

- **A.** Neurotmesis
- **B.** Axonotmesis
- **C.** Neurapraxia
- **D.** A and B
- **E.** None of the above

246. No structural problem with the axon; nerve conduction often returns within 6 to 8 weeks

247. Loss of axon continuity, but soma remains continuous

248. Associated with Wallerian degeneration

249. Usually best managed by early surgical repair

End of set

250. A 67-year-old male underwent an anterior cervical fusion in the remote past and presents with a 3-month history of new-onset neck pain and deltoid weakness on the right. His sagittal T2-weighted MRI is depicted on the next page (Figure 8.250Q). What is shown on this sagittal MRI scan that may account for this new clinical picture?

- **A.** Pseudoarthrosis
- **B.** Osteomyelitis
- **C.** End-fusion degenerative changes
- **D.** Spondylolysis
- **E.** Subsidence

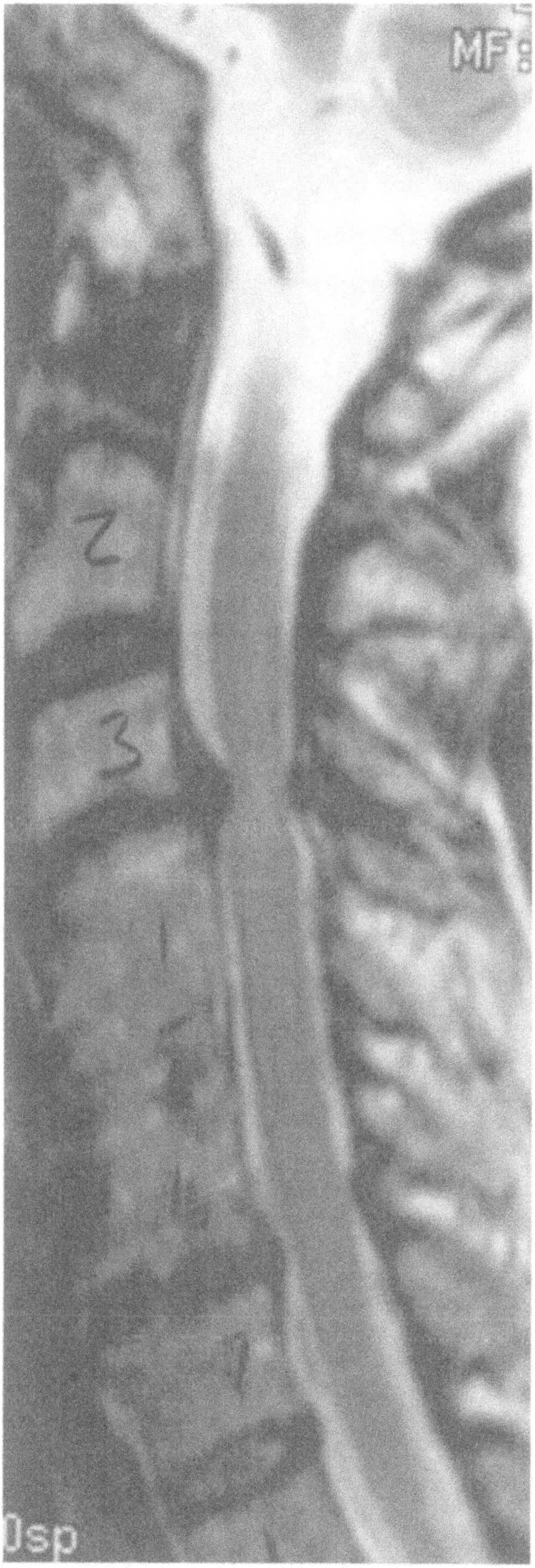

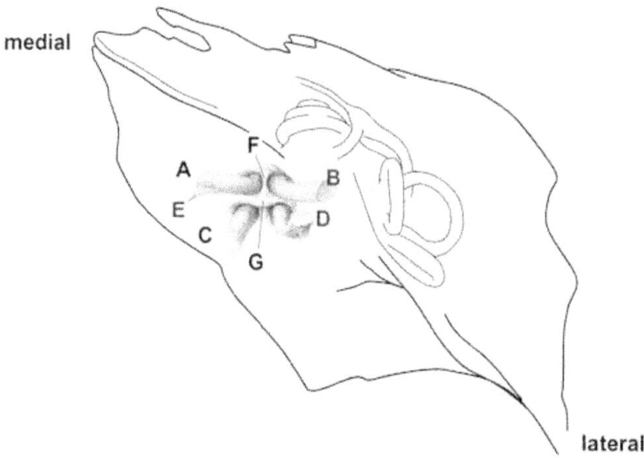

FIGURE 8.250Q

QUESTIONS 251–257

Directions: Figure 8.251–8.257Q depicts the right internal auditory canal and surrounding petrous temporal bone. Match the following anatomic structures with the appropriate letterhead, using each answer only once.

FIGURE 8.251–257Q

251. Superior division of vestibular nerve

252. Cochlear nerve

253. Inferior division of vestibular nerve

254. Facial nerve

255. Nervous intermedius

256. Bill's bar

257. Transverse crest

End of set

QUESTIONS 258–260

Scenario: A 5-year-old male is referred to your office for evaluation of urinary incontinence and a sacral dimple. The dimple was explored shortly after birth and was amputated after it was found to track to the level of the lumbodorsal fascia. On examination, notable findings include a smaller left foot with a high plantar arch, a small scar overlying the coccyx, hypoactive deep tendon reflexes in the legs, and mild scoliosis. His MRI is most consistent with a lipomyelomeningocele with a tethered cord.

258. What process of embryologic development is usually disrupted to produce this abnormality?

A. Disjunction
B. Migration
C. Myelination
D. Cleavage
E. Transverse segmentation

259. Where are the dorsal roots usually located in relation to the fatty stalk in patients with dorsal lipomyelomeningocele?

A. Posterior
B. Dorsolateral
C. Ventrolateral
D. Dorsomedial
E. Rostral

260. Dorsal lipomas may be safely resected by staying in what relationship to the dorsal root entry zone?

A. Ventromedial
B. Dorsolateral
C. Dorsomedial
D. Rostral
E. Ventrolateral

End of set

261. The primary bones that make up the nasal septum include the

1. Vomer   A. 1, 2, and 3 are correct
2. Nasal   B. 1 and 3 are correct
3. Ethmoid   C. 2 and 4 are correct
4. Frontal   D. Only 4 is correct
                E. All of the above

262. What is the most common organism that causes viral (aseptic) meningitis?

A. Arbovirus
B. Myxovirus
C. Enterovirus
D. Arenavirus
E. Togavirus

263. What stage(s) of sleep is associated with night terrors?

A. Stage 1
B. Stage 3
C. Stage 4
D. REM
E. B and C

264. A 77-year-old male presents to your office with a 4-month history of unilateral epistaxis and nasal discharge. His MRI is depicted below (Figure 8.264Q). Histopathologic analysis of the tumor revealed uniform small cells with round nuclei, scant cytoplasm, a prominent reticular core, and scattered Homer-Wright rosettes. Immunohistochemistry was positive for neuron-specific enolase and S-100 but was cytokeratin, CD20, and CD79a negative. What is the most likely diagnosis?

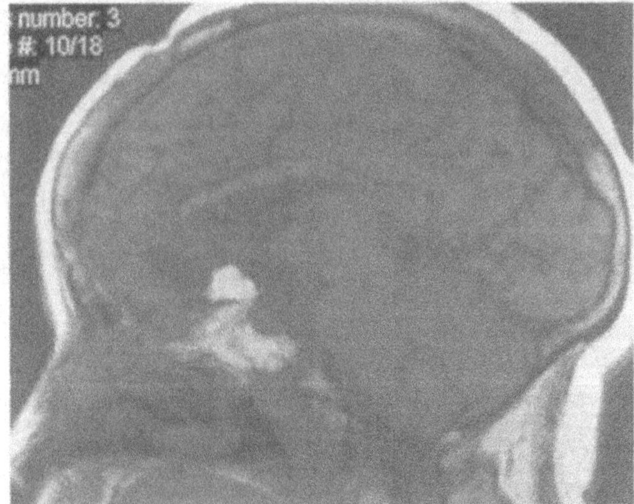

FIGURE 8.264Q

A. Lymphoma
B. Squamous cell carcinoma
C. Esthesioneuroblastoma
D. Adenocarcinoma
E. Rhabdomyosarcoma

265. An abducens palsy associated with an ipsilateral Horner's syndrome suggests a lesion in what location?

- **A.** Pontine tegmentum
- **B.** Dorello's canal
- **C.** Prepontine cistern
- **D.** Cavernous sinus
- **E.** Region of the ligament of Grüber

266. The principal premotor structure concerned with voluntary vertical saccades is the

- **A.** Paramedian pontine reticular formation (PPRF)
- **B.** Rostral interstitial nucleus of the medial longitudinal fasciculus (MLF)
- **C.** Rostral interstitial nucleus of Cajal
- **D.** Nucleus of Roller
- **E.** Nucleus of Collier

QUESTIONS 267–276

Directions: The observation of various adverse effects during deep brain stimulation (DBS) often characterizes the extent of current spread to adjacent structures. For each stimulation-induced adverse effect, match the associated direction of current spread, using each answer once, more than once, or not at all.

- **A.** Anterior
- **B.** Posterior
- **C.** Medial
- **D.** Lateral
- **E.** Anterior and lateral
- **F.** Inferior and medial
- **G.** Posterior and medial
- **H.** None of the above

267. Flushing and perspiration after STN DBS

268. Dysarthria after STN DBS

269. Paresthesias after GPi DBS

270. Photopsia and nausea after Gpi DBS

271. Diplopia after STN DBS

272. Tonic contraction after Vim DBS

273. Blepharospasm after STN DBS

274. Dysequilibrium and gait ataxia (without limb ataxia) after STN DBS

275. Tonic contraction after STN DBS

276. Paresthesias after Vim DBS

End of set

277. What histological finding is pathognomonic for denervation followed by reinnervation of muscle fibers?

- **A.** Atrophic muscle fibers
- **B.** Angular fibers
- **C.** Eosinophilic infiltration
- **D.** Target cells
- **E.** Type-specific grouping of muscle fibers

278. The photomicrograph depicted below (Figure 8.278Q) is most consistent with what diagnosis?

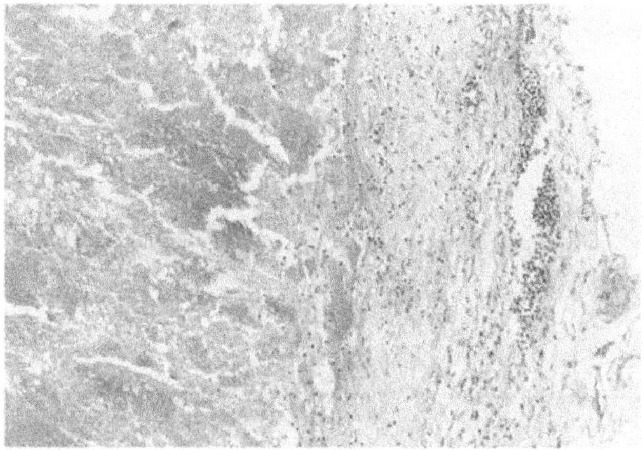

FIGURE 8.278Q

- **A.** Tuberculosis
- **B.** Chronic infarct
- **C.** Multiple sclerosis
- **D.** Histoplasmosis
- **E.** Pilocytic astrocytoma

279. The gross specimen depicted below (Figure 8.279Q) reveals?

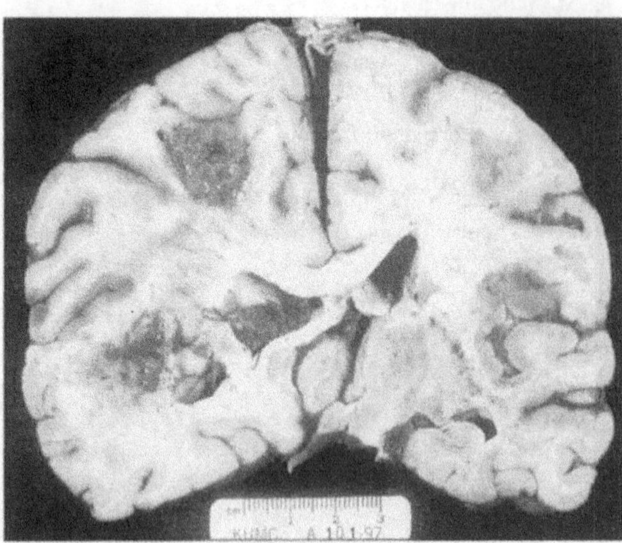

FIGURE 8.279Q

A. Neurocysticercosis
B. Third ventricular tumor
C. Metastatic disease
D. Toxoplasmosis
E. Multiple sclerosis

280. Which of the following muscles abduct the vocal cords?

1. Lateral cricoarytenoid
2. Transverse arytenoid
3. Cricothyroid
4. Posterior cricoarytenoid

A. 1, 2, and 3 are correct
B. 1 and 3 are correct
C. 2 and 4 are correct
D. Only 4 is correct
E. All of the above

281. Installation of cold water in the right ear elicits what type of response?

A. Left beating nystagmus
B. Eye deviation to the left
C. Right beating nystagmus
D. Convergence retraction nystagmus
E. WEBINO response

QUESTIONS 282–286

Directions: Match the following, using each answer only once.

A. Dilute (1/8%) pilocarpine
B. 1% Hydroxyamphetamine
C. 10% Cocaine
D. Atropine
E. Dilute epinephrine (1:1000)

282. No effect on Horner's pupil

283. Dilates second-order Horner's pupil

284. Dilates third-order Horner's pupil

285. Dilates normal pupil

286. Constricts Adie's pupil

End of set

QUESTIONS 287–291

Directions: Match the following questions with the appropriate diagnostic technique, using each answer once, more than once, or not at all.

A. B-mode ultrasonography
B. Doppler ultrasonography
C. Both
D. None of the above

287. Based on reflection of sound waves off of moving targets

288. Best used to evaluate flow dynamics

289. Based on reflection of sound waves off of tissue interfaces that are stationary

290. Typically shows the carotid system as a pulsatile luminal structure with a thin echogenic line representing the intimal surface

291. Can sample blood flow within a vessel while simultaneously displaying vessel wall anatomy

End of set

292. What gene is abnormal in spinobulbar muscular atrophy (Kennedy's disease)?

A. Androgen receptor gene
B. Dystrophin gene
C. Superoxide dismutase gene
D. TGF-β receptor gene
E. Mitochondrial complex 1 gene

293. All of the following are true about levodopa EXCEPT?

A. Vitamin B_6 decreases effective dose of levodopa
B. MAO inhibitors can exaggerate the central dopamine effects by decreasing metabolism of dopamine
C. Can cause orthostatic hypotension
D. Carbidopa can increase the effectiveness of levodopa by inhibiting a peripheral decarboxylase inhibitor
E. Antipsychotics increase the efficacy of levodopa

294. Ramsay Hunt syndrome usually involves which cranial nerve?

A. Central seventh cranial nerve
B. Lower seventh cranial nerve
C. Olfactory nerve
D. Mandibular division of the trigeminal nerve
E. Trochlear nerve

295. The positive symptoms of schizophrenia are a result of increased dopamine activity in which of the following pathways?

A. Nigrostriatal
B. Tuberoinfundibular
C. Mesocortical
D. Mesolimbic
E. Tuberolimbic

296. What muscles are involved with elevation of the mandible or mouth closure?

1. Medial pterygoid muscle
2. Masseter muscle
3. Temporalis muscle
4. Buccinator muscle

A. 1, 2, and 3 are correct
B. 1 and 3 are correct
C. 2 and 4 are correct
D. Only 4 is correct
E. All of the above

297. What is depicted on the CT scan below (Figure 8.297Q)?

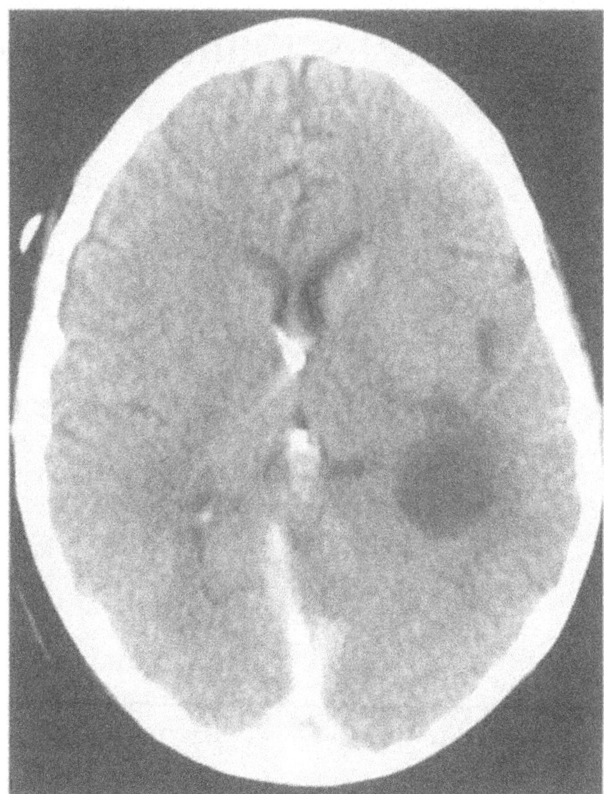

FIGURE 8.297Q

A. Evidence of posterior interhemispheric blood after head trauma
B. Empty delta sign of superior sagittal thrombosis associated with a cystic tumor
C. Pineocytoma
D. A hyperdense MCA sign
E. A left posterior temporal infarct

298. All of the following are true of hyperosmolar hyperglycemic nonketotic diabetic ketoacidosis syndrome (HHNS) EXCEPT?

A. Most patients are mildly hypernatremic
B. HHNS is often accompanied by severe prerenal azotemia
C. HHNS is associated with an anion gap
D. Most patients are hypokalemic
E. Insulin is always administered in the initial management period

QUESTIONS 299–300

Directions: Match the medication with the potential toxicity, using each answer only once.

A. Methotrexate
B. Vincristine
C. Bleomycin
D. None of the above

299. Raynaud's phenomenon, pulmonary fibrosis

300. Leukoencephalopathy

End of set

Multidisciplinary Self-Assessment Answer Key

1. D	42. A	83. D	124. C	165. C
2. A	43. A	84. D	125. D	166. E
3. E	44. C	85. D	126. A	167. D
4. E	45. B	86. C	127. D	168. D
5. F	46. E	87. D	128. E	169. C
6. D	47. B	88. C	129. A	170. B
7. A	48. A	89. G	130. B	171. B
8. C	49. E	90. I	131. B	172. C
9. B	50. C	91. E	132. A	173. E
10. A	51. D	92. H	133. A	174. C
11. D	52. D	93. B	134. D	175. D
12. A	53. C	94. A	135. E	176. B
13. D	54. A	95. J	136. C	177. C
14. B	55. C	96. A	137. A	178. B
15. C	56. A	97. E	138. A	179. D
16. C	57. A	98. B	139. B	180. C
17. F	58. B	99. D	140. E	181. E
18. H	59. A	100. E	141. B	182. A
19. E	60. A	101. A	142. C	183. B
20. A	61. C	102. A	143. G	184. B
21. D	62. D	103. C	144. F	185. B
22. G	63. C	104. B	145. C	186. B
23. B	64. C	105. C	146. E	187. E
24. I	65. B	106. C	147. B	188. B
25. A	66. A	107. E	148. A	189. C
26. C	67. D	108. A	149. B	190. A
27. D	68. E	109. D	150. D	191. C
28. E	69. F	110. G	151. B	192. B
29. D	70. C	111. B	152. C	193. D
30. C	71. A	112. F	153. A	194. B
31. C	72. A	113. C	154. E	195. C
32. D	73. I	114. E	155. E	196. E
33. C	74. J	115. H	156. B	197. C
34. C	75. F	116. I	157. E	198. C
35. D	76. B	117. E	158. D	199. E
36. C	77. G	118. C	159. A	200. B
37. E	78. C	119. C	160. F	201. A
38. C	79. I	120. D	161. H	202. E
39. E	80. H	121. D	162. E	203. C
40. A	81. B	122. B	163. A	204. B
41. C	82. C	123. B	164. G	205. E

206. D	**225.** A	**244.** D	**263.** E	**282.** C
207. A	**226.** D	**245.** C	**264.** C	**283.** B
208. C	**227.** E	**246.** C	**265.** D	**284.** D
209. B	**228.** F	**247.** B	**266.** B	**285.** D
210. B	**229.** C	**248.** D	**267.** A	**286.** A
211. D	**230.** A	**249.** A	**268.** D	**287.** B
212. C	**231.** B	**250.** C	**269.** G	**288.** B
213. C	**232.** C	**251.** B	**270.** A	**289.** A
214. E	**233.** B	**252.** C	**271.** F	**290.** A
215. A	**234.** D	**253.** D	**272.** D	**291.** D
216. C	**235.** A	**254.** A	**273.** H	**292.** A
217. C	**236.** C	**255.** E	**274.** C	**293.** E
218. C	**237.** C	**256.** F	**275.** E	**294.** B
219. B	**238.** D	**257.** G	**276.** B	**295.** D
220. A	**239.** B	**258.** A	**277.** E	**296.** A
221. E	**240.** E	**259.** C	**278.** A	**297.** B
222. A	**241.** C	**260.** C	**279.** C	**298.** E
223. B	**242.** D	**261.** B	**280.** D	**299.** C
224. D	**243.** C	**262.** C	**281.** A	**300.** A

Multidisciplinary Self-Assessment Answers

1. D. Refer to Table 8.1A (DeMyer, p. 137; Greenberg, p. 700; Youmans, pp. 272, 4397, 4872).

2. A. Note the "picket fence" arrangement (pseudopalisading) of the nuclei surrounding a region of necrosis in this photomicrograph, which depicts a glioblastoma (Ellison, pp. 628–631).

3. E. Complete white blood cell count, peripheral eosinophil level, and serum anticysticercal antibody levels should be obtained in all patients suspected of having NCC. Patients requiring ventriculostomy placement should have cerebrospinal fluid (CSF) analyzed for eosinophil and anticysticercal antibody levels. Stool testing for ova and parasites is helpful in patients with simultaneous intestinal tapeworm infection but is insensitive and nonspecific for *T. solium* species and is found in less than 33% of cases. Several laboratory methods have been developed to detect host antibodies against circulating cysticercal antigens. From the many tests performed, current data indicate that enzyme-linked immunosorbent assay (ELISA) and electroimmunotransfer blot (EITB) tests are the most effective. Studies comparing these diagnostic modalities have shown that the EITB assay is more sensitive overall than ELISA, especially when serum is being tested. Both techniques are more sensitive in cases with multiple cysts than in cases with solitary or confined lesions. Additionally, no global difference among cases was found with parasites located in different compartments (ventricles, subarachnoid space, parenchyma) of the central nervous system (Greenberg, pp. 236–238; Proano-Narvaez et al., p. 2118).

4-E; 5-F; 6-D; 7-A; 8-C; 9-B. Refer to Table 8.4–8.9A (DeMyer, p. 135; Brazis, pp. 85–95; Merritt, pp. 136–137, 186, 710–713, 715–717).

10. A. The differential diagnosis of oligodendroglial tumors includes clear cell ependymoma, central neurocytoma, and dysembryoplastic neuroepithelial tumor. All of these entities exhibit the presence of neoplastic cells with a uniform round nucleus and clear cytoplasm. A rare differential diagnosis of oligodendroglioma is clear cell meningioma (not fibrous meningioma), which can be differentiated from oligodendroglioma by abundant diastase-sensitive PAS positivity and immunoreactivity for EMA. Note the prominent calcification, "chicken wire" capillaries (prominent branching), "fried egg" cells with round monomorphic nuclei, and perinuclear halos arranged in a back-to-back fashion in this photomicrograph depicting an oligodendroglioma (Ellison, pp. 641–644; WHO, p. 59).

11. D. The anterior abdominal wall consists of the epidermis, superficial layer of superficial fascia (of Camper), the deep layer of superficial fascia (of Scarpa), the deep fascia (investing fascia of musculature), the external and internal oblique muscles, the transverse abdominis muscle, transversalis fascia, loose extraperitoneal connective tissue, and peritoneum. Camper's fascia is predominately an adipose

TABLE 8.1A   Clinical features of spinal cord hemisection (Brown-Séquard syndrome)

CLINICAL FINDINGS	ANATOMIC CORRELATION
Contralateral loss of pain and temperature sensation caudal to lesion Preserved light (crude) touch due to redundant ipsilateral and contralateral pathways (anterior spinothalamic tracts)	Spinothalamic tract injury
Acute: Ipsilateral paralysis of voluntary movements caudal to level of lesion Delayed onset: UMN signs including hyperreflexia, spasticity, and extensor toe sign	Lateral corticospinal tract injury
Ipsilateral loss of vibration sense, position sense, form perception, and two-point discrimination	Dorsal column injury
Segmental weakness and atrophy	Injury to ventral motor neurons at level of lesion
Segmental numbness	Disruption of dorsal rootlets at level of lesion
Loss of sweating caudal to lesion; if lesion is cervical, ipsilateral Horner's syndrome	Descending autonomic fiber disruption

TABLE 8.4–9A   Clinical syndromes of various spinal cord lesions

SYNDROME	CLINICAL FINDINGS
Poliomyelitis	Usually follows acute inflammatory viral infection Results from a cell-mediated immunologic reaction against motor fibers Virus has predilection for lower motor neurons, which results in segmental demyelination and Wallerian degeneration Selective atrophy of associated muscles
Familial spastic paraplegia	Pyramidal neurons undergo "dying back" process in a distal to proximal fashion (lower followed by upper extremity paralysis; corticobulbar paralysis) Results in gradual development of spastic weakness of the legs with gait abnormality
Amyotrophic lateral sclerosis (Lou Gehrig's disease)	Involves both upper and lower motor neurons Involves astrocytic proliferation and scarring/sclerosis of the lateral columns
Tabes dorsalis (syphilis)	Dorsal column degeneration Lower extremity > upper extremity involvement Leg fiber degeneration > arm fiber involvement
Subacute combined degeneration (B_{12} deficiency)	Combined upper motor neuron (lateral corticospinal tract) and dorsal column sensory loss early in disease course Also demyelination of spinocerebellar tracts
Syringomyelia	Cavitating process in central canal Pain and temperature fibers affected first Lesions may extend out to involve corticospinal tracts or motor neurons

layer that contains most of the fat of the subdermis. It continues over the pubis as the superficial layer (of Cruveilhier) of the superficial perineal fascia, crosses the inguinal ligament to merge with the superficial fascia of the thigh, and continues over the chest as the superficial layer of superficial thoracic fascia. Scarpa's fascia is a fibrous layer that will best hold sutures (highest tensile strength). It continues over the pubis as the deep layer of superficial perineal fascia (of Colles) and passes into the upper thigh, where it attaches to the fascia lata. The deep fascia is the investing fascia of the musculature, aponeuroses, and large neurovascular structures and is not easily separated from the underlying epimysium of muscle. It extends into the penis as Buck's fascia, continues over the spermatic cord as the external spermatic fascia, and passes over the pubis and perineal musculature as the deep perineal fascia of Gallaudet (April, p. 173).

12. A. Note the cord tethering and fatty filum on this sagittal MRI (Ramsey, pp. 104–106).

13. D. This angiogram depicts the classic "caput medusae" pattern of a venous angioma, which is an extreme anatomic variant of medullary (white matter) venous drainage. The precise etiology of this lesion remains unclear, although some authors have proposed that it results from arrested development of parts of the venous vasculature at a time when normal arterial development is nearly complete. This results in the retention of primitive venous channels that typically empty into a single large draining vein (Osborn, pp. 294–295).

14. B. The stria medullaris thalami contains projections that originate in the septal nuclei, anterior thalamic nuclei, and hypothalamus (preoptic region) and terminate in the habenular nuclei. The habenular nuclei then project to the raphe nuclei of the midbrain via the fasciculus retroflexus. In this manner, the stria medullaris thalami act as a relay point for limbic system information that is transmitted to the midbrain (Carpenter, p. 252; Martin, p. 473).

15. C. Visual information flows vertically from photoreceptor cells (outer nuclear layer) to bipolar cells (inner nuclear layer) to ganglion cells (ganglion cell layer) as well as laterally via horizontal cells (outer plexiform layer) and amacrine cells (inner plexiform layer). Light produces opposite effects on the rate of bipolar cell firing depending on whether it stimulates the center or surrounding part of the cell's receptive field. Additionally, a lateral network of horizontal cells that directly interconnect neighboring groups of photoreceptor cells helps mediate this antagonist property. Hence, horizontal cells provide a mechanism for mediating opposite responses in adjacent photoreceptor cells, which is used to enhance luminance contrast. The precise role of amacrine cells remains unclear, although some amacrine cells function like horizontal cells. They mediate antagonistic inputs between bipolar cells and ganglion cells in the inner plexiform layer. Other amacrine cells have been implicated in shaping the complex receptive field properties of various types of ganglion cells, such as M-type cells that process orientation information (Pritchard, pp. 292–302; Kandel, p. 515).

16. C. Exner's area lies superior to Broca's area, in Brodmann's area 8, and if damaged may result in pure agraphia without aphasia (Brazis, pp. 515–516).

17-F; 18-H; 19-E; 20-A; 21-D; 22-G; 23-B; 24-I. These three axial CT scans (Figures 8.17–8.24 Q a, b, c) illustrate critical portions of the petrous temporal bone and progress sequentially in a superior-inferior direction. In these figures, A represents the lateral semicircular canal, B the superior semicircular canal, C the internal auditory canal, D the vestibular aqueduct, E the posterior semicircular canal, F the vestibule, G the facial nerve, H the cochlea, and I the endolymphatic sac. Notice the labyrinthine and anterior tympanic portions of the facial nerve, separated by the geniculate ganglion, in figure B. Figure C depicts the horizontal segment of the facial nerve and the vestibular aqueduct joining the endolymphatic sac at the posterior aspect of the petrous temporal bone (Som, pp. 1319–1325).

25. A. Some of the valves currently used in clinical practice include the static (Holter-Hausner valve, Denver shunt, Codman Uni-Shunt) and programmable (Codman Medos, Sophy valve) differential pressure valves, flow-regulated valves (Orbis Sigma), and gravity-actuated valves (Cordis horizontal-vertical valve). The PS Medical Delta valve consists of an antisiphoning device just distal to a differential pressure valve. More recently Codman has introduced the Hakim programmable valve with a Siphon-Guard valve, while Medtronic has introduced the Strata valve, a programmable valve with variable pressure settings that can be coupled with their Delta valve antisiphoning device. The valves described above all use different approaches to control flow through the valve system and limit overshunting. Differential pressure valves open when the pressure at the inlet is higher than that the outlet by a preselected amount. Programmable differential pressure valves act in a similar fashion except that the surgeon can change the opening pressure with an external device, which often obviates the need for surgical shunt revision. Flow-regulated valves use a three-stage resistance mechanism to keep the flow rate through the valve constant. Gravity-actuated valves attempt to decrease siphoning by increasing opening pressure with the assistance of gravity when a patient sits or stands. Cordis horizontal-vertical valves are gravity-actuated valves that have traditionally been used with lumboperitoneal shunts (Youmans, pp. 3376–3379; Albright, pp. 79–80; Wilkins, pp. 3647–3651; American Society of Pediatric Neurosurgeons, pp. 506–508; Committee on Education in Neurological Surgery, pp. 137–138).

26-C; 27-D. The process of cellular migration typically occurs between the second and fifth gestational months. Faulty cellular migration can result in heterotopias, callosal agenesis, lissencephaly, pachygyria/polymicrogyria, and open- or closed-lip schizencephaly. Note the prominent cleft (open-lip) that is lined entirely by gray matter on this sagittal MRI. Porencephalic clefts are predominately lined by gliotic white matter (Osborne DN, pp. 52–55).

28. E. Proopiomelanocortin (POMC) gives rise to beta-lipotropin and ACTH. The sequences of beta-endorphin and melanocyte-stimulating hormone are contained in beta-lipotropin (Kandel, p. 487).

29. D. This patient has developed diabetes insipidus (DI). Criteria frequently used to make the diagnosis include: urine osmolarity 50 to 150 mOsm/L, specific gravity 1.001 to 1.005, urine output ≥ 250 to 300 cc/hr for 3 consecutive hours, and progressively increasing Na$^{.}$ levels on serial lab draws. This patient should receive aqueous vasopressin (Pitressin) (IVP/IM/SQ), as the lipid-soluble form is poorly absorbed compared to the aqueous form. This patient would likely not tolerate oral DDAVP due to her nausea, and a nasogastric tube is generally contraindicated after a transsphenoidal operation. Fludrocortisone acetate acts directly on the renal tubules to increase sodium absorption. This medication, along with urea, would be more applicable for patients with cerebral salt wasting or SIADH. Complications with fludrocortisone acetate include pulmonary edema, hypokalemia, and hypertension (Greenberg, pp. 20–23; Committee on Education in Neurological Surgery, p. 99).

30. C. This EEG depicts normal posterior dominant rhythm ("alpha rhythm") in a healthy adult man, maximal in the posterior head regions when the eyes are closed (Rowan, pp. 25–26).

31. C. A number of extracranial-to-intracranial anastomoses exist that may potentially provide collateral blood flow to the orbit and preserve vision after occlusion of the internal carotid or ophthalmic arteries. This collateral flow is mainly supplied by branches of the external carotid artery, including the internal maxillary (most important) and facial arteries, via their extensive ethmoid, ophthalmic, and cavernous carotid collaterals. Although this collateral filling is not always evident on angiography, this patient's angiogram is more likely to show poor collateral flow to the globe from the maxillary or facial arteries, considering her symptomatology. The ascending pharyngeal artery does not usually provide collateral blood supply to the globe, while vasospasm would be highly unlikely in this setting. There should be other accompanying neurologic deficits if there was complete occlusion of the right internal carotid artery with inadequate collateral feeding of that hemisphere (Osborn DN, p. 397).

32-D; 33-C. One of the hallmarks of pilocytic astrocytomas is their relatively indolent growth rate with low mitotic activity. Management typically includes gross total resection, if possible, followed by radiation therapy for recurrence. In some cases, invasion of the brainstem and/or cranial nerves precludes gross total resection. Macroscopic features common to these tumors include the formation of a cyst with a solid mural nodule. Tumors without cyst wall enhancement are typically adequately treated with mural nodule excision alone, while tumors with a thickened, enhancing cyst wall are best managed with gross total excision. Microscopically, these tumors show a biphasic pattern consisting of bipolar, highly fibrillated (or piloid) cells with Rosenthal fibers and a loose-knit cystic component associated with granular bodies or protein droplets. The arrow depicts Rosenthal fibers, which are ubiquitin $\alpha\beta$ crystallin, and GFAP-positive (Greenberg, pp. 401–403; Ellison, pp. 630–635; WHO, pp. 45–51).

34. C. A 6-month-old infant is able to transfer objects from hand to hand, support most of his weight, lift his head off the table prior to being pulled up, turn his head to voice, and reach for objects (Rudolph, p. 15).

35. D. The suck reflex can be elicited in infants below 4 months of age and consists of bursts of upward tongue pressure and buccinator contraction when the examiner places a clean finger or pacifier into the infants mouth. The tonic neck reflex (typically disappears by 6 months) involves turning the head of a supine infant to one side. The opposite arm should extend 90 degrees from the trunk and the opposite leg should extend downward ("fencing position"). Placing a finger in an infant's hand or under the toes can elicit the palmar grasp or plantar reflex, respectively. The palmar grasp reflex usually disappears by 6 months, while the plantar reflex is often present until 10 months of age. The stepping/placing reflex is produced when the baby is held upright and the dorsal edge of the foot is allowed to brush against an object such as a bed or table. Infants less than 6 weeks of age should flex the knee and lift the foot. The ventral suspension (Landau) reflex results in extension of the head, trunk, and hips and knee flexion when an infant is supported on the examiner's hand in a prone position. This reflex does not usually disappear until the age of 2 years. The Moro reflex occurs when the baby is placed in the supine position and the examiner lifts the baby's head by placing his or her hand under it. Sudden release of the head a few centimeters toward the bed should elicit a complete Moro response in infants less than 3 to 4 months of age. It consists of abduction of the arms at the shoulder, extension of the forearms at the elbow, and extension of the fingers, followed by arm adduction at the shoulders. Additional reflexes include the crossed adductor (disappears by 7 months), parachute, and neck righting (disappears by 2 years) reflexes (Rudolph, p. 15).

36-C; 37-E. Extensive removal of the anterior clinoid process and optic strut (roof of the optic canal), as well as sectioning of the falciform ligament and distal dural ring is often required for successful clipping of large ophthalmic segment aneurysms. Attempts to clip large and giant paraclinoid/ophthalmic artery aneurysms with broad necks without this degree of exposure may place the ophthalmic and internal carotid arteries in jeopardy of clip-induced stenosis/occlusion. Ophthalmic segment aneurysms typically arise beneath the lateral aspect of the optic nerve, which initially results in compression of temporal fibers and an ipsilateral monocular superior nasal quadrantanopsia. With aneurysmal enlargement, the optic nerve is deflected further medially and superiorly against the rigid falciform ligament, which causes superior fiber compression and a monocular inferior nasal field cut (Greenberg, p. 783; Wilkins, pp. 2291–2299; Samson, pp. 41–53).

38. C. Identification of the oligodendroglial component on permanent section is usually aided by the classic "fried egg" appearance of the perinuclear halo. This develops as a consequence of the fixation process; it is not evident on smear or frozen examination and may be absent in rapidly fixed tissue and in paraffin sections made from frozen material (Ellison, pp. 641–645; WHO, pp. 56–61).

39. E. The spinocerebellar tracts convey unconscious proprioception from Golgi tendon organs, muscle spindles, and joint receptors in the periphery to the CNS. Dorsal spinocerebellar fibers (C8-L2) enter the medial aspect of the dorsal roots and synapse in the dorsal nucleus of Clarke. Second-order neurons in Clarke's nucleus then project to the vermis and paramedian lobule of the cerebellum via the inferior cerebellar peduncle, where they terminate as mossy fibers. Above the level of C8, Ia and Ib afferents enter the fasciculus cuneatus and synapse in the accessory cuneate nucleus of the medulla (the equivalent of Clarke's nucleus of the spinal cord). Second-order neurons then enter the cerebellum (cuneocerebellar fibers) via the inferior cerebellar peduncle before synapsing in the cerebellum. The ventral spinocerebellar tract is a crossed tract that originates in Rexed laminae V to VII in the lower lumbar and coccygeal levels. This tract then decussates a second time in the pons before entering the cerebellum as mossy fibers via the superior cerebellar peduncle (Carpenter, pp. 90–94).

40. A. The cortical representation for macular retinal vision is located in the occipital poles. The primary visual cortex (area 17) is located along the upper and lower banks of the calcarine sulcus. Layer IV of the primary visual cortex is particularly prominent and is known as the "band of Gennari." The occipital poles often receive collateral blood flow from the middle cerebral arteries, which is thought to account for macular sparing with field cuts that originate from cortical infarctions secondary to posterior cerebral artery occlusions. Moreover, the area of cortex subserving central or macular vision is relatively large (compared to peripheral vision), so that a single infarction or other pathologic process rarely destroys it entirely (Martin, pp. 193–194).

41. C. The superior olivary nuclei receive the ventral acoustic striae and contain third-order auditory neurons that subsequently project to the contralateral lateral lemniscus. The superior olives are the initial sites of binaural convergence within the auditory pathway (Kandel, pp. 606–608).

42. A. The angiogram depicts a right posterior carotid wall aneurysm as well as extravasation of contrast dye from the aneurysm in a patient about to be treated with GDC embolization (microcatheter evident in internal carotid artery). Intraprocedural aneurysmal rupture is reported to occur in 2 to 8% of patients treated with GDC embolization. It seems to be more prevalent during treatment of smaller aneurysms, especially in the acute phase following SAH. It may occur during several phases of the embolization procedure. When the microcatheter is responsible for the rupture, it is important to avoid withdrawing the device prematurely, as the offending device often plugs the ruptured site and prevents additional extravasation of blood. Similarly, if the aneurysm ruptures during the coiling phase, it is important that the clinician deploy the coil in an attempt to seal the leak. In general, once rupture occurs, the remaining aneurysmal sac should be packed as quickly as possible. In refractory cases, temporary or permanent balloon occlusion of the parent vessel or immediate surgical clipping may be warranted (Youmans, pp. 2071–2072).

43. A. Note the prominent ST-segment elevation in leads V_1 through V_6 on this ECG, depicting an anterior wall myocardial infarction. In general, ST-segment and T-wave changes appear over the first minutes to hours of an infarction, and Q waves appear over hours to days. An evolving myocardial infarction may first manifest with peaked T waves followed by ST segment elevation and T-wave inversion. Eventually Q waves may appear. In a large anterior wall infarction, these changes are most apparent in leads V_1 through V_6, while in an inferior infarction, these changes often occur in leads II, III, and aVF. Of note, if a patient's T waves are chronically inverted, the peaking may make them appear normal—a process referred to as pseudonormalization. T waves are the least reliable of ST- and T-wave segment abnormalities because many noncardiac events may influence them (i.e., elevated K^+). Dying myocardial cells release their enzymes into the bloodstream, and the increased concentration should be confirmed in the peripheral blood (Fishman, pp. 9–24; Marino, pp. 301–313).

44-C; 45-B. The clinical history and MRI are most consistent with a cystic craniopharyngioma. The modestly elevated prolactin level is likely the result of the "stalk effect," whereby injury of the hypothalamus or pituitary stalk (i.e., from large tumors) results in modest elevations of prolactin from reduced prolactin inhibitory factor levels (dopamine). As a general rule, prolactin levels > 150 ng/mL are rarely secondary to a stalk effect, whereas levels < 90 usually suggest a stalk injury. Large components of this tumor extend inferiorly into the sphenoid sinus and superiorly into the suprasellar space. Moreover, the optic chiasm appears draped over the rostral margin of the tumor. Although these are worrisome findings that warrant special concern, they are not uncommon with craniopharyngioma. This sagittal MRI shows that the posterior component of this tumor has eroded through a significant portion of the tuberculum sella and clivus, a relatively rare but significant finding. This latter detail is especially concerning, since failure to recognize this degree of bony erosion on preoperative MRI may result in inadvertent injury to major posterior fossa structures (basilar artery, perforating vessels) during transsphenoidal tumor resection. Thyroxin (T_4) is generally preferred over thyroid extract (T_3) because blood levels are often more predictable. This is especially true for patients with concomitant liver injury, as T_3 is converted to T_4 in the liver. Patients with cirrhosis may remain hypothyroid even while taking T_3. Although it is preferable to correct hypothyroidism preoperatively, it is important to correct any cortisol deficiency as well, as premature thyroid replacement can precipitate an adrenal crisis in this group of patients. Thyroxine has been shown to decrease phenytoin levels (Committee on Education in Neurological Surgery, p. 102; Greenberg, pp. 419–436).

46. E. Sarcoidosis, not Behçet's syndrome, is associated with elevated levels of angiotensin-converting enzyme (Merritt, pp. 121–122).

47-B; 48-A; 49-E; 50-C; 51-D. Refer to Table 8.47–8.51A (Merritt, pp. 613, 711, 723–724, 727–728, 766; Greenberg, pp. 72–75, 78–79).

52-D; 53-C; 54-A. Note the abnormally thickened stalk with high signal intensity on this coronal MRI depicting Langerhans' cell histiocytosis. The etiology of this condition is unknown, but it is believed to result from overproliferation of an antigen-presenting dendritic cell of bone marrow origin. Although it is usually treated as a neoplastic process, some speculate that it is due to malfunction of the immune system. Other manifestations of this disease may include lytic skull lesions (approximately 80% of cases) as well as hematopoietic, hepatic, and pulmonary abnormalities. A pathognomic finding of this condition on electron microscopy is the presence of Birbeck granules, a unique organelle of the Langerhans' cell (Ramsey, pp. 381–385; Merritt, p. 872).

55-C; 56-A. Acoustic neuroma. Note the palisading of nuclei (picket fence–like arrangement) separated by an anuclear area (arrow) on this photomicrograph, which depicts a Verocay body (Ellison, pp. 695–699).

57. A. A lesion of the MLF does not allow for transfer of information from the abducens nucleus (CN VI) to the opposite

TABLE 8.47–51A   Disorders and their common EMG abnormalities

DISORDER	EMG FINDING
Carpal tunnel syndrome	Sensory > motor latencies
Polymyositis	Myopathic motor units, fibrillations, pseudomyotonia
Amyotrophic lateral sclerosis	Proximal and distal denervation with fasciculations and giant units in at least two extremities; denervation of tongue or thoracic paraspinous muscles
Guillain-Barré syndrome	Reduction in motor unit firing pattern. After 3–5 days, marked slowing in conduction velocities. After 14–21 days, spontaneous denervation activity (positive sharp waves and fibrillations) indicates Wallerian degeneration (axonal loss). Greater axonal loss implies "prolonged disability"
Myotonia	"Dive bomber" frequency
Eaton-Lambert syndrome	Postexercise facilitation
Myasthenia gravis	Decremental response (10% or greater)

oculomotor nucleus (CN III) and results in internuclear ophthalmoplegia (INO). It is characterized by deficient adduction during attempted conjugate gaze away from the side of the MLF lesion and monocular nystagmus of the abducting eye. An MLF lesion is on the same side as the eye with the adduction weakness, and INO is named for the side of the MLF lesion. A lesion in the nucleus of CN III would paralyze volitional movements and convergence (Kline, pp. 63–64).

58-B; 59-A; 60-A; 61-C; 62-D; 63-C. Compressive lesions of the ulnar nerve at the level of the elbow, forearm, or wrist can produce a "claw hand" (A) in severe cases. The ulnar half of the flexor digitorum profundus, lumbricals 3 and 4, the dorsal and palmar interossei, and the hypothenar muscles are typically paralyzed. When the metacarpophalangeal joints are extended, the distal and proximal interphalangeal joints cannot be extended because the interossei and half the lumbricals are not functional, which results in a "claw-like" posture. Laceration of the ulnar nerve in the wrist leaves the innervation of the ulnar side of the flexor digitorum profundus intact but can also result in a claw hand. There is also loss of abduction of the thumb, so that a piece of paper cannot be held between the side of the thumb and the index finger.

Lesions of the median nerve near the elbow can produce paralysis of the flexor digitorum superficialis, the flexor digitorum profundus I and II, the flexor pollicis longus, as well as the thenar muscles and lumbricals 1 and 2. This produces the "sign of benediction," in which the index and middle fingers cannot flex and the thumb cannot be opposed. In addition, there may be numbness over the radial side of the palm and of the digits lateral to the center of the ring finger.

C8 nerve root or anterior interosseous nerve injury causes weakness of the long flexors of the thumb (flexor pollicis longus), index and middle fingers (weak flexor digitorum profundus I and II), and the pronator quadratus. In trying to pinch the index finger and thumb, the terminal phalanges extend and instead of the tips, the pulps touch ("pinch sign," C) (April, pp. 98–100; Patten, pp. 285–296; Greenberg, p. 540).

64-C; 65-B; 66-A; 67-D; 68-E; 69-F. Apraxia is defined as the inability to execute a normal volitional act despite the fact that the motor systems and mental status are relatively intact. Speech apraxia often results from a lesion near the posterior part of the inferior frontal gyrus (approximately area 44), while writing apraxia or dysgraphia results from damage in the left angular gyrus. Dressing apraxia results from damage in the posterior right parietal lobe, while gait apraxia is usually associated with diffuse cerebral disease such as Alzheimer's disease. Lesions that affect the inferomedial part of the temporo-occipital region tend to cause an inability to recognize facial features (prosopagnosia), while lesions of either parietal lobe may produce astereognosis, in which patients fail to recognize the forms of objects when felt but not when viewed (Brazis, pp. 481–508).

70. C. The muscle stretch reflex is a monosynaptic circuit that is dependent on two neurons. Afferent axons serving the muscle stretch reflex synapse directly with ventral motoneurons (Carpenter, p. 79).

71. A. After a complete spinal cord injury, all voluntary movements and sensation below the level of the lesion are lost, but a number of visceral reflexes may be preserved in some cases. A patient with a complete C2 spinal cord injury is unlikely to be able to breathe, since the spinal cord does not contain intrinsic circuitry for breathing. Retained reflexes may include micturition, defecation, peristalsis, and possibly even ejaculation, although there may be no sensation of the sexual act (Brazis, pp. 85–88; DeMyer, pp. 142–143).

72. A. The most important cranial nerve for palatal elevation is generally CN X. Interruption of the left CN X can cause paralysis of palatal elevation on the left side. Taste, swallowing, and phonation are also partially subserved by CN X; therefore an insult to this cranial nerve may result in problems with speech, swallowing, and taste. Salivation problems may be evident with deficits in CN VII and IX (Carpenter, pp. 137–144, 172–173).

73-I; 74-J; 75-F; 76-B; 77-G; 78-C; 79-I; 80-H. The major ascending tracts of the spinal cord (left) are the dorsal columns, spinothalamic tract, dorsal spinocerebellar tract, and ventral spinocerebellar tract. The dorsal columns convey tactile discrimination (Meissner corpuscles), vibration (pacinian corpuscle), joint position sense (muscle spindles and Golgi tendon organs), and conscious proprioception. First-order neurons give rise to axons that ascend in the fasciculus cuneatus (A, upper extremity fibers) and gracilis (B, lower extremity), which terminate in the gracile and cuneate nuclei of the medulla. Second-order neurons, known as arcuate fibers, cross to the contralateral side as the medial lemniscus and ascend to the ventral posterolateral (VPL) nucleus of the thalamus. Synaptic connections are then made in the thalamus with third-order neurons, which travel through the posterior limb of the internal capsule to reach the postcentral gyrus of the cerebral cortex.

Four groups of fibers have been distinguished in the anterolateral system (I) on the basis of their anatomic projections: spinothalamic, spinoreticular, spinomesencephalic, and spinotectal. First-order neurons of the lateral spinothalamic tract (pain and temperature sensation) project axons via the dorsolateral tract of Lissauer to second-order neurons in the substantia gelatinosa of the dorsal horn. Second-order neurons then decussate in the ventral white commissure, ascend in the ventral half of the lateral funiculus, and synapse in the VPL nucleus of the thalamus. Third-order neurons from the thalamus are then relayed to the somatosensory cortex of the postcentral gyrus (areas 3, 1, and 2) through the posterior limb of the internal capsule. A number of collateral fibers from the spinothalamic tract are relayed to the reticular formation (spinoreticulothalamic tract), which transmits nociceptive fibers to the intralaminar nuclei of the thalamus. Additional fibers of the anterolateral system terminate in either the periaqueductal gray (spinomesencephalic) or the deep layers of the superior colliculus (spinotectal). The periaqueductal gray sends descending projections to serotonergic neurons of the raphe nucleus of the pons and nucleus gigantocellularis (noradrenergic neurons) of the medulla. Both of these areas, in turn, send projections to the dorsal horn and inhibit postsynaptic responses to nociceptive input. The spinotectal pathway directs visual attention to areas of the body that experience intense somatosensory input. Other pathways, such as the dorsal spinocerebellar (K) and ventral spinocerebellar tracts (J), transmit unconscious proprioception from the lower limbs and inferior half of the body to the cerebellum, while the cuneocerebellar and rostrocerebellar tracts convey

similar information from the upper body and limbs (not shown).

The corticospinal tract arises predominately from three cortical areas (approximately 30% each): the premotor cortex (area 6), the precentral motor cortex (area 4), and the postcentral sensory cortex (areas 3, 1, and 2). It undergoes a 90% decussation in the caudal medulla and travels in the dorsal quadrant of the lateral funiculus of the spinal cord. The ventral corticospinal tract (H) is a small, uncrossed tract that decussates in the ventral white commissure and is mainly concerned with control of axial musculature. The vestibulospinal tract (F) arises from the lateral vestibular nucleus (Dieter's) and influences extensor tone. The medial longitudinal fasciculus (G) carries fibers from medial and inferior vestibular nuclei, tectospinal tract, and interstitial nucleus of Cajal and coordinates eye movements, mediates nystagmus, and helps control conjugate gaze (Carpenter, pp. 83–106; Pritchard, pp. 114–125; Brazis, pp. 80–85; DeMyer, pp. 120–132).

81. B. Facial nerve displacement by an acoustic neuroma is most commonly (in decreasing order of frequency) anterior, followed by superior, inferior, and posterior. The facial nerve is often stretched during microdissection and is most susceptible to injury at the proximal rim of the porus acusticus (Connolly, p. 475).

82. C. Paralysis of pelvic floor muscles, early sphincter and bladder dysfunction, symmetric saddle anesthesia, impaired erection and ejaculation, constipation, and minimal pain best characterize the conus medullaris syndrome. A tethered cord may present with a combination of neurologic, urologic, orthopedic, and dermatologic manifestations. Commonly patients present with numb feet, muscle atrophy, upper motor neuron signs, bowel and bladder dysfunction, foot deformities, scoliosis, and cutaneous stigmata of spinal dysraphism. Compression of the lumbar and sacral roots below L3 often results in cauda equina syndrome, which is characterized by early pain, asymmetric saddle anesthesia, and a variable patellar reflex response. Sphincter changes are often similar to those of the conus medullaris syndrome but tend to occur late in the clinical course. With S1 lesions, there is weakness of the triceps surae, flexor digitorum longus (FDL), flexor hallucis longus (FHL), and small foot muscles. The Achilles reflexes are absent, whereas the patellar reflexes are preserved. There is complete sensory loss over the sole, heel, and outer part of the foot and ankle. The gastrocnemius and soleus muscles are stronger with S2 segmental lesions, however, the FDL, FHL, and foot muscles remain weak. The sensory loss tends to involve the upper part of the dorsal calf, dorsolateral thigh, and the saddle area (Brazis, pp. 99–100).

83. D. This CT demonstrates a subarachnoid hemorrhage (SAH), which is most commonly seen after trauma. Although the blood pattern may vary, traumatic SAH often involves the convexities of the cerebral hemispheres, while aneurysmal subarachnoid hemorrhages generally have a preponderance of blood in the basal cisterns (Greenberg, p. 754).

84. D. Experimental studies indicate the orbitofrontal cortex is a key region involved with the conscious perception of smell, as lesions in this region have been shown to result in failure to discriminate between various odorants (Kandel, p. 633).

85-D; 86-C. This T2-weighted image shows the hyperintense and thickened folia in a characteristic laminated pattern that is most consistent with Lhermitte-Duclos disease. It is associated with hypertrophy of granular cell neurons and axonal hypermyelination in the molecular layer (Osborn DN, pp. 69–70).

87. D. This T2-weighted MRI shows a right temporal lobe mass with signal loss (flow void), which is most consistent with a large middle cerebral artery aneurysm (Osborn DN, pp. 266–268).

88-C; 89-G; 90-I; 91-E; 92-H; 93-B; 94-A; 95-J. Refer to Table 8.88–95A (Brazis, pp. 221–232; Wilkins, pp. 118–125).

96. A. Orbital injuries often impair the action of the superior oblique muscle because of displacement of the trochlea, which attaches to the anterior rim of the orbit and acts as a sling for the recurrent course of the trochlear tendon. Looking down and to the left typically involves the right superior oblique (trochlear nerve, IV) and left inferior rectus (oculomotor nerve, III) muscles. When the eyes look conjugately toward any object, the muscle that is the prime mover

works in unison with the muscle of the opposite eye (Kline, pp. 105–114).

97. E. Note the numerous capillaries and cells with a vacuolated appearance in this photomicrograph depicting a hemangioblastoma. This tumor is associated with VHL in about 25% of cases, is carried in an autosomal dominant fashion (chromosome 3p25), and is associated with retinal angioma, renal cell carcinoma, renal and pancreatic cysts, pheochromocytoma, or epididymal papillary cystadenoma. This tumor may cause polycythemia in about 10% of cases due to inappropriate production of erythropoietin (Ellison, pp. 736–738).

98-B; 99-D. Acute hemolytic transfusion reactions are uncommon and are rarely life-threatening. They are produced by antibodies in the recipient that bind to ABO surface antigens or erythrocytes of mismatched donor blood. These antibodies fix complement and can produce rapid cell lysis within minutes. Lysis then provokes a severe inflammatory reaction, which can lead to hypotension, multiorgan dysfunction, and a host of other clinical findings. This type of transfusion reaction is often the result of identification errors, leading to ABO mismatched blood. The transfusion should be stopped immediately; the volume status, urine output, and blood pressure should be monitored and maintained; and the patient's blood sent for free hemoglobin, haptoglobin levels, and a Coombs' test. Treatment includes supportive care with maintenance of good urine out.

Febrile nonhemolytic reactions are the most common acute transfusion reactions, appearing in about 1% of all transfusions. These reactions occur when antibodies in the recipient react against leukocytes in the donor blood. The antileukocyte antibodies develop in response to prior

TABLE 8.88–95A   Nystagmus and associated lesion sights

TYPE OF NYSTAGMUS	LESION SIGHTS
Seesaw	Posterior diencephalon/pretectum (interstitial nucleus of Cajal), para/suprasellar lesions, lateral medulla
Spasmus mutans	Seen in infants, etiology/lesion site unclear; associated with following triad: head nodding, nystagmus, head turning
Lid nystagmus	Lateral medulla, cerebellum
Brun's nystagmus	Pontomedullary junction, vestibular pathways
Ocular bobbing	Central pons
Ocular myoclonus	Ipsilateral inferior olive, red nucleus, contralateral dentate nucleus (Guillain-Mollaret triangle) (also associated with palatal myoclonus)
Upbeat nystagmus	Medulla, ventral tegmentum, cerebellar pathways (anterior vermis)
Downbeat nystagmus	Cervicomedullary junction (Chiari malformation), cerebellum, nuclei prepositus hypoglossi, medial vestibular nuclei
Ocular flutter	Cerebellar pathways, brainstem
Abducting nystagmus	Pons (MLF)
Convergence-retraction nystagmus	Dorsal midbrain, pretectum (pineal tumors)

transfusions or pregnancies and are most often seen in multiparous women or in patients with prior blood transfusions. More than 50% of patients who develop febrile nonhemolytic reactions will not experience a similar reaction during subsequent transfusions; therefore no special precautions are necessary. If a second febrile reaction occurs, leukocyte-poor red blood cell preparations are advised.

Allergic or hypersensitivity reactions are the result of sensitization to plasma proteins in prior transfusions. Patients with IgA deficiency are particularly prone to hypersensitivity reactions, and these can occur without prior exposure to plasma products (Marino, pp. 700–703; Nwariaku, pp. 54–55).

100. E. The presence of multiple intradural spinal cord tumors is relatively common with NF-2 and may include ependymomas (most common), schwannomas, and meningiomas (Greenberg, p. 478).

101. A. The pyramidal neurons of the hippocampus (Ammon's horn) send numerous fiber projections to the subiculum and entorhinal cortex (area 28), which form the anterior part of the parahippocampal gyrus (Carpenter, pp. 369–382).

102. A. Note the "staghorn" vascular channel in this grade II hemangiopericytoma. These tumors are vimentin-positive, EMA-negative, have a dense arrangement of sheet-like cells, and have a high nuclear-cytoplasmic ratio. Other characteristics include focal lobularity, paucicellular areas, and dense pericellular reticulin (Ellison, pp. 736–738).

103. C. Lesions that occupy the anterior part of the left parasylvian fissure may cause a nonfluent type of aphasia (Broca's). This region may abut the parts of the motor cortex that supply the upper motor neuron fibers for the contralateral facial nucleus. Therefore a patient with right-sided upper motor neuron facial deficit may also have an expressive-type of aphasia originating from Broca's area (Brazis, pp. 511–516).

104. B. A coronal section through the genu of the internal capsule would almost exclusively bisect the globus pallidus, which is triangle-shaped, with its apex fitting into the genu of the internal capsule (Carpenter, pp. 337–344).

105. C. The middle cerebral artery (MCA) is divided anatomically into four major segments: M1 (horizontal) segment, M2 (insular segment), M3 (opercular segment), and M4 (cortical) segment. The anterior temporal artery typically arises from the M1 segment of the MCA before the bifurcation. It passes directly anteriorly and inferiorly over the temporal tip and usually does not course toward the sylvian fissure. Although relatively uncommon, aneurysms can form at the origin or further distally along this vessel (as

depicted here). An accessory middle cerebral artery is an MCA branch that arises from either the ACA (more common) or the ICA and parallels the M1 segment toward the sylvian fissure. The lenticulostriate arteries are divided into a smaller medial group and a larger lateral group that originate from the distal half of the M1 segment and project superiorly to enter the anterior perforated substance to supply parts of the lentiform nuclei, caudate nucleus, and internal capsule. The posterior temporal artery usually originates from the M4 segment of the MCA and supplies the posterior temporal lobe. The frontopolar artery is a branch of the anterior cerebral artery (A2 portion), which originates below the rostrum or genu of the corpus callosum and extends anteriorly to supply the frontal pole (Osborn DCA, pp. 135–137).

106. C. Most patients develop some degree of vessel narrowing after aneurysmal subarachnoid hemorrhage. About 70% will develop angiographic vasospasm, and approximately 30% will go on to develop symptomatic vasospasm (Youmans, p. 1545).

107. E. Over the past few decades a variety of medical, surgical, and radiation interventions have evolved that have proven effective in reducing GH levels. No one treatment is uniformly effective, and often a combination of interventions is required. When a macroadenoma is surgically resected transsphenoidally, endocrine remission rates vary between 65 and 90%. When a macroadenoma is resected, immediate postoperative remission is reported to be even lower (30 and 79%). The rate of remission is adversely affected by a higher preoperative GH level and larger invasive tumors. Therefore biochemical cure with surgery for large GH-secreting macroadenomas is typically not expected. Conventional radiation therapy can usually shrink pituitary tumors when up to 50 Gy is delivered in 1.8-Gy fractions over 6 weeks, but a decrease or normalization of GH levels usually takes many years. When initial GH levels are > 100 µg/mL, only 60% of patients will attain GH levels < 5 µg/mL after 18 years following radiation, and about 50% will develop hypopituitarism within 10 years. Radiosurgery has the same disadvantages as conventional radiation and would add increased risk in this patient due to the proximity of the lesion to the optic nerves and chiasm. Although perhaps controversial, some endocrinologists are advocating primary drug therapy in patients with GH-secreting macroadenomas (especially with normal vision). Bromocriptine, a dopamine agonist, has been documented to lower GH levels in up to 71% of patients, and octreotide, a somatostatin analogue, has achieved similar results. If there is no shrinkage of the tumor after 16 weeks of therapy, further use of medication has been shown to have little impact. Patients with rapidly deteriorating vision or other neurologic problems related to the lesion (unlike our patient) are often not good candidates for a trial of medical therapy and often require more urgent surgical intervention. Nevertheless, the most effective treatment strategy for acromegaly secondary to a GH-secreting macroadenoma usually requires a combination of surgical and medical options (Berger, pp. 405–406).

108-A; 109-D; 110-G; 111-B; 112-F; 113-C; 114-E; 115-H; 116-I. Figure 8.108–8.116Q demonstrates the surgical anatomy of the right lateral and anterior third ventricle during endoscopic third ventriculostomy for aqueductal stenosis. The ventriculostomy site is depicted in the floor of the third ventricle in this figure. The veins of the third ventricular system collect into deeper veins that course in a subependymal location as they travel through the margins of the choroidal fissure to empty into the internal cerebral, basal, and great veins. In general, the veins draining the frontal horn and body of the third ventricle drain into the internal cerebral vein (not depicted here) as it courses through the velum interpositum; those draining the temporal horn drain into a segment of the basal vein of Rosenthal coursing through the ambient cistern; and the veins from the atrium drain into segments of the basal, internal cerebral, and great veins coursing through the quadrigeminal cistern. Of note, the thalamostriate vein passes forward in the sulcus between the caudate nucleus and thalamus toward the foramen of Monro (FOM), where it turns sharply posterior to enter the velum interpositum to join the internal cerebral vein. The angle formed by the junction of the internal cerebral vein and thalamostriate vein, referred to as the venous angle, approximates the level of the FOM on the lateral view of a cerebral angiogram (Wilkins, pp. 1427–1429; Youmans, pp. 1237–1240).

117. E. Occlusion or injury of the thalamostriate vein may cause drowsiness, hemiplegia, mutism, and hemorrhagic infarction of the basal ganglia (Wilkins, pp. 1427–1429).

118. C. Acute microscopic changes after DAI typically include axonal retraction balls and perivascular hemorrhages, while in later stages there can be astrogliosis, endothelial proliferation, and accumulation of hemosiderin-laden macrophages (Marion, pp. 40–45; Ellison, pp. 249–257; Ramsey, pp. 431–434).

119. C. In approaching the posterior ilium during autogenous iliac bone graft harvesting, a limited incision that stays within 8 cm of the posterior superior iliac spine typically avoids the superior cluneal nerves. Dissection is then carried down to the gluteal fascia, which should be opened directly above the iliac crest to facilitate fascial closure. During subcrestal exposure, the lateral subperiosteal dissection should be carried to the gluteus medius and tensor fascia lata muscles. Subperiosteal dissection usually avoids damage to the superior gluteal artery, which courses through the musculature. The sciatic notch usually lies approximately 7 to 8 cm below the iliac crest and must not be violated, as it harbors the main trunk of the sciatic artery, the sciatic nerve, and the

ureter, which runs ventral to the superior gluteal artery. Medially, the dissection should extend to the iliacus muscle, which prevents injury to the iliohypogastric and ilioinguinal nerves (Connolly, pp. 819–820).

120-D; 121-D; 122-B. Note the absence of the corpus callosum and the high-riding third ventricle on this sagittal MRI depicting agenesis of the corpus callosum. This condition is usually not associated with Chiari I malformation but rather with the Chiari II malformation (Osborn DN, pp. 29–33).

123. B. Stability at the atlantoaxial unit is mainly provided by the horizontal portion of the cruciate ligament (transverse atlantal ligament), and the paired alar ligaments (atlantoalar portion) that connect the dens with the lateral masses of C1. With disruption of these ligaments, the remaining cruciate and apical ligaments are insufficient to maintain stability. Ligaments that connect the axis to the occiput include the tectorial membrane (rostral continuation of the posterior longitudinal ligament), occipitoalar portion of the alar ligament, and the apical ligament (connects the tip of dens to the foramen magnum), while the ligaments connecting the atlas to the occiput include the tectorial membrane and anterior longitudinal ligament (Greenberg, p. 701; Youmans, pp. 3528–3551).

124-C; 125-D. This patient harbors a glomus jugulare tumor, which often presents with unilateral hearing loss or pulsatile tinnitus. Intracranial extension usually affects multiple cranial nerves, which may result in a number of clinical problems including dysphagia. Angiography is essential because it helps with surgical planning. It helps delineate the blood supply to the tumor as well as collateral blood flow to the brain. Often preoperative embolization is a useful adjunct for these highly vascular and locally invasive tumors. Although observation with serial imaging studies to determine tumor progression may be an appropriate option for medically frail patients, gross total resection is considered the treatment of choice for symptomatic lesions (Youmans, pp. 1295–1308).

126-A; 127-D. The fracture-pattern (Jefferson fracture) depicted on this axial CT scan most often results from an axial load on a neutral neck. These patients are usually neurologically intact due to the large diameter of the spinal canal at this level. If the sum of overhang of both lateral masses on C2 is ≥ 7 mm, the transverse ligament is probably disrupted, which requires rigid immobilization (usually with a halo vest) or surgical fixation if additional fractures are present (Greenberg, pp. 702–703).

128-E; 129-A. A lesion of the facial nerve distal to the geniculate ganglion but proximal to the stylomastoid foramen typically results in complete paralysis of all ipsilateral facial muscles, a diminished corneal reflex (with preserved corneal sensation, CN V), impaired sublingual and submandibular salivary gland secretions, hyperacusis, and frequently loss of taste in the anterior two-thirds of the tongue ipsilaterally. Hyperacusis results from paralysis of the stapedius muscle, while salivary secretions are impaired due to the interruption of preganglionic parasympathetic fibers. Lesions proximal to the geniculate ganglion produce all of the disturbances described above and invariably loss of taste in the anterior two-thirds of the tongue and decreased lacrimation. This lesion interrupts all SVA fibers that course centrally and all preganglionic (GVE) fibers as they pass to the pterygopalatine and submandibular ganglia. Taste is permanently lost and no regeneration of sensory fibers takes place. Preganglionic parasympathetic fibers may regenerate, but this may occur in an aberrant fashion. Fibers that previously projected to the submandibular ganglion may regrow and enter the greater petrosal nerve, which may result in lacrimation after a salivary stimulus ("crocodile tears") (Carpenter, pp. 172–173).

130. B. Mammillary fibers projecting from the medial mammillary nucleus and, to a lesser extent, intermediate and lateral mammillary nuclei form a fiber bundle called the fasciculus mammillaris princes, which divides into two components: the mammillothalamic tract and mammillotegmental tract. The mammillothalamic tract contains fibers that originate from the medial mammillary nucleus and project to the anterior thalamic nucleus. Fibers from the hippocampus are also superimposed on this fiber bundle as they travel to the anterior thalamic nucleus through the fornix. The mammillotegmental tract terminates in the dorsal and ventral tegmental nuclei (Carpenter, p. 309).

131. B. Crossed fibers from the fastigial nucleus emerge from the cerebellum through the uncinate fasciculus of Russell, which arches around the superior cerebellar peduncle. Uncrossed fastigial efferents project to the brainstem in the juxtarestiform body. The largest number of fastigial efferents project to structures in the lower brainstem (nucleus reticularis gigantocellularis, central pontine reticular formation, dorsal paramedian reticular nucleus). A small number of fibers ascend in the dorsolateral brainstem and send collaterals to the superior colliculus and nuclei of the posterior commissure prior to terminating in various thalamic regions (VLc and VPLo) (Carpenter, pp. 241–243).

132. A. Some excitatory effects of the sympathetic nervous system that lack parasympathetic opposition include splenic capsule contraction, sweating and piloerection, and elevation of the upper eyelid by the superior tarsal muscle of Muller. Gastrointestinal peristalsis, bladder wall contraction, bronchial size, pupillary diameter, heart rate, and blood pressure can all be oppositionally altered by the sympathetic and parasympathetic nervous system (DeMyer, p. 92).

133-A; 134-D. The mechanism of most modern hangman's fractures results from hyperextension and axial loading (diving and motor vehicle accidents), while judicial hangings often resulted in hyperextension and distractive forces from submeatal knot placement. Patients rarely require surgical intervention for this type of fracture, which is typically reserved for irreducible fractures, failure of external immobilization, traumatic C2-3 disc herniation (with canal compromise and progressive neurologic deficit), and established nonunion. All fusion techniques typically involve fusing C2 to C3, although the majority of patients can be successfully treated with a cervical collar, SOMI brace, or halo vest (most common) (Greenberg, pp. 704–706).

135. E. Klippel-Feil syndrome ranges from fusion of only a few vertebral bodies to fusion of the entire spine. It results from failure of somite segregation between 3 and 8 weeks' gestation. The classic triad (usually present in < 50% of people) includes low posterior hairline, shortened neck (brevicollis), and limited neck motion. It may occur in conjunction with various other abnormalities including basilar impression, atlantoaxial fusion, facial asymmetry, torticollis, pterygium colli (neck webbing), scoliosis, and Sprengel's deformity (25% of cases). Sprengel's deformity results in a raised scapula due to failed migration from its region of formation in the neck. Systemic congenital abnormalities may also occur, including deafness (30%), unilateral absence of a kidney, and cardiopulmonary complications. Treatment is usually directed at detecting and managing the systemic anomalies, which typically consists of a cardiac evaluation (ECG), CXR, and a renal ultrasound. Nevus flammeus is usually seen in patients with tethered cord syndrome (Greenberg, p. 158).

136-C; 137-A, 138-A, 139-B. The anterior fontanelle, the largest fontanelle, is diamond-shaped and normally closes by 2.5 years of age. The posterior fontanelle is triangle-shaped and closes by 2 to 3 months. The sphenoid and mastoid fontanelles are smaller, more irregular, and usually close by 2 to 3 months and 1 year, respectively (Greenberg, p. 138).

140. E. Blood supply to the dura originates from the middle meningeal artery, which is a branch of the maxillary artery. It enters the skull through the foramen spinosum. The ophthalmic artery (anterior meningeal branches) and occipital and vertebral arteries (posterior meningeal arteries) also provide meningeal branches to the dura (Carpenter, pp. 1–2).

141. B. The typical order of the three great vessels that originate from the aortic arch is the brachiocephalic trunk (innominate artery) followed by the left common carotid artery (LCCA) and then left subclavian artery (LSCA). This configuration is found in approximately two-thirds of all cases. A shared origin of the brachiocephalic trunk and left common carotid artery is seen in 27% (most frequent variant) of cases, while in 7% of cases the left common carotid artery arises from the proximal brachiocephalic artery instead of the aortic arch. In 1 to 2% of cases, the LCCA and LSCA share a common origin and form a left-sided brachiocephalic trunk (Osborn DCA, p. 16).

142. C. Formal diagnosis of myasthenia gravis depends on demonstration of response to cholinergic medications, EMG evidence of abnormal neuromuscular transmission ("jitter," "blocking"), and identification of circulating antibodies to Ach receptors or myofibrillar proteins such as actin, titin, myosin, and actinomycin (in approximately 85 to 90% of cases). In single-muscle-fiber EMG studies, an electrode measures the interval between evoked potentials of muscle fibers in the same unit. This interval normally varies by "jitter", for which the temporal limits have been defined. In myasthenia gravis, "jitter" is increased. If muscle fibers are not activated due to abnormal neuromuscular transmission, it is called "blocking." Myasthenia gravis is characterized by both "blocking" and increased "jitter," although these findings are not specific for myasthenia gravis, as other disorders may show a similar response on EMG studies. Signs of denervation are almost never seen in disorders of ACh release unless other conditions supervene. Cholinergic medications should be stopped once an endotracheal tube has been placed to reduce the amount of pulmonary secretions. Prednisone, plasmapheresis, and IVIG therapy have all been used in patients with generalized disease and/or respiratory crisis. Thymectomy is generally recommended for patients with generalized myasthenia gravis, not ocular myasthenia (Merritt, pp. 723–726).

143-G; 144-F; 145-C; 146-E; 147-B; 148-A. Refer to Table 8.143–8.148A (Merritt, p. 525).

149. B. The largest quantity of afferents projecting to the striatum originate in the cerebral cortex, although the amygdala, intralaminar nuclei of the thalamus, the substantia nigra, and dorsal raphe nucleus send fibers to various parts of the striatum as well (Carpenter, pp. 332–336).

150-D; 151-B; 152-C; 153-A; 154-E. Athetoid movements are slow, writhing movements predominately of the hand and wrist, while dystonia characteristically affects the axial muscles. The lesion "status marmoratus" characterizes one form of cerebral palsy, which consists of a marbled appearance of the corpus striatum and thalamus secondary to perinatal hypoxia. Hypoxic damage in these areas results in overgrowth of astrocytes as part of the healing process. Oligodendrocytes then mistakenly myelinate astrocytic processes, which causes white patches to appear in the nuclei, giving them a marbled appearance. Damage to the striatum and thalamus from other causes such as infarcts may also result in athetosis. Lesions of the substantia nigra can result in rigidity and resting tremor, which are some of the hallmarks of Parkinson's disease. Lesions of the subthalamic

TABLE 8.143–148A   Mucopolysaccharidoses

SYNDROME	ENZYME DEFICIENCY	CLINICAL FEATURES
Hurler's	α-L-Iduronidase	Death usually by age 10, corneal clouding, mental retardation, coarse facial features, dwarfism, organomegaly, deafness, urinary excretion of dermatan sulfate and heparan sulfate
Hunter's	Iduronate-2-sulfate sulfatase	Similar to Hurler's with the exception of pebbling of skin and absence of corneal clouding, death usually by age 15, urinary excretion of dermatan sulfate and heparan sulfate
Sanfilippo A	Sulfamidase (heparan sulfate N-sulfatase)	Mild coarsening of facial features, organomegaly, hirsutism, joint stiffness, dysostosis multiplex, dementia, spastic paraparesis, seizures, athetosis, corneal clouding absent, slight dwarfing
Sanfilippo B	α-N acetylglucosamidase	Similar to Sanfilippo A with urinary excretion of heparan sulfate
Morquio A	Galactose-6-sulfate sulfatase	Severe skeletal disorder, little neurologic abnormality, urinary excretion of keratan sulfate, cardiac or respiratory disease may cause death in third or fourth decade
Morquio B	β-Galactosidase	Urinary excretion of keratan sulfate and oligosaccharides as well
Marateaux-Lamy syndrome	Sulfatase B	Resembles Hurler's syndrome with normal intelligence, dermatan sulfate excretion
Scheie	α-L-Iduronidase	Milder form of Hurler's, corneal clouding, dysostosis multiplex, pigmentary retinopathy, carpal tunnel syndrome, life span may be normal except in cases of cardiac disease
Sly	β-Glucuronidase	Mental retardation, dwarfing, dysostosis multiplex, cardiac disease, organomegaly, hydrocephalus

nucleus can produce hemiballism, while terminal tremor, ataxia, and CN III palsy usually result from injury in the vicinity of the red nucleus. Bilateral lesions of the amygdala can produce the Klüver-Bucy syndrome, which is characterized by visual agnosia, oral-exploratory behavior, hypersexuality, hypomotility, and hypermetamorphosis (tendency to take notice and attend to every visual stimulus) (Brazis, pp. 433–436, 439–442, 552; Merritt, pp. 681–682).

155. E. The thalamus receives its arterial supply from the anterior choroidal artery (ICA) and thalamoperforating arteries (PComA and basilar artery) as well as the thalamogeniculate and posterior choroidal arteries (PCA). Infarctions may occur in each of these thalamic territories and cause various clinical syndromes, depending on which thalamic nuclei are involved (Carpenter, pp. 441–450).

156. B. Note the prominent diffuse plaques traversed by neuronal processes in this patient with Alzheimer's disease. Diffuse amyloid plaques are extracellular, ill-defined focal aggregates of amyloid and preamyloid material and are approximately 60 to 300 mm in diameter. Neuronal cell processes traversing the plaque typically appear normal and do not contain tau protein (Ellison, pp. 553–557).

157-E; 158-D; 159-A; 160-F; 161-H; 162-E; 163-A; 164-G. Occipital condylar and burst fractures are often the result of purely axial compressive forces on a neutral neck, while teardrop and compression-wedge fractures result from compressive force on a flexed neck. Other injury or fracture patterns in the cervical spine include unilateral (axial rotation, flexing) and bilateral locked (hyperflexion and distraction) facets, Chance fracture (flexion, distraction), and unilateral facet fracture (lateral bending, compression). Odontoid fractures usually result from hyperflexion injuries and result in anterior displacement of C2 on C3. (Greenberg, pp. 702–714; Youmans, pp. 517–523, 4896–4897, 4927; Harris, pp. 69–91).

165. C. Note the squamous cells, peripheral palisading of nuclei, and nodules of wet keratin in this adamantinomatous craniopharyngioma (Ellison, pp. 724–727; WHO, pp. 244–246).

166. E. Approximately 90% of cases of vertigo are likely secondary to lesions of the vestibular end organs or vestibular nerves, while the rest usually originate from the central nervous system, including craniocervical junction abnormalities (Merritt, pp. 28–30).

167. D. The supratentorial dura is innervated primarily by branches of the trigeminal nerve, while the infratentorial dura is innervated by branches of the vagus and lower cervical spinal nerves (Carpenter, p. 2).

168-D; 169-C. Depicted here is an axial and parasagittal MRI showing a soft (mainly disc material) posterolateral disc herniation of the cervical spine that is eccentric to the left. Considering that this disc herniation is not purely central, it may be amenable to a posterolateral procedure in an attempt to preserve vocal cord function (posterior keyhole laminotomy) in this wedding singer. Over 90% of patients with acute cervical radiculopathy will improve with nonsurgical therapy including adequate pain medication and anti-inflammatories. Surgery is indicated for those who fail to improve or develop progressive neurologic deficits while undergoing nonsurgical therapy. A number of large series have reported good or excellent results in 90 to 96% of patients who underwent a posterior approach for such disc herniations (Greenberg, pp. 310–314).

170. B. Yolk sac tumor is a germ cell tumor that exhibits loosely arranged cells with clear cytoplasm and prominent eosinophilic bodies. Yolk sac tumors are positive for AFP, and they often exhibit Schiller-Duval bodies (Ellison, p. 683).

171. B. Meticulous preoperative anesthetic workup is extremely important for acromegalic patients, since they frequently exhibit cardiomyopathy and macroglossia, which can be associated with a difficult airway (Youmans, p. 569).

172. C. HD primarily affects the GABA/enkephalin projections from the striatum to the external segment of the globus pallidus (indirect pathway), resulting in thalamic facilitation of motor cortical areas and hyperkinesia (Merritt, pp. 659–662).

173. E. Note the prominent lobules of cells with an intervening vascular network of sinusoids in this photomicrograph of a normal adenohypophysis (Ellison, p. 716).

174. C. Meckel-Gruber syndrome typically includes encephalocele, microcephaly, microphthalmia, cleft lip, polydactyly, polycystic kidneys, congenital heart disease, and ambiguous genitalia; it is most often associated with maternal hyperthermia on gestational days 20 to 26 (Rudolph, p. 156).

175. D. The release of a single quantum of acetylcholine (10,000 molecules of ACh) produces a miniature endplate potential (MEPP) in the postsynaptic membrane, which is not significant enough to generate an action potential. The summation of several quanta is required to induce enough depolarization in the postsynaptic cell membrane to result in an action potential (Kandel, pp. 255–262).

176. B. Nitric oxide (NO) is produced in neurons by the Ca^{2+}/calmodulin-dependent enzyme NO synthase. NO, in turn, stimulates the synthesis of cGMP through the action of guanylyl cyclase, an enzyme that converts GTP to cGMP. NO acts locally and is primarily released from endothelial cells to induce smooth muscle relaxation and blood vessel dilation (Kandel, p. 239).

177. C. Neuronal cytoplasmic organelles include rough and smooth endoplasmic reticulum, endosomes, secretory vesicles, lysosomes, peroxisomes, mitochondria, and the Golgi apparatus. Proteins and phospholipids destined for secretion are initially synthesized in the rough endoplasmic reticulum (rER). These products are then transported to the Golgi apparatus via transport vesicles for processing (although N-linked glycosylation and glycolipid conjugation are initiated in the rER). The Golgi complex further modifies these proteins by adding polysaccharides, which can direct specific proteins to secretory vesicles, lysosomes, and the plasma membrane. Golgi processing includes glycosylation reactions (O-linked and N-linked glycosylation), proteoglycan formation, polysaccharide phosphorylation, attachment of fatty acids, and sulfation of tyrosine (not arginine) and sugar residues. This processing increases the hydrophilicity (solubility) of these proteins, increases their biological activity, or helps delay their degradation by proteases. Clathrin coats facilitate the budding of vesicles from the Golgi complex. Secretory vesicles (dense-core vesicles) are targeted primarily to axon terminals, where they participate in calcium-regulated exocytosis after action potential propagation (Kandel, pp. 67–71, 94–97).

178. B. The BBB is primarily composed of tight junctions between nonfenestrated endothelial cells. These endothelial cells are also deficient in vesicular transport compared to endothelial cells elsewhere in the body, which further contributes to the selectivity of the BBB. The resistance provided by the tight junctions between endothelial cells in the brain is extremely high. Substances may cross the BBB by diffusion, active transport, carrier-mediated transport, and through ion channels. Lipid-soluble substances readily diffuse across endothelial cell membranes into the brain; hence the permeability of many substances is directly related to their lipid-solubility. Specific carrier-mediated transport is responsible for the entry of most substances into the brain. The glucose transporter (Glut1) is energy-independent, thus transporting only glucose down its concentration gradient from the bloodstream into the brain. There are also three distinct carrier systems for amino acid transport across the BBB. The L system transports large neutral branched-chain amino acids and L-DOPA into the brain. A transport system that is a member of the multiple-drug-resistance (MDR) transporter family found in tumor cells removes a wide range of hydrophobic toxins and chemotherapeutic agents from the brain. Additionally, specific ion channels allow the movement of electrolytes across the BBB. A metabolic BBB also exists due to the presence of certain enzymes that rapidly metabolize substances as they enter the CNS. An example is the high concentration of DOPA decarboxylase in epithelial cells that rapidly metabolize L-DOPA as it enters the brain

unless a DOPA decarboxylase inhibitor (carbidopa) is also administered (Kandel, pp. 1288–1294).

179. D. The substantia nigra has the highest concentration of substance P in the brain. Striatonigral projections from the caudate nucleus and putamen contain GABA, substance P, and enkephalin (Carpenter, pp. 215–221).

180-C; 181-E. Note that the anterior cerebral arteries are being pushed upward on this lateral angiogram, depicting an olfactory groove meningioma. These lesions often grow insidiously, causing gradual compression of the frontal lobes; thus they are quite large and bilateral by the time of presentation. Common signs/symptoms may include headaches, personality changes, visual loss, anosmia, and seizures. A bifrontal transbasal approach is frequently used in resecting these tumors, although a unilateral subfrontal or frontotemporal (pterional) craniotomy can also be used. The anterior and posterior ethmoid arteries typically supply olfactory groove meningiomas (Kaye and Black, pp. 523–532; Youmans, pp. 1115–1115).

182-A; 183-B; 184-B; 185-B; 186-B. Charcot-Marie-Tooth (CMT) disease, or peroneal muscular atrophy, accounts for about 90% of all hereditary neuropathies, of which there are three types. CMT-1, the most common, is autosomal dominant and is a demyelinating disease that results in a distal sensorimotor neuropathy. It results from mutations in peripheral myelin protein 22 (PMP-22), exhibits slowed nerve conduction velocities, and exhibits onion-bulb formations on histopathologic studies. CMT-2 resembles CMT-1 but results in axonal degeneration instead of demyelination. CMT-3, also known as Dejerine-Sottas syndrome, is autosomal dominant and results in a hypertrophic demyelinating neuropathy. DMD is an X-linked recessive condition that results from mutation of the dystrophin gene, located at Xp21. Patients often have difficulty rising from the ground and rely heavily on the arms to raise the torso and legs (Gowers' sign). These patients may also exhibit toe-walking and develop an exaggerated lumbar lordosis or scoliosis as well as pseudohypertrophy of the calves from fibrosis and fatty infiltration of degenerating muscle. MD is a trinucleotide repeat disorder that results from mutation of the dystrophia myotonica protein kinase gene on chromosome 19. It is a pleiotropic, autosomal dominant disorder affecting the skeletal muscle, heart, eyes, and exocrine glands. The myopathy of MD affects several cranial nerves (ptosis, dysarthria, dysphagia) and the distal extremities (finger flexors and extensors). Patients exhibit myotonia (impaired muscle relaxation), cataracts, frontal balding, testicular atrophy, retinal degeneration, cardiomyopathy, and an increased incidence of mental retardation. FSHMD is an autosomal dominant disorder that results in scapular winging, facial weakness, shoulder girdle weakness, and lower extremity weakness (Merritt, pp. 737–746).

187. E. The common peroneal nerve (L4-S2) innervates the extensors and adductors of the leg (and part of the biceps femoris) and gives rise to the lateral sural cutaneous nerve (to the inferolateral leg), the deep peroneal nerve, and the superficial peroneal nerve. The deep peroneal nerve innervates the tibialis anterior, extensor hallucis longus, and extensor digitorum longus muscles. The superficial peroneal nerve innervates the peroneus longus/brevis (foot eversion) and the skin of the distal anterior leg, dorsum of the foot, and digits. Lesions of the common peroneal nerve mainly result in paralysis of dorsiflexion (footdrop) and foot eversion (Patten, p. 311; Greenberg, pp. 522, 545).

188. B. Hippocampal sclerosis usually has a very characteristic pattern in patients with mesial temporal lobe epilepsy. The greatest amount of damage is usually seen in the CA1 and CA4 sectors, while the least amount of damage occurs in CA2. Synaptic reorganization of granule cell mossy fibers is usually a characteristic feature of hippocampal sclerosis (Committee on Education in Neurological Surgery, pp. 20, 110; Mathern et al., pp. 105–113).

189. C. Nephrocalcinosis frequently accompanies type I, or distal, renal tubular acidosis (RTA). In type 1 RTA, the proximal reabsorption of HCO_3^- is adequate, but the ability of the distal tubule to secrete H^+ ions is inadequate. The urine pH remains above 5.5, and hypokalemia, hypercalcemia, nephrocalcinosis, and osteomalacia frequently accompany this abnormality. Moderate amounts of bicarbonate therapy may correct the acidosis. With type II RTA, the ability of the proximal tubule to reabsorb HCO_3^- is compromised; HCO_3^- is lost in the urine and acidemia develops secondary to the inability of the distal tubule to reabsorb the flood of HCO_3^-. Eventually, the serum HCO_3^- decreases to a point where the proximal renal tubule can reabsorb most of the reduced HCO_3^- load, while the remainder is reclaimed in the distal tubule. This maintains the urine pH < 5.5. K^+ is frequently low with proximal type II RTA. Type IV RTA is seen with hyporeninemic hypoaldosteronism, which is characterized by a mild acidosis associated with increased K^+ levels compared to the low levels seen with types I and II RTA. The elevated K^+ suppresses ammonia production, which sustains the acidosis (Fishman, pp. 138–139).

190-A; 191-C; 192-B. This lesion is most consistent with a DNT (WHO grade I). Patients usually present with long-standing drug-resistant partial seizures that begin before the age of 20. They are usually found in the temporal lobe or other supratentorial location and typically encompass the cerebral cortex. On occasion, they appear to deform the overlying calvarium, a finding that further supports the diagnosis of DNT. The histologic hallmark of this tumor is the glioneuronal element, which is shown here to consist of a free-floating neuron in a microcyst surrounded by oligodendroglial-like cells (Ellison, pp. 659–661; WHO, pp. 103–106).

193. D. Although the MCV progressively decreases as the anemia becomes more severe, the MCHC usually remains normal until the hematocrit values drop below 30%. As the anemia becomes more marked, the red blood cells become progressively more distorted (poikilocytosis), the TIBC begins to increase, the ferritin levels drop, the serum iron stores begin to fall, and the bone marrow iron stores become depleted. Causes of anemia with low MCV include iron deficiency (pregnancy, GI bleeding), thalassemia, anemia of chronic inflammation, sideroblastic anemia, and aluminum toxicity (Fishman, pp. 345–347; Barker, pp. 620–623).

194. B. The addition of phenytoin and phenobarbital most often increases the serum concentration of valproate (Geyer, p. 213).

195. C. IBM affects proximal limb muscles, but in contrast to polymyositis, is much more likely to affect the distal muscles of the legs. It commonly occurs in men after the age of 50 and has less of an association with autoimmune and collagen vascular diseases than polymyositis. Whereas polymyositis does respond to steroids, IBM has no widely accepted therapy, as steroids have shown minimal benefit (Merritt, pp. 767–768).

196. E. Graves' disease (hyperthyroidism) does not typically cause carpal tunnel syndrome but is more likely to produce ophthalmopathy, including a "stare" and "lid lag," and thyroid exophthalmos from mucinous and cellular infiltration of the extraocular muscles (inferior and medial recti most commonly affected). Common etiologies of carpal tunnel syndrome include rheumatoid arthritis, pregnancy, acromegaly, amyloidosis, myxedema, and birth control pills (Greenberg, pp. 536–539).

197. C. This constellation of signs/symptoms is most consistent with the lateral medullary syndrome (of Wallenberg). In a young patient who was subjected to strenuous exercise and extreme neck movements, the most likely diagnosis is vertebral artery dissection (Greenberg, pp. 849–850).

198. C. EGF and TGF-α bind to EGFR with equal affinity; however, whereas EGFR is commonly upregulated in high-grade malignancies, EGF is rarely over-expressed. In contrast, TGF-α is frequently expressed in gliomas, which binds to EGFR and stimulates tyrosine kinase–specific activity, leading to further cell transformation. Thus, it is believed that TGF-α is the primary ligand binding to EGFR in malignant gliomas (Youmans, pp. 726–727).

199. E. TNF-α, IL-1b, IL-6, and potassium levels have been shown to increase after DAI, while magnesium—which is involved in glycolysis, oxidative phosphorylation, cellular respiration, and the synthesis of DNA, RNA, and proteins—has been shown to decrease after severe head injury (Marion, pp. 40–45).

200. B. Denervation of muscle results in fibrillation potentials and positive sharp waves within approximately 2 to 3 weeks and 8 days, respectively. These findings persist until the muscle fibers are reinnervated (usually 3 to 4 months after mild insults) or until the denervated muscle undergoes complete atrophy (Youmans, p. 3856).

201. A. Note the multiple prominent irregularities and loculations located circumferentially around the margins of the dura on this CT myelogram, which is most consistent with arachnoiditis (Ramsey, pp. 739–741).

202. E. Sarcoidosis is a systemic granulomatous disease that involves the nervous system in 5% of patients (neurosarcoidosis). CNS granulomas in neurosarcoidosis can involve the cranial nerves, meninges, hypothalamus, brain parenchyma, and spinal cord. The skull base is frequently affected, and granulomas in this location may result in obstructive hydrocephalus. Cranial nerve palsies may also occur; the facial nerve is most commonly involved. Hypothalamic granulomas can result in diabetes insipidus, galactorrhea, amenorrhea, and changes in behavior, sleep patterns, and appetite. Sarcoidosis can also cause peripheral neuropathies, such as mononeuropathy multiplex. MRI often reveals the presence of CNS granulomas, and CSF exhibits a lymphocytic pleocytosis with elevations in IgG and the IgG index. Oligoclonal bands and elevated angiotensin-converting enzyme (ACE) levels can also be found in the CSF. Neurosarcoidosis can present as a self-limited monophasic illness or a chronic disease with relapses and remissions. Treatment of neurosarcoidosis involves corticosteroids (prednisone), with immunosuppressant drugs added in refractory cases (azathioprine, methotrexate, cyclosporine) (Merritt pp. 180–181).

203. C. Electrocerebral inactivity is consistent with brain death in the setting of a detailed brain death exam. It is defined as no cerebral electrical potentials greater than $2\,\mu V$. It is not required to pronounce brain death and is used as an ancillary test when the diagnosis is not clear. Drug intoxication (e.g., phenobarbital) and hypothermia may result in reversible electrocerebral inactivity (Greenberg, p. 130).

204. B. The most potentially serious complication of hyperkalemia is slowing of electrical heart conduction. The ECG begins to change when the serum K^+ reaches approximately 6.0 mEq/L and is always abnormal when it is > 8.0 mEq/L. The earliest ECG abnormality is a tall, tapering T wave that is most evident in the precordial leads V_2 and V_3. As K^+ levels increase further, the P-wave amplitude decreases and the PR interval lengthens. The P waves may eventually disappear and the QRS complex widen. The final event is ventricular asystole (Marino, pp. 654–655).

205-E; 206-D; 207-A; 208-C; 209-B. Occlusion of the anterior choroidal artery causes a homonymous defect in the upper and lower quadrants, with sparing of the horizontal sector (quadruple sectoranopia, B), which is usually characteristic of a lateral geniculate body infarct that is supplied by the anterior choroidal artery. The central portion of the lateral geniculate body receives blood flow primarily from the lateral posterior choroidal artery. Interruption of this vessel causes a horizontal homonymous sector defect (wedge-shaped, D). Superior homonymous quadrantic defects ("pie-in the sky," E) may result from a lesion along Meyer's loop (after temporal lobectomy) or along the inferior bank of the calcarine fissure. The anterior chiasm or junctional syndrome results in a unilateral optic nerve defect of one eye and a superior temporal defect in the other eye (A) due to the loop made by the inferonasal retina of the other eye (Willebrand's knee). Lesions located in the most anterior portion of the calcarine cortex cause a crescent-shaped defect restricted to the temporal field of the contralateral eye (monocular temporal crescent, C). This is the only retrochiasmatic lesion that may result in a strictly unilateral visual field defect (Brazis, pp. 132–140).

210. B. The musculocutaneous nerve innervates the biceps, brachialis, and coracobrachialis muscles, which control elbow flexion and forearm supination (Brazis, p. 60).

211. D. Where the pyramidal tract decussates at the cervicomedullary junction with segregation of arm fibers (rostral) and leg fibers (caudal), a lesion can cause the unique combination of ipsilateral arm weakness and contralateral leg paresis (cruciate paralysis) (Brazis, p. 95; Greenberg, p. 95).

212-C; 213-C. Hydranencephaly describes a brain replaced by CSF rather than compressed by expansion of the ventricles, as in severe hydrocephalus. Moreover, with severe hydrocephalus, there is usually a thin mantle of brain, which is absent in hydranencephaly. The absence of a cortical mantle with hydranencephaly is most often associated with angiographic evidence of supraclinoid occlusion of the carotid arteries, which strongly suggests a vascular pathogenesis. The posterior fossa and thalami are often preserved due to preserved posterior circulation. The cranium of afflicted children usually fails to grow and remains small. The incidence is estimated to be 1 in 6000, and affected infants rarely live longer than a year (Albright, pp. 155–156).

214. E. DPL is considered positive if greater than 10 mL of gross blood is aspirated from the peritoneal cavity or if 1 L of lactated Ringer's solution is infused into the peritoneal cavity and microscopic evaluation reveals red blood cells > 100,000/mm^3, white blood cells > 500/mm^3, or the presence of bile, particulate matter, or amylase greater than the normal serum value. It can be used for penetrating stab wounds after positive local exploration or suspected hollow viscus injury, following an abnormal ultrasound examination, or following a normal ultrasound when the patient exhibits hemodynamic instability or signs and symptoms suggestive of an intra-abdominal injury (Nwariaku, pp. 64–65).

215. A. Note the large, glassy eosinophilic cell bodies with an angular shape on this photomicrograph, which depicts a gemistocytic astrocytoma (Ellison, p. 627; WHO, p. 25).

216. C. In conductive hearing loss on the right, the Weber test lateralizes to the right, the Rinne test is negative (bone conduction is better than air conduction), and the Schwabach test is normal or prolonged (the patient can hear the tuning fork longer than the examiner can) (Brazis, pp. 298–299).

217. C. With peripheral lesions, severe rotational vertigo associated with nausea and vomiting and nystagmus appear approximately 2 to 15 seconds after performing the Nylén-Bárány maneuver. There is usually habituation of response with repeated maneuvers, and the reproducibility of abnormalities with this maneuver becomes inconsistent with repeated testing. Cochlear and other neurologic symptoms are usually absent. The vertigo and nystagmus typically resolve within 10 to 15 seconds after their appearance; after the patient is rapidly brought back to a sitting position, vertigo recurs and nystagmus develops in the opposite direction (Brazis, pp. 305–306).

218. C. Note the occlusion of the blood vessel, which is due to the presence of many ghost-like red blood cells that contain parasites on this H & E section depicting malaria. Patients with this disease can present with seizures, headache, somnolence, confusion, photophobia, and almost any focal neurologic deficit. Without urgent treatment, these patients usually progress to coma and brain death (Ellison, pp. 653–656).

219. B. This photomicrograph depicts a subependymal giant cell astrocytoma. This lesion is usually located adjacent to the foramen of Monro and is associated with tuberous sclerosis (dominant mutation in TSC 1 on 9p or TSC 2 on 16p). It usually resembles gemistocytic astrocytoma, but is not infiltrative. Note the abundant cytoplasm, abundant perivascular fibrillar zone, and prominent nucleolus in this section. The nuclei are eccentric, which distinguishes this from gemistocytic astrocytoma (Ellison, pp. 637–639).

220. A. This constellation of clinical findings is most consistent with Parinaud's syndrome, which is often associated with pineal region masses causing direct compression of the tectal plate or from compression of the mesencephalic tectum by a dilated suprapineal recess in cases of hydrocephalus (Greenberg, p. 87).

221. E. SII lies along the superior bank of the lateral sulcus and extends posteriorly into the parietal lobe; it has representation of body parts in the reverse sequence to that found in the primary somesthetic area, with the two face areas being adjacent. Representation of the body is bilateral in SII (although contralateral predominates), and the efferent cortical projections are mainly to SI and the primary motor cortex (Carpenter, pp. 404–405).

222. A. The corpus callosum functions to transfer information from one hemisphere to the other. After sectioning, the patient cannot execute a command with the left hand but will do so consistently with the right. The left hemisphere understands the command but is unable to transfer that information to the right side of the brain. The right hemisphere does not typically understand the command because it lacks the ability to understand language. Therefore a patient presented with an object with the right hand should be able to reliably name it, since these fibers are relayed to the contralateral cerebral cortex (DeMyer, pp. 316, 319).

223. B. The most common locations for hypertensive intracranial hemorrhage include the putamen, followed by the thalamus, pons, cerebellum, and lobar regions. The origin of some "hypertensive" putaminal hemorrhages are believed to result from microaneurysms of "Charcot-Bouchard," but this is somewhat controversial (Greenberg, p. 815).

224. D. Hydrocephalus, gait disturbance ("magnetic gait" with short, shuffling steps), dementia (primarily memory impairment with bradyphrenia or slowness of thought), incontinence, and transient elevations in intracranial pressure (with monitoring) may all occur with normal pressure hydrocephalus (NPH). Headache and papilledema are typically not seen in patients with NPH; their presence should raise suspicion of another diagnosis (Greenberg, pp. 191–194).

225. A. The seizure spikes are over a fairly wide area of the right parasagittal region (maximal F4, C4) consistent with a right frontal onset corresponding with a right parasagittal meningioma. In order to localize seizure foci, it is imperative for clinicians to memorize standard electrode placement and designations. Note that by convention, electrodes designated with odd numbers are on the left, while with even numbers on the right. The standard electrode designations are as follows: Fp1/Fp2 = frontopolar or prefrontal; F3/F4 = mid-frontal; C3/C4 = central (roughly over central sulcus); P3/P4 = parietal; O1/O2 = occipital; F7/F8 = inferior frontal (sometimes called anterior frontal); T3/T4 = midtemporal (records activity over anterior and midtemporal activity, important for temporal lobe epilepsy); T5/T6 = posterior temporal; Fz, Cz, Pz = midline electrodes in frontal and parietal regions (record mesial surfaces of hemispheres); A1/A2 = ear reference electrodes (while used for references also record midtemporal activity); T1/T2 = so-called true anterior temporal electrodes; Sp1/Sp2 = sphenoidal electrodes (record activity from inferomesial surface of the temporal lobes) (Rowan, pp. 4–7).

226-D; 227-E; 228-F; 229-C; 230-A; 231-B. Fibers of the ansa lenticularis (D) leave the outer part of the medial globus pallidus, pass around the internal capsule, and enter the prerubral field (field H of Forel, not labeled) prior to merging with the lenticular fasciculus (H2). Fibers of the lenticular fasciculus originate from the inner part of the medial globus pallidus, traverse the posterior limb of the anterior capsule, and pass medially, dorsal to the subthalamic nucleus, to also enter the prerubral field. The ansa lenticularis and lenticular fasciculus then travel together dorsal to the zona incerta as components of the thalamic fasciculus (A). The subthalamic fasciculus (C) is comprised of pallidosubthalamic fibers originating from the lateral or external pallidal segment and subthalamopallidal fibers that terminate in the medullary lamina of both pallidal segments. Both components of the subthalamic fasciculus cross the internal capsule. Thalamostriate fibers from the centromedian nucleus project to the putamen (E) (Carpenter, pp. 337–345).

232. C. Note the prominent ring enhancement of this spinal epidural abscess, with compression of the adjacent spinal cord. The most likely causative organism in a patient with a history of intravenous drug abuse is *Staph. aureus* (Ramsey, pp. 498–502).

233. B. Necrotizing wound infections are produced by *Clostridium* and β-hemolytic streptococcal species. Unlike other wound infections that may appear a few days to 1 week after surgery, necrotizing infections are evident in the first few postoperative days; they are characterized by skin crepitance and fluid-filled bullae. Spread to deeper tissues is a major concern, as this may result in rhabdomyolysis and myoglobinuric renal failure (Marino, p. 489).

234. D. There are three main branches that originate from the intracavernous portion of the ICA: the meningohypophyseal trunk, the artery of the inferior cavernous sinus, and the artery of McConnell. The meningohypophyseal trunk trifurcates into the tentorial artery (of Bernasconi and Cassinari), the dorsal meningeal artery (supplies dura over dorsum sellae), and the inferior hypophyseal artery, which supplies the posterior pituitary gland and sellar floor. McConnell's artery runs along the dura covering the sellar floor to supply the anterior pituitary gland, while the artery of the inferior cavernous sinus provides blood supply to the third, fourth, and sixth cranial nerves as well as the gasserian ganglion and cavernous sinus dura. The vidian artery originates from the petrous ICA (Osborn DCA, pp. 86–87).

235. A. Patients with entrapment or trauma to the suprascapular nerve often complain of shoulder pain centered over the lateral scapula and posterior shoulder, which is most often aggravated by arm abduction during the first 15 degrees (supraspinatus muscle) and external arm rotation when the elbow is flexed at 90 degrees (infraspinatus muscle). Atrophy of the supraspinatus and infraspinatus muscles may also be apparent on inspection. EMG reveals denervation potentials in the supraspinatus and infraspinatus muscles and is the best diagnostic test. Conservative treatment measures include shoulder exercises and local injections of steroids and analgesics. Operative decompression usually includes sectioning of the suprascapular ligament (Youmans, pp. 3932–3933).

236. C. Patients with osteoid osteoma involving the lumbar spine typically present with back pain that is exacerbated at night. This condition is believed to result from prostaglandin production by the tumor. Aspirin has classically been shown to relieve the pain (Youmans, p. 4297).

237. C. Atonic seizures, also called "drop attacks," are characterized by total loss of muscle tone. When they are preceded by a brief myoclonic seizure or tonic spasm, an acceleratory force is added to the fall, further contributing to the high rate of self-injury with this type of seizure. Most patients referred for corpus callosotomy have severe, medically refractory seizures usually accompanied by mental retardation and a severely abnormal EEG. Unlike lesionectomy, corpus callosotomy is palliative, not curative. Nevertheless, this procedure can be highly effective for generalized seizures, with 80% of patients experiencing complete or nearly complete cessation of atonic, tonic, and tonic-clonic attacks in some reports (Merritt, pp. 814, 827).

238-D; 239-B. The spinal accessory nerve is at particular risk during lymph node biopsies involving the posterior triangle of the neck. Patients typically present within a week with a shoulder droop or inability to raise the arm. An additional sensory complaint is noted in some patients from injury to the greater auricular and lesser occipital nerves, which course behind the sternocleidomastoid muscle in close proximity to the spinal accessory nerve. Fortunately, most patients exhibit spontaneous resolution of symptoms (Committee on Education in Neurological Surgery, p. 113; Donner et al., pp. 907–910).

240. E. MEG has several advantages over EEG recording. First, unlike EEG-based techniques, which measure electrical potentials mainly from extracellular volume currents, the magnetic fields measured with MEG primarily reflect intracellular current flow and are not attenuated by the inhomogeneously conducting layers of bone, scalp, and other extracerebral tissue. This provides excellent spatial and temporal resolution for localization of neuronal activity, and it more accurately represents the localization of eloquent cortex than EEG. Second, mass lesions or other pathologic changes in the brain, which may significantly distort the signal detected by EEG, do not affect the signal detected by MEG. Third, because MEG includes only a tangential component of neuronal current, as opposed to EEG recording (which uses both tangential and radial component), the signal detected is less complex than the signal detected by EEG. And finally, whereas EEG reflects only surface recordings, MEG includes data points below the surface of the brain as well.

Magnetic source imaging (MSI) is a technique that allows the mapping of brain function onto brain structure by combining the functional data obtained by MEG with the neuroanatomic data obtained by MRI studies. By mapping the neurophysiologic data acquired by MEG onto the neuroanatomic data acquired by MRI, the functional measures can be given an accurate anatomic reference, which can often help guide surgery. Nevertheless, despite the obvious advantages of MEG and MSI, these strategies are not widely employed. The high financial cost of acquiring such units and the labor-intensive effort that is required by both patients and clinicians during data analysis are just two of the more noteworthy reasons these techniques have not gained universal favor (American Society of Pediatric Neurosurgeons, pp. 1048–1049).

241-C; 242-D. Note the expansion of bone (sphenoid) and "ground glass appearance" on this noncontrasted CT scan in a patient with fibrous dysplasia. Malignant degeneration, usually to osteosarcoma, has been reported to occur in approximately 0.5% of patients with fibrous dysplasia (Albright, pp. 456–457).

243. C. The stylopharyngeus muscle is innervated by the glossopharyngeal nerve (IX) and is the only muscle derived from the third brachial arch. The muscles of facial expression are all innervated by the facial nerve (VII) and are derived from the second brachial arch, whereas the thyroarytenoid muscle and intrinsic laryngeal musculature (except cricothyroid muscle, fourth arch derivative) are derived from the sixth brachial arch. The muscles of mastication are derived from the first brachial arch and are innervated by the mandibular division of the trigeminal nerve (April, p. 556).

244. D. Note the paucity of blood flow in the distal internal carotid and cerebral artery vasculature and the presence of prominent collaterals that resemble a "puff of smoke" on this lateral angiogram, which depicts moyamoya (Albright, pp. 1053–1069).

245. C. The ganglion cells in the retina gives rise to the optic nerve. The ganglion cells receive impulses from the bipolar cells, which, in turn, receive signals from the light-sensitive rods and cones (Kandel, pp. 517–521).

246-C; 247-B; 248-D; 249-A. With neurotmesis, there is complete anatomic transection of the nerve accompanied by

Wallerian degeneration. These injuries almost always require surgical repair, although the timing remains unclear. For sharply divided nerves, immediate repair appears to be ideal, whereas for bluntly injured nerves, some advocate waiting approximately 3 to 4 weeks prior to intervening surgically to allow for better proximal and distal nerve stump delineation. With axonotmesis, there is a loss of axonal continuity, but the soma remains continuous. Wallerian degeneration also occurs with this type of insult. With neurapraxia, conduction ceases without structural damage to the nerve. There is a physiologic transection, which is often accompanied by defective axonal transport. This type of nerve injury frequently recovers by 6 to 8 weeks on average. Stimulating distal to a nerve lesion at about 1 week postinjury results in no action potentials if Wallerian degeneration occurs (Greenberg, p. 532; Youmans, pp. 3825–3826).

250. C. The acquisition of bony spinal fusion increases motion and stress at adjacent motion segments, which can accelerate degenerative changes. This process is further enhanced by failure to repair sagittal balance during surgery. Although not the ideal study to evaluate bony fusion, this MRI does not demonstrate pseudoarthrosis at the prior fusion site, subsidence, basilar invagination, or osteomyelitis. It shows end-fusion degenerative changes and loss of the normal lordotic curve of the cervical spine, which may be contributing to this patients' new clinical problems (Benzel, p. 130).

251-B; 252-C; 253-D; 254-A; 255-E; 256-F; 257-G. This diagram shows the structures that traverse the internal auditory canal (IAC). The facial nerve (A) and nervus intermedius are separated from the superior vestibular nerve by a vertical crest of bone known as Bill's bar (F). Bill's bar arises from the transverse crest (G) within the lateral aspect of the IAC. The cochlear nerve (C) and inferior vestibular nerve enter the IAC inferior to the transverse crest, as depicted in the diagram (Wilkins, pp. 1063–1071, 1101–1114).

258-A; 259-C; 260-C. Three forms of lipomyelomeningocele have been described that have clinical relevance: dorsal, caudal (terminal), and transitional. They are believed to arise from faulty disjunction of the neuroectoderm from the overlying ectoderm, which leaves gaps between these two developing layers. Subsequently, mesenchymal cells are believed to ingress through these defective areas into the central canal, where they are induced to form a bulk of lipomatous tissue, which subsequently prevents fusion or complete closure of the neural tube.

With dorsal lipomas, the rootlets generally lie ventrolateral to the dorsal root entry zone, a crucial anatomic landmark during surgical procedures. Embryologically, this is related to the fact that neural crest cells lie immediately ventrolateral to the point of disjunction of cutaneous and neuroectoderm. Therefore, for many of the dorsal lipomas, if surgeons stay dorsomedial to the dorsal root entry zone, they will likely avoid neurologic injury. Transitional and/or caudal lipomas may be more challenging: as the anatomy is usually distorted, the lipoma-cord interface is usually less predictable, and the exiting roots may be enmeshed with lipoma. SSEP, EMG, or other monitoring procedures may serve as useful adjuncts during these challenging procedures (Youmans, pp. 3229–4243; American Society of Pediatric Neurosurgeons, pp. 289–301; Kaye and Black, pp. 2026–2037).

261. B. The ethmoid bone (vertical plate) and vomer contribute to the anterosuperior and posteroinferior portions of the nasal septum, respectively. The nasal bones and nasal crests of the frontal bones make smaller contributions (Moore, p. 945).

262. C. Viral infections of the CNS can result in meningitis, ventriculitis, encephalitis, and myelitis. CSF in patients with viral syndromes of the CNS reveals increased pressure, lymphocytic pleocytosis, mild elevations in protein, and normal glucose levels. Viral (aseptic) meningitis usually peaks in the summer and fall seasons, whereas bacterial meningitis is more common during the winter. The most common causes of viral meningitis are the enteroviruses, but togaviruses are also frequent pathogens. Encephalitis often results from infections with herpes simplex virus, mumps, or arboviruses (Merritt, pp. 134–138).

263. E. Night terrors most commonly occur during stages 3 and 4 of deep sleep. During a night terror, the child appears extremely frightened and agitated and, although seemingly awake, is actually in deep sleep (stage 3 or 4) and is difficult to rouse. Upon awakening, the child has no apparent memory of the event. Although concerning to parents, night terrors are felt to be benign and self-limited (Rudolph, p. 28; Merritt, p. 15).

264. C. The clinical history of this patient and destructive MRI appearance of this lesion are highly suggestive of a malignant neoplasm involving the paranasal sinuses. The histologic and immunohistochemical markers are most consistent with esthesioneuroblastoma (Kaye and Laws, pp. 885–889).

265. D. Sympathetic nervous system fibers (traveling with the internal carotid artery) and cranial nerve VI are in close proximity in the cavernous sinus. Tumors or other lesions in this location may produce oculosympathetic paralysis (without anhidrosis) (Brazis, p. 265).

266. B. Vertical and torsional saccadic eye movements are generated by the rostral interstitial nucleus of the MLF (riMLF), located in the prerubral field of the ventral diencephalomesencephalic junction, rostral to the tractus retroflexus and ventral to the nucleus of Darkschewitsch. Although cells involved with downward saccades are different from the ones involved with upward saccades, they are dispersed throughout the riMLF without separation of upward and downward pools (Brazis, pp. 199–200).

267-A; 268-D; 269-G; 270-A; 271-F; 272-D; 273-H; 274-C; 275-E; 276-B. Refer to Table 8.267–8.276A (Tarsy, pp. 192–193, 206).

277. E. Denervation typically causes atrophy of muscle fibers, which eventually become angulated, as well as the formation of distinctive fibers with three unique zones often referred to as "target cells." Reinnervation is characterized by type-specific grouping of fibers, which is in contrast to the

TABLE 8.267–276A   Comparison of adverse effects after Gpi, STN, and Vim DBS

ADVERSE EFFECT	GPI DBS	VIM DBS	STN DBS
Photopsias and nausea	Optic tract (anterior)		
Tonic contraction	Internal capsule (posterior and medial)	Internal capsule (lateral)	Corticospinal tract (anterior or lateral)
Paresthesias	Medial lemniscus (posterior and medial)	VPL nucleus (posterior)	Medial lemniscus (posterior)
Diplopia			Fascicles of cranial nerve III or supranuclear oculomotor system (inferior and medial)
Ataxia		Cerebellothalamic fibers (anterior)	Red nucleus (medial)
Flushing and perspiration			Hypothalamus (anterior)
Blepharospasm			STN (typically indicates highly effective stimulation)
Dysarthria			Corticobulbar tract (lateral)

mixed, "checkerboard" pattern of types 1 and 2 skeletal fibers and the atrophic, angulated cells of denervated fibers. Eosinophils in muscle cells are often seen with parasitic infections (Merritt, p. 736).

278. A. Within this tuberculoma, note the prominent region of caseating necrosis (left), in which no cellular detail can be ascertained. A peripheral rim of lymphocytes and a fibrous capsule surround the granuloma, and an occasional histiocyte is observed (Ellison, pp. 339–342).

279. C. Note the multiple lesions at the gray-white junction, which is most consistent with metastatic disease (Ellison, pp. 743–750).

280. D. The right and left posterior cricoarytenoid muscles abduct the vocal cords (Moore, p. 1060).

281. A. Injecting cold water into the right ear causes the endolymph to move away from the ampulla of the horizontal canal. This causes a decreased tone of input into the left abducens nucleus, which results in slow conjugate eye movements toward the right due to right lateral rectus and left medial rectus contraction. Subsequently, there will be compensatory fast eye movements (left-beating nystagmus) to the left. Warm water injected into the right ear will produce the opposite response. The mnemonic COWS (cold opposite; warm same) helps define the fast phase of eye movements during caloric testing (Kline, pp. 57–59).

282-C; 283-B; 284-D; 285-D; 286-A. Refer to discussion questions 55–58, neuroanatomy chapter (Geyer, p. 274; Greenberg, pp. 576–578).

287-B; 288-B; 289-A; 290-A; 291-D. Brightness modulation ultrasonography (B mode), based on reflection of sound waves off tissue interfaces, is better used to view anatomic detail and can be used to measure blood vessel diameter and evaluate plaques. It typically shows the carotid system as a pulsatile luminal structure, with a thin echogenic line representing the intimal surface. The basic principle underlying this mode of imaging is the variable impedance that different body tissues naturally possess. Doppler shift ultrasonography is based on the reflection of sound waves off moving targets such as red blood cells. It is better for evaluating flow dynamics such as blood velocity, which typically increases in segments of stenosis. Although the combination of B-mode and Doppler ultrasonography improved the ability to localize the source of the reflected signal when it was involved with complicated blood velocity patterns (vasospasm, atherosclerosis), the signal was still quit difficult to interpret. More recently, through the use of fast Fourier transformations, the complex signal was separated into a number of single-frequency components, which made it easier to interpret. These technologies were later integrated,

and duplex ultrasonography was born. The advantage of duplex scanning compared to the pre-existing technology is that it could sample flow within a vessel while simultaneously displaying vessel wall anatomy (Youmans, pp. 1561–1565).

292. A. Spinobulbar muscular atrophy (SBMA), or Kennedy's disease, is a trinucleotide repeat disorder (CAG) that involves mutations of the androgen receptor gene, which is located on the X chromosome. It is an X-linked recessive disorder that typically affects adult males in the third decade of life and results in lower motor neuron degeneration only. Symptoms are similar to ALS and include dysarthria, dysphagia, limb weakness, hyporeflexia, and tongue fasciculations. SMBA progresses much more slowly than ALS, and patients may survive for extended periods after initial symptom onset (Merritt, pp. 709–710).

293. E. Antipsychotics decrease the efficacy of levodopa by inhibiting D2 receptors. Dose-related, reversible side effects include nausea, vomiting, orthostatic hypotension, dyskinesias, restlessness, anxiety, athetosis, insomnia, hallucinations, mania, nightmares, and dystonia (Merritt, pp. 689–691).

294. B. The Ramsay Hunt syndrome is associated with herpetic infections of the geniculate ganglion. Herpetic eruptions may appear in the pinna, EAC, and possibly on the tympanic membrane. It is most often associated with a lower seventh cranial nerve palsy, although there may also be decreased hearing, tinnitus, and/or vertigo from involvement of CN VIII (Greenberg, p. 381).

295. D. The positive symptoms of schizophrenia, such as hallucinations, are the direct result of dopamine overactivity in the mesolimbic pathway. Most antipsychotics work by blocking the dopamine receptors in this pathway and often work well for the positive symptoms of schizophrenia. The negative symptoms (flat affect, decreased motivation) are the result of decreased dopamine in the mesocortical system and are often not improved with the commencement of antipsychotics (Kandel, p. 1203).

296. A. The masseter, temporalis, and medial pterygoid muscles are the prime elevators of the mandible, whereas the buccinator muscle compresses the cheek (April, pp. 496, 504).

297. B. Note the empty delta sign, representing an occluded superior sagittal sinus. This abnormality may be associated with pregnancy, dehydration, infections, hypercoagulable states, and tumors (as in this case) (Merritt, pp. 269–271).

298. E. Insulin may or may not be used initially in patients with HHNS. Serum glucose levels may drop precipitously with fluid replacement alone. Insulin is required for patients who are acidotic, hyperkalemic, or in renal failure. If insulin is used, it must be administered in a low-dose regimen as a continuous infusion. To avoid overcorrection, glucose levels must be monitored frequently and the insulin drip stopped once glucose levels fall below 300 mg/dL or so. At this point 5% dextrose should be added to the infusion. Treatment of HHNS focuses primarily on replacing fluid losses, which may be up to 9 to 12 L in some cases, as well as correcting the hyperosmolarity and any electrolyte imbalance (Merritt, pp. 292–293).

299-C; 300-A. Methotrexate may cause leukoencephalopathy, myelosuppression, nephrotoxicity, and mucositis; if administered intrathecally, it can cause arachnoiditis. Bleomycin is associated with Raynaud's phenomenon, myelosuppression, and pulmonary fibrosis, while vincristine can cause a peripheral neuropathy (Kay and Laws, pp. 381–383).

References

Adams: Adams RD, Victor M. Principles of Neurology. 4th ed. New York: McGraw-Hill, 1989.

Alberts: Alberts B, Bray D, Lewis J, et al. The Cell. 3rd ed. New York: Garland Publishing, 1994.

Albright: Albright AL, Pollack IF, Adelson PD. Principles and Practice of Pediatric Neurosurgery. New York: Thieme, 1999.

Alexander: Alexander E III, Loeffler JS, Lunsford LD. Stereotactic Radiosurgery. New York: McGraw-Hill, 1993.

American College of Surgeons Committee on Trauma: Advanced Trauma Life Support for Doctors. 6th ed. Chicago: American College of Surgeons, 1999.

American Society of Pediatric Neurosurgeons: American Society of Pediatric Neurosurgeons: Section of Pediatric Neurosurgery of the AANS. In: McClone DG, ed. Pediatric Neurosurgery. Philadelphia: WB Saunders, 2001.

April: April EW. Anatomy. 2nd ed. Baltimore: Williams & Wilkins, 1990.

Barker: Barker LR, Burton JR, Zieve PD. Principles of Ambulatory Medicine. 5th ed. Baltimore: Williams & Wilkins, 1999.

Bear: Bear MF, Connors BW, Paradiso MA. Neuroscience: Exploring the Brain. Baltimore: Williams & Wilkins, 1996.

Benzel: Benzel EC. Biomechanics of Spine Stabilization. Rolling Meadows, IL: American Association of Neurological Surgeons, 2001.

Berger: Berger M, Wilson C. The Gliomas. Philadelphia: WB Saunders, 1999.

Bernstein: Bernstein M, Berger MS. Neuro-Oncology: The Essentials. New York, Thieme, 2000.

Black PM. Solitary brain metastases: radiation, resection, or radiosurgery. Chest 1993:103;367S–369S.

Brazis: Brazis PW, Masdeu JC, Biller J. Localization in Clinical Neurology. 3rd ed. Boston: Little, Brown, 1996.

Brown SD, Gutierrez G. Does gastric tonometry work? Yes. Critical Care Clinics 1996:12;569–585.

Carmel PW, Grief LK. The aseptic meningitis syndrome: a complication of posterior fossa surgery. Pediatric Neurosurgery 1993:19;276–280.

Carpenter: Carpenter MB. Core Text of Neuroanatomy. 4th ed. Baltimore: Williams & Wilkins, 1991.

Carroll RS, Zhang J, Dasher K, et al. Progesterone and glucocorticoid receptor activation in meningiomas. Neurosurgery 1995:37;92–97.

Carson WL, Duffield RC, Arendt M, et al. Internal forces and moments in transpedicular spine instrumentation: the effect of pedicle screw angle and transfixation—the 4R-4Bar linkage concept. Spine 1990:15;893–901.

Castillo M, Kwock L, Mukherji SK. Clinical applications of proton MR spectroscopy. AJNR Am J Neuroradiol 1996:17;1–5.

Cecil: Goldman L, Bennett JC, eds. Cecil Textbook of Medicine. 21st ed. Philadelphia: WB Saunders, 2000.

Committee on Education in Neurological Surgery: Hadley MN, ed. Self-Assessment in Neurological Surgery (SANS). Park Ridge, IL: Committee on Education in Neurological Surgery, 1997.

Connolly: Connolly, ES, McKhann GM II, Huang, J, Choudri TF. Fundamentals of Operative Techniques in Neurosurgery. New York: Thieme 2002.

Curtis J, Daneman D, Hoffman HJ, et al. The endocrine outcome after surgical removal of craniopharyngioma. Pediatr Neurosurg 1994:21(supp);24–27.

DeMyer: DeMyer W. Neuroanatomy. Mediz, PA: Williams and Wilkins, 1988.

Donner TR, Kline DG. Extracranial spinal accessory nerve injury. Neurosurgery 1993:32;907–910.

Ellison: Ellison D, Love S, et al. Neuropathology. 2nd ed. St Louis: Mosby, 2004.

Executive Committee for ACAS: Endarterectomy for asymptomatic carotid artery stenosis. Executive committee for the Asymptomatic Carotid Atherosclerosis Study. JAMA 1995:273;1421–1428.

Fishman: Fishman MC, Hoffman AR, Klausner RD, Thaler MS. Medicine. 4th ed. Philadelphia: Lippincott-Raven, 1996.

Fitzgerald: Fitzgerald RH, Kaufer H, Malhani AL, eds. Orthopaedics. St. Louis: Mosby, 2002.

Fix: Fix JD. Neuroanatomy. Philadelphia: Harwal, 1992.

Friedman WA, Bova FJ. Linear accelerator radiosurgery: current spectrum and results. Journal of Neurosurgery 77: 832–841; 1992.

Geyer: Geyer JD, Keating JM, Potts DC. Neurology for the Boards. Philadelphia: Lippincott-Raven, 1998.

Grant: Agur A, ed. Grant's Atlas of Anatomy. 9th ed. Baltimore: Williams & Wilkins, 1991.

Greenberg: Greenberg MS. Handbook of Neurosurgery. 5th ed. New York: Thieme, 2001.

Harris: Harris JH, Edeiken-Monroe E. The Radiology of Acute Cervical Spine Trauma. 2nd ed. Baltimore: Williams & Wilkins, 1987.

Juhasz C, Chugani HT. Imaging of epileptic brain with positron emission tomography. Neuroimaging Clin N Am 2003:13;705–716.

Kandel: Kandel ER, Schwartz JH, Jessel TM, eds. Principles of Neural Science, 4th ed. New York: McGraw-Hill, 2000.

Katzung: Katzung BG, ed. Basic and Clinical Pharmacology. 7th ed. Stamford, CT: Appleton & Lange, 1998.

Kaye and Black: Kaye AH, Black PM, eds. Operative Neurosurgery. Edinburgh: Churchill Livingstone, 1999.

Kaye and Laws: Kaye AH, Laws ER Jr, eds. Brain Tumors. Edinburgh: Churchill Livingstone, 1995.

Kline: Kline LB, Bajandas FJ. Neuro-Ophthalmology: Review Manual. 5th ed. Thorofare, NJ: Slack, 2001.

Kopitnik: Kopitnik T Jr, Samson D, White J, et al. Posterior Circulations Aneurysms. Practical Course. San Antonio, TX: Congress of Neurological Surgeons, 2000.

Kosmorsky GS. Spontaneous intracranial hypotension. J of Neuroophthalmol 1995:15;79–83.

Levin: Levin DL, Morriss FC. Essentials of Pediatric Intensive Care. St. Louis: Quality, 1990.

Lunsford LD, Kondziolka D, Flickinger JC. Stereotactic radiosurgery: current spectrum and results. Clin Neurosurg 1992:38;405–444.

Marino: Marino PL. The ICU Book. 2nd ed. Baltimore: Williams & Wilkins, 1998.

Marion: Marion DW. Traumatic Brain Injury. New York: Thieme, 1999.

Martin: Martin JH. Neuroanatomy. 2nd ed. Stamford, CT: Appleton & Lange, 1996.

Mathern GW, Babb TL, Vickrey BG, et al. The clinical-pathogenic mechanisms of hippocampal neuron loss and surgical outcomes in temporal lobe epilepsy. Brain 1995:118;105–113.

Merritt: Rowland LP, ed. Merritt's Neurology. 10th ed. Philadelphia: Lippincott, Williams & Wilkins, 1998.

Moore: Moore KL. Clinically Oriented Anatomy. 3rd ed. Baltimore: Williams & Wilkins, 1992.

Naidich TP, Brightbill TC. Systems for localizing fronto-parietal gyri and sulci on axial CT and MRI. International Journal of Neuroradiology 1996:2;313–338.

NASCET: Beneficial effect of carotid endarterectomy in symptomatic patients with high-grade carotid stenosis.

North American Symptomatic Carotid Endarterectomy Trial Collaborators. N Engl J Med 1991:325;445–453.

Nwariaku: Nwariaku F, Thal E. Parkland Trauma Handbook. St. Louis: Mosby, 1999.

Osborn DCA: Osborn AG. Diagnostic Cerebral Angiography. 2nd ed. Philadelphia: Lippincott, Williams & Wilkins, 1999.

Osborn DN: Osborn AG. Diagnostic Neuroradiology. St. Louis: Mosby, 1994.

Overbeeke R, Steffens-Nakken, Vermes I, et al. Early features of apoptosis detected by four different flow cytometry assays. Apoptosis 1998:3;115–121.

Patten: Patten J. Neurological Differential Diagnosis. 2nd ed. London, Springer-Verlag, 1996.

Pattisapu JV, Walker ML, Myers GG, et al. Use of helmets for positional molding. Concepts Pediatr Neurosurgery 1989:9;178–184.

Pritchard: Pritchard TC, Alloway KD. Medical Neuroscience. Madison, CT: Fence Creek, 1999.

Proano-Narvaez JV, Meza-Lucas A, Mata-Ruiz O, et al. Laboratory diagnosis of human neurocysticercosis: double-blind comparison of enzyme-linked immunosorbent assay and electroimmunotransfer blot assay. J Clin. Microbiol 2002:40;2115–2118.

Ramsey: Ramsey RG. Teaching Atlas of Spine Imaging. New York: Thieme, 1999.

Robbins: Cotran RS, Kumar V, Robbins SL. Robbins Pathologic Basis of Disease. 4th ed. Philadelphia: WB Saunders, 1989.

Rolak: Rolak LA. Neurology Secrets. 2nd ed. Philadelphia: Hanley & Belfus, 1998.

Ross GM. Induction of cell death by radiotherapy. Endocrine-Related Cancer 1999:6;41–44.

Rowan: Rowan AJ, Tolunsky E. Heinmann B. Primer of EEG with a Mini-Atlas. Philadelphia: Elsevier, 2003.

Rudolph: Rudolph AM, Kamei RK, eds. Rudolph's Fundamentals of Pediatrics. Norwalk, CT: Appleton & Lange, 1994.

Samson: Samson DS, Batjer HH. Intracranial Aneurysm Surgery. Mount Kisco, NY: Futura Publishing, 1990.

Schwartz PS, Waxman DJ. Cyclophosphamide induces caspase 9–dependent apoptosis in 9L tumor cells. Molecular Pharmacology 2001:60;1268–1279.

Simmons: Simmons RL, Steed DL. Basic Science Review for Surgeons. Philadelphia: WB Saunders, 1992.

Som: Som PM, Curtin HD. Head and Neck Imaging. 3rd ed. St. Louis, Mosby, 1996.

Tarsy: Tarsy D, Vitek JL, Lozano AM, eds. Surgical Treatment of Parkinson's Disease. Totowa, NJ: Humana, 2003.

Tew: Tew JM, van Loveren HR, Keller JT. Atlas of Operative Microneurosurgery: Brain Tumors. 2 Vols. Philadelphia: WB Saunders, 2001.

Wheater: Wheater PR, Burkitt HG, Daniels VG. Functional Histology. 2nd ed. New York: Churchill Livingstone, 1987.

WHO: Kleihues P, Cavenee WK. World Health Organization (WHO) Classification of Tumours: Pathology and Genetics; Tumors of the Nervous System. Lyon, France: IARC Press, 2000.

Wilkins: Wilkins RH, Rengachery SS, eds. Neurosurgery. 2nd ed; 3 vols. New York: McGraw-Hill, 1996.

Wilson-Pauwels: Wilson-Pauwels L, Akesson EJ, Stewart PA. Cranial Nerves: Anatomy and Clinical Comments. Philadelphia: BC Decker, 1988.

Youmans: Winn RH, eds. Youmans Neurological Surgery. 5th ed; 4 vols. Philadelphia: WB Saunders, 2004.

Zaatreh: Zaatreh M, Finkel A. Spontaneous intracranial hypotension. Southern Medical Journal 2002: 95;1342–1346.

Index

9 781405 104791